Cardiac Pacemakers and Resynchronization Step-by-Step

AN ILLUSTRATED GUIDE

Companion Website

With this book you are given free access to a companion resources site:

www.wiley.com/go/barold/cardiac

The website includes more than **300 images** taken from this book

You are free to download these images and use them for your own presentations to students*

How to access the website:

Look under the label below to see your access code.
Go to **www,wiley.com/go/barold/cardiac** and enter the code when prompted.

*Please note that these images are for your own use for study and instruction. If you are using these images in a presentation, the reference to the book should always be displayed along with the image. See website for full copyright information.

Cardiac Pacemakers and Resynchronization Step-by-Step

AN ILLUSTRATED GUIDE

Second Edition

S. Serge Barold
MD, FRACP, FACP, FACC, FESC, FHRS
University of South Florida and Florida Heart Rhythm Institute
Tampa, Florida, USA

Roland X. Stroobandt
MD, PhD
Professor of Medicine
Heart Center, Department of Electrophysiology
University Hospital, Ghent
Ghent, Belgium

Alfons F. Sinnaeve
ing., MSc
Professor Emeritus of Electronic Engineering
Technical University KHBO, Department of Electronics
Oostende, Belgium

WILEY-BLACKWELL
A John Wiley & Sons, Ltd., Publication

This edition first published 2010, © 2010 by S. Serge Barold, Roland X. Stroobandt, and Alfons F. Sinnaeve

Blackwell Publishing was acquired by John Wiley & Sons in February 2007. Blackwell's publishing program has been merged with Wiley's global Scientific, Technical and Medical business to form Wiley-Blackwell.

Registered office:
John Wiley & Sons Ltd, The Atrium, Southern Gate, Chichester, West Sussex, PO19 8SQ, UK

Editorial offices:
9600 Garsington Road, Oxford, OX4 2DQ, UK
The Atrium, Southern Gate, Chichester, West Sussex, PO19 8SQ, UK
111 River Street, Hoboken, NJ 07030-5774, USA

For details of our global editorial offices, for customer services and for information about how to apply for permission to reuse the copyright material in this book please see our website at www.wiley.com/wiley-blackwell.

Library of Congress Cataloging-in-Publication Data

Barold, S. Serge.
Cardiac pacemakers and resynchronization therapy step-by-step : an illustrated guide / S. Serge Barold, Roland X. Stroobandt, Alfons F. Sinnaeve. – 2nd ed.
p. ; cm.
Rev. ed. of: Cardiac pacemakers step-by-step. c2004.
Includes bibliographical references and index.
ISBN 978-1-4051-8636-0
1. Cardiac pacemakers–Pictorial works. I. Stroobandt, R. (Roland) II. Sinnaeve, Alfons F. III. Barold, S. Serge. Cardiac pacemakers step-by-step. IV. Title.
[DNLM: 1. Cardiac Pacing, Artificial–methods–Handbooks. 2. Pacemaker, Artificial–Handbooks. 3. Electrocardiography–methods–Handbooks. WG 39 B264c 2010]
RC684.P3B365 2010
617.4'120645–dc22 2010010756

ISBN: 9781405186360

A catalogue record for this book is available from the British Library.

Set in 9.5/12 pt Palatino by Aptara® Inc., New Delhi, India

Printed and bound by CPI Group (UK) Ltd, Croydon CR0 4YY

C9781405186360_200524

Contents

Preface to the first edition

The impetus for writing this book came from our observations that many healthcare professionals and young physicians working in emergency rooms, intensive and coronary care units were unable to interpret simple pacemaker electrocardiograms correctly. Over the years we also heard many complaints from beginners in the field of cardiac pacing that virtually all, if not all, the available books are too complicated and almost impossible to understand. Indeed, the ever-changing progress in electrical stimulation makes cardiac pacing a moving target. Therefore we decided to take up the challenge and write a book for beginners equipped with only a rudimentary knowledge of electrocardiography and no knowledge of cardiac pacing whatsoever. Because many individuals first see the pacemaker patient after implantation, the book contains little about indications for pacing and implantation techniques. The book starts with basic concepts and progressively covers more advanced aspects of cardiac pacing including troubleshooting and follow-up.

As one picture is worth a thousand words, this book tries to avoid unnecessary text and focuses on visual learning. We undertook this project with the premise that learning cardiac pacing should be enjoyable. Cardiac pacing is a logical discipline and should be fun and easy to learn with the carefully crafted illustrations in this book. The artwork is simple for easy comprehension. Many of the plates are self-explanatory and the text in the appendix only intends to provide further details and a comprehensive overview.

Many of the images used to create the illustrations in this book are taken from CorelDraw and Corel Mega Gallery clipart collections.

We are grateful to Charlie Hamlyn of Blackwell Publishing and Tom Fryer of Sparks for their superb work in the production of this book.

S. Serge Barold
Roland X. Stroobandt
Alfons F. Sinnaeve

Preface to the second edition

The first edition of the book has been well received all over the world and translated into Japanese, Chinese and Polish. The same format has been retained in the second edition because of its wide popularity and the frequent positive feedback that it facilitates learning and understanding. Many new plates were added. A few plates were upgraded and a few were deleted when the message was no longer relevant. We have reviewed the advances in cardiac pacing over the last seven years and introduced an important new presentation on cardiac resynchronization, which is a rapidly growing field. The incorporation of many suggestions from readers has also contributed to the increased size of the second edition. For example, the latter now includes an expanded text (including a large section on cardiac resynchronization), a discussion of indications, and a list of pertinent references. As before, we omitted the technical details of pacemaker implantation and lead extraction. We are grateful to Thomas V. Hartman, Kate Newell, and Cathryn Gates from Wiley-Blackwell Publishing for their outstanding work in the production of this book.

S. Serge Barold
Roland X. Stroobandt
Alfons F. Sinnaeve

Abbreviations

A ampere
ACC American College of Cardiology
AEGM atrial electrogram
AEI atrial escape interval
AF atrial fibrillation
AFR atrial flutter response
Ah amperehour
AH atrial–His
AHA American Heart Association
AHR atrial high rate
AMS automatic mode switching
AP atrial paced event
APC atrial premature complex
AR atrial event sensed in the refractory period
As amperesecond
AS atrial sensed event
AT atrial tachycardia
ATP antitachycardia pacing
ATR atrial tachycardia response
AV atrioventricular
AVE atrioventricular extension
AVI atrioventricular interval (also called AV delay)
AVI-U atrioventricular interval, unblanked
BiV biventricular
BLR basic lower rate
BOL beginning-of-life
BP biventricular paced event
BP blood pressure
bpm beats per minute
BV biventricular
C coulomb
CAD coronary artery disease
CHF congestive heart failure
CO cardiac ouput
CRT cardiac resynchronization therapy
CRT-D cardiac resynchronization therapy device and defibrillator
CS coronary sinus
CSNRT corrected sinus node recovery time
CT computed tomography
ECG electrocardiogram
EGM electrogram
ELT endless loop tachycardia
EMI electromagnetic interference
EOL end-of-life
EOS end-of-service
ER evoked response
ERI elective replacement indicator
ERT elective replacement time
ESCI escape interval
ESCR escape rate
FARI filtered atrial rate interval
FCC Federal Communications Commission
HCM hypertrophic cardiomyopathy
HF heart failure
HR heart rate
HRS Heart Rhythm Society
HRV heart-rate variability
HV His–ventricular
Hz hertz
I current (in amps, A)
IACD intraatrial conduction delay
ICD implantable cardioverter-defibrillator
IV interventricular
LA left atrium
LBBB left bundle branch block
LBT listen before talk
LRI lower rate interval
LRL lower rate limit
LV left ventricle
LVEF left ventricular ejection fraction
LVESV left ventricular end-systolic volume
LVOT left ventricular outflow tract
μA microampere
mA milliampere
mEq milliequivalent
MI myocardial infarction
MICS Medical Implant Communications System
MRI magnetic resonance imaging
ms millisecond
MSDR maximum sensor-driven rate
MTR maximum tracking rate
mV millivolt
MV minute volume
MVP managed ventricular pacing
NYHA New York Heart Association
OVI open ventricular interval
PAVB postatrial ventricular blanking period
pAVI AV interval after a paced event
PM pacemaker
PMT pacemaker-mediated tachycardia

ppm	pacing per minute
PR	peripheral resistance
PVAB	postventricular atrial blanking period
PVARP	postventricular atrial refractory period
PVARP-U	postventricular atrial refractory period, unblanked
PVC	premature ventricular complex (= VPC)
PVE	premature ventricular event
pVRP	ventricular refractory period after pacing
R	resistance (in ohms, Ω)
RA	right atrium
RAM	random-access memory
RBBB	right bundle branch block
RF	radiofrequency
RNRVAS	repetitive non-reentrant VA synchrony
ROM	read-only memory
RR	respiratory rate
RRT	recommended replacement time
RV	right ventricle
RVA	right ventricular apex
RVOT	right ventricular outflow tract
SAI	spontaneous atrial interval
SAR	spontaneous atrial rate
SAS	synchronous atrial stimulation
sAVI	AV interval after a sensed event
SDI	sensor-driven interval
SDR	sensor-driven rate
SND	sinus node dysfunction
SV	stroke volume
sVRP	ventricular refractory period after sensing
SVT	supraventricular tachycardia
TARP	total atrial refractory period
TCL	tachycardia cycle length
TDI	tissue Doppler imaging
TEE	transesophageal echocardiography
TV	tidal volume
U	voltage (in volts, V)
URI	upper rate interval
URL	upper rate limit
V	volt
VA	ventriculoatrial
VB	ventricular blanking period
VEGM	ventricular electrogram
VF	ventricular fibrillation
VHR	ventricular high rate
VP	ventricular paced event
VPC	ventricular premature complex
VPI	ventricular paced interval
VPR	ventricular paced rate
VR	ventricular event sensed in the refractory period
VRP	ventricular refractory period
VRP-U	ventricular refractory period, unblanked
VS	ventricular sensed event
VSP	ventricular safety pacing
VT	ventricular tachycardia
WI	Wenckebach interval

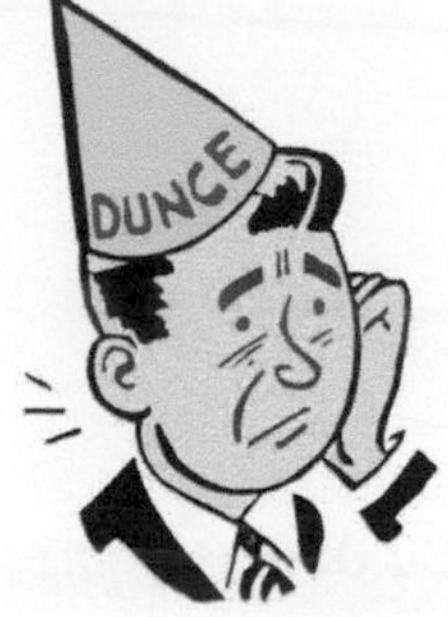

WHAT IS A PACEMAKER ???

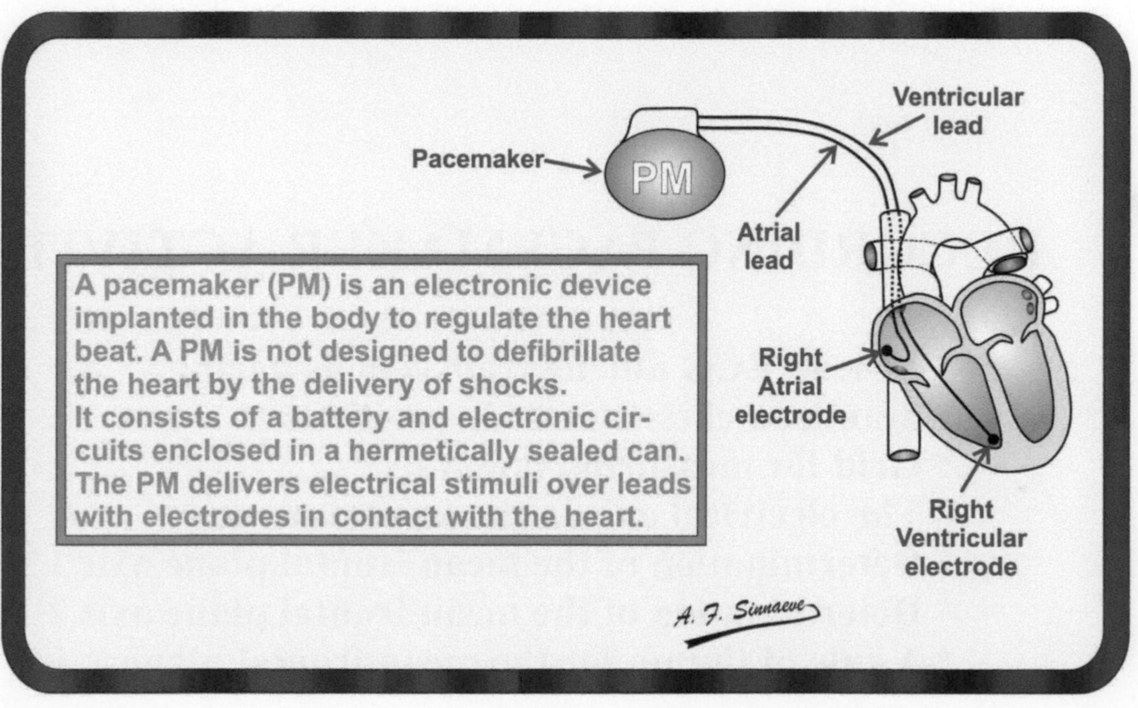

A pacemaker (PM) is an electronic device implanted in the body to regulate the heart beat. A PM is not designed to defibrillate the heart by the delivery of shocks.
It consists of a battery and electronic circuits enclosed in a hermetically sealed can. The PM delivers electrical stimuli over leads with electrodes in contact with the heart.

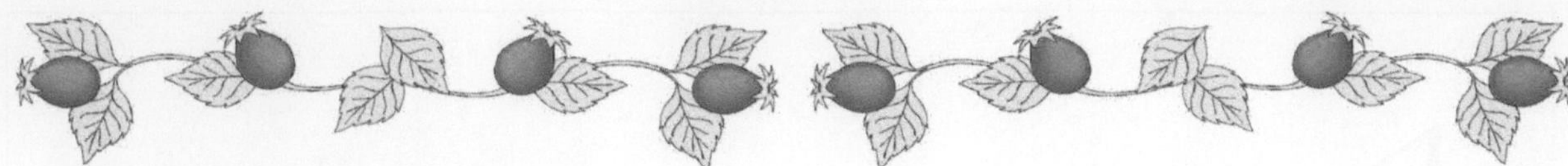

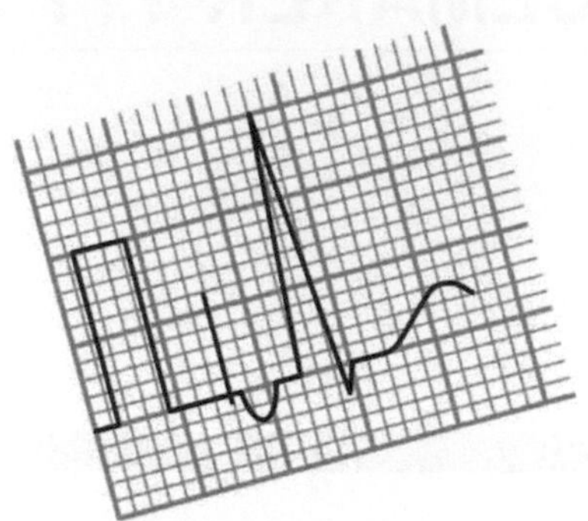

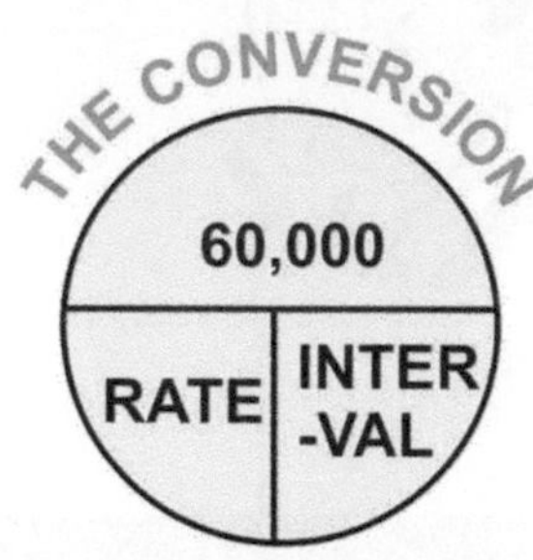

RECORDING PACEMAKER ACTIVITY

* 12-lead ECG during transvenous pacing
* Standard chest electrode positions
* Grid for measuring intervals
* The electrical axis in the frontal plane
* Determination of the mean frontal plane axis 1
* Determination of the mean frontal plane axis 2
* A rule of thumb for the mean frontal plane axis

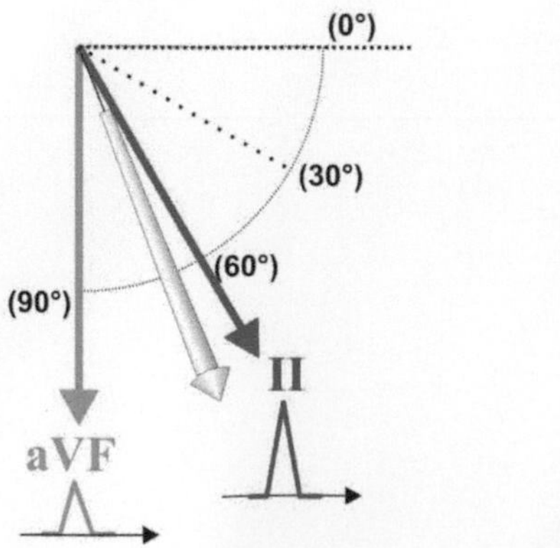

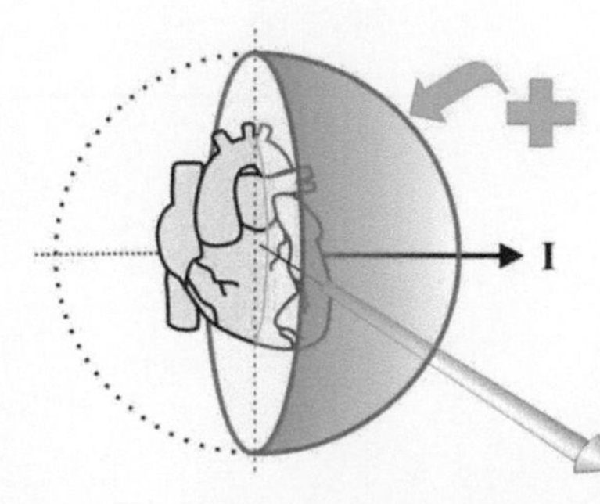

A. F. Sinnaeve

CONFIGURATION OF 12- LEAD ECG DURING TRANSVENOUS PACING

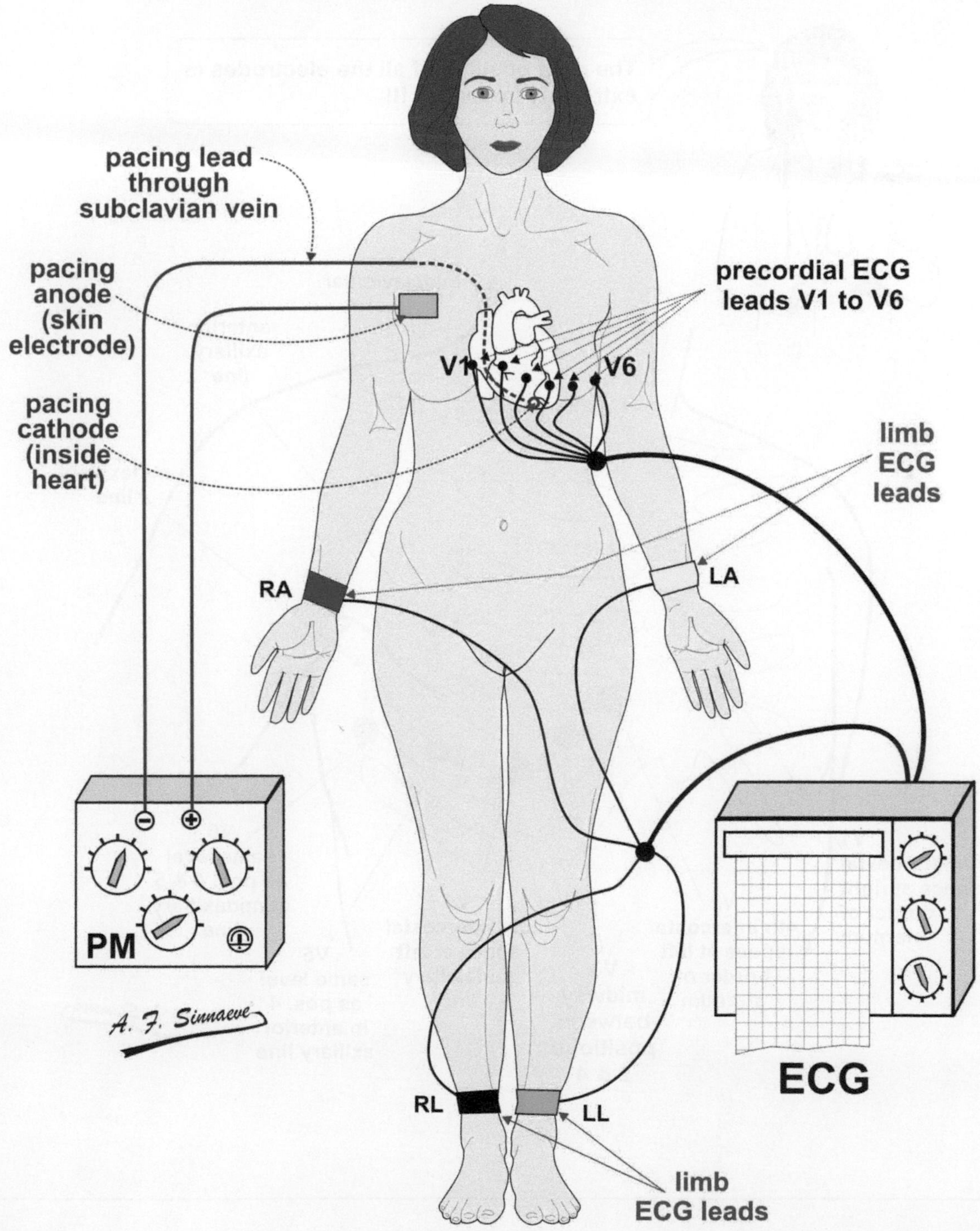

pacing lead through subclavian vein

pacing anode (skin electrode)

pacing cathode (inside heart)

precordial ECG leads V1 to V6

V1

V6

limb ECG leads

RA

LA

PM

ECG

RL

LL

limb ECG leads

A. F. Sinnaeve

4

STANDARD CHEST ELECTRODE POSITIONS

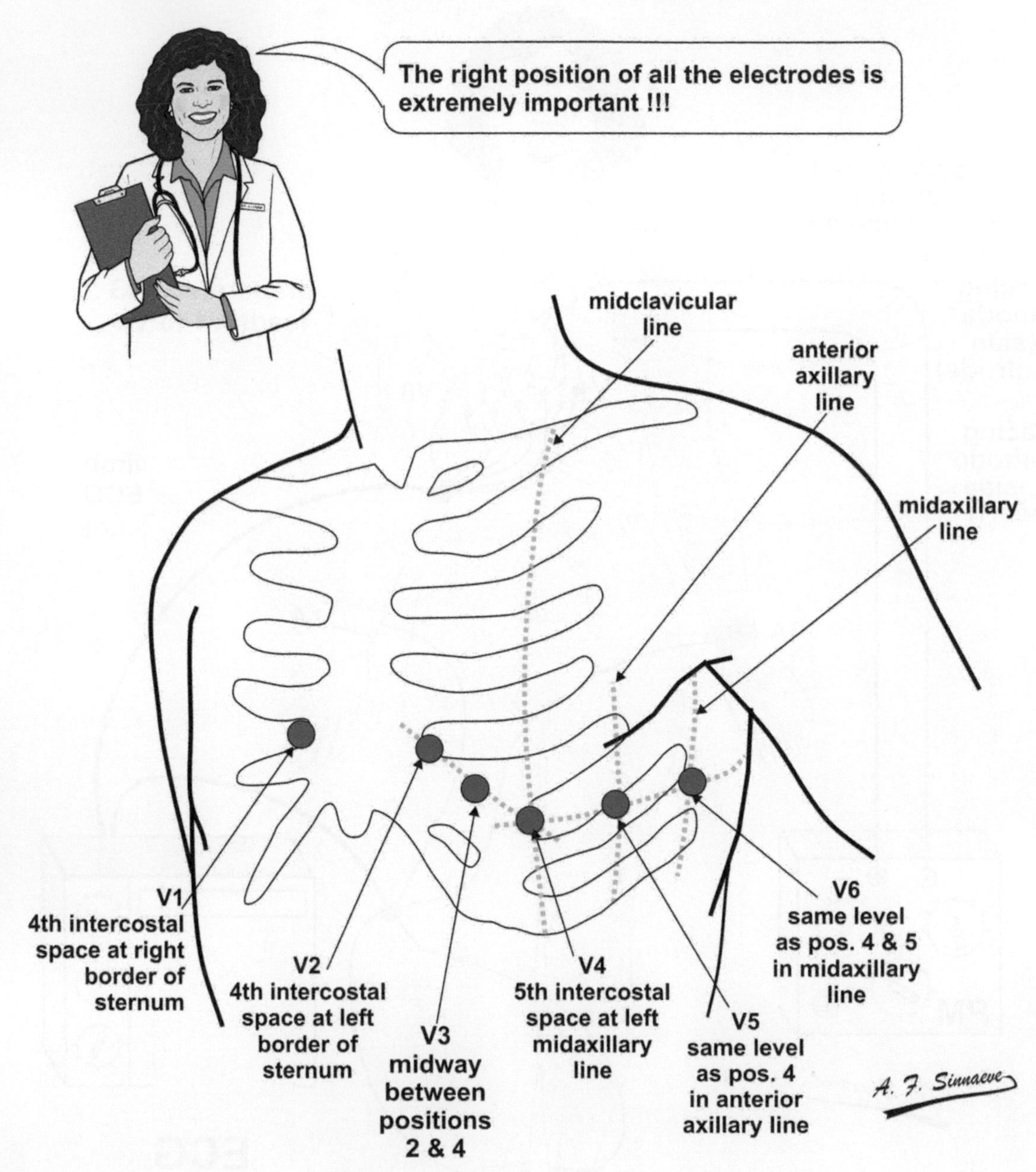

The right position of all the electrodes is extremely important !!!
midclavicular line
anterior axillary line
midaxillary line
V1 4th intercostal space at right border of sternum
V2 4th intercostal space at left border of sternum
V3 midway between positions 2 & 4
V4 5th intercostal space at left midaxillary line
V5 same level as pos. 4 in anterior axillary line
V6 same level as pos. 4 & 5 in midaxillary line
A. F. Sinnaeve

TIMING INTERVALS VERSUS RATE

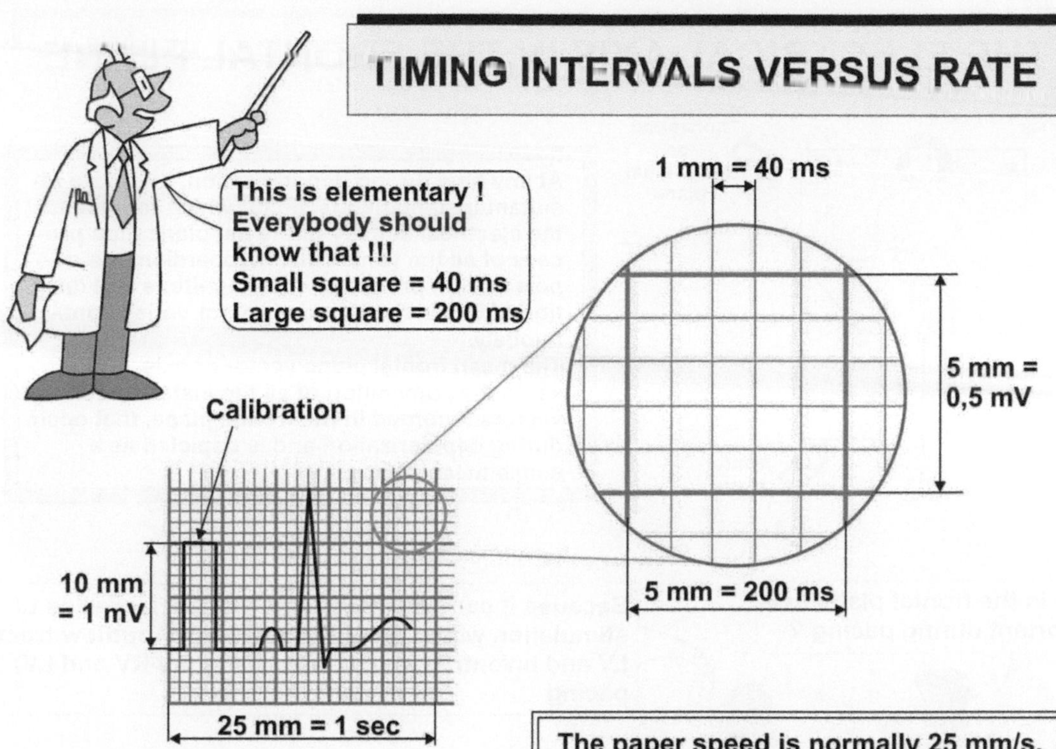

The paper speed is normally 25 mm/s, thus 1 mm on the paper corresponds with 1/25 s = 0.04 s = 40 ms

THE CONVERSION

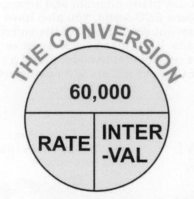

60,000

RATE | INTER-VAL

UNITS OF TIME

1 minute = 60 seconds
or 1 min = 60 s
1 second = 1,000 milliseconds
or 1 s = 1,000 ms
1 minute = 60,000 milliseconds
or 1 min = 60,000 ms

RATE **is expressed in beats per minute or bpm**

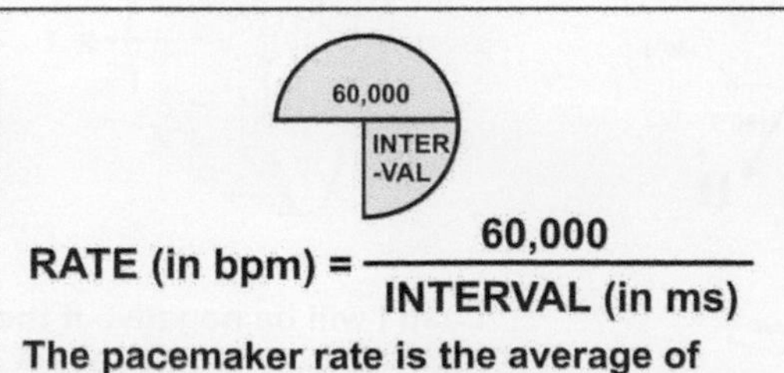

$$\text{RATE (in bpm)} = \frac{60{,}000}{\text{INTERVAL (in ms)}}$$

The pacemaker rate is the average of several intervals calculated for 1 minute of time

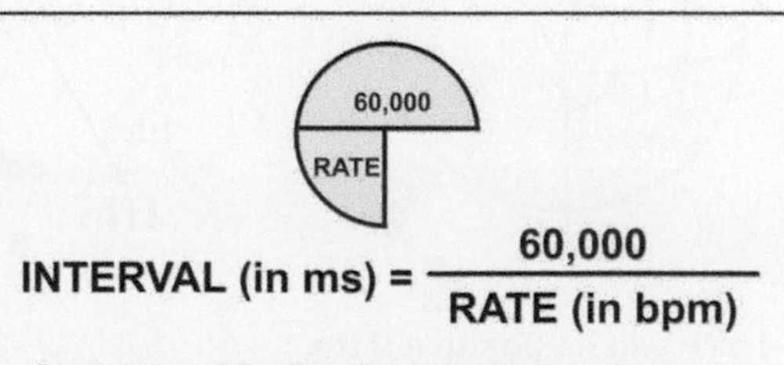

$$\text{INTERVAL (in ms)} = \frac{60{,}000}{\text{RATE (in bpm)}}$$

An interval is the time between two consecutive events, e.g. Vp-Vp or Vs-Vs

Abbreviations : min = minute ; mm = millimeter ; ms = millisecond ; mV = millivolt ; s = second ; Vp = ventricular paced event ; Vs = ventricular sensed event

THE ELECTRICAL AXIS IN THE FRONTAL PLANE

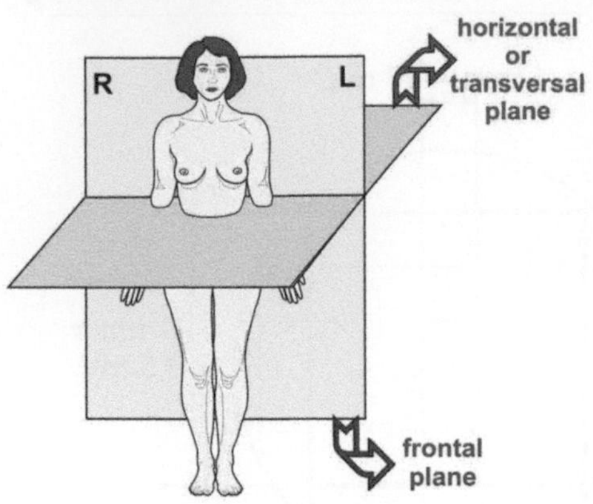

At any time during depolarization, there is a resultant instantaneous vector which represents the electrical activity of the depolarization process of all the ventricular myocardium. As depolarization proceeds, the magnitude and direction of this instantaneous vector varies continuously.
The mean frontal plane vector or axis, represents the summation of all the instantaneous vectors recorded in the frontal plane, that occur during depolarization and is depicted as a single mean vector.

Why is the frontal plane axis important during pacing ?

Because it can help locate the 4 important sites of stimulation which are the RV apex, RV outflow tract, LV and biventricular (i.e. simultaneous RV and LV) pacing.

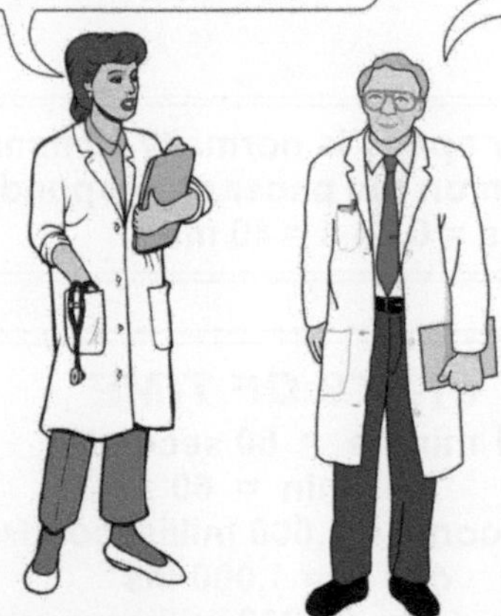

To determine the mean frontal plane axis, you have to understand the frontal plane diagram and arrangement of the frontal plane ECG leads. You also have to understand the hemisphere concept of the various frontal plane ECG leads. If the mean QRS vector or axis is situated in the positive (+) hemisphere of a particular lead, this ECG lead will show a positive (+) deflection

Lead aVF will be negative if the mean QRS vector is in this hemisphere

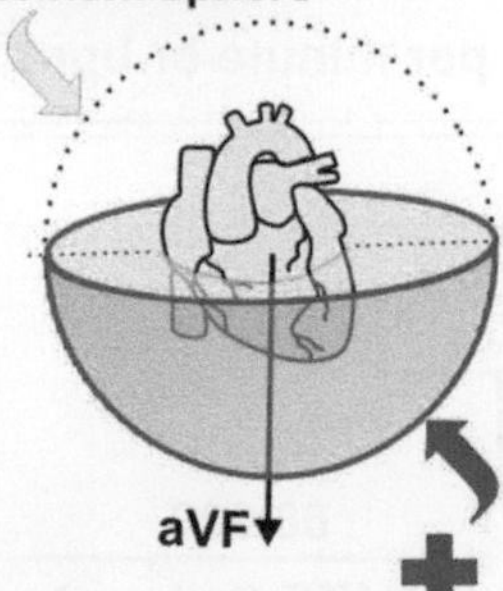

Lead aVF will be positive if the mean QRS vector is situated in this hemisphere

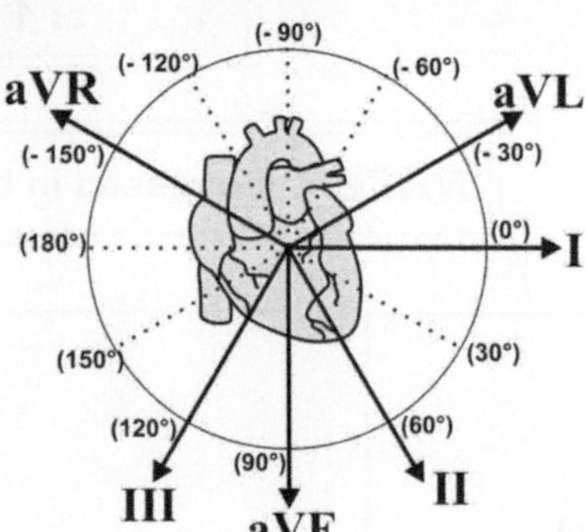

A. F. Sinnaeve

Lead I will be positive if the mean QRS vector is situated in this hemisphere

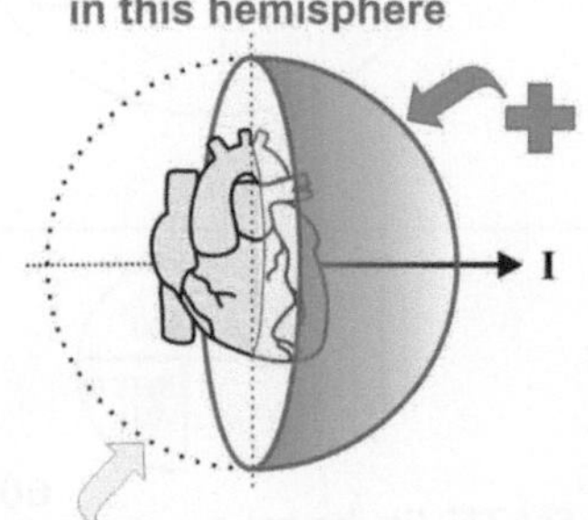

Lead I will be negative if the mean QRS vector is in this hemisphere

DETERMINATION OF THE MEAN FRONTAL PLANE AXIS

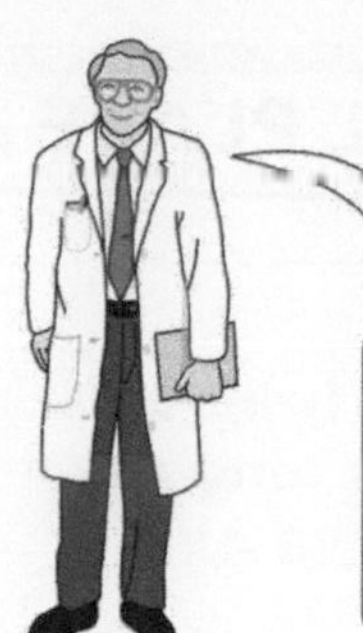

JUST REMEMBER 3 IMPORTANT QUESTIONS :
* In which quadrant is the QRS vector situated ?
* Which of the adjacent leads has the tallest R wave or the deepest S wave ?
* Which is the most equiphasic lead (or zero lead)?

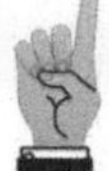

STEP 1 : LOOK AT LEADS I & aVF TO DETERMINE IN WHICH QUADRANT THE FRONTAL PLANE AXIS IS SITUATED

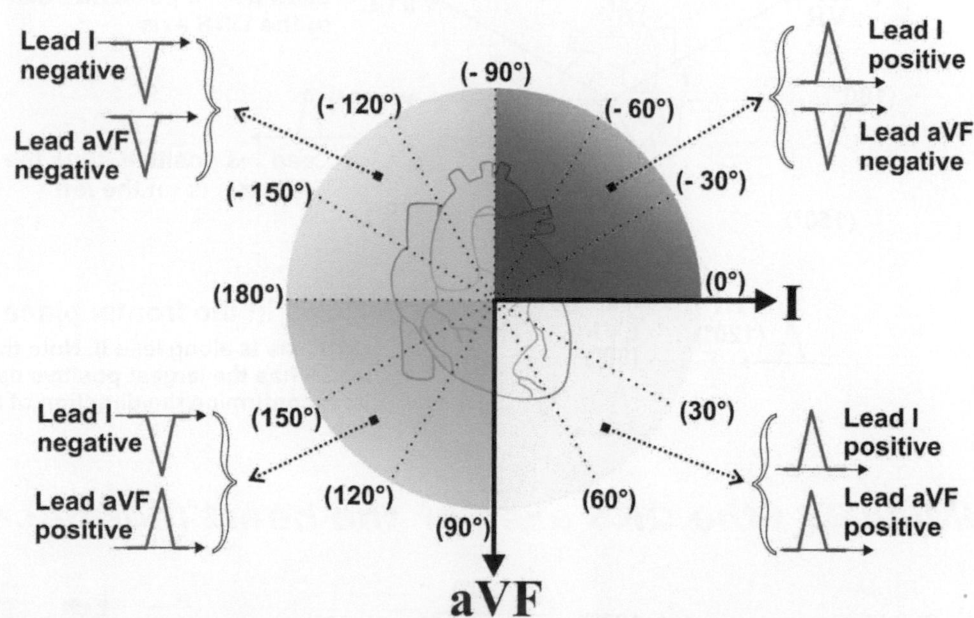

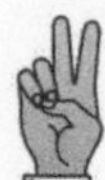

STEP 2 : LOOK IN THE APPROPRIATE QUADRANT FOR THE TALLEST R WAVE OR THE DEEPEST S WAVE

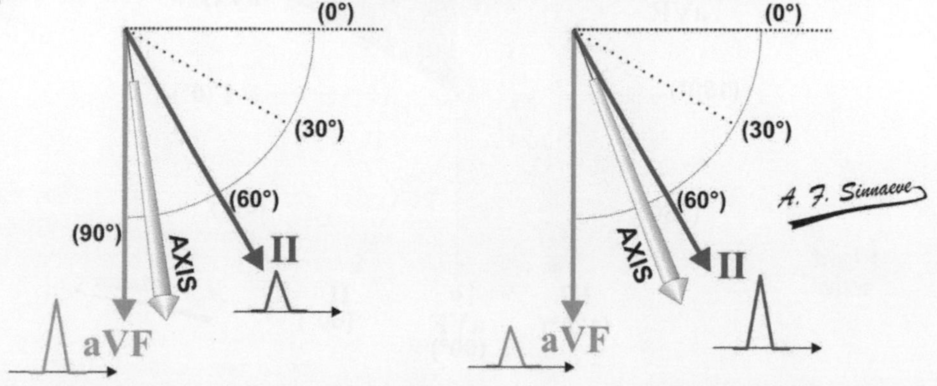

The lead nearest to (or parallel along) the QRS axis has the largest positive deflection. If two leads have equal positive deflections, the axis is exactly in the middle between these two leads.

DETERMINATION OF THE MEAN FRONTAL PLANE AXIS CONT'D

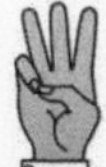

STEP 3 : LOOK FOR THE MOST EQUIPHASIC LEAD (where the positive minus the negative defection is closest to zero)
THIS LEAD IS PERPENDICULAR TO THE QRS AXIS

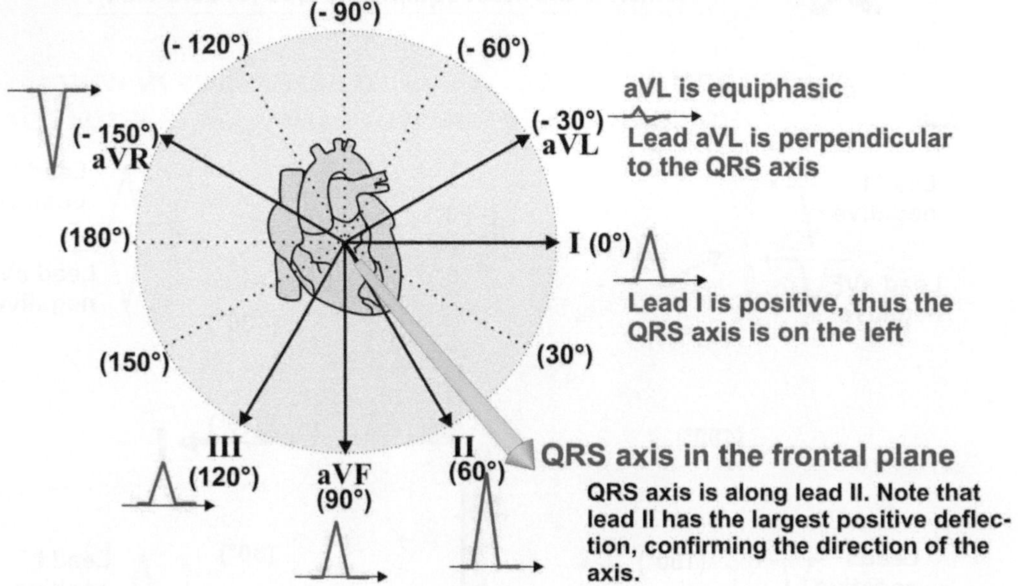

SUMMARY : the QRS axes of the heart (not paced)

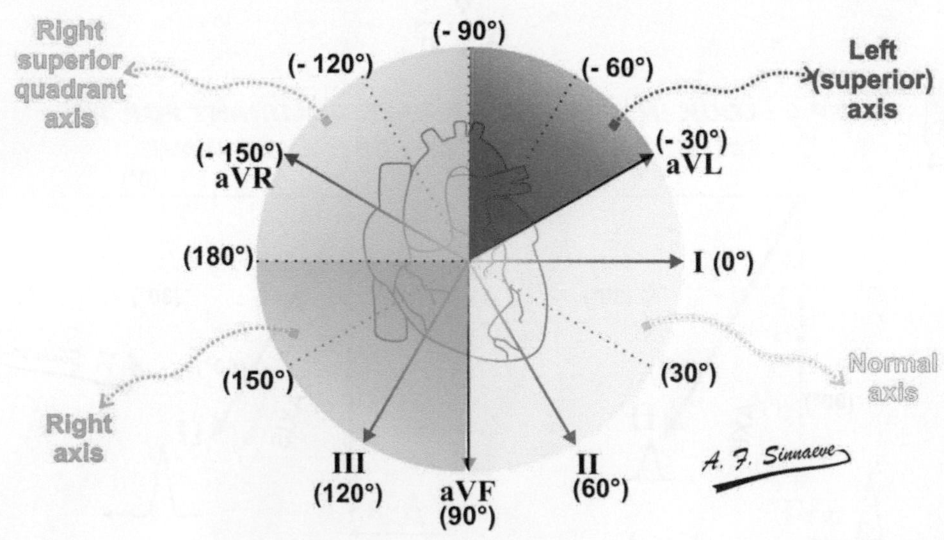

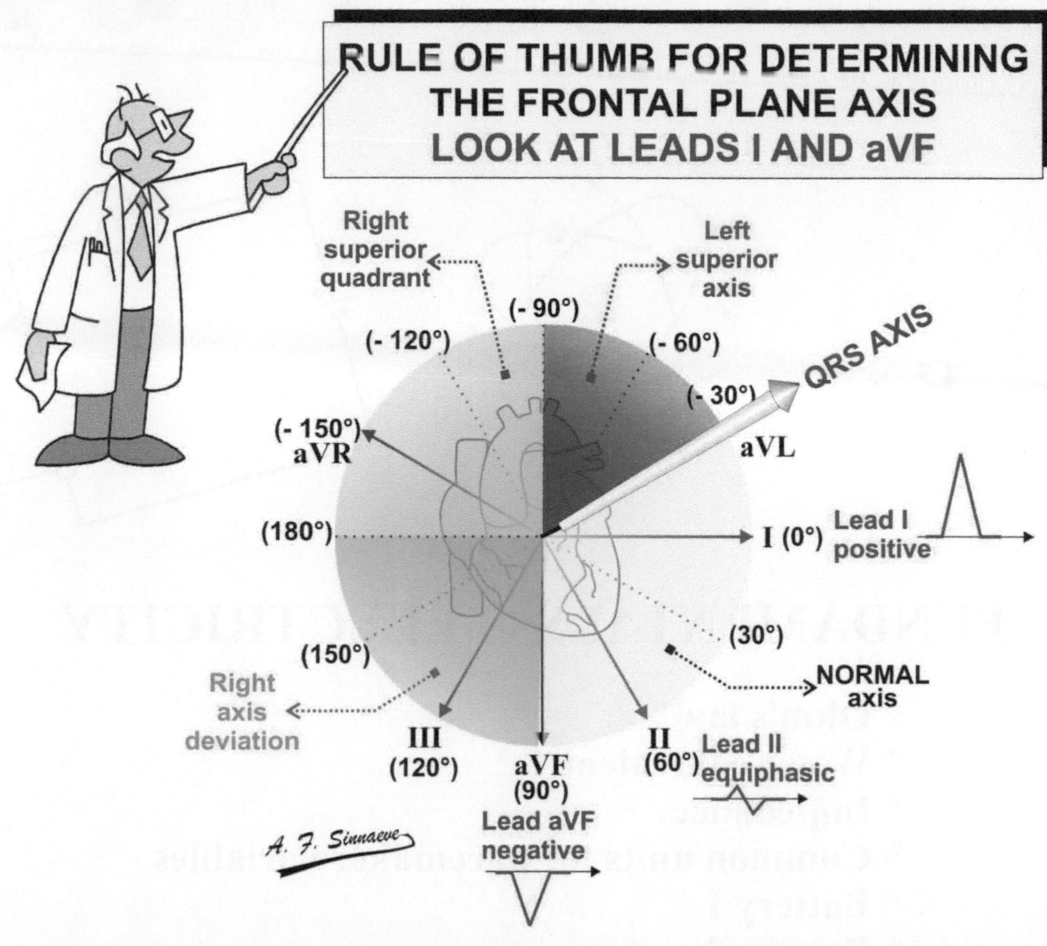

1/ If both leads I and aVF are positive (dominant R wave), the axis is normal (yellow area)

2/ If lead I is positive and lead aVF is negative, you must look at lead II

a. If lead II is equiphasic (positivity is equal to negativity so that the algebraic sum is zero), the axis is directed along lead aVL. This because an equiphasic lead (lead II in this case) is perpendicular to the axis (along lead aVL)

b. If lead II is more positive than negative, the axis is below -30° and normal (yellow area)

c. If lead II is more negative than positive, the axis is more negative than -30° and is in the left superior quadrant (red area)

3/ If lead I is negative (down) and aVF is positive (up) the axis is in the right inferior quadrant (green area - right axis deviation)

4/ If leads I and aVF are negative (down), the axis is in the right superior quadrant (blue area). The axis is simply described as being in the right superior quadrant. It is called neither extreme right nor extreme left axis deviation.

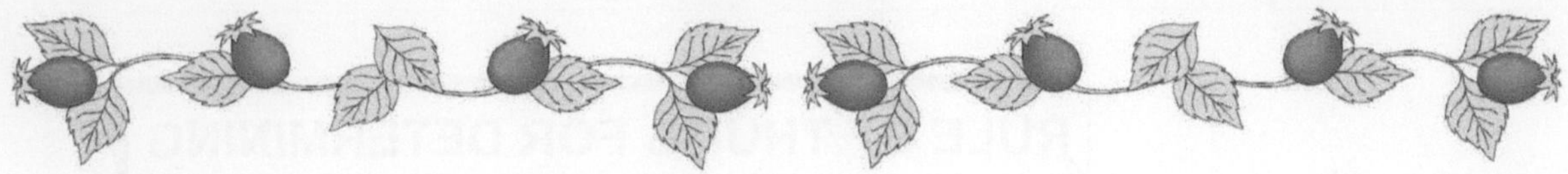

10

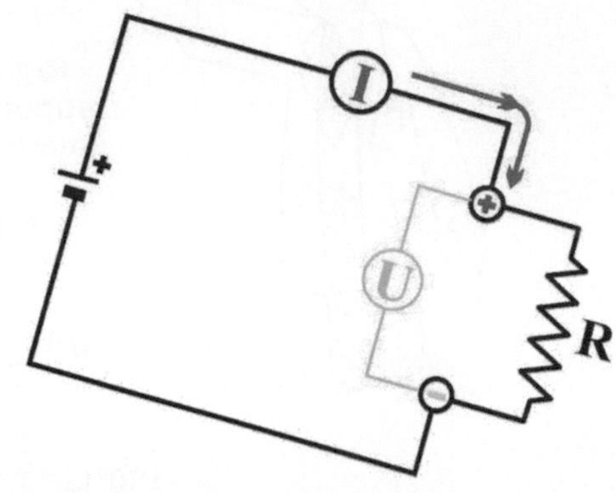

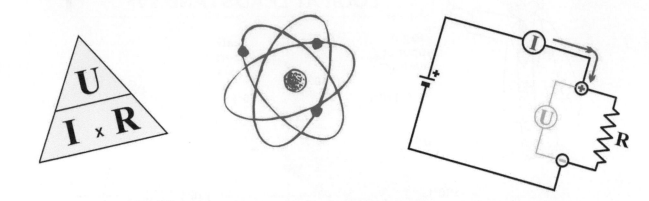

FUNDAMENTALS of ELECTRICITY

- **Ohm's law**
- **Water equivalent**
- **Impedance**
- **Common units for pacemaker variables**
- **Battery 1**
- **Battery 2**
- **Battery impedance and battery voltage**
- **Battery capacity**

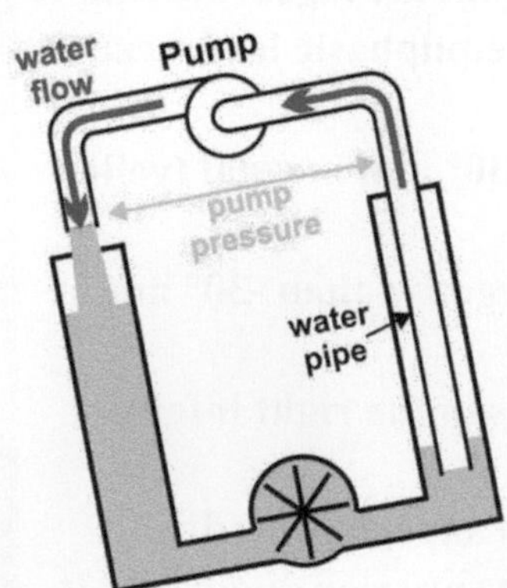

Ω

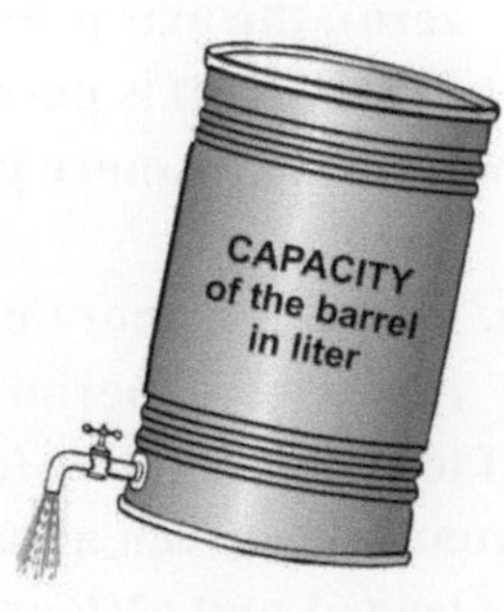

OHM's LAW

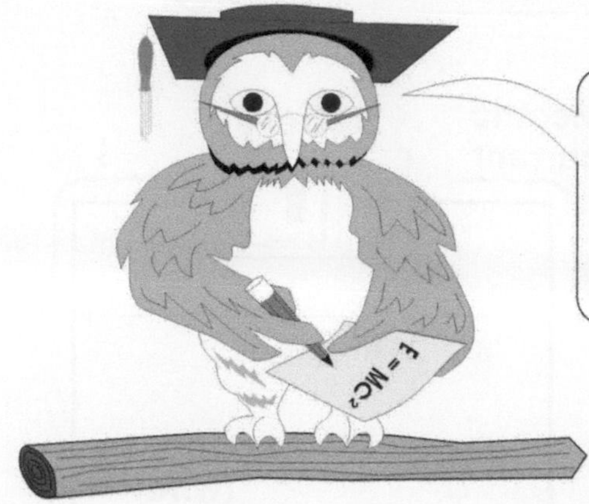

This is the most important law of electricity !!!
Everybody should be familiar with these three variables, their relation and their units !

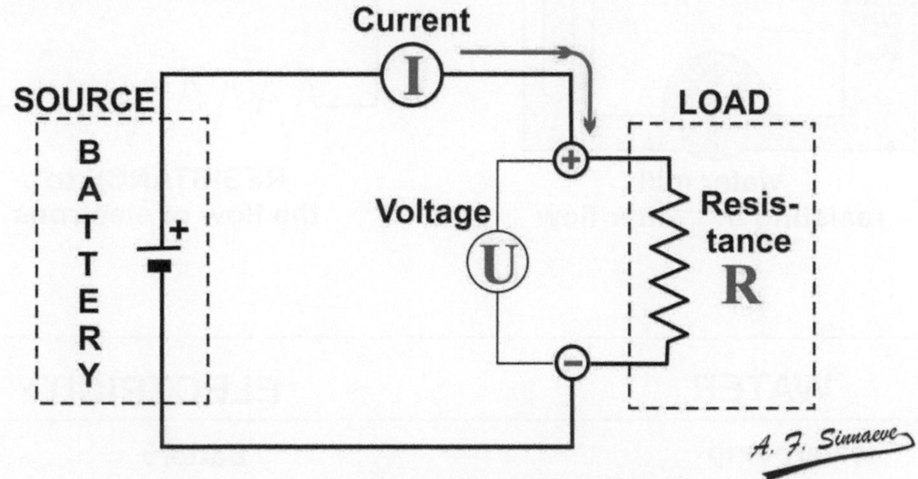

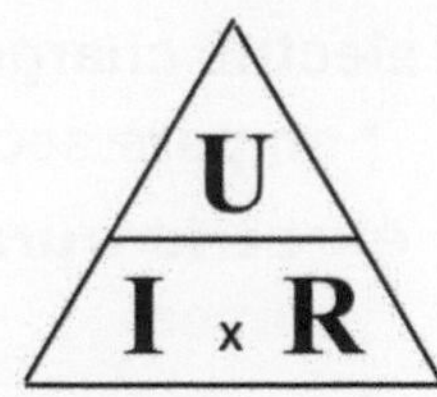

U = voltage (in volt V)

I = current (in ampere A)

R = resistance (in ohm Ω)

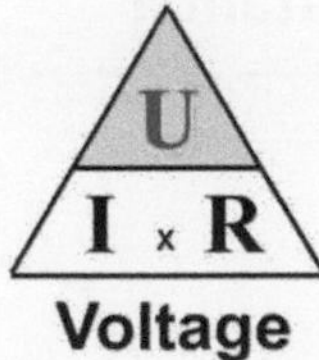

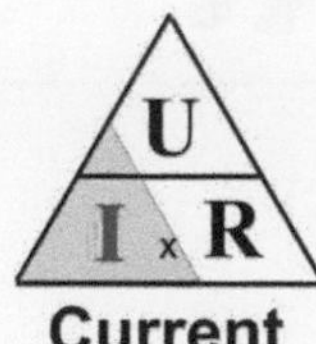

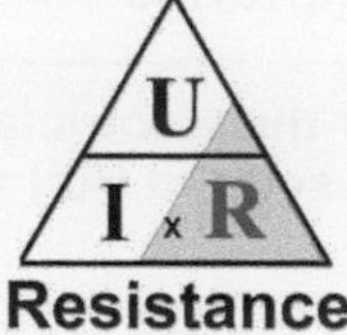

Look at the triangle and hide the variable that you are looking for : the rest of the triangle shows the formula that has to be used !

THE WATER EQUIVALENT

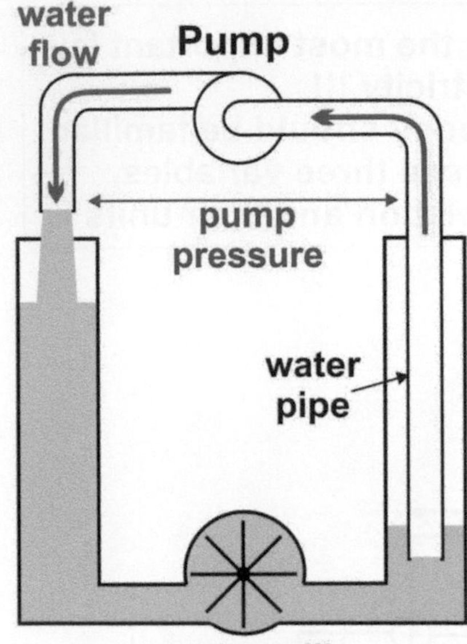

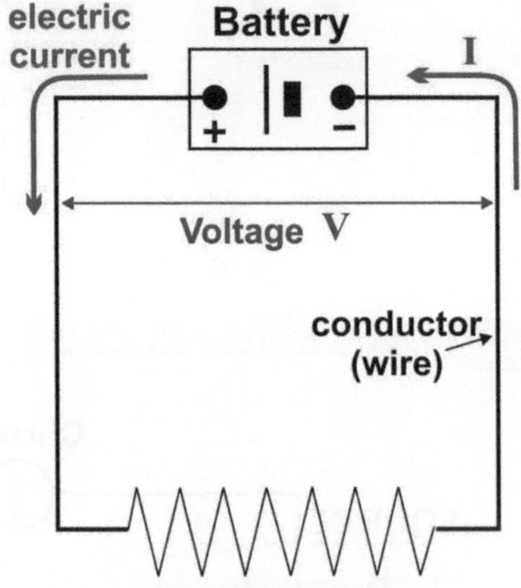

WATER	ELECTRICITY
* waterpump	* battery
* pump pressure	* voltage
* quantity of water	* electric charge
* liter	* ampere.second
* ***flow of water***	* ***electric current***
* liter per sec	* ampere
* water pipe	* wire
* resistance	* resistance

Note for the electricians :
ampere.second (As) = coulomb (C)

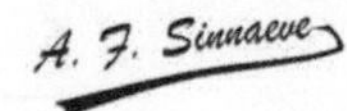

PACING IMPEDANCE

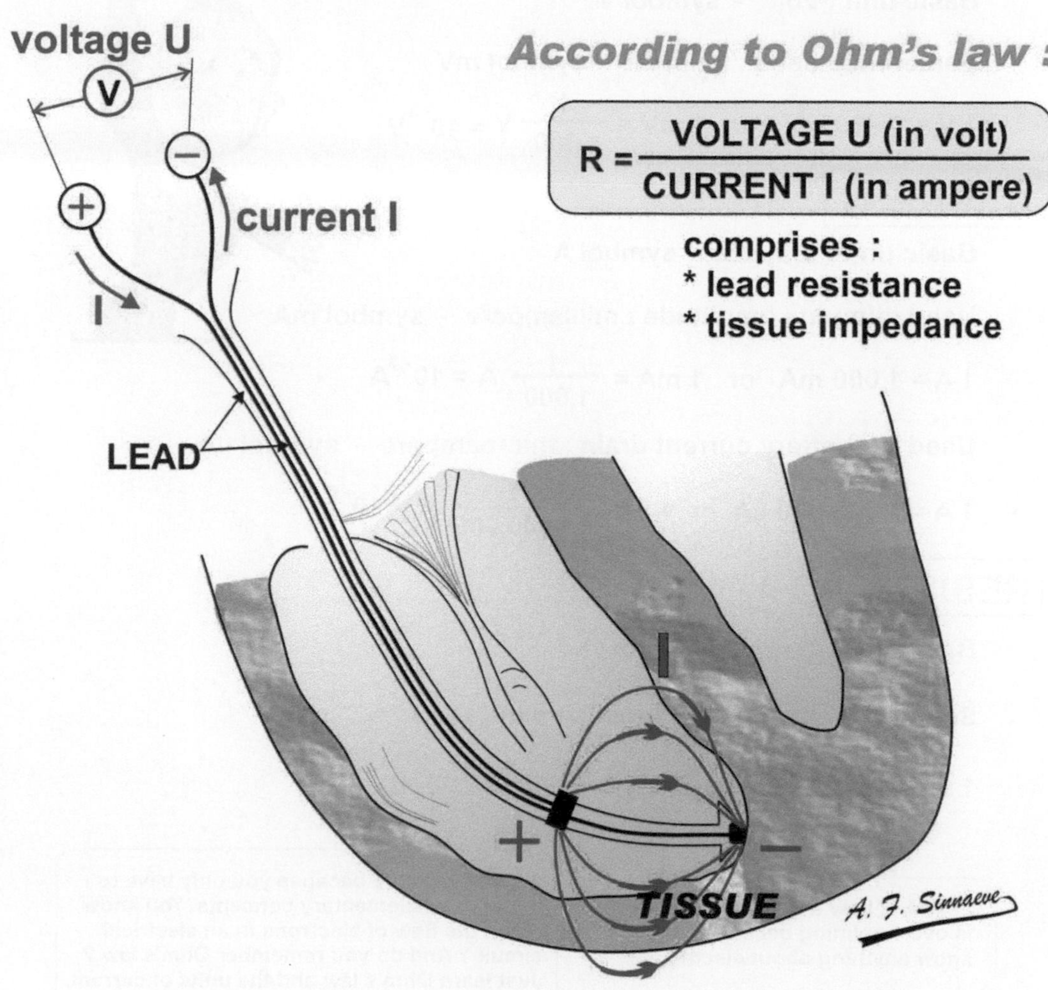

According to Ohm's law :

$$R = \frac{\text{VOLTAGE U (in volt)}}{\text{CURRENT I (in ampere)}}$$

comprises :
* lead resistance
* tissue impedance

INSULATION DEFECT < 250Ω	NORMAL PACING IMPEDANCE ca. 500Ω	LEAD FRACTURE > 1000Ω

Note for electricians :
The pacing impedance is not purely resistive (the tissue impedance is capacitive) and should be indicated by a Z. In the clinical practice only the absolute value or magnitude of the pacing impedance is considered and since it is expressed in "OHM" according to Ohm's law, most people are calling it simply "resistance"

COMMON UNITS FOR PACEMAKERS

VOLTAGE

Basic unit : volt - symbol V

Sometimes used : millivolt - symbol mV

$$1\ \text{V} = 1{,}000\ \text{mV} \quad \text{or} \quad 1\ \text{mV} = \frac{1}{1{,}000}\ \text{V} = 10^{-3}\text{V}$$

CURRENT

Basic unit : ampere - symbol A

Used stimulus amplitude : milliampere - symbol mA

$$1\ \text{A} = 1{,}000\ \text{mA} \quad \text{or} \quad 1\ \text{mA} = \frac{1}{1{,}000}\ \text{A} = 10^{-3}\text{A}$$

Used for battery current drain : microampere - symbol μA

$$1\ \text{A} = 1{,}000{,}000\ \mu\text{A} \quad \text{or} \quad 1\ \mu\text{A} = \frac{1}{1{,}000{,}000}\ \text{A} = 10^{-6}\text{A}$$

RESISTANCE

Basic unit : ohm - symbol Ω

Sometimes used : kilo-ohm - symbol kΩ

$$1\ \Omega = \frac{1}{1{,}000}\ \text{k}\Omega \quad \text{or} \quad 1\ \text{k}\Omega = 1{,}000\ \Omega = 10^{3}\ \Omega$$

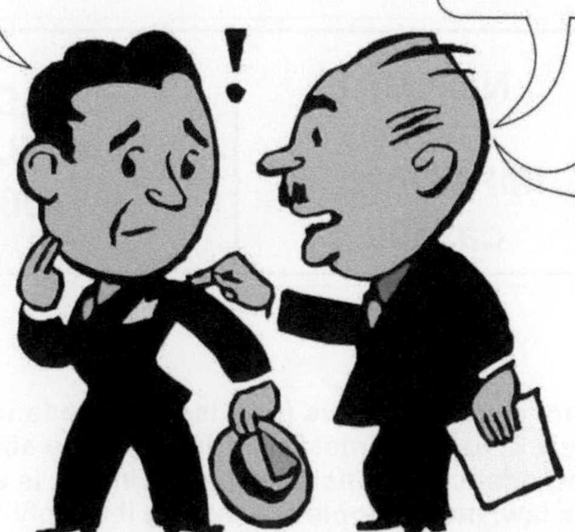
Learning how a pacemaker works is overwhelming because I don't know anything about electricity !
It's really simple because you only have to understand elementary concepts. You know about the flow of electrons in an electrical circuit ? And do you remember Ohm's law ? Just learn Ohm's law and the units of current, voltage and resistance used in Ohm's law.
You can forget parameters like energy (joules) and charge (coulombs) because they are not strictly needed in the day-to-day practice of pacemaker follow-up.
A. F. Sinnaeve

ANODE - CATHODE & ELECTRIC CURRENT

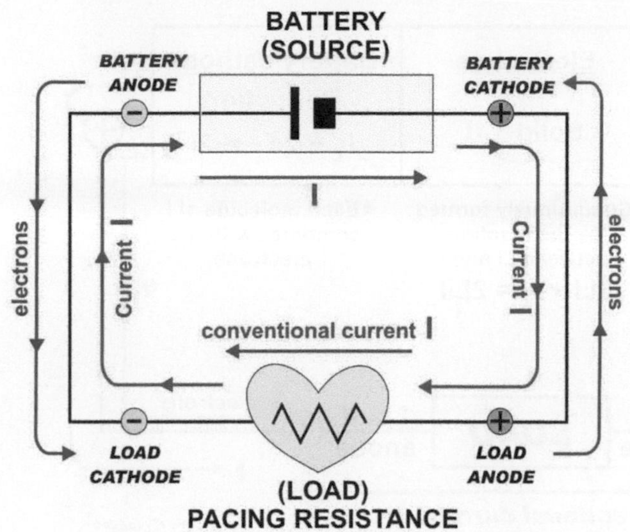

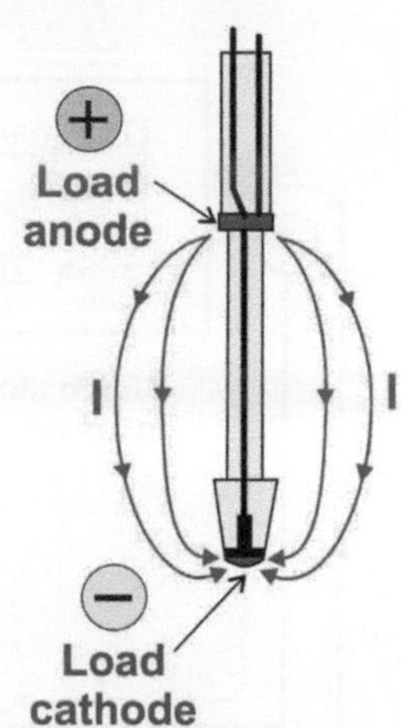

It's not difficult at all ! There are only a few facts to remember. Let me explain....

The arrangement of a circuit with a battery and a load is confusing ! Is the anode not always positive and the cathode always negative ???

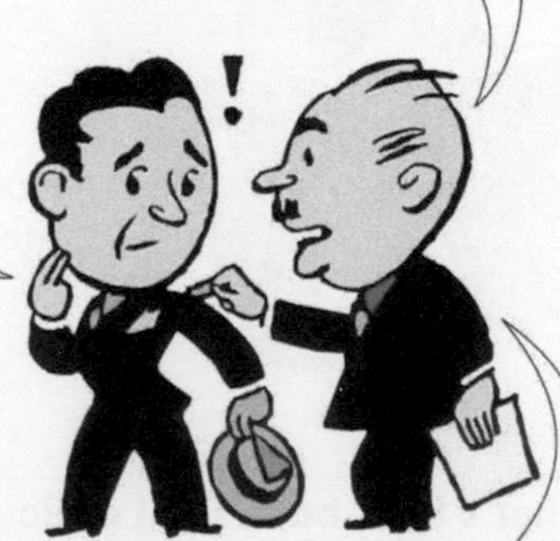

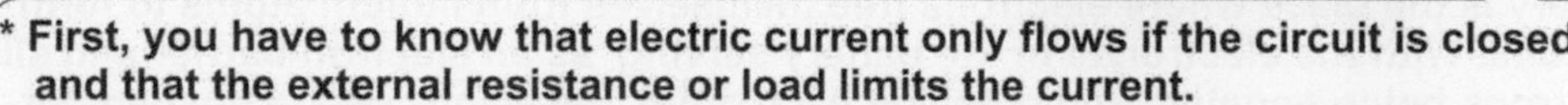

* First, you have to know that electric current only flows if the circuit is closed and that the external resistance or load limits the current.
* Second, you have to understand that in a closed circuit the ***electrons*** flow from the negative pole of the battery, through the load and back to the positive pole of the battery. However, ***conventional electric current*** flows in the opposite direction from the + pole of the battery via the load to its - pole. That's a historical convention dating from the time electrons weren't yet discovered.
* Third, just remember that the battery is the source delivering electricity while the load consumes electricity. If you follow the circuit, you will see that the anode is always the electrode by which the electrons leave (A for anode in "Away"). The cathode on the contrary, is always the electrode into which the electrons enter or come (C for cathode in "Come"). That's easy isn't it ? This terminology applies to both the battery and the load !

The Lithium - Iodine battery

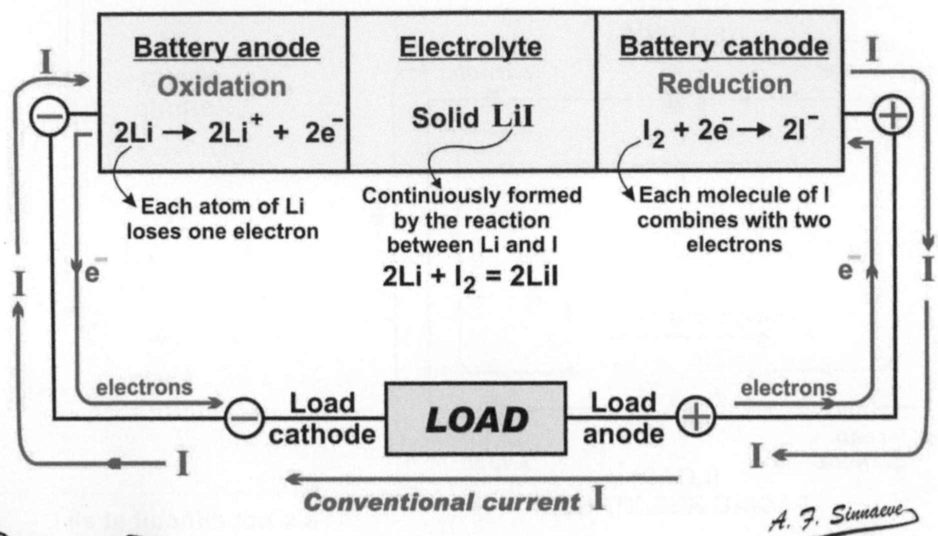

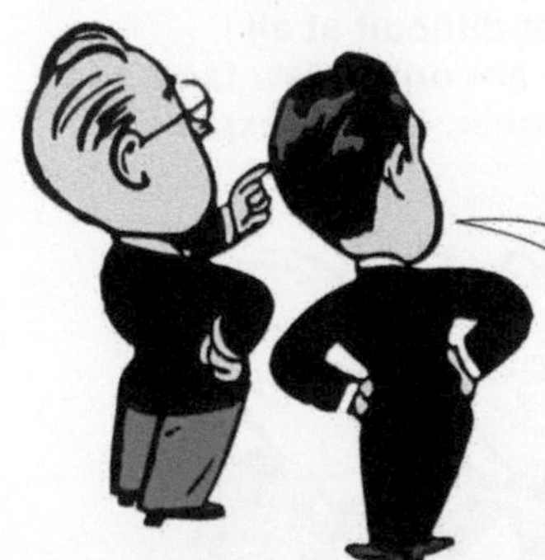

How about the lithium-iodine battery ? Someone told me that no electrons can flow through that battery ?

Yes, that's true, but it isn't difficult to understand. The anode of a lithium- iodine battery is the place where electrons free themselves from lithium atoms to form Li^+ ions. With the electrolyte of the battery serving as an electron barrier and all electrons being negative and repelling each other, the electrons are pushed outside the battery to start their journey through the electrical circuit.
Following the electrical conductors, the electrons enter the load via its cathode. Just as a liquid, electricity cannot be compressed. So, an equal amount of electrons is leaving the load via its anode, being attracted by the positive pole of the battery. The electrons enter the battery cathode where they combine with iodine I_2 to form $2I^-$ ions.
Inside the battery, the electrical circuit is closed by the flow of the Li+ and I^- ions. These ions attract each other and diffuse through the electrolyte. When the two kinds of ions meet each other, they combine to form lithium- iodide LiI.
However, the lithium- iodide is not a good electrical conductor and so the buildup of this LiI increases the internal resistance of the battery.

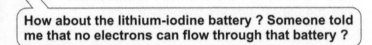

The Lithium - Iodine battery

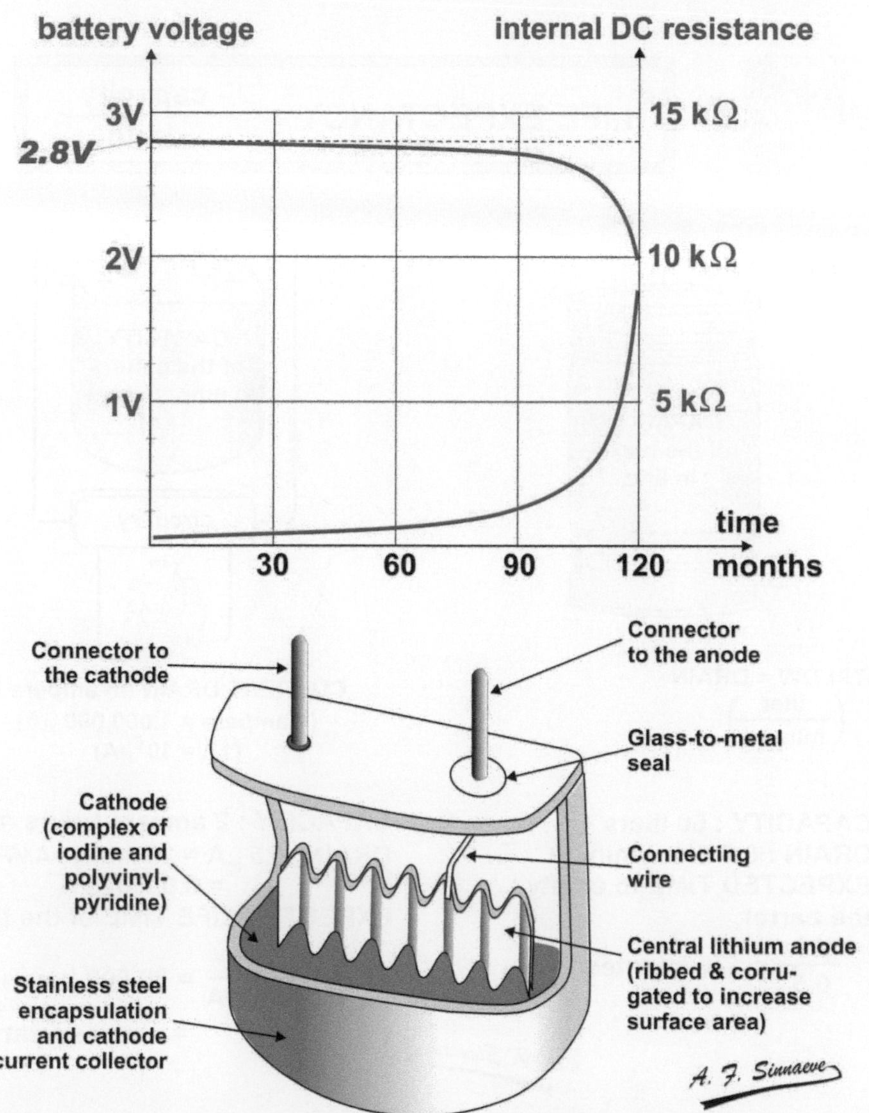

The anode of the battery produces lithium ions, while the cathode is producing iodine ions. These ions are moving to the other pole of the battery and are recombining to lithium iodide (LiI). This discharge product forms a barrier for the further movement of ions and thus an internal battery resistance is built up.
At the BOL the electrolyte barrier is thin with a low normal impedance. However, at the EOL the layer becomes thick and when the cathode material is almost depleted, the internal resistance is very high.

BOL = beginning-of-life ; **EOL** = end-of-life

BATTERY CAPACITY & LONGEVITY

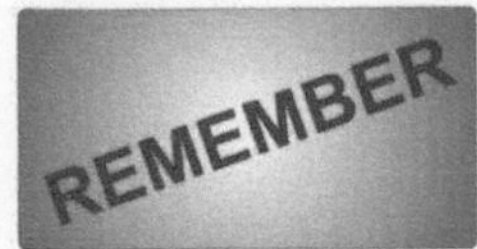

$$\text{LIFE EXPECTANCY} = \frac{\text{capacity}}{\text{drain}}$$

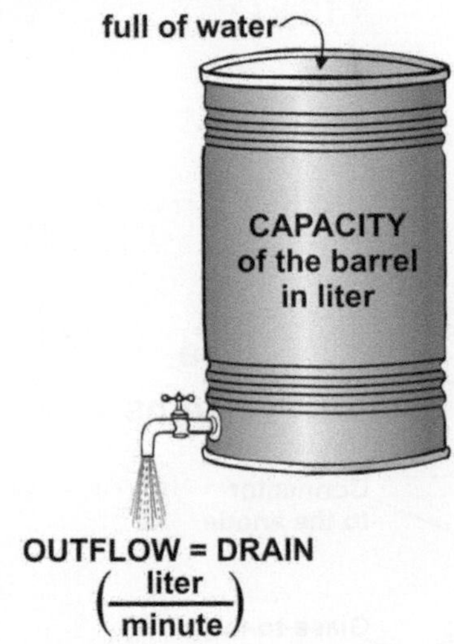

OUTFLOW = DRAIN $\left(\frac{\text{liter}}{\text{minute}}\right)$

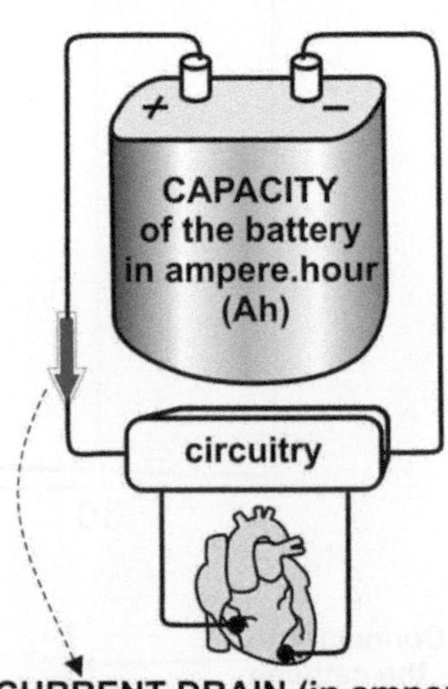

CURRENT DRAIN (in ampere A)
(1 ampere = 1,000,000 μA)
($1A = 10^6 \mu A$)

e.g. CAPACITY : 60 liters
DRAIN : 0.5 liters/minute
EXPECTED TIME to empty the barrel:

$$\frac{60}{0.5} = 120 \text{ minutes} = 2 \text{ hours}$$

e.g. CAPACITY : 2 ampere.hours = 2 Ah
DRAIN : 25 μA = 25 *MICROAMPERE* = 0.000025 A
EXPECTED LIFE TIME of the battery :

$$\frac{2 \text{ Ah}}{0.000025 \text{ A}} = 80{,}000 \text{ hours} = \text{about 9 years}$$

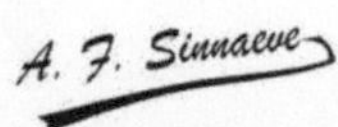

Battery life expectancy increases if the current drain decreases by using :
- pulses with a smaller voltage amplitude
- pulses with a shorter duration

Hence the importance of determining the chronic pacing threshold so as to program the output voltage and pulse duration to provide an adequate safety margin and also conserve battery capacity to extend battery life

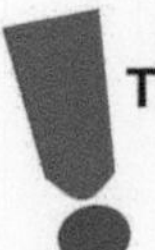

The output current of the pulses to the heart is expressed in mA (1 mA = 1/1,000 A)
The current drain of the battery is expressed in μA (1 mA = 1/1,000.000 A)
1 milliampere (mA) = 1,000 microampere (μA)

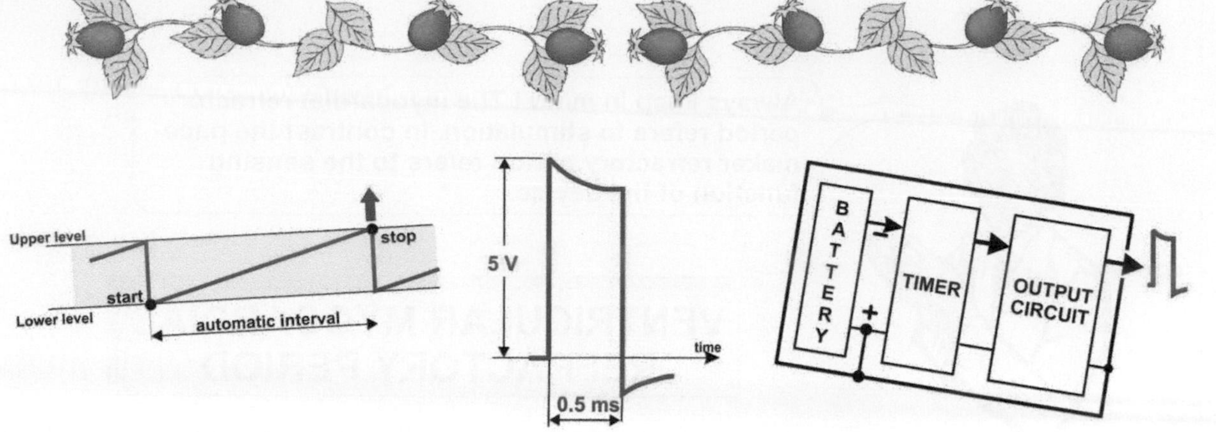

VENTRICULAR STIMULATION

* Myocardial refractory period
* Asynchronous ventricular pacing (VOO)
* Ventricular depolarization by pacing
* The output pulse of the pacemaker
* Programming and telemetry
* Wireless programming
* Panic button
* Determination of pacing threshold with constant pulse width
* Determination of pacing threshold with constant voltage
* Strength-duration curve
* Safety margin for capture
* Autocapture
* Bipolar vs unipolar pacing -
    - stimulus on analog recorder
* Variable stimulus appearance on digital recorder

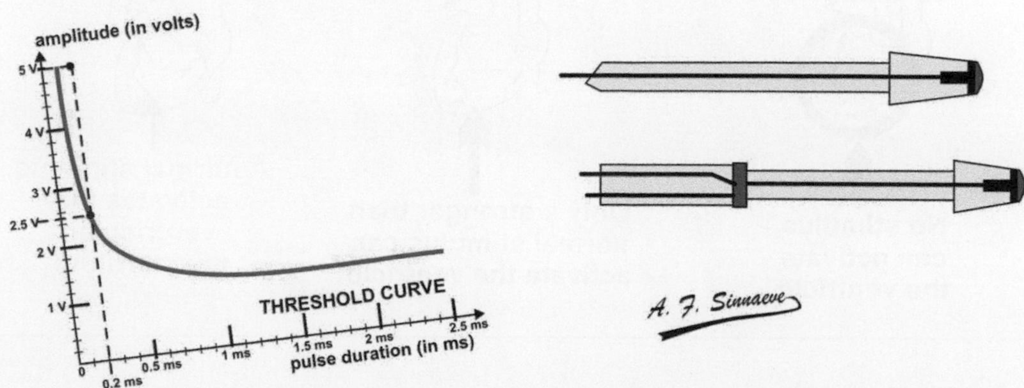

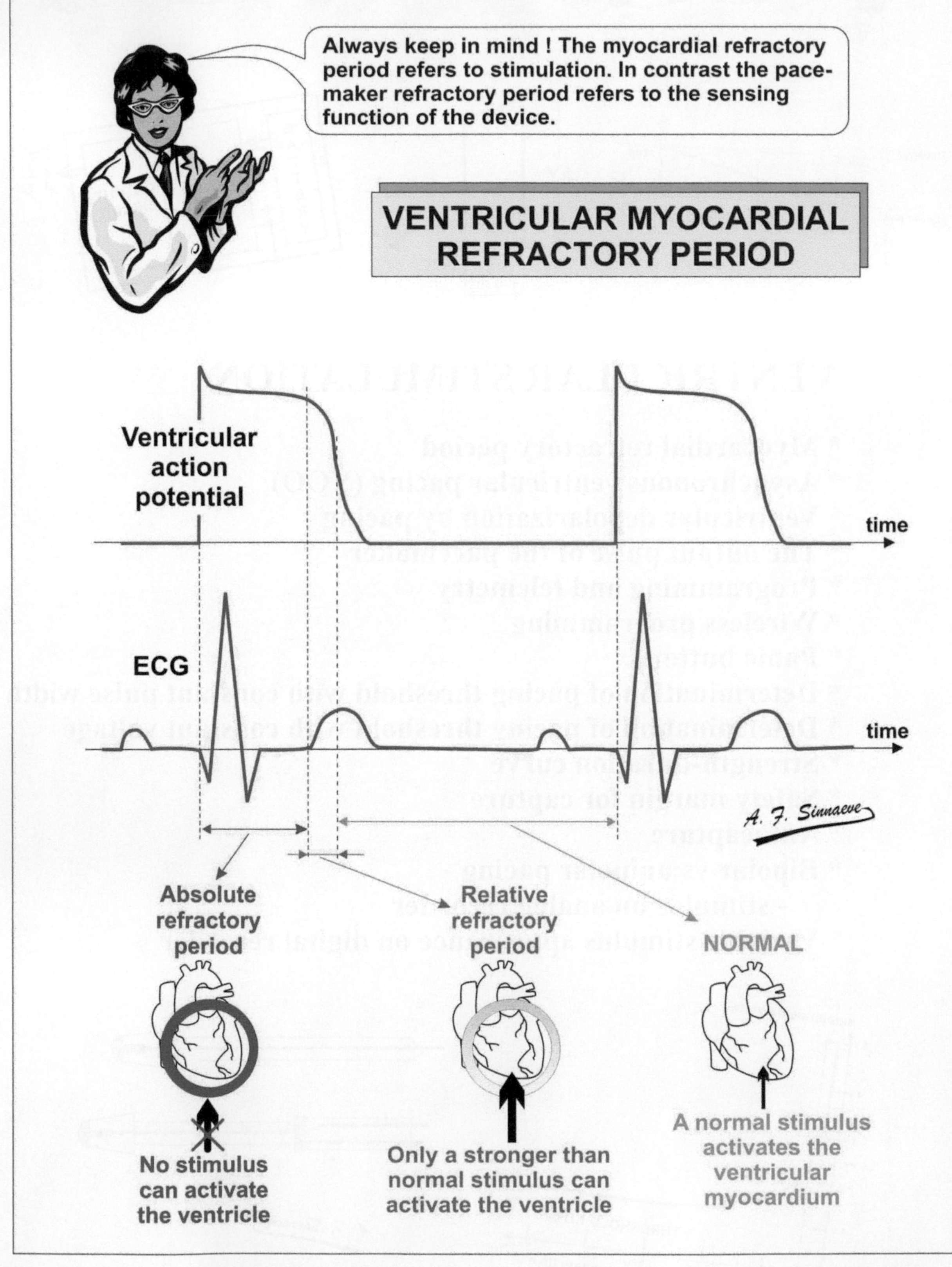
Always keep in mind ! The myocardial refractory period refers to stimulation. In contrast the pace-maker refractory period refers to the sensing function of the device.
VENTRICULAR MYOCARDIAL REFRACTORY PERIOD
Ventricular action potential
time
ECG
time
A. F. Sinnaeve
Absolute refractory period
Relative refractory period
NORMAL
No stimulus can activate the ventricle
Only a stronger than normal stimulus can activate the ventricle
A normal stimulus activates the ventricular myocardium

ASYNCHRONOUS VENTRICULAR PACING (VOO)

Note that the VOO mode causes a competitive rhythm because there is no sensing of spontaneous ventricular activity. Only stimuli beyond the ventricular myocardial refractory period cause successful capture !

UNIPOLAR PACEMAKER

connector

stimulus

lead

pacemaker can

BATTERY TIMER OUTPUT CIRCUIT

defines the time interval between the stimuli

determines amplitude & duration of the stimuli

electrode

TIMER ACTION

the timer activates the output circuit

Upper level

start

stop

Lower level

automatic interval

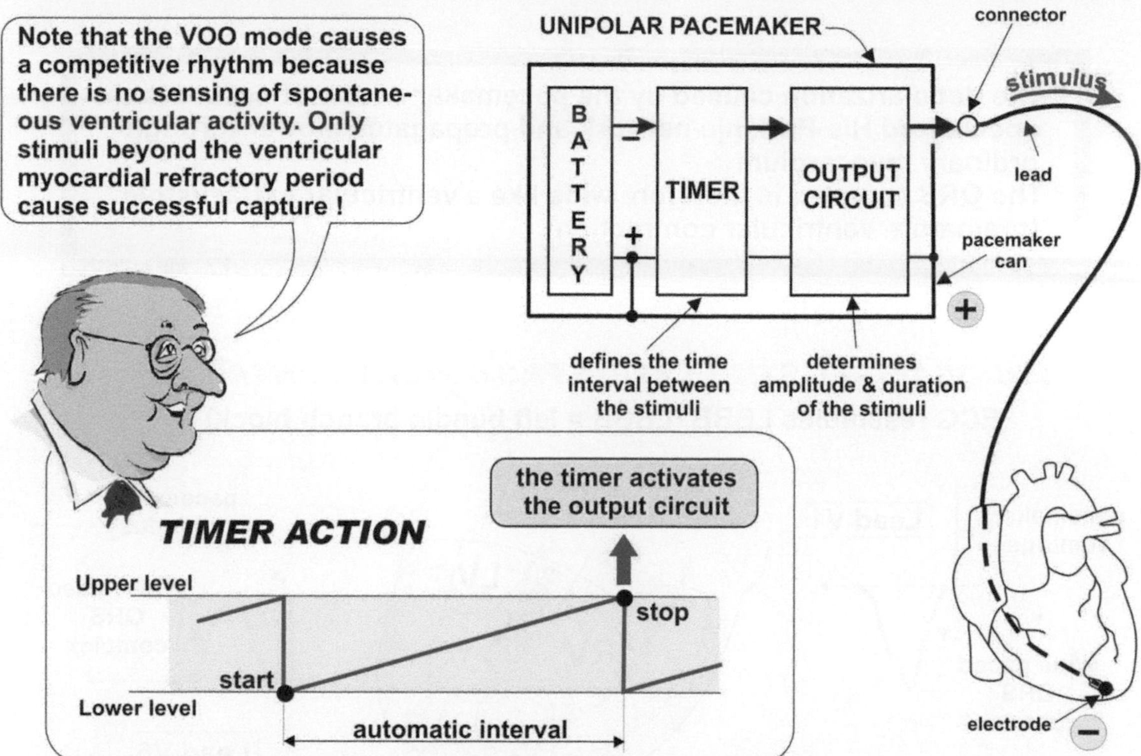

ASYNCHRONOUS PACING with COMPETITIVE RHYTHM !!!

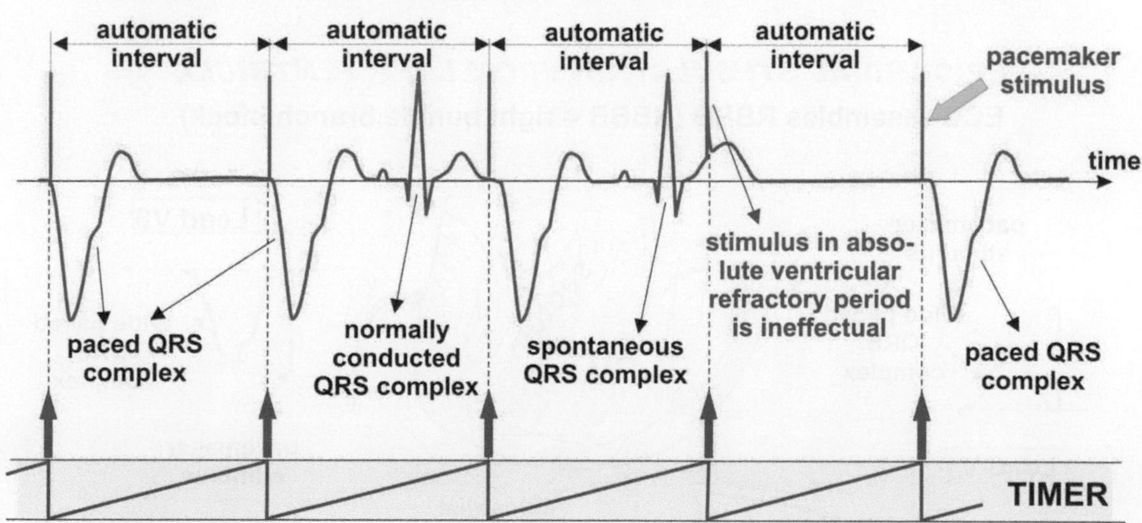

CAUTION

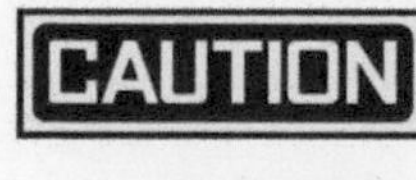

Modern pacemakers are non-competitive but assume asynchronous function only as long as a special magnet is placed over the pacemaker

VENTRICULAR DEPOLARIZATION BY PACING

* The depolarization caused by the pacemaker does not occur via the specialized His-Purkinje network and propagates slower through ordinary myocardium
* The QRS complex is therefore wide like a ventricular extrasystole (premature ventricular contraction)

ENDOCARDIAL STIMULATION FROM RIGHT VENTRICLE

ECG resembles LBBB (LBBB = left bundle branch block)

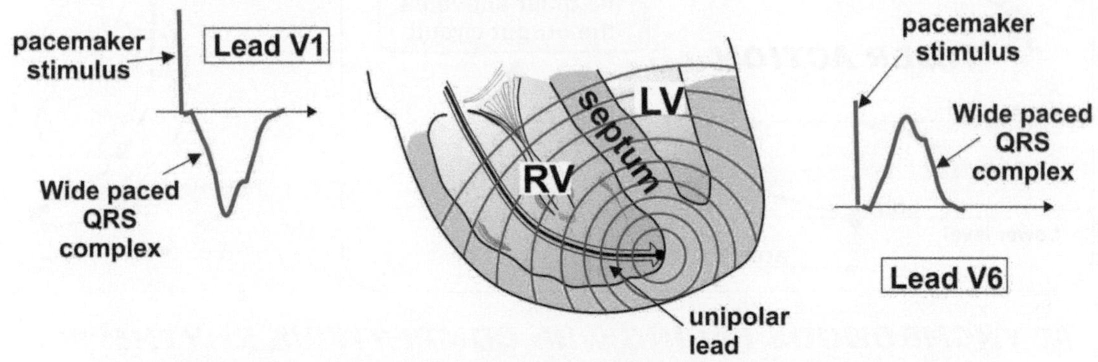

EPICARDIAL STIMULATION FROM LEFT VENTRICLE

ECG resembles RBBB (RBBB = right bundle branch block)

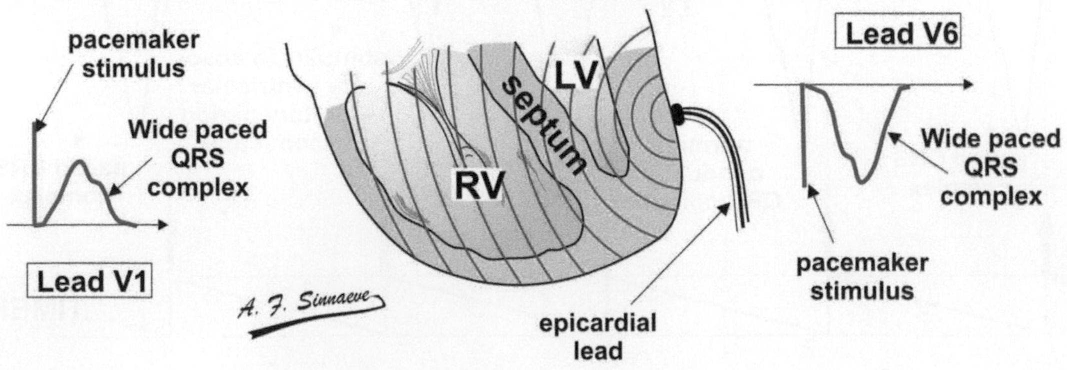

THE OUTPUT PULSE OF THE PACEMAKER

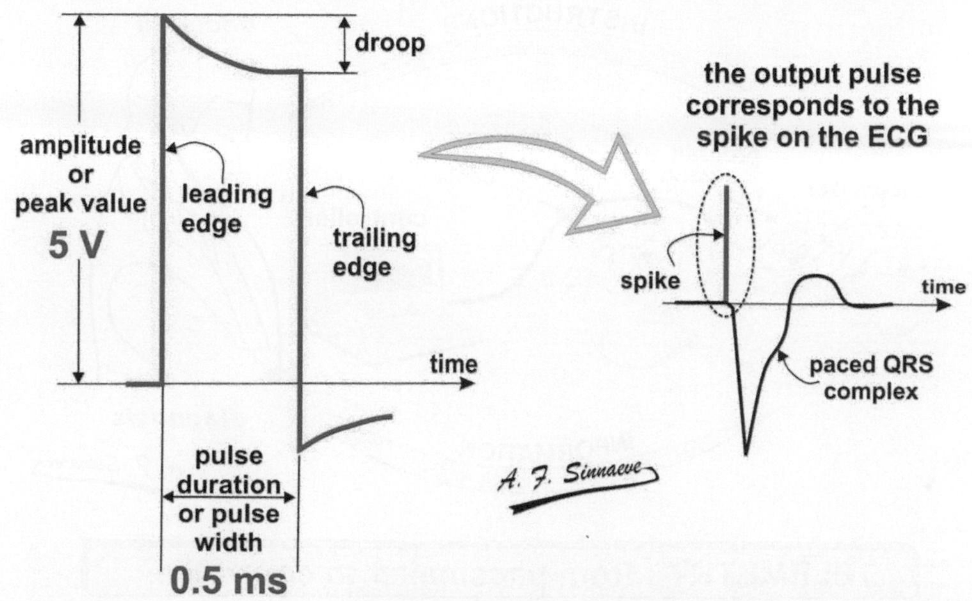

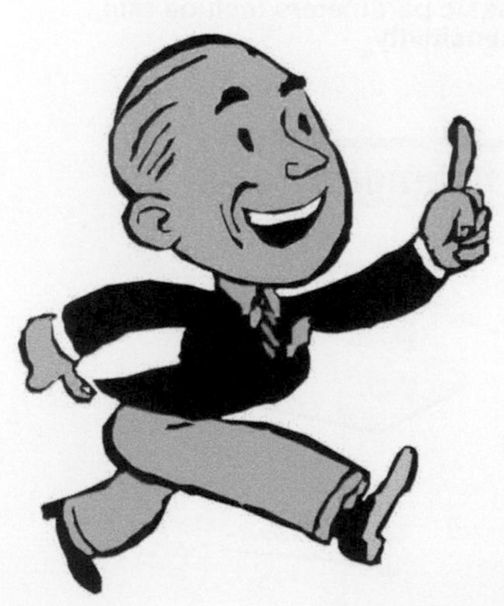

The voltage of a permanent pacemaker refers to the amplitude of the leading edge, which is always constant. It is actually closer to 5.4 V because the lithium iodine cell generates a voltage of 2.8 V which is then doubled electronically.
The droop is influenced by a variety of factors but visualization of the droop and trailing edge are not required for the management of patients. The process does not terminate with the trailing edge. The pacemaker stimulus charges the electrode-tissue interface to a large voltage (polarization voltage) which is subsequently dissipated over a much longer period than the brief pacemaker stimulus. One must understand the existence of this "afterpotential" because it can play a role in problems associated with oversensing, i.e. unintended sensing of certain events.

PROGRAMMING : from controller to pacemaker

Pacemakers have many programmable functions that can be altered noninvasively with a special programmer and a wand positioned over the pacemaker. Unfortunately there is no universal programmer and each manufacturer provides programmers that will work only with their own pacemakers.

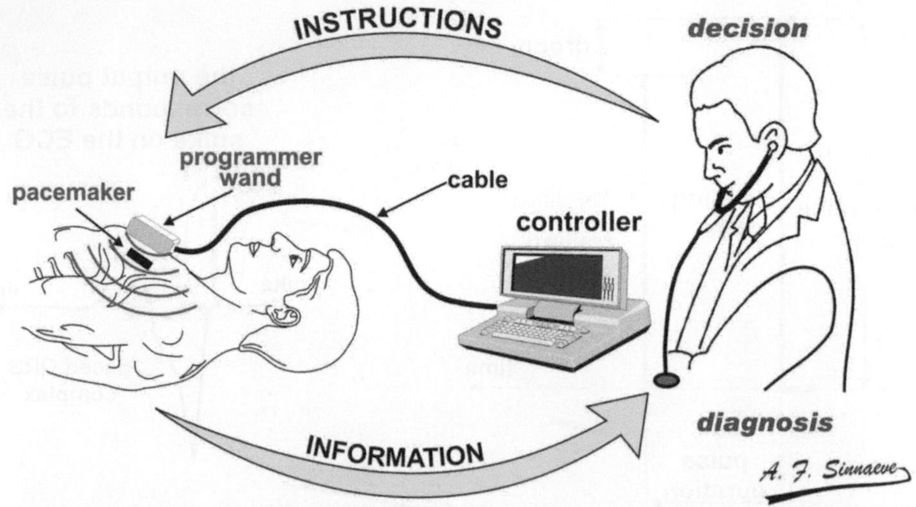

TELEMETRY : from pacemaker to controller

The stored parameters and/or instructions to the pacemaker can be retrieved by interrogation with a special programming head placed over the pacemaker. The data is then sent to the programmer which automatically delivers a printout. Basic parameters include rate, output (amplitude in volts and pulse duration in ms) and sensitivity.

WIRELESS Programming and telemetry

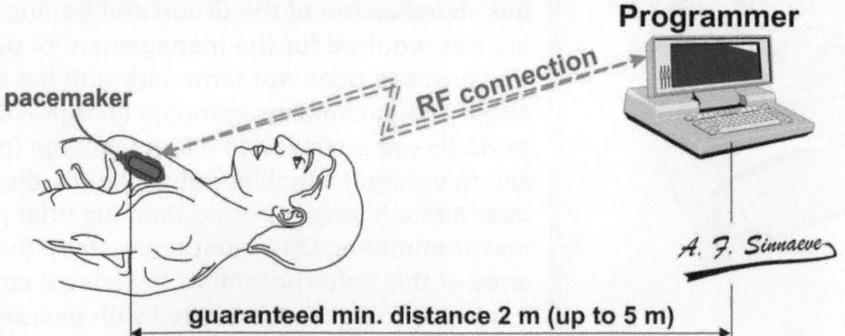

Contemporary pacing systems do not need a wand and a cable for programming and telemetry. Due to the amazing progress of electronics, they are able to communicate with the programmer from a distance. They contain a more powerful transceiver and an antenna working very efficiently at a much higher frequency (RF = radio frequency). Nevertheless, the same basic principles of transmitting information by coded messages are still valid !

N.B. : a **transceiver** (transmitter-receiver) is an electronic component, coupled to an antenna, which is able to transmit signals to the outside world and also can receive signals from that world

THE EMERGENCY BUTTON

WARNING

* Asystole can occur when programming the output. In an emergency use the panic button to restore pacing with a preset combination of parameters.
* Always have 2 programmers in case one malfunctions or breaks down

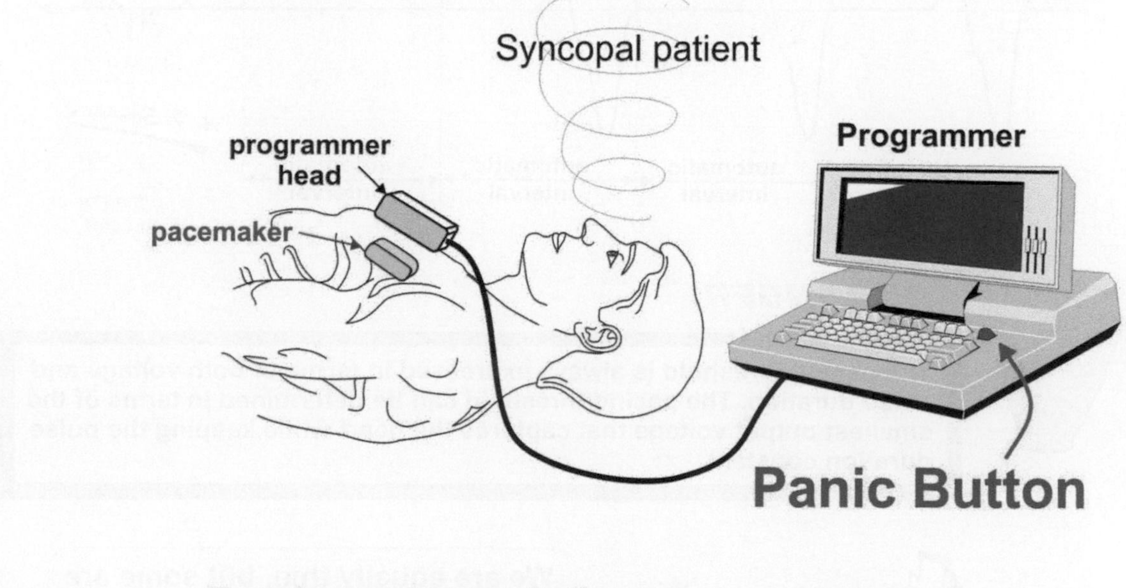

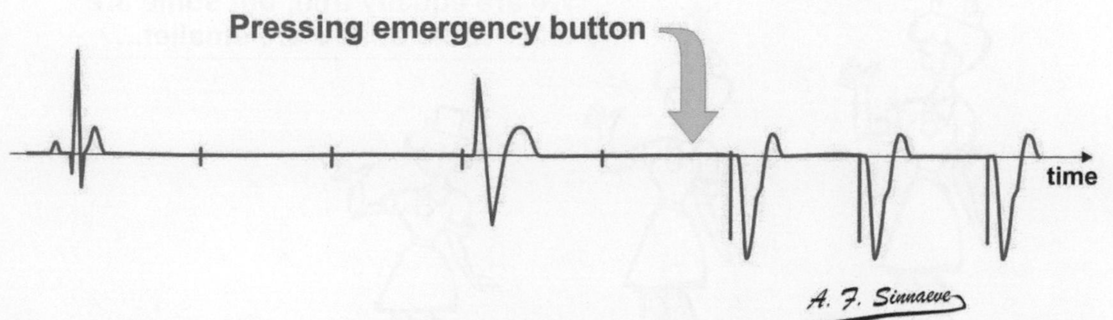

DETERMINATION OF PACING THRESHOLD

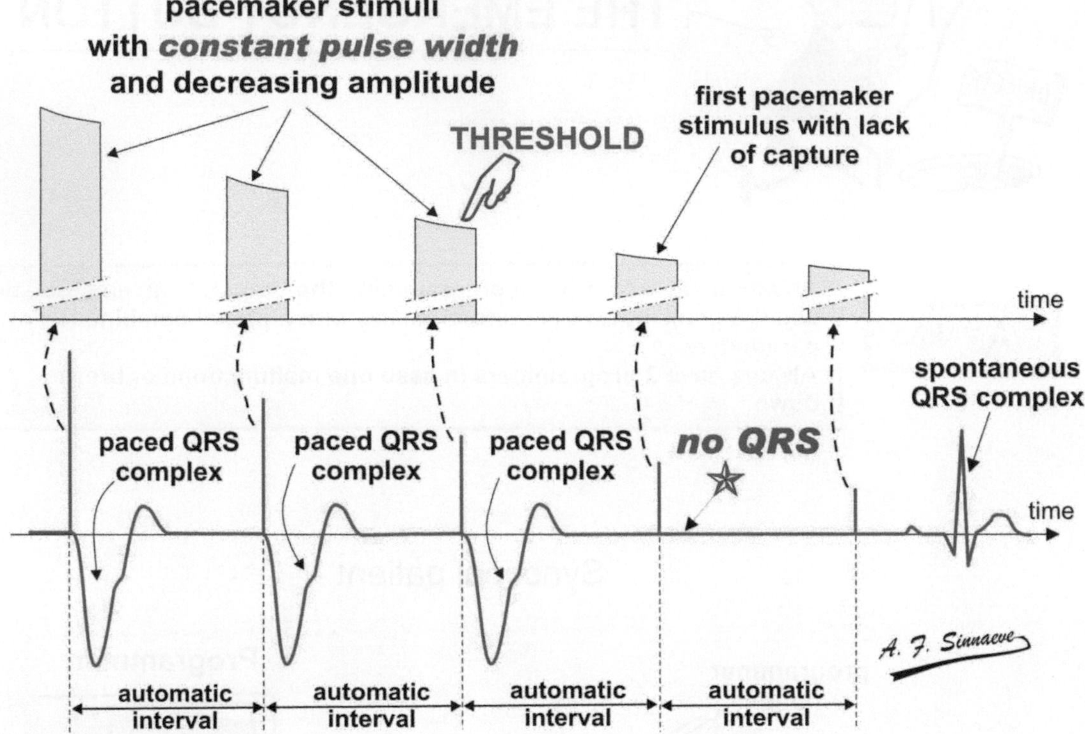

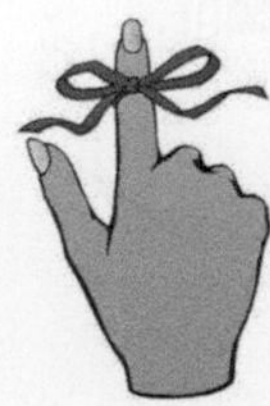

REMINDER

The pacing threshold is always expressed in terms of both voltage and pulse duration. The pacing threshold can be determined in terms of the smallest output voltage that captures the heart while keeping the pulse duration constant.

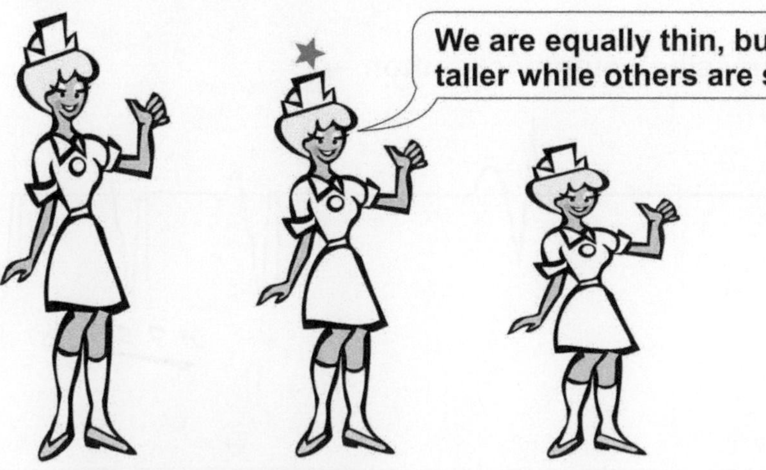
We are equally thin, but some are taller while others are smaller...

DETERMINATION OF PACING THRESHOLD

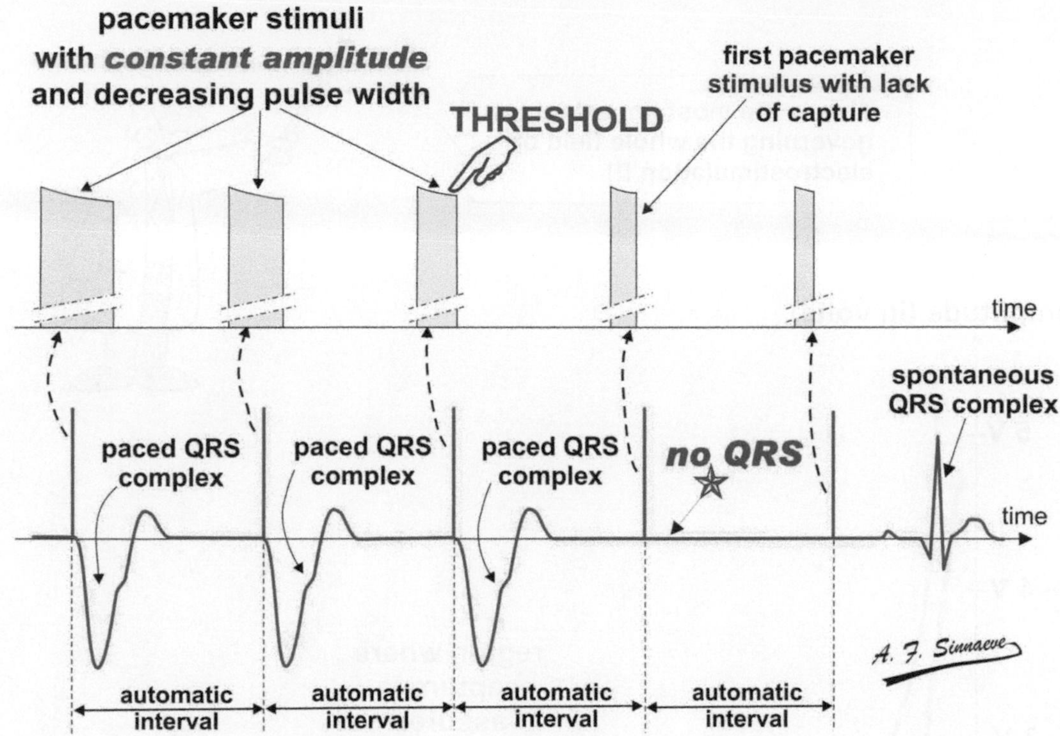

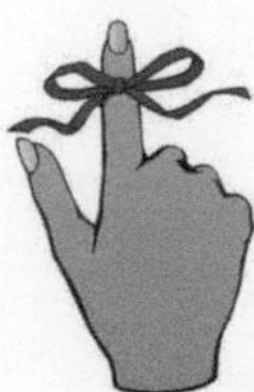

REMINDER

The pacing threshold is always expressed in terms of both voltage and pulse duration. The pacing threshold can be determined in terms of the shortest pulse duration that captures the heart while keeping the output voltage constant.

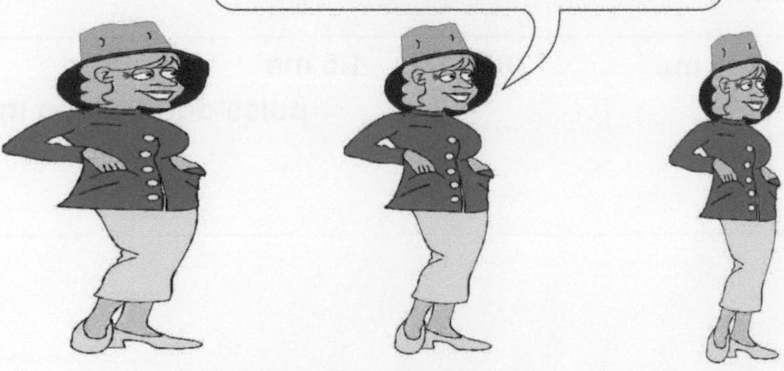
Equal height, but not otherwise equal !
Some are too wide, others are too thin...

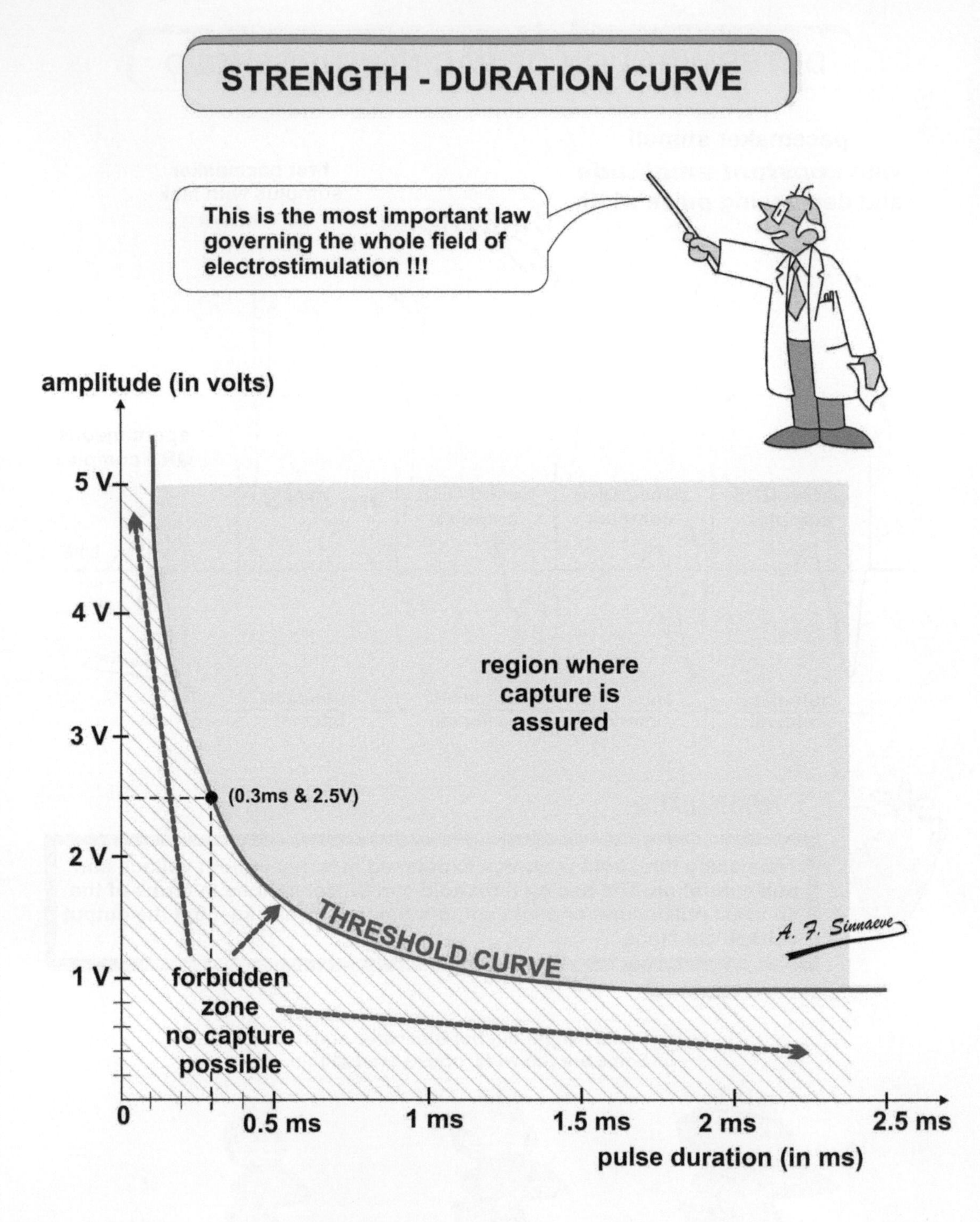
STRENGTH - DURATION CURVE
This is the most important law governing the whole field of electrostimulation !!!
amplitude (in volts)
5 V
4 V
3 V
2 V
1 V
0
0.5 ms
1 ms
1.5 ms
2 ms
2.5 ms
pulse duration (in ms)
region where capture is assured
(0.3ms & 2.5V)
THRESHOLD CURVE
forbidden zone no capture possible
A. F. Sinnaeve

SAFETY RATIO CONCEPT FOR CAPTURE

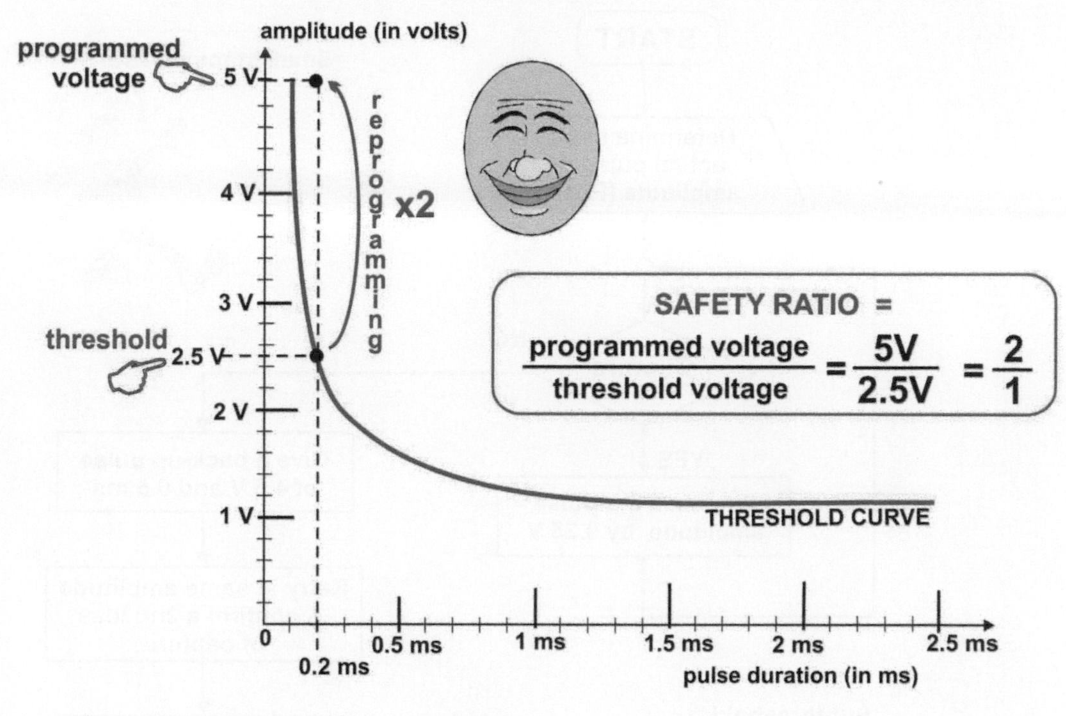

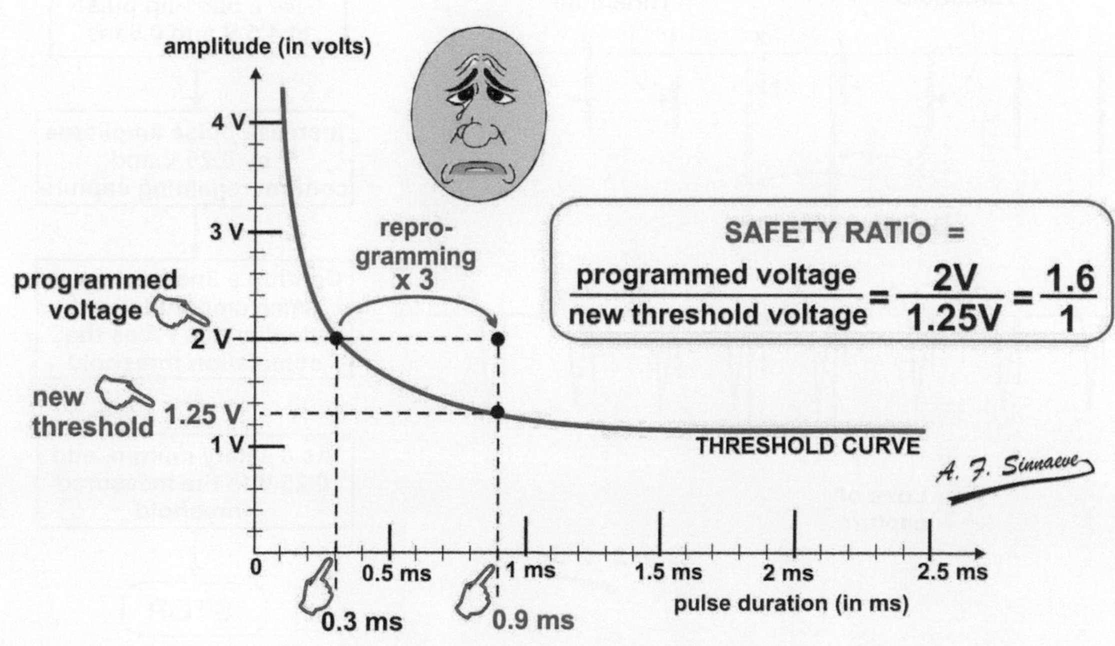

AUTOMATIC STIMULATION THRESHOLD SEARCH

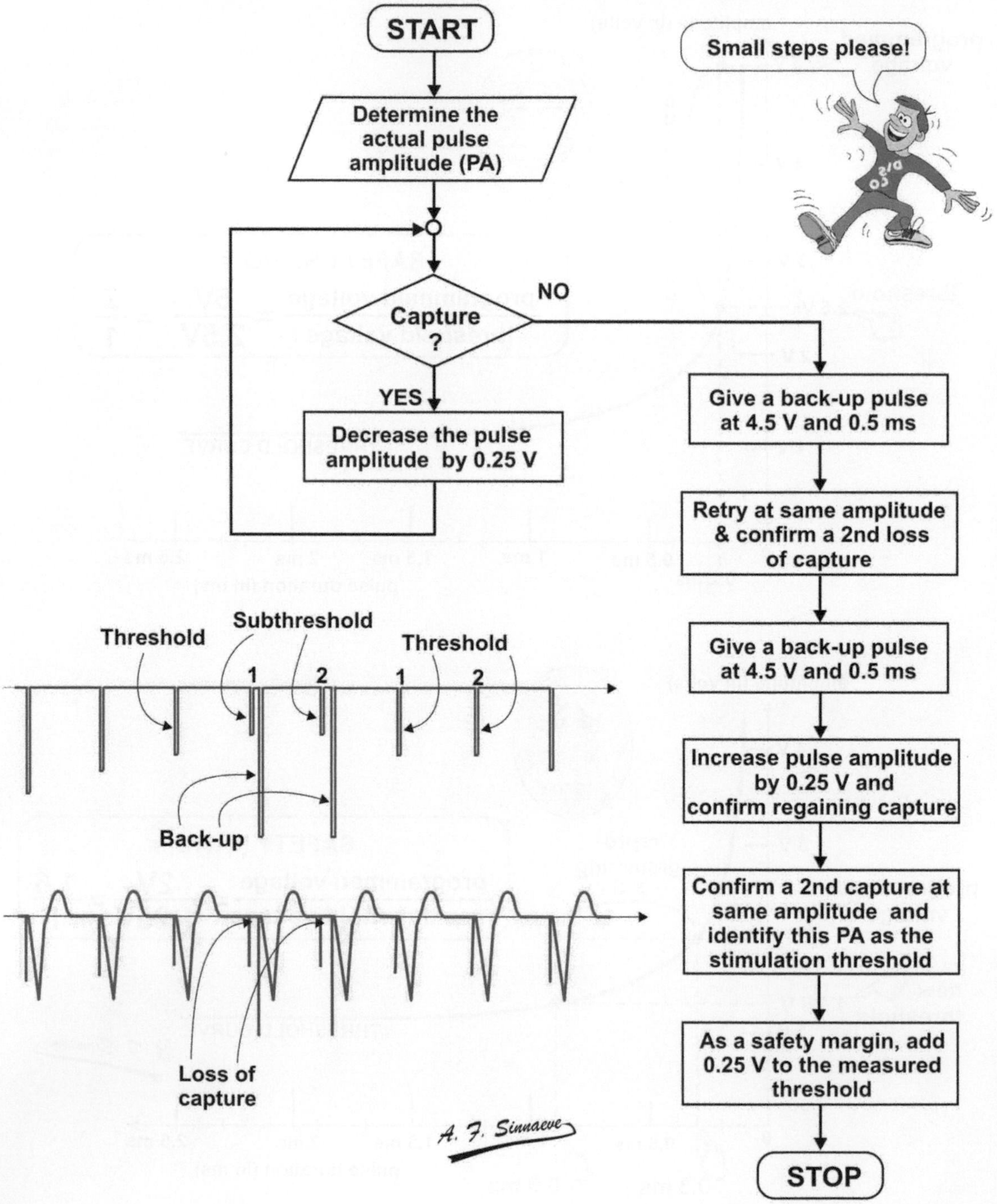

START

Determine the actual pulse amplitude (PA)

Capture ?

YES

Decrease the pulse amplitude by 0.25 V

NO

Give a back-up pulse at 4.5 V and 0.5 ms

Retry at same amplitude & confirm a 2nd loss of capture

Give a back-up pulse at 4.5 V and 0.5 ms

Increase pulse amplitude by 0.25 V and confirm regaining capture

Confirm a 2nd capture at same amplitude and identify this PA as the stimulation threshold

As a safety margin, add 0.25 V to the measured threshold

STOP

Small steps please!

Threshold

Subthreshold

1

2

Threshold

1

2

Back-up

Loss of capture

A. F. Sinnaeve

BIPOLAR vs UNIPOLAR PACING SIZE OF THE STIMULUS ON ECG

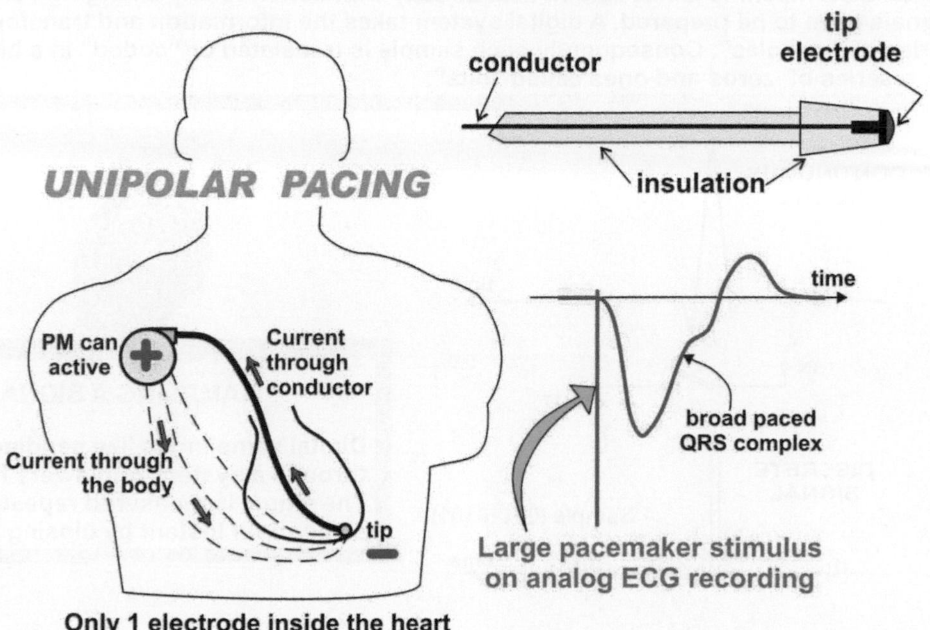

Only 1 electrode inside the heart

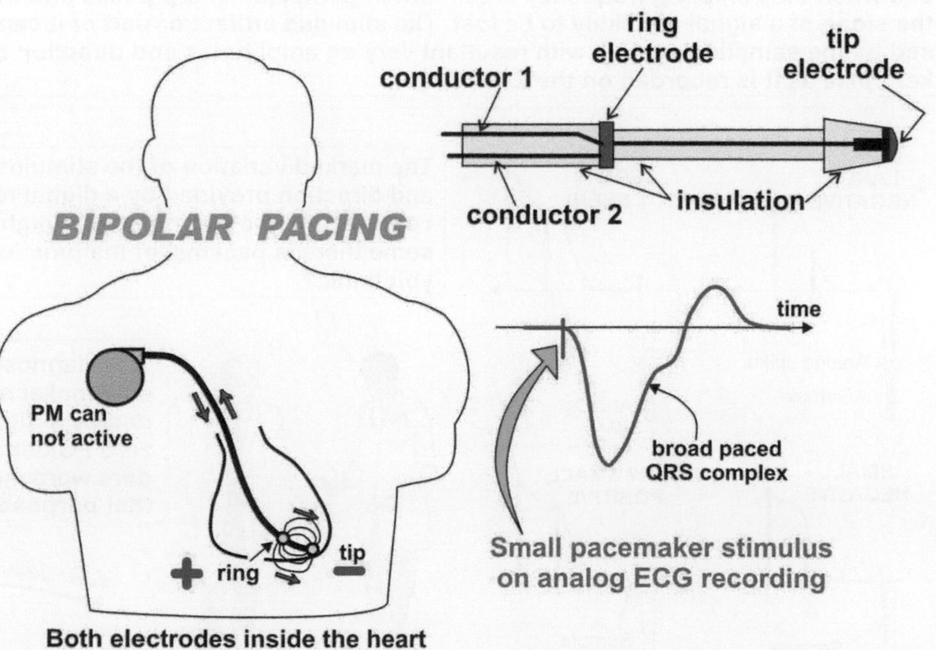

Both electrodes inside the heart

VARIABILITY OF THE STIMULUS ARTIFACT ON A DIGITAL ELECTROCARDIOGRAPH

An analog recording system attempts to recreate the information as it actually happens. A digital ECG machine is not able to deal directly with continuously changing voltages, so the signals have to be prepared. A digital system takes the information and transforms it into a series of "samples". Consequently each sample is translated or "coded" in a binary number i.e. a series of zeros and ones called "bits".

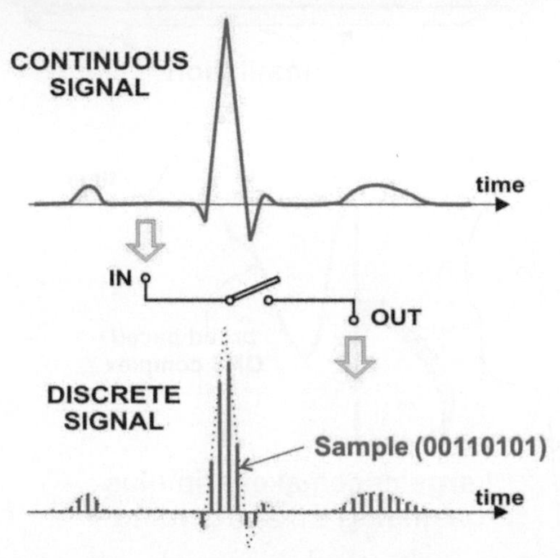

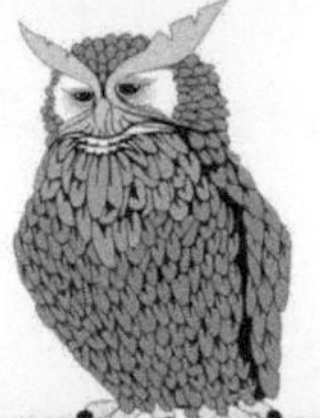

SAMPLING A SIGNAL

Digital sampling is like sending the signal through a system with a very fast switch. The signal is measured repeatedly during a very brief instant by closing the switch.

Since the signal is only sampled at discrete points in time, some information may be missed when the sampling frequency is too low. In particular, sharp peaks and transitions in the slope of a signal are likely to be lost. The stimulus artifact or part of it can be easily missed by the sampling system with resultant varying amplitudes and direction of the pacemaker spike as it is recorded on the ECG.

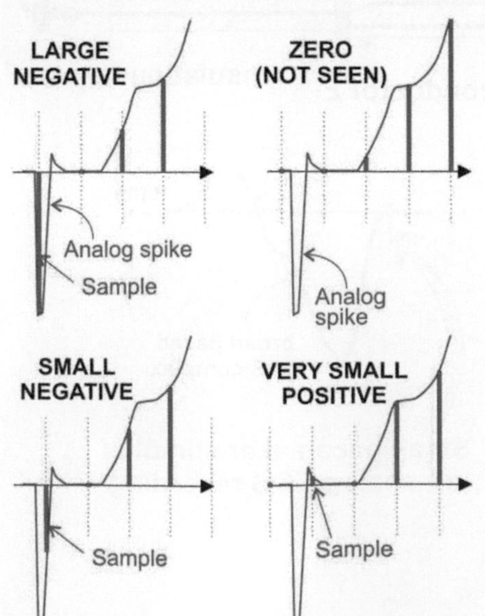

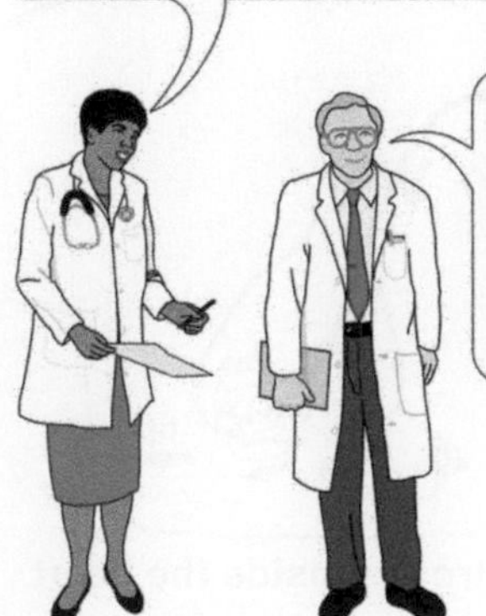

The marked variation of the stimulus in amplitude and direction provided by a digital recorder may be confusing to the beginner who might wrongly assume there is pacemaker malfunction. What do you think ?
The diagnostic value of the pacemaker stimulus recorded by a digital recorder is zero ! Older analog recorders were more useful for that purpose

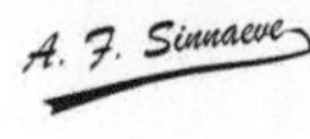

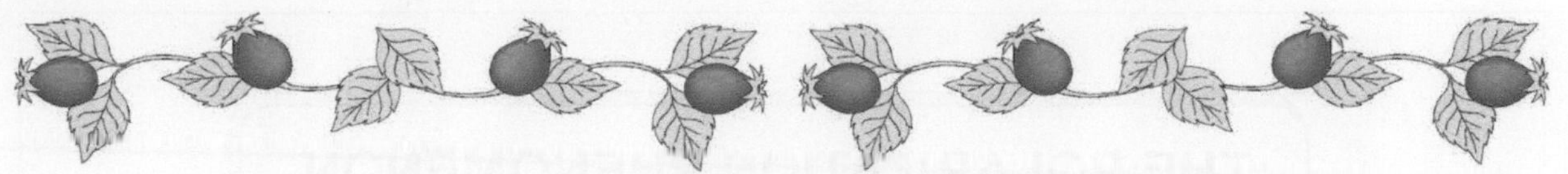

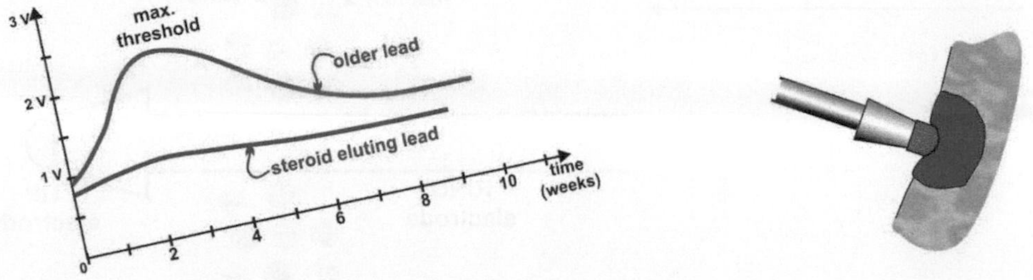

PACING LEADS

* The polarization phenomenon
* Fixation and conductors
* Evolution of the pacing threshold
* The porous electrode
* Low impedance vs high impedance electrode
* Lead displacement

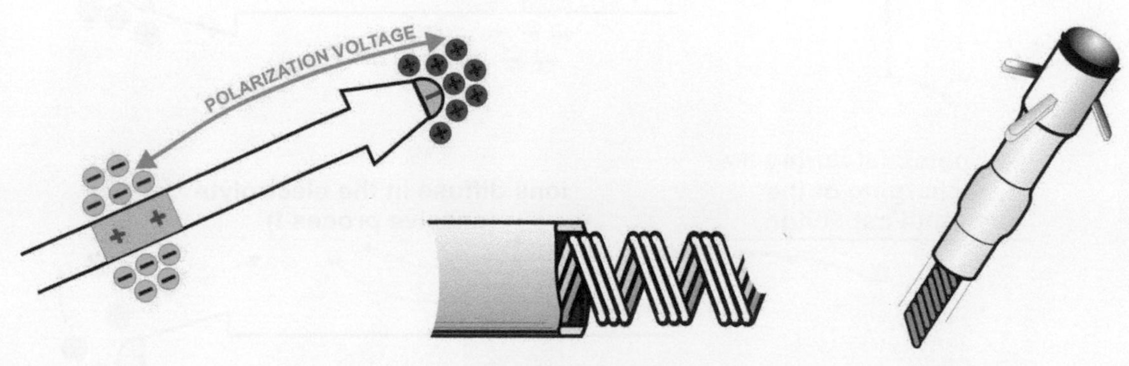

A. F. Sinnaeve

THE POLARIZATION PHENOMENON

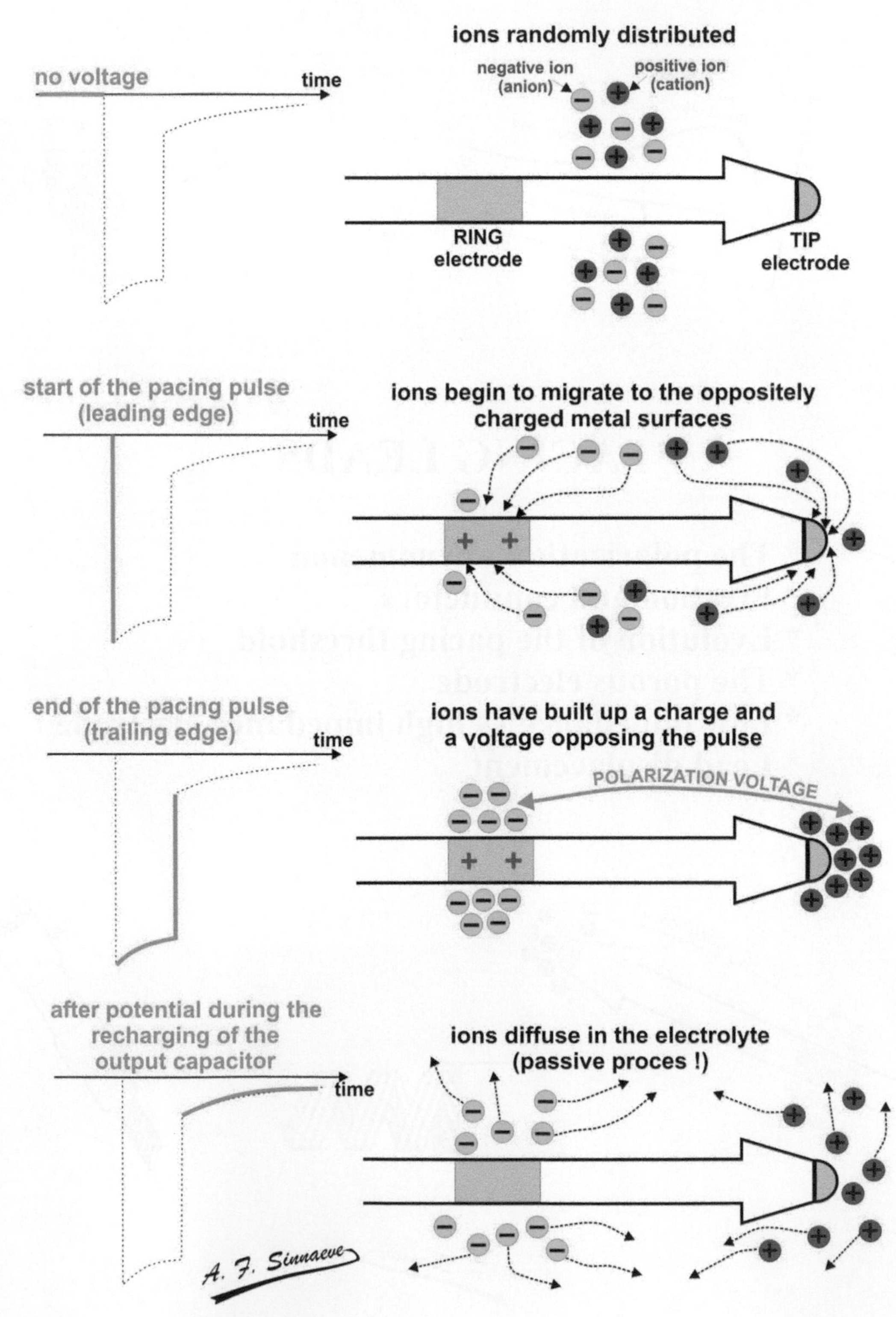

PASSIVE LEAD FIXATION

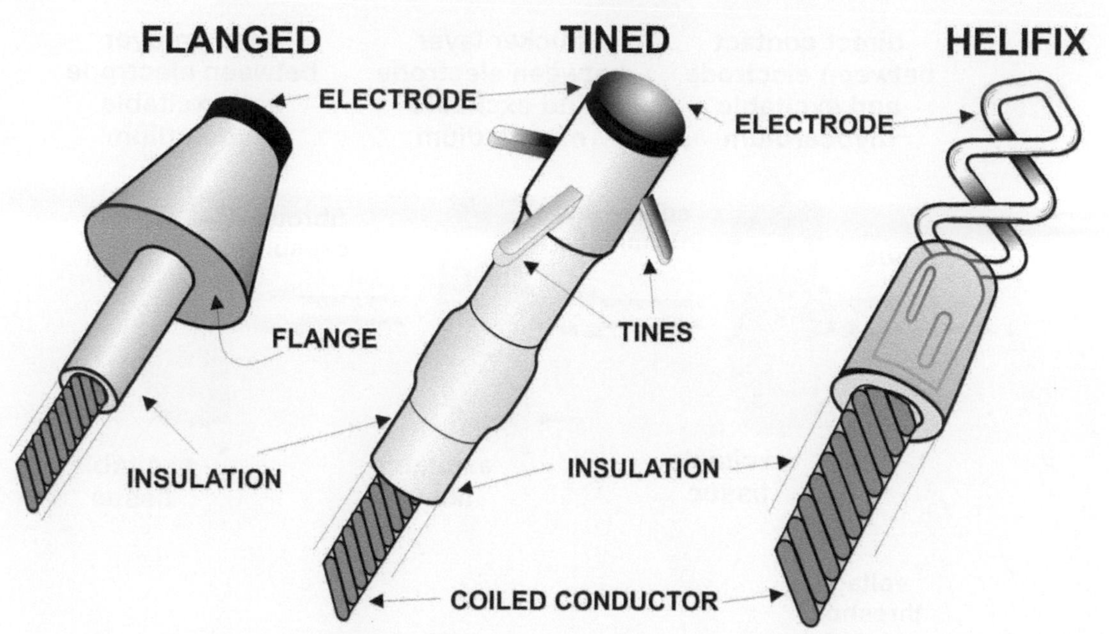

ACTIVE LEAD FIXATION

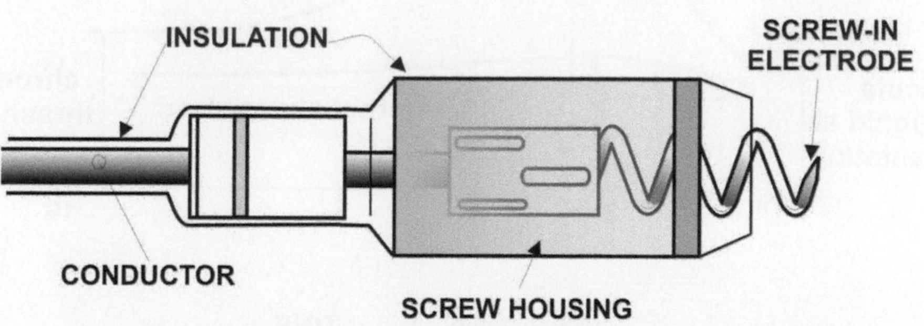

A TRI-FILAR CONDUCTOR COIL

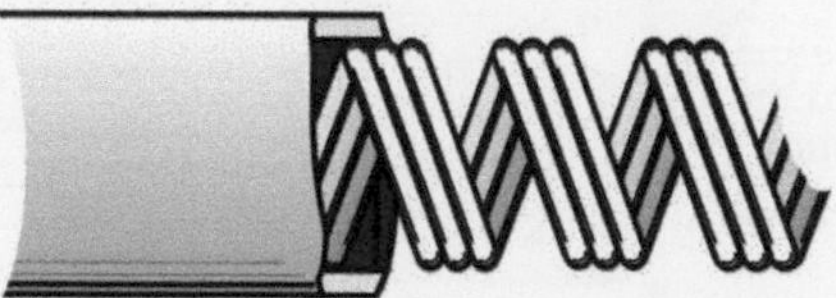

A. F. Sinnaeve

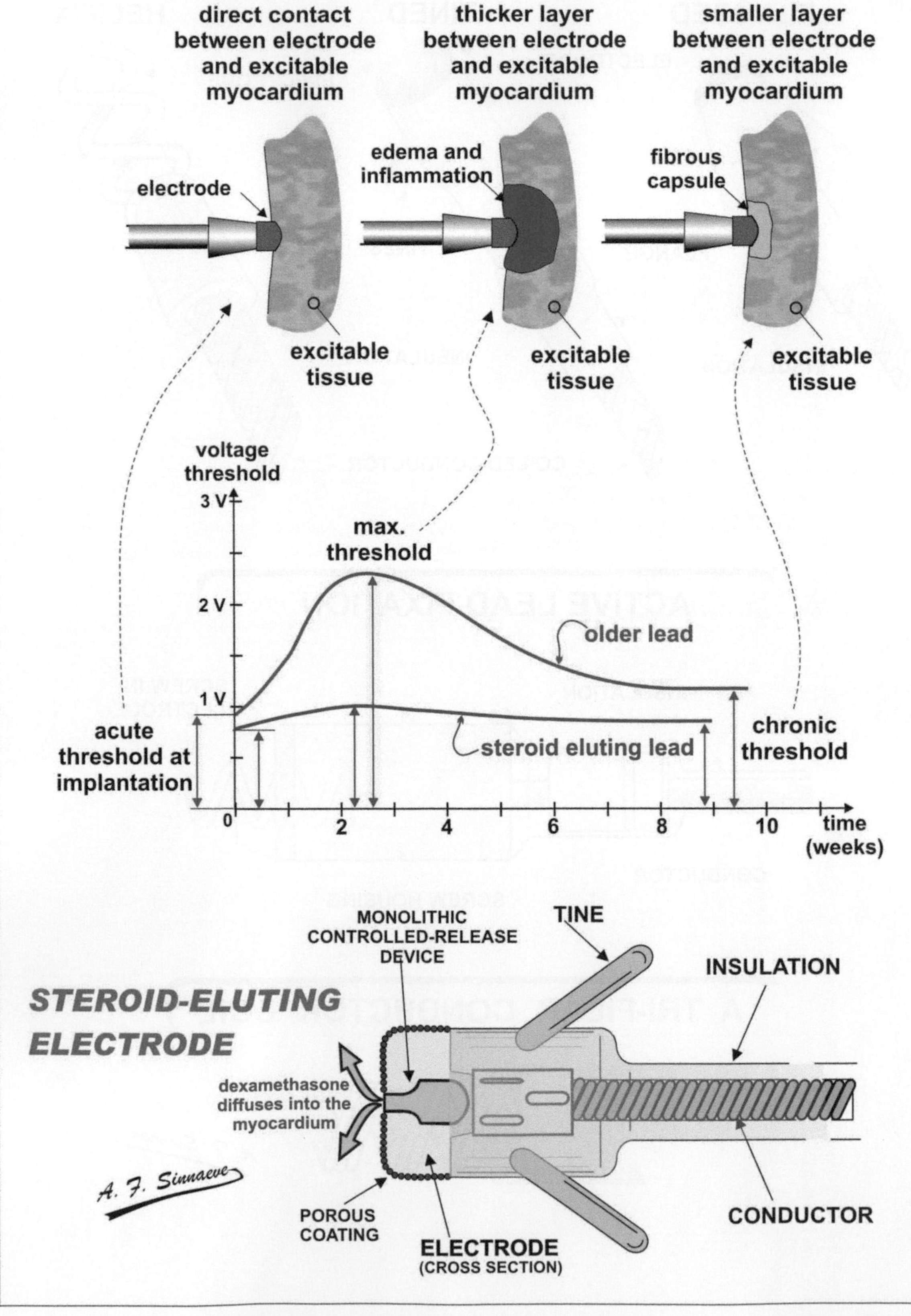

EVOLUTION OF PACING THRESHOLD
direct contact between electrode and excitable myocardium
thicker layer between electrode and excitable myocardium
smaller layer between electrode and excitable myocardium
electrode
edema and inflammation
fibrous capsule
excitable tissue
excitable tissue
excitable tissue
voltage threshold
3 V
2 V
1 V
max. threshold
older lead
steroid eluting lead
acute threshold at implantation
chronic threshold
0
2
4
6
8
10
time (weeks)
STEROID-ELUTING ELECTRODE
MONOLITHIC CONTROLLED-RELEASE DEVICE
TINE
INSULATION
dexamethasone diffuses into the myocardium
POROUS COATING
ELECTRODE (CROSS SECTION)
CONDUCTOR
A. F. Sinnaeve

THE POROUS ELECTRODE

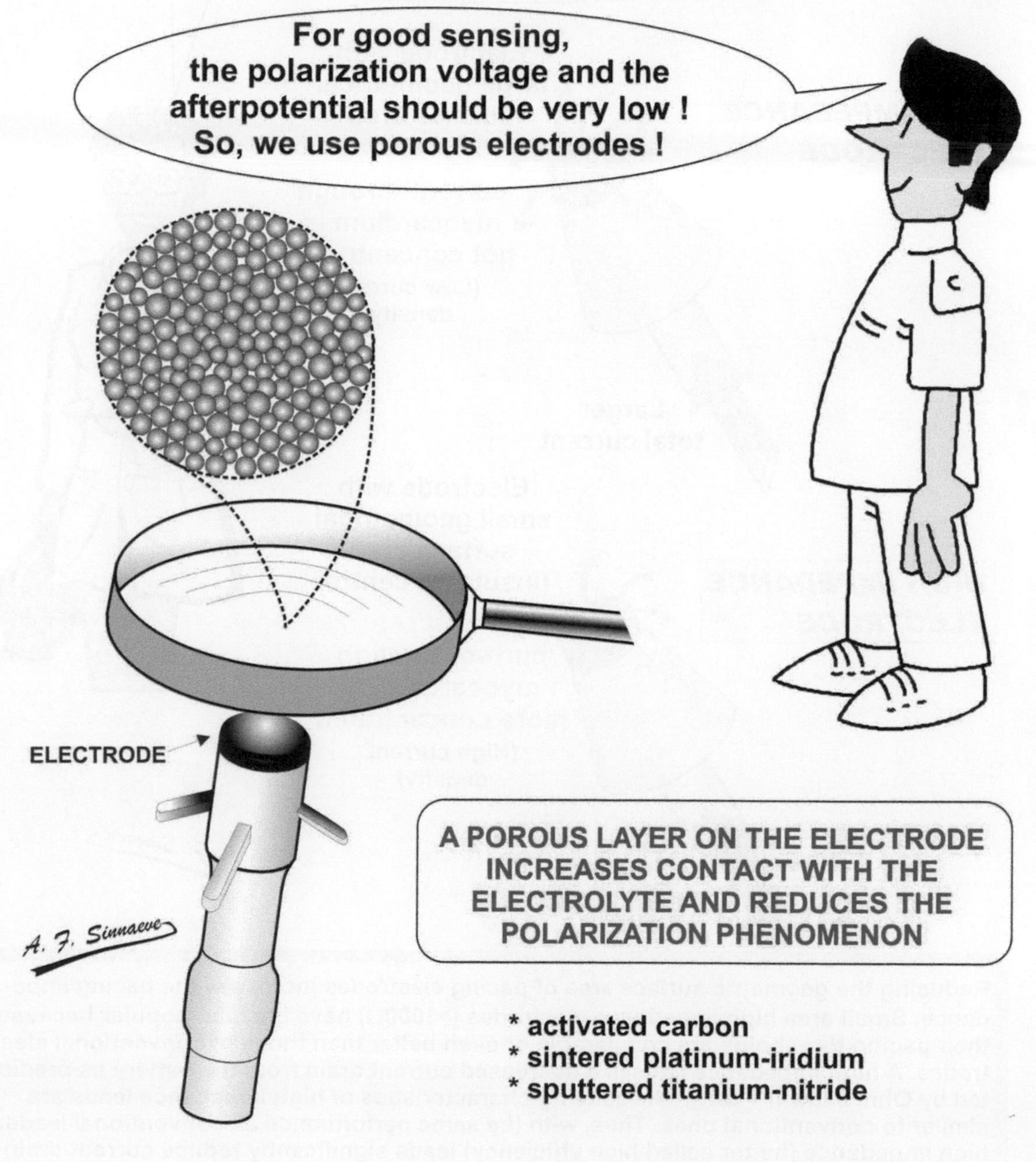

* activated carbon
* sintered platinum-iridium
* sputtered titanium-nitride

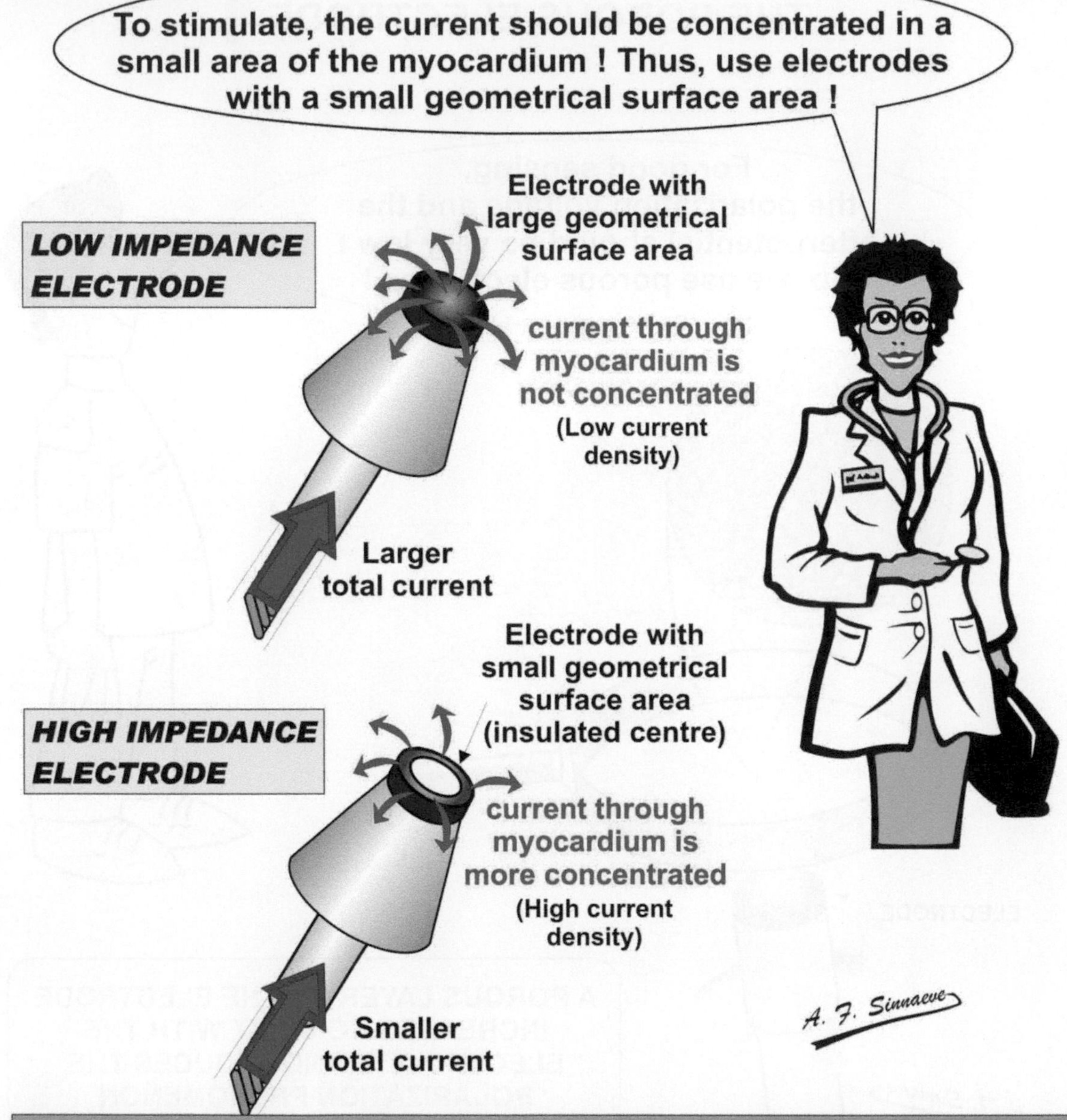

Reducing the geometric surface area of pacing electrodes increases the pacing impedance. Small area high impedance electrodes (>1000Ω) have become popular because their pacing thresholds are comparable or even better than those of conventional electrodes. A high impedance causes a decreased current drain from the battery as predicted by Ohm's law (I = U/R). The sensing characteristics of high impedance leads are similar to conventional ones. Thus, with the same performance as conventional leads, high impedance (better called high efficiency) leads significantly reduce current drain from the battery for stimulation and thereby increase battery longevity.

LEAD DISPLACEMENT

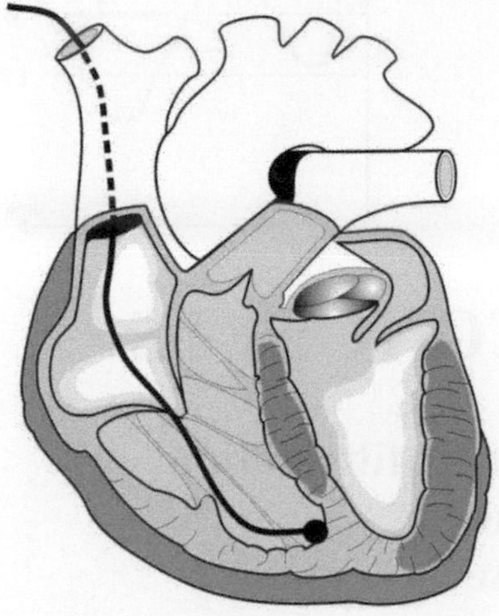

Normally positioned lead at right ventricular apex

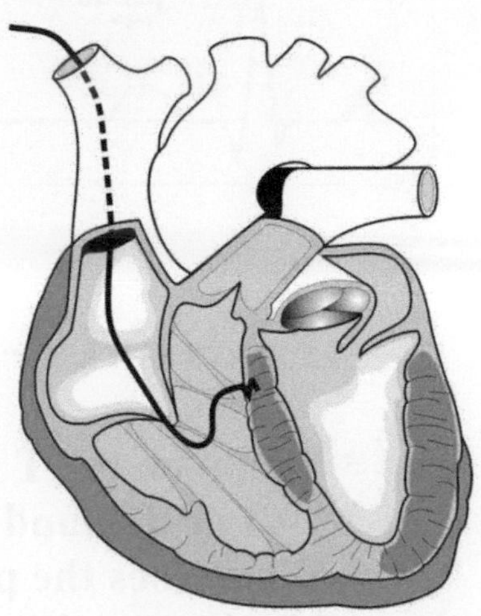

Normally positioned screw-in lead at RV outflow tract

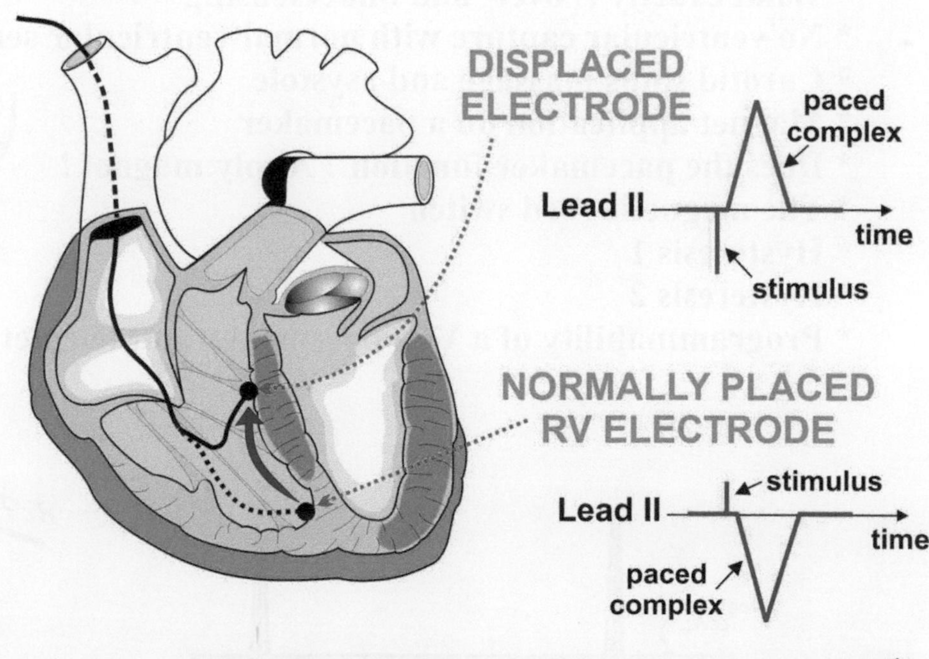

A. F. Sinnaeve

Abbreviations : RV = right ventricle (right ventricular)

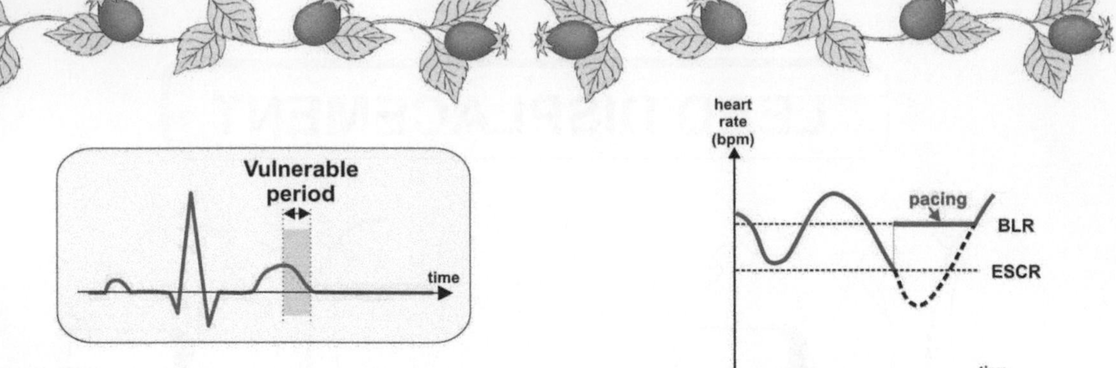

SENSING - BASIC CONCEPTS

* Firing on the T wave - Ventricular fibrillation
* VVI or demand ventricular pacing
* What does the pacemaker sense ?
* Markers and symbols
* Three-letter code for single chamber pacemakers
* The intracardiac electrogram - Sensing 1
* The intracardiac electrogram - Sensing 2
* Undersensing by the demand pacemaker
* What exactly is over- and undersensing
* No ventricular capture with normal ventricular sensing
* Carotid sinus massage and asystole
* Magnet application on a pacemaker
* Does the pacemaker function ? Apply magnet !
* The magnetic reed switch
* Hysteresis 1
* Hysteresis 2
* Programmability of a VVI pacemaker and telemetry

A. F. Sinnaeve

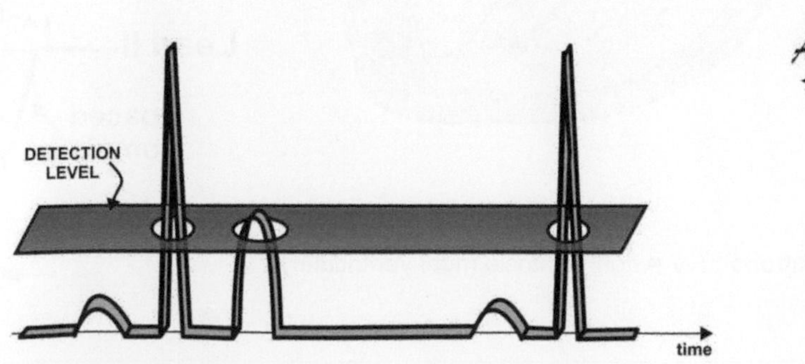

ASYNCHRONOUS PACING & STIMULUS ON T-WAVE

There must be a risk of firing a pacemaker stimulus into the ventricular vulnerable period !?

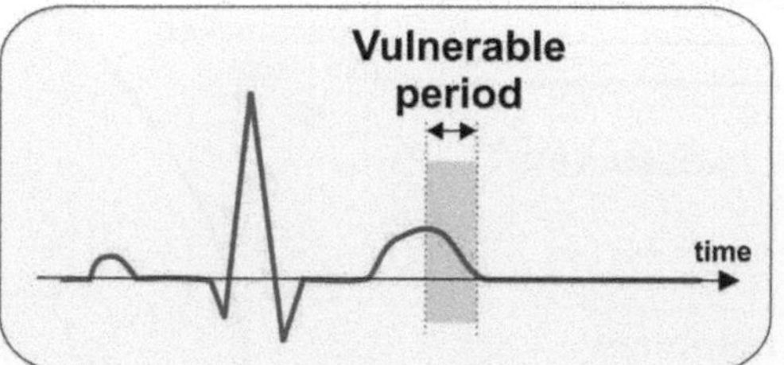

The risk is very small in the usual clinical situations. Countless patients transmit their ECG safely over the phone during follow-up when the magnet is placed over the pacemaker with the creation of a competitive ventricular rhythm and firing of the pacemaker on the T wave. The risk is confined to patients with serious metabolic (electrolyte) abnormalities or acute myocardial infarction or ischemia.

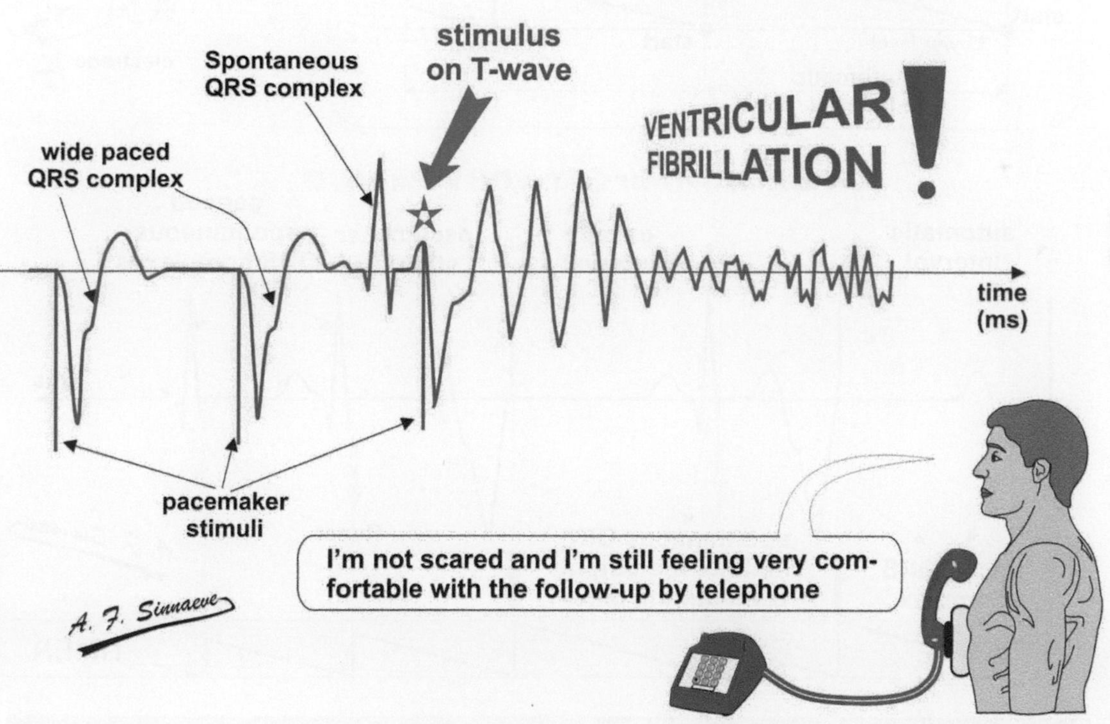

I'm not scared and I'm still feeling very comfortable with the follow-up by telephone

A. F. Sinnaeve

VENTRICULAR DEMAND PACING (VVI)

Note that in the VVI mode, a competitive rhythm is not possible. Moreover the lifetime of the battery is extended because the pacemaker is not pacing during long periods of time when it is standby.

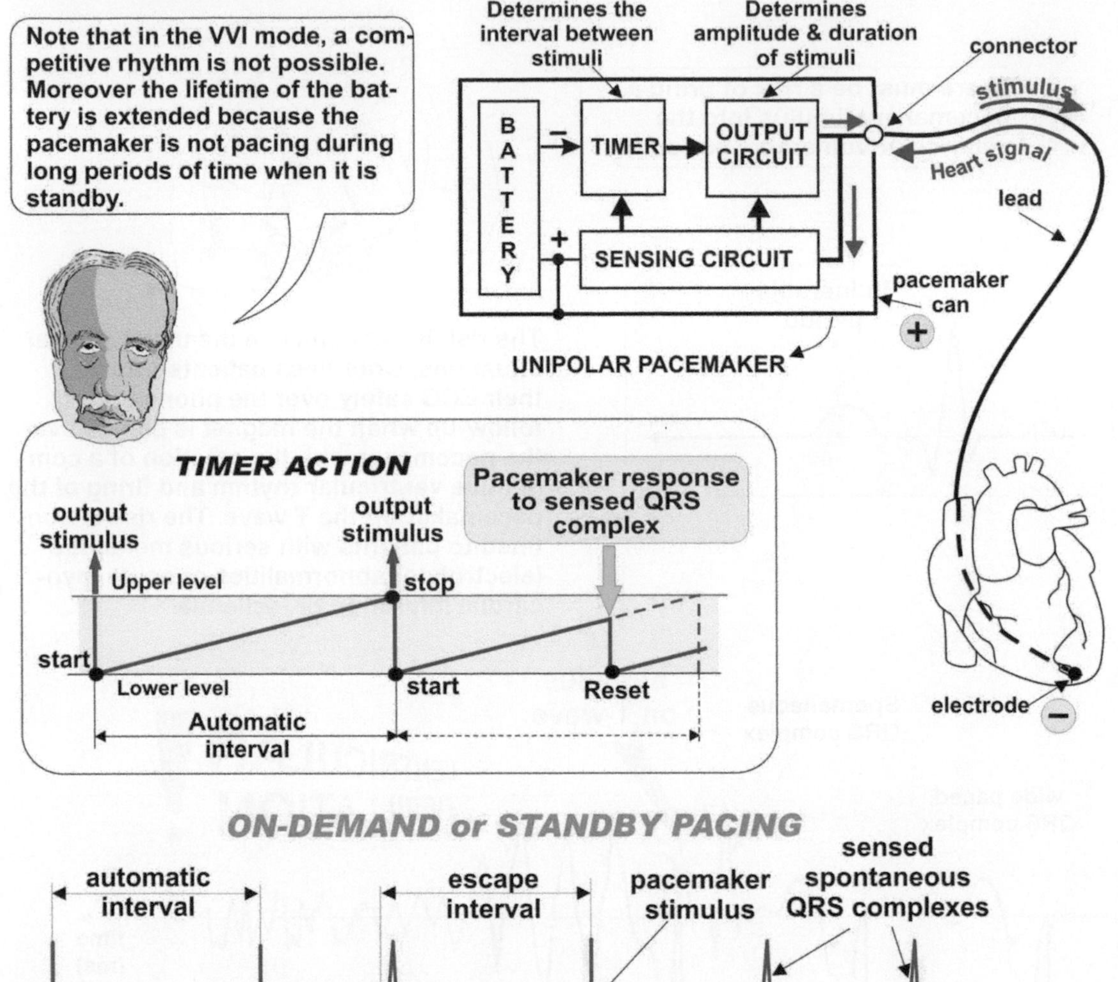

ON-DEMAND or STANDBY PACING

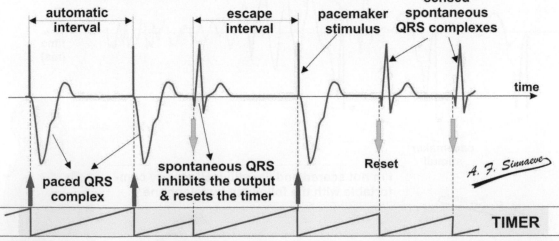

The electronic escape interval (starting at the time of intracardiac sensing) is equal to the automatic interval. The escape interval is measured on the surface ECG from the onset of the QRS complex because the time of intracardiac sensing cannot be determined accurately. Therefore the escape interval so measured will be slightly longer than the automatic interval because intracardiac sensing occurs later than the beginning of the surface QRS complex.

WHAT DOES THE PACEMAKER SENSE ?

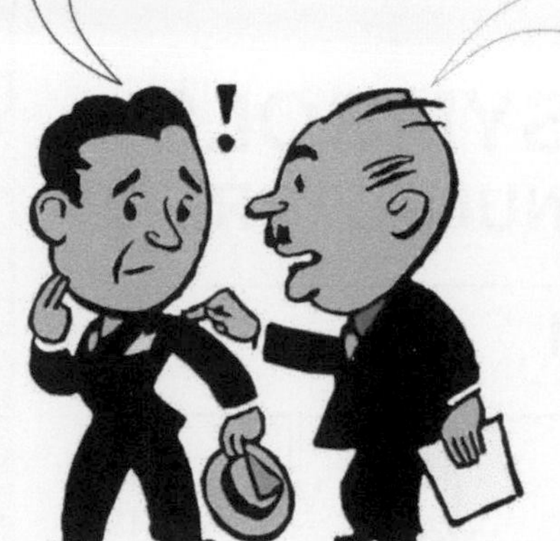
How does a demand pacemaker know when to deliver a stimulus ? Does it recognize the ECG ?
The pacemaker does not sense the surface ECG nor the ECG near the pacemaker can. It detects what is going on inside the heart itself by measuring the potential difference (voltage) between the two electrodes used for pacing. The voltage of intracardiac depolarization is larger than that of the surface ECG and is called an electrogram rather than electrocardiogram.
Therefore, the time of electronic sensing the intracardiac electrogram does not correspond with the onset of the surface ECG because it takes a finite time for the activation to reach the electrodes (for example in the right ventricle) and generate the electrogram

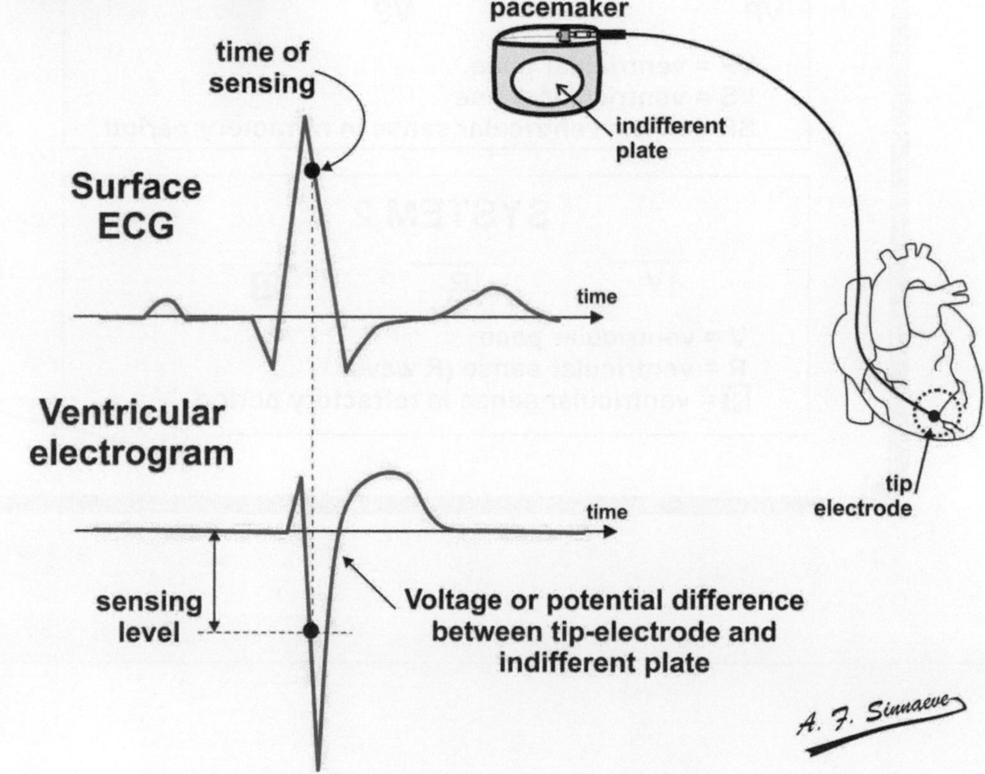

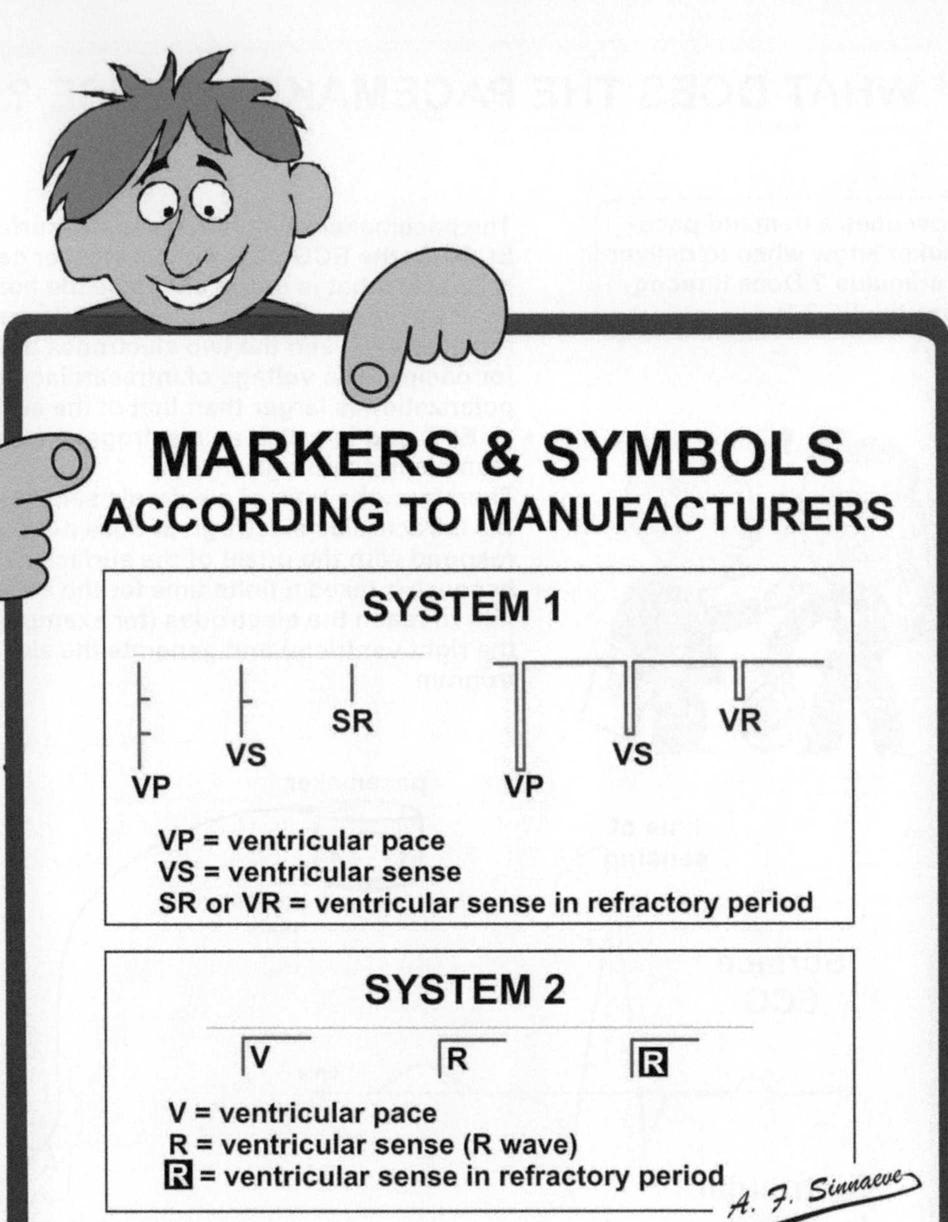
MARKERS & SYMBOLS
ACCORDING TO MANUFACTURERS
SYSTEM 1
VP
VS
SR
VP
VS
VR
VP = ventricular pace
VS = ventricular sense
SR or VR = ventricular sense in refractory period
SYSTEM 2
V
R
R
V = ventricular pace
R = ventricular sense (R wave)
R = ventricular sense in refractory period
A. F. Sinnaeve

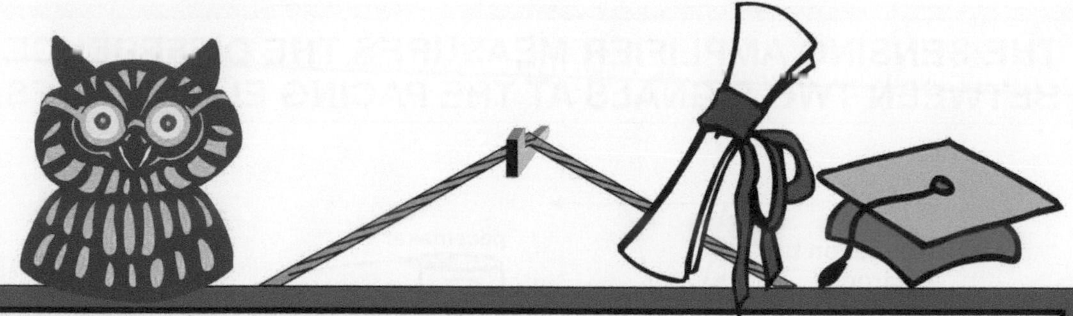

THREE-LETTER PACEMAKER CODE (ICHD)

POSITION	1st	2nd	3rd
CATEGORY	CHAMBER(S) PACED	CHAMBER(S) SENSED	MODE OF RESPONSE
LETTERS	V = VENTRICLE A = ATRIUM S = SINGLE	V = VENTRICLE A = ATRIUM S = SINGLE O = NONE	T = TRIGGERED I = INHIBITED O = NONE

EXAMPLES :

AAI = a pacemaker pacing and sensing in the atrium, being inhibited by spontaneous electrical activation of the atrium

VVT = a pacemaker pacing and sensing in the ventricle and working in the triggered mode (each sensed ventricular event elicits a pacemaker stimulus)

A. F. Sinnaeve

THE SENSING AMPLIFIER MEASURES THE DIFFERENCE BETWEEN TWO SIGNALS AT THE PACING ELECTRODES

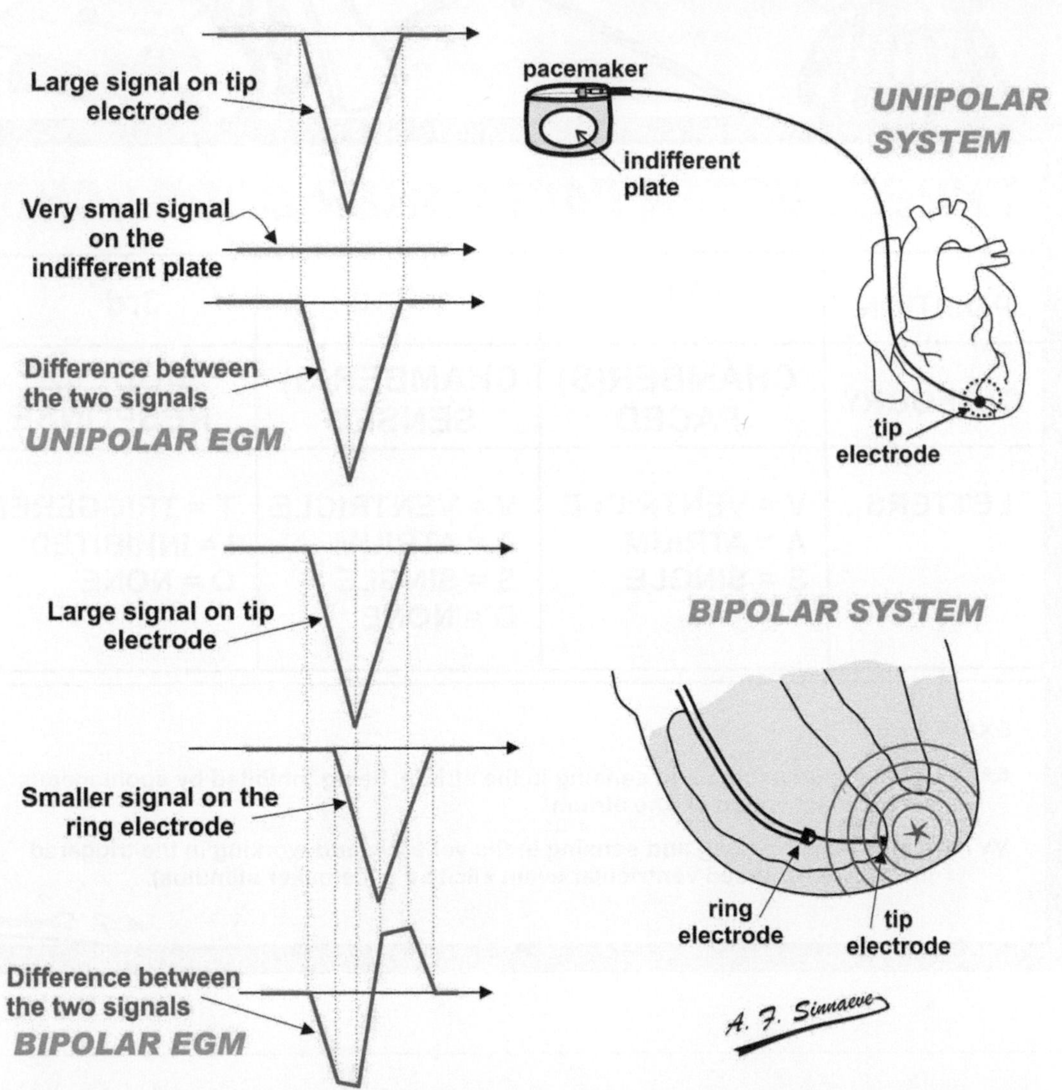

Note that on each instant of time, the bipolar electrogram (EGM) is the difference between the EGMs recorded at the tip and ring electrodes. The EGMs arrive at different times and this timing or phase difference generates the bipolar EGM.

VARIABILITY OF BIPOLAR SENSING

* The sensed signal to the pacemaker is the voltage or potential difference between the two intracardiac electrodes
* The bipolar EGM depends on both the amplitude and timing (phase difference) of the electrograms registered at each of the two intracardiac electrodes

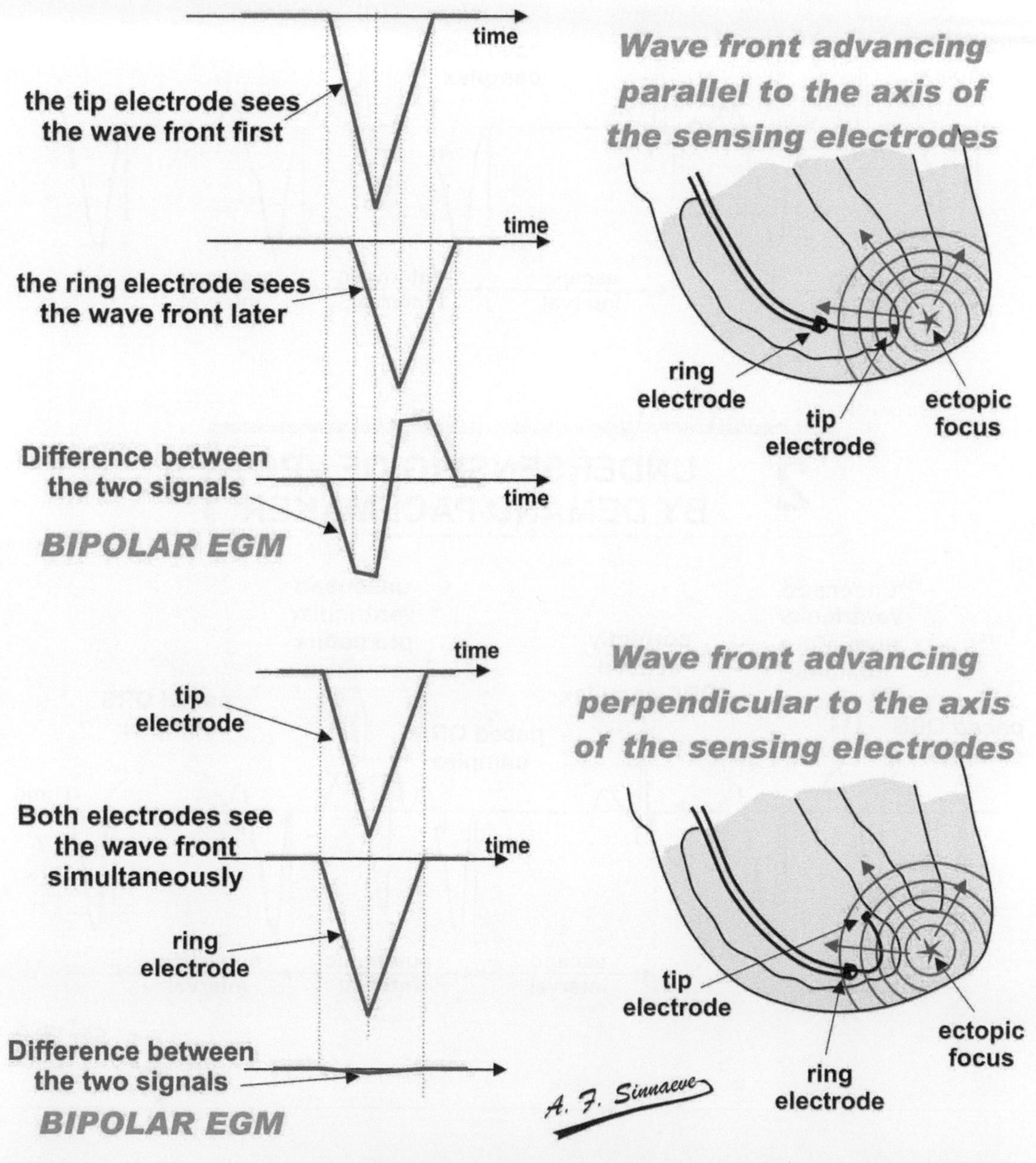

Identical signals arriving exactly at the same time at the two electrodes will yield a zero bipolar electrogram (EGM). Although this is theoretical, it is possible for two large unipolar EGMs to generate a relatively small bipolar EGM. In this situation, if there is undersensing, the bipolar sensing mode can be reprogrammed to the unipolar sensing mode.

1 INTERMITTENT UNDERSENSING OF A DEMAND PACEMAKER

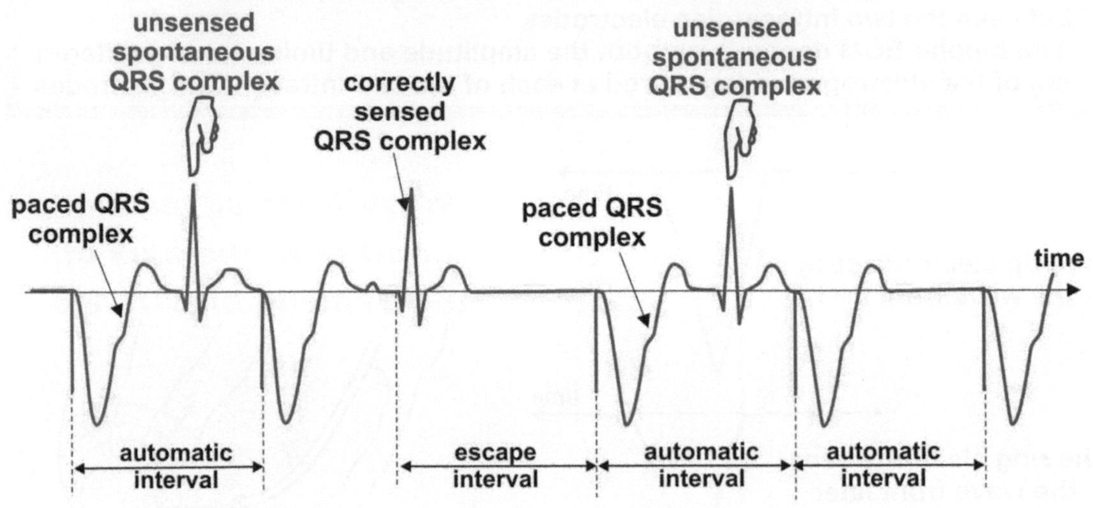

2 UNDERSENSING OF VPC BY DEMAND PACEMAKER

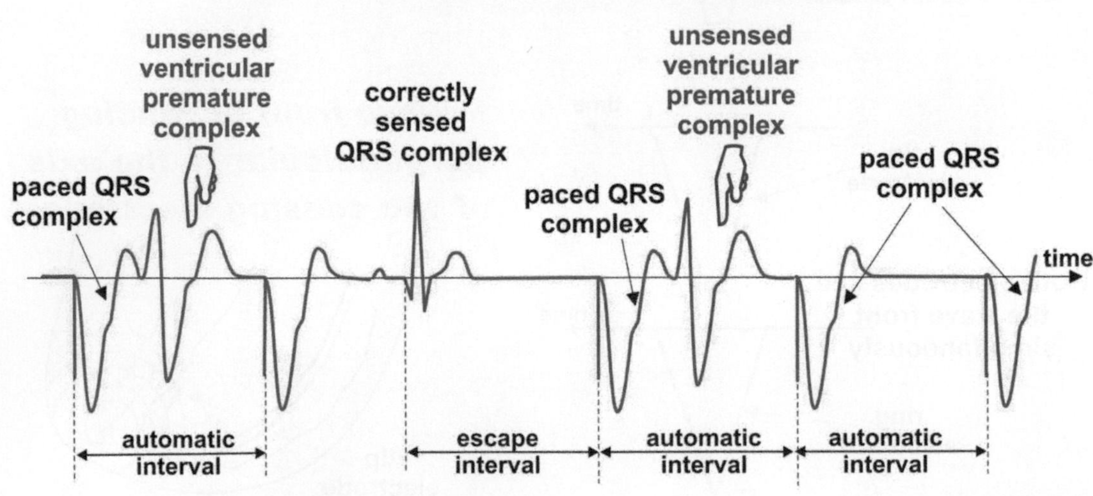

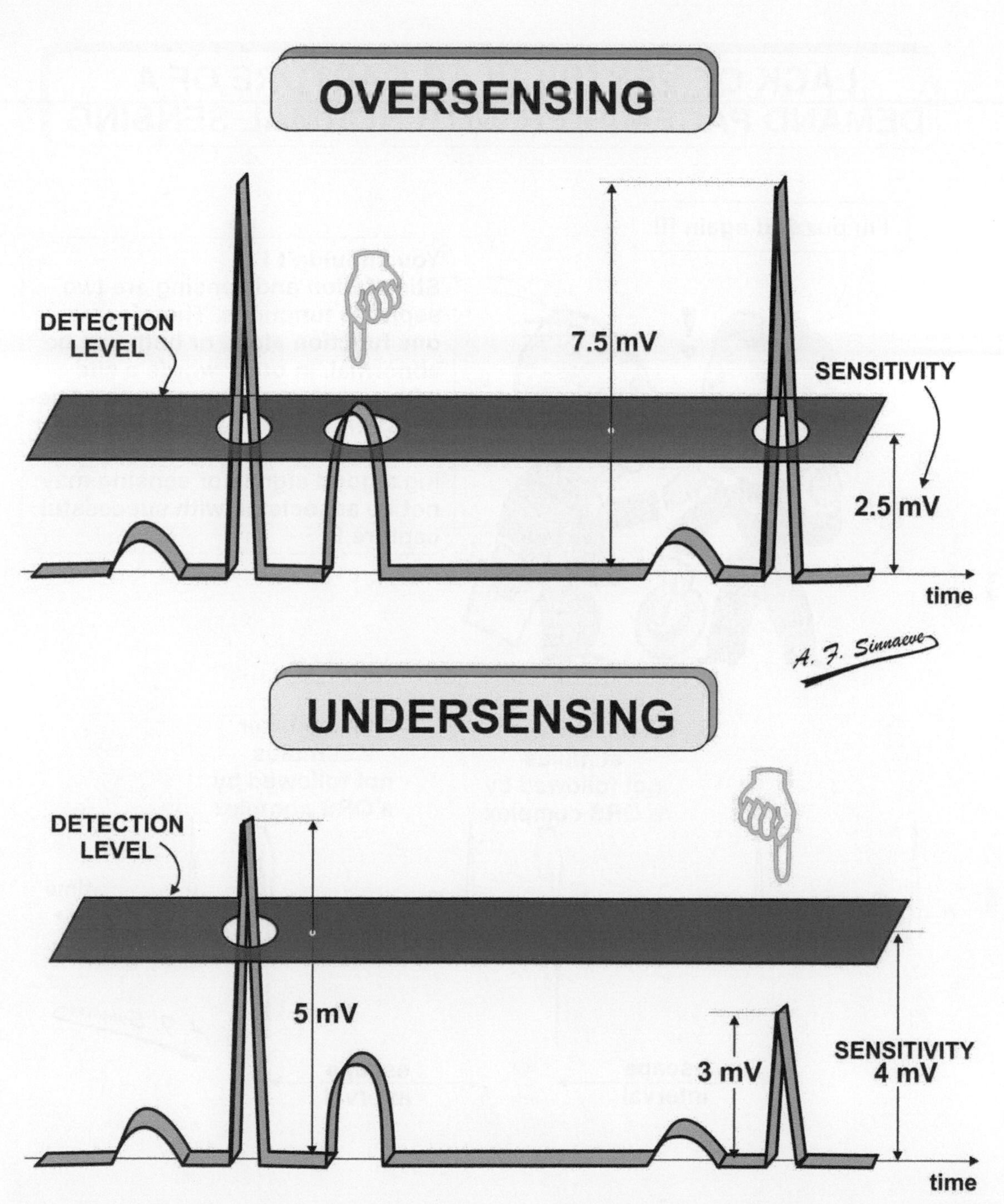

The voltage refers to the intracardiac electrogram and not the surface QRS complex. Sensitivity refers to a programmable parameter of the pacemaker. A sensitivity of 4 mV means that the pacemaker can only sense a signal equal to or greater than 4 mV. It will sense a signal of 5 mV but not a signal of 3 mV.

LACK OF VENTRICULAR CAPTURE OF A DEMAND PACEMAKER WITH NORMAL SENSING

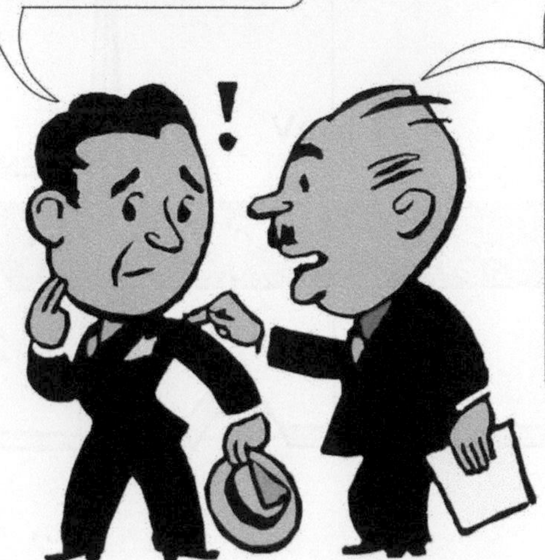

I'm puzzled again !!!
You shouldn't ! Stimulation and sensing are two separate functions. Therefore one function alone or both can be abnormal. In other words a site with excellent capture does not necessarily provide a good signal for sensing. Alternatively a site yielding a good signal for sensing may not be associated with successful capture !

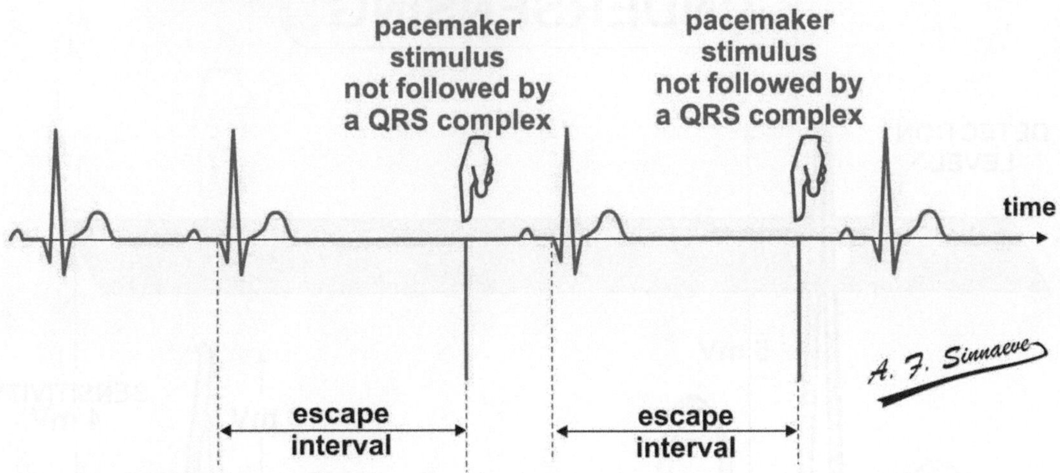

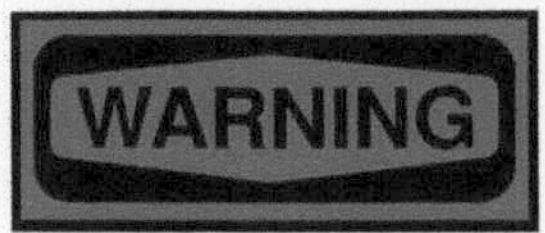

WARNING

Capture and sensing must be tested separately

CAROTID SINUS MASSAGE

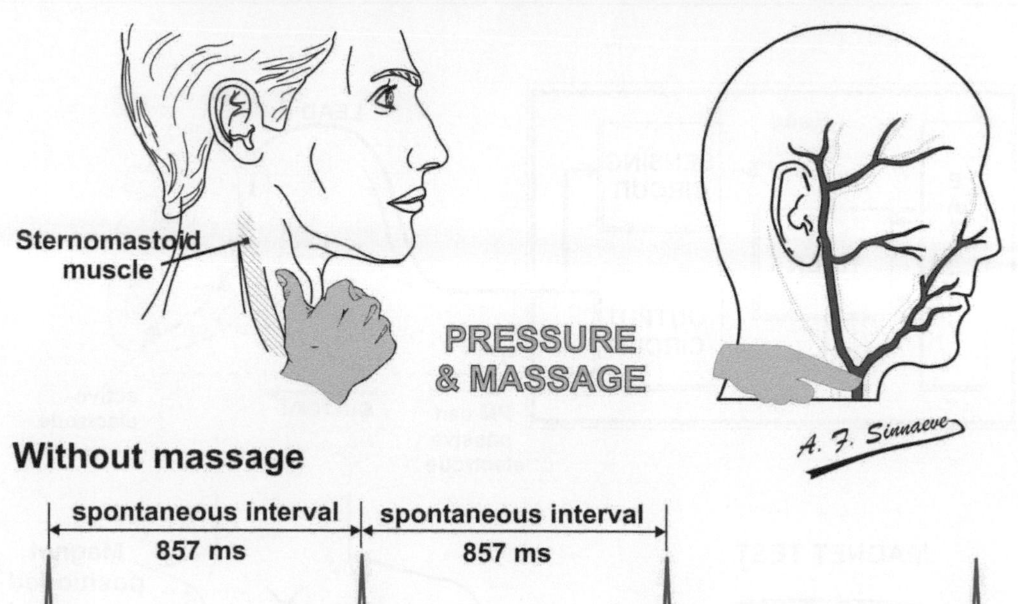

During massage (CSP =carotid sinus pressure)

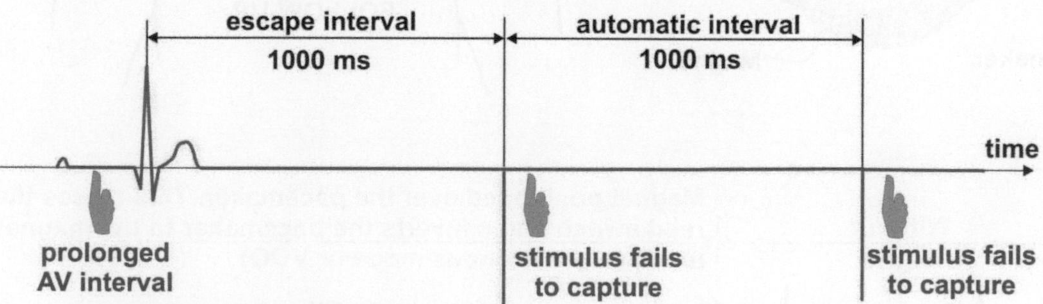

WARNING !!!

When a patient presents with an ECG showing no pacemaker stimuli, do not perform carotid sinus massage to test the pacemaker because it may cause prolonged bradycardia. The pacemaker will then deliver its stimuli that may or may not capture the heart. The pacing function should be tested first by the application of a pacemaker magnet, which converts any pacemaker to the fixed-rate or asynchronous mode (VVI to VOO).

MAGNET APPLICATION ON A DEMAND PACEMAKER

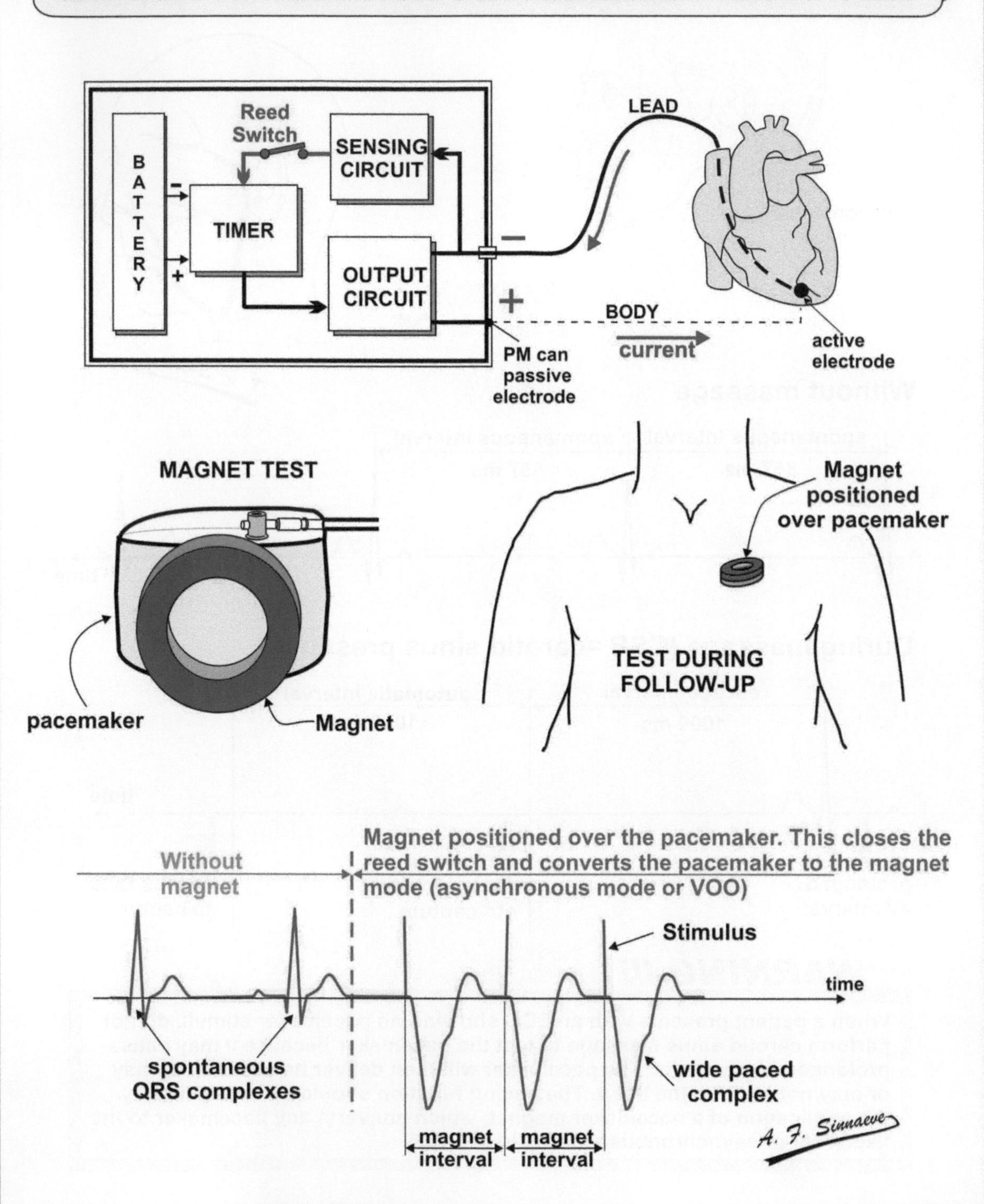

Reed Switch
SENSING CIRCUIT
BATTERY
TIMER
OUTPUT CIRCUIT
LEAD
BODY
current
PM can passive electrode
active electrode
MAGNET TEST
pacemaker
Magnet
Magnet positioned over pacemaker
TEST DURING FOLLOW-UP
Without magnet
Magnet positioned over the pacemaker. This closes the reed switch and converts the pacemaker to the magnet mode (asynchronous mode or VOO)
Stimulus
time
spontaneous QRS complexes
wide paced complex
magnet interval
magnet interval
A. F. Sinnaeve

DOES THE PACEMAKER FUNCTION ?

Spontaneous rhythm of the patient 80 bpm (beats per minute)

(or spontaneous R-R interval = $\frac{60{,}000}{80}$ **= 750 ms)**

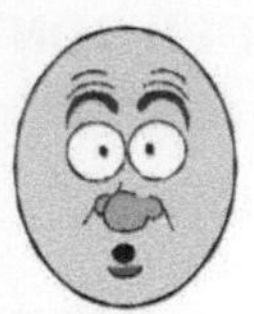

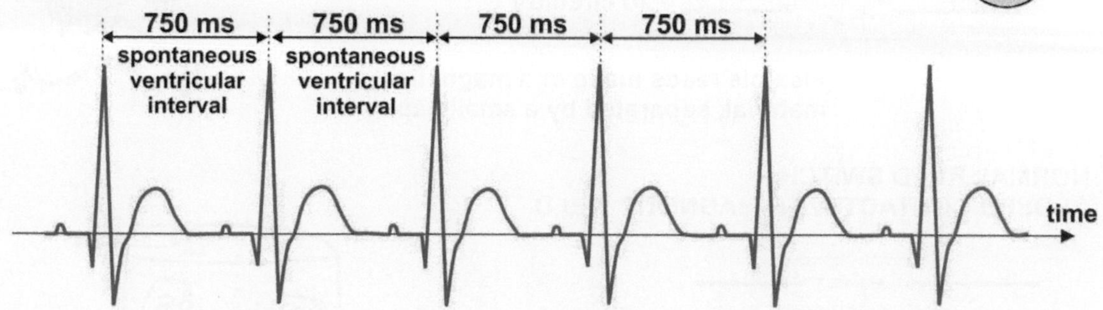

After magnet application, showing the pacemaker programmed at 60 bpm (or an automatic interval = $\frac{60{,}000}{100}$ **= 1,000 ms also equal to the magnet interval of this pacemaker)**

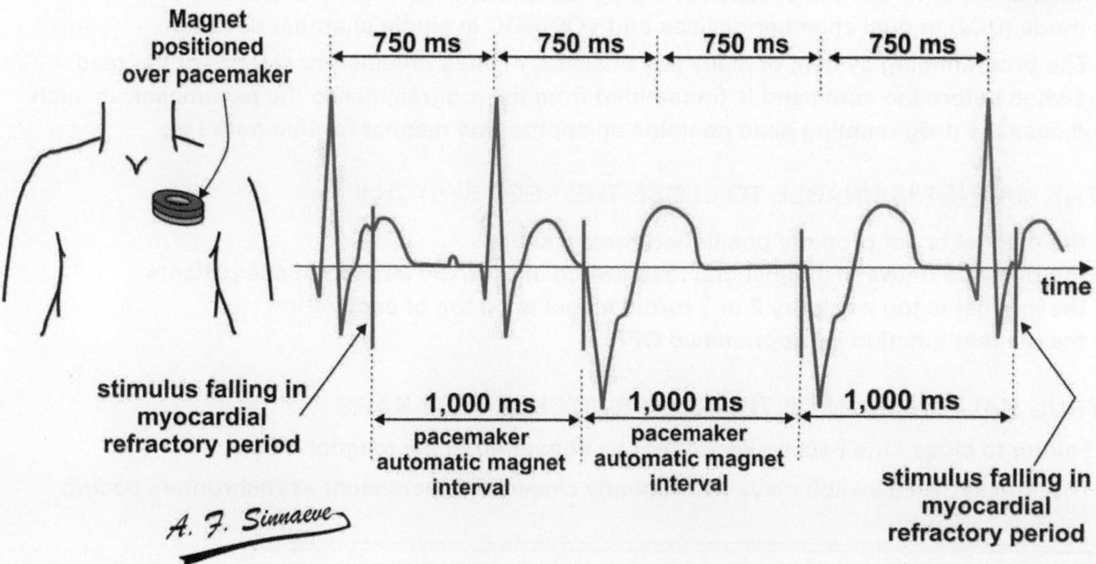

THE MAGNETIC REED SWITCH

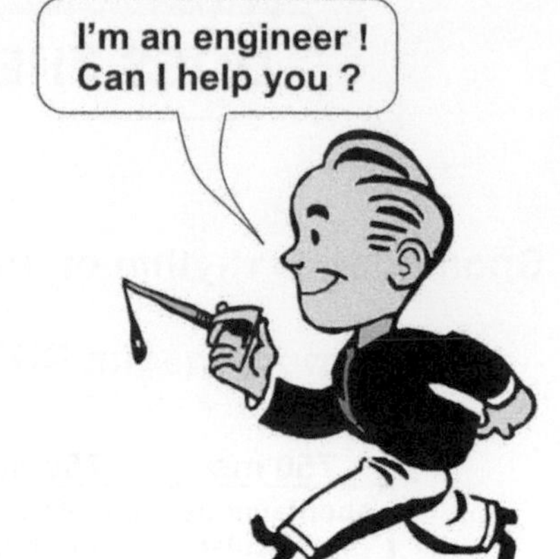

NORMAL REED SWITCH
OPEN CONTACT WITHOUT MAGNETIC FIELD

Sealed glass envelope

Connector

Inert gas

Connector
to circuitry

Flexible reeds made of a magnetic
material, separated by a small gap

NORMAL REED SWITCH
CLOSED CONTACT WITH MAGNETIC FIELD

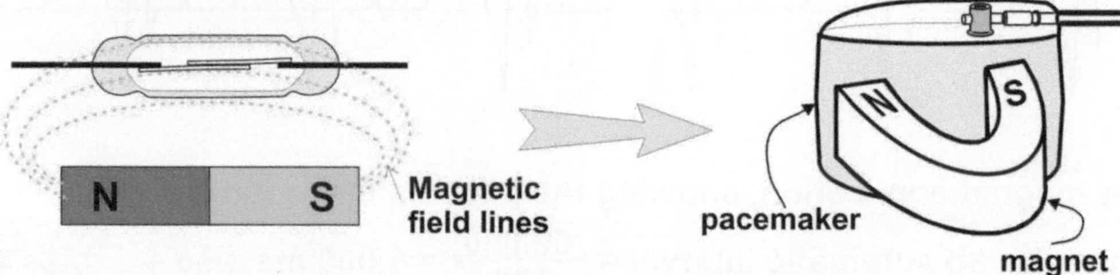

A MAGNET AND A REED SWITCH ARE NEEDED FOR TESTING

* Magnet mode forces the pacemaker's programmed operation to an asynchronous mode (DOO in dual chamber devices and VOO/AOO in single chamber devices)
* The programming system of many pacemakers requires preliminary closure of the reed switch before the command is transmitted from the programmer to the pacemaker; in such a case the programming head contains an appropriate magnet for this purpose.

THE MAGNET IS UNABLE TO CLOSE THE REED SWITCH IF

° the magnet is not properly positioned (wrong site)
° the distance between magnet and reed switch may be too large in obese patients
° the magnet is too weak (try 2 or 3 toroid magnets on top of each other)
° the magnet function is programmed OFF

TRUE MALFUNCTION OF THE REED SWITCH IS VERY RARE

* Failure to close : the pacemaker cannot be converted to the magnet mode
* The "sticky" reed switch stays permanently closed with persistent asynchronous pacing

Caution : as a rule , application of a magnet on an ICD, deactivates tachycardia therapy but not its pacing and sensing function for bradycardia therapy.

A. F. Sinnaeve

HYSTERESIS 1

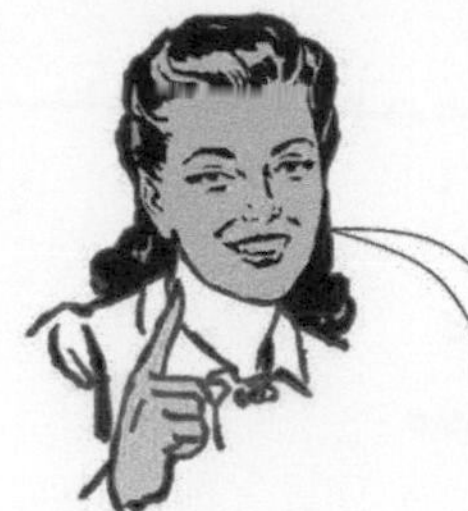

Hysteresis has some fine advantages :
* the spontaneous AV synchrony can be maintained as long as possible
* it prevents symptomatic retrograde VA conduction
* allowing a lower rate increases the longevity of the battery

WITHOUT HYSTERESIS
the automatic interval equals the escape interval

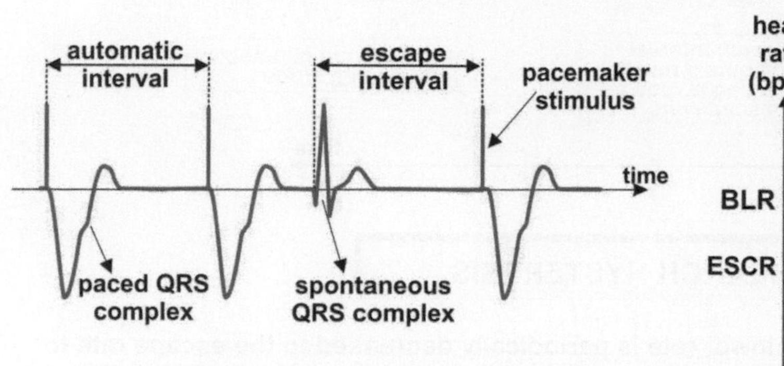

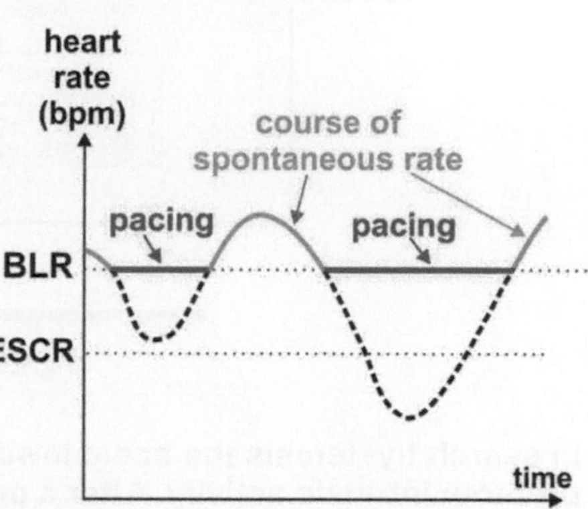

WITH HYSTERESIS
the escape interval is longer than the automatic interval

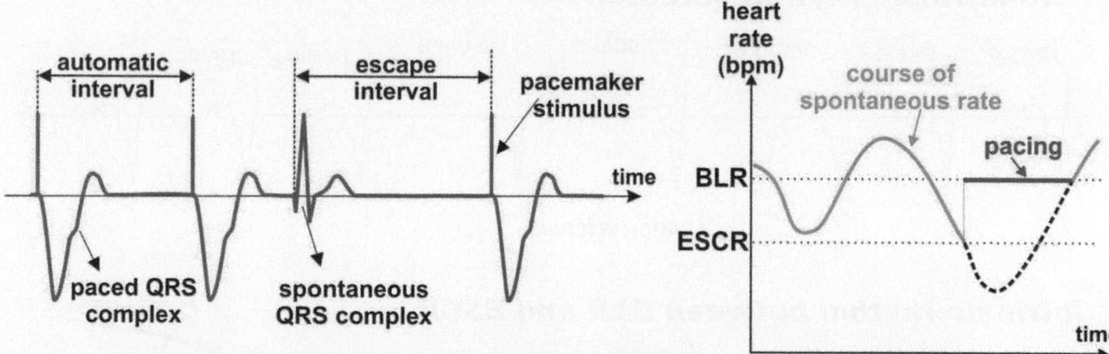

LRI = basic lower rate interval = automatic interval (in ms)

ESCI = escape interval (in ms)

BLR = basic lower rate = $\frac{60\,000}{\text{LRI}}$ (in bpm)

ESCR = escape rate = $\frac{60\,000}{\text{ESCI}}$ (in bpm)

A. F. Sinnaeve

HYSTERESIS 2

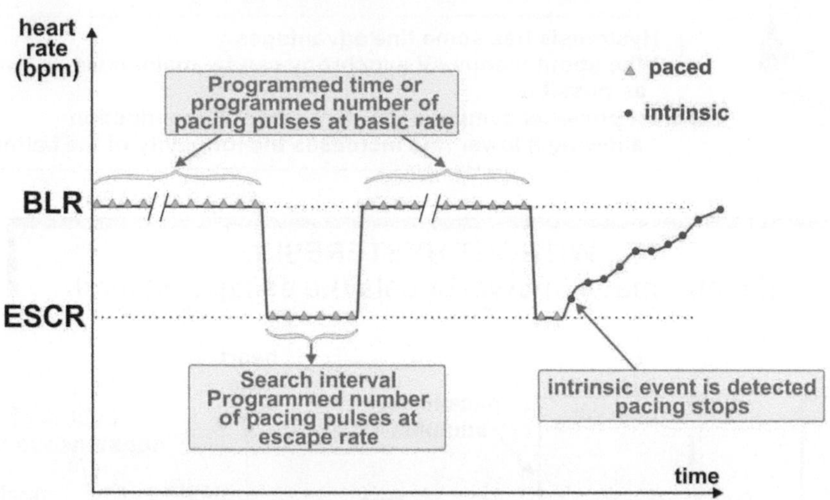

SEARCH HYSTERESIS

In search hysteresis the basic lower rate is periodically decreased to the escape rate to promote intrinsic activity. After a programmable number of successive pacing cycles at basic lower rate or after a programmable time, the device reduces its rate to the escape rate (or hysteresis rate) for a programmable number of cycles, called the search interval. If no intrinsic event is detected during search intervals, pacing resumes at basic lower rate, however if an intrinsic event is detected, pacing stops.

No intrinsic rhythm detected

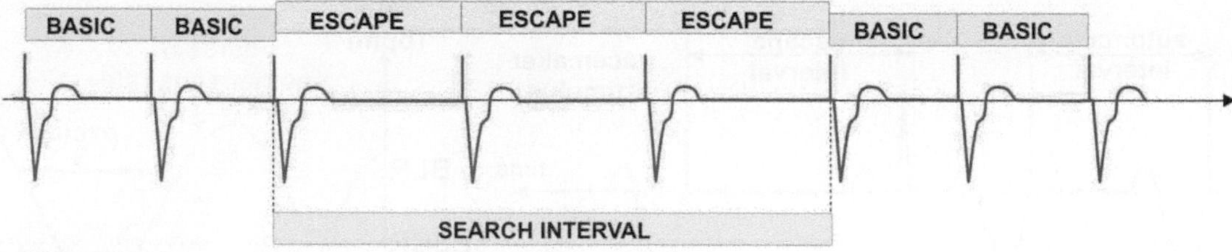

Intrinsic rhythm between BLR and ESCR

A. F. Sinnaeve

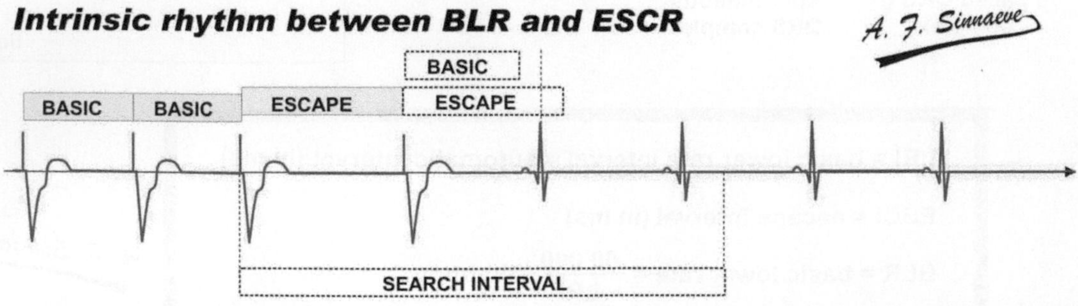

Abbreviations : BLR = basic lower rate ; ESCR = escape rate ;

PROGRAMMABILITY & TELEMETRY

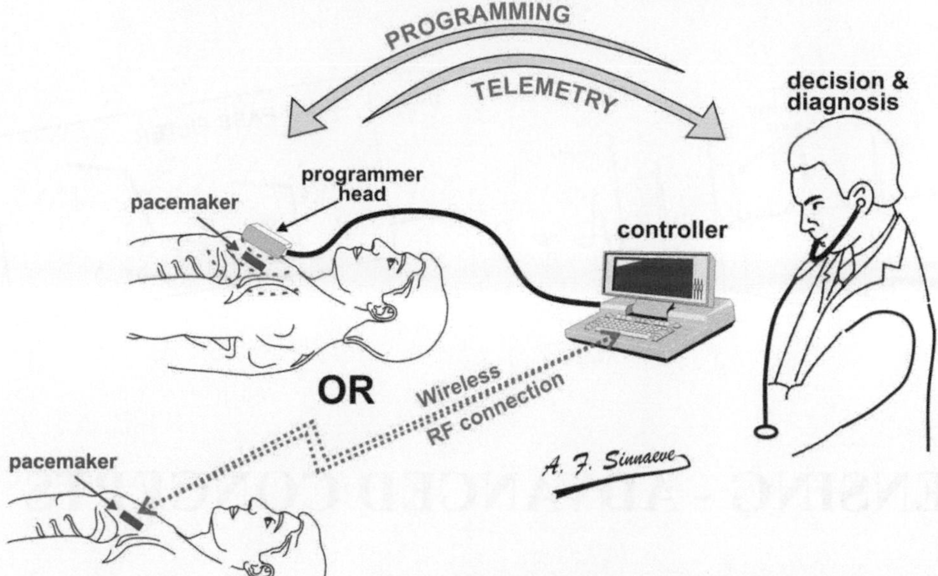

Programming :
The programmer is the transmitter, the pacemaker is the receiver

Telemetry :
The pacemaker is the transmitter, the programmer is the receiver

PROGRAMMABLE PARAMETERS IN VVI PACEMAKERS

* Rate
* Pulse width
* Voltage amplitude
* Sensitivity of the sensing circuit
* Refractory period
* Hysteresis
* Mode of pacing

IMPORTANT DATA OBTAINABLE BY TELEMETRY

* ADMINISTRATIVE DATA (model, serial number, patient's name, date of implantation, indication for implantation)
* PROGRAMMED DATA (mode, rate, refractory period, hysteresis on/off, pulse amplitude & width, sensitivity)
* MEASURED DATA (rate, pulse amplitude, pulse current, pulse energy, pulse charge, lead impedance, battery impedance, battery voltage, battery current drain)
* STORED DATA (Holter function, rhythm histogram, ...)
* MARKER SIGNALS for ECG interpretation
* INTRACARDIAC ELECTROGRAM

A. F. Sinnaeve

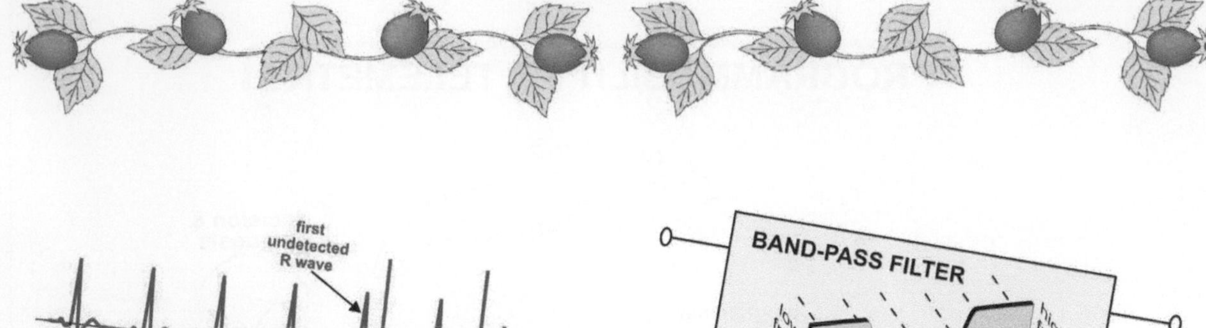

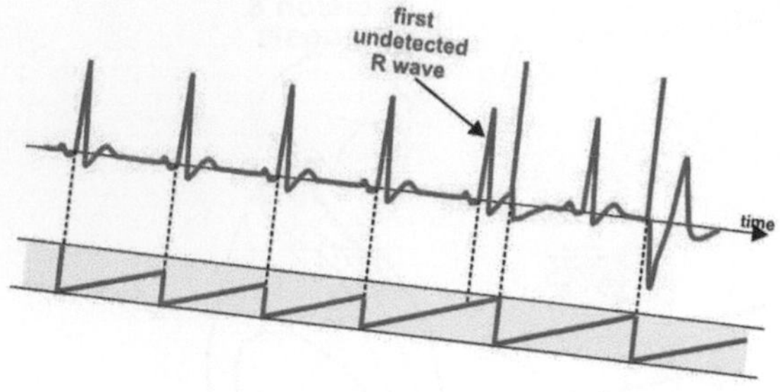

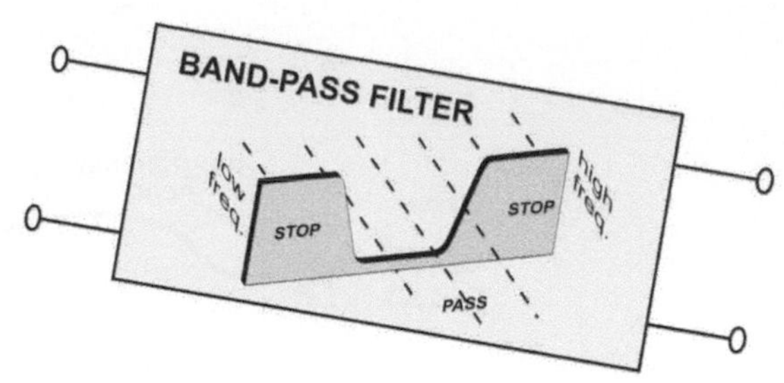

SENSING - ADVANCED CONCEPTS

- **Sensing circuit - Basic block diagram**
- **Intrinsic deflection and slew rate**
- **Filtering the endocardial signal 1**
- **Filtering the endocardial signal 2**
- **Traditional ventricular refractory period (VRP)**
- **Functions of VRP**
- **The pacemaker VRP**
- **The blanking period**
- **Programming lower sensitivity**
- **Programming higher sensitivity**
- **Sensing threshold - nonautomatic determination**
- **Electrographic (EGM) signal recording with ECG machine**

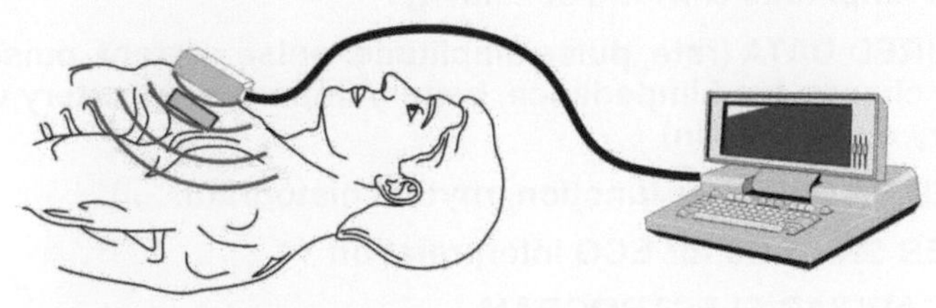

A. F. Sinnaeve

THE SENSING FUNCTION

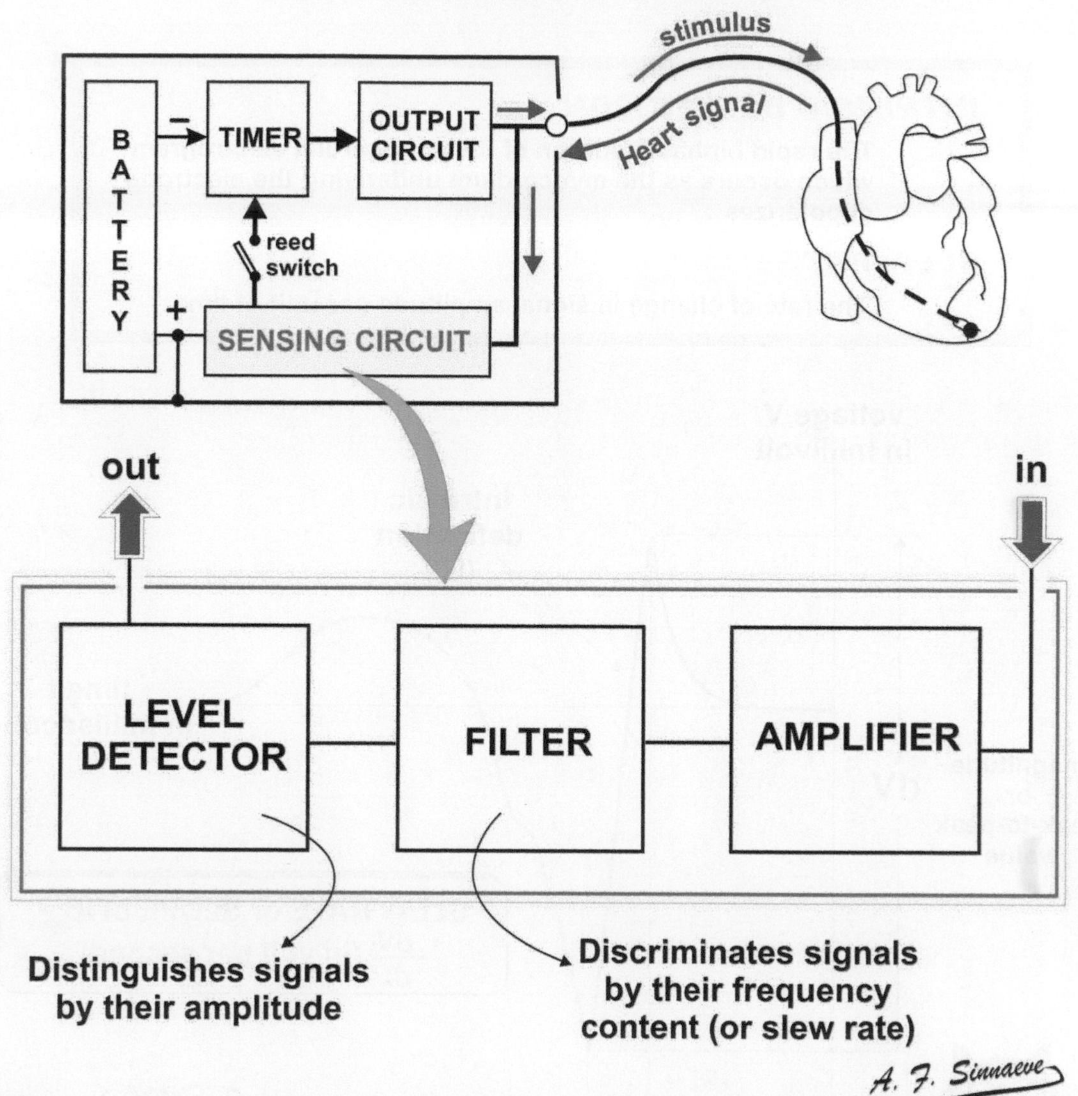

!

"Amplifier" and "Level Detector" determine the SENSITIVITY expressed in millivolts

* high sensitivity is characterized by a small number of mV (i.e. the sensing circuit already reacts on small signals)
* low sensitivity is expressed by a large number of mV (i.e. the sensing circuit only reacts upon large signals)

VENTRICULAR ELECTROGRAM INTRINSIC DEFLECTION & SLEW RATE

INTRINSIC DEFLECTION :

The rapid biphasic portion of the endocardial electrogram which occurs as the myocardium underlying the electrode depolarizes

SLEW RATE :

The rate of change in signal amplitude per unit of time

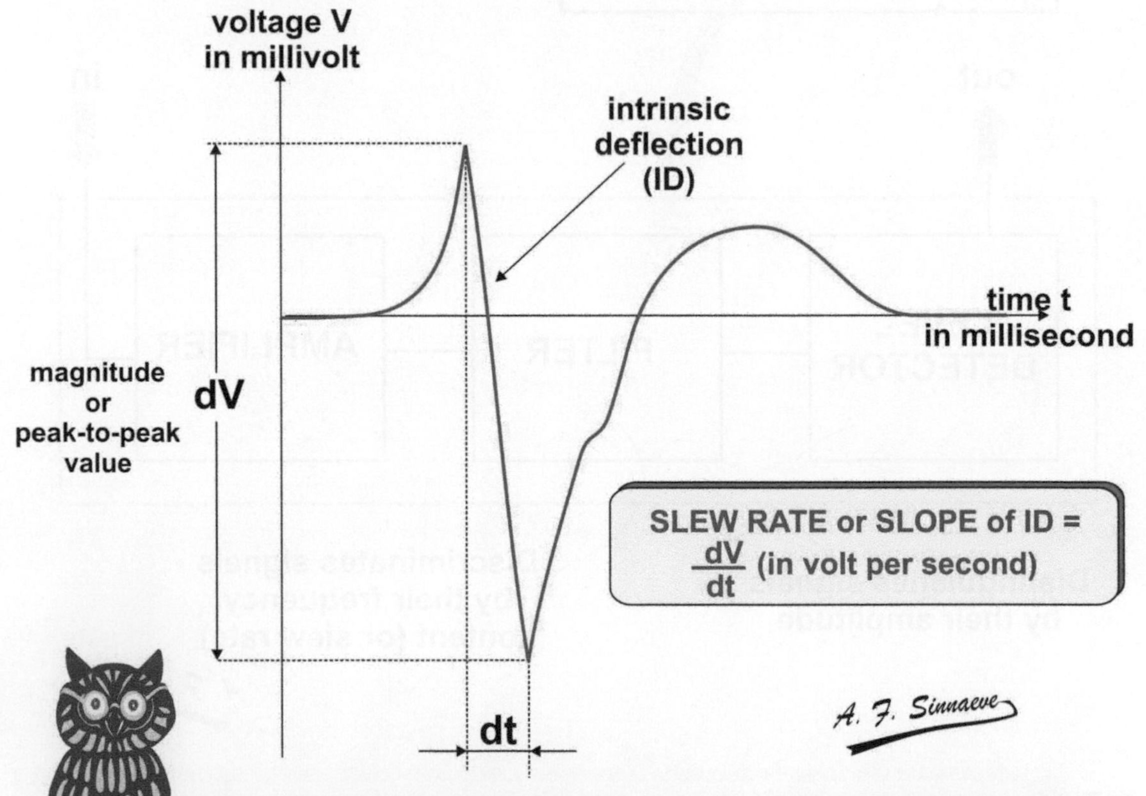

A large intracardiac signal (electrogram or EGM) almost always has a good (i.e. sharp rising) slew rate for sensing. The slew rate becomes important in relatively small signals : in this situation a pacemaker may not be able to sense an EGM with a slow-rising slope. The slew rate can be determined at the time of implantation. Although the EGM can be visualized noninvasively after implantation, the slew rate cannot !

FILTERING OF THE ENDOCARDIAL SIGNAL

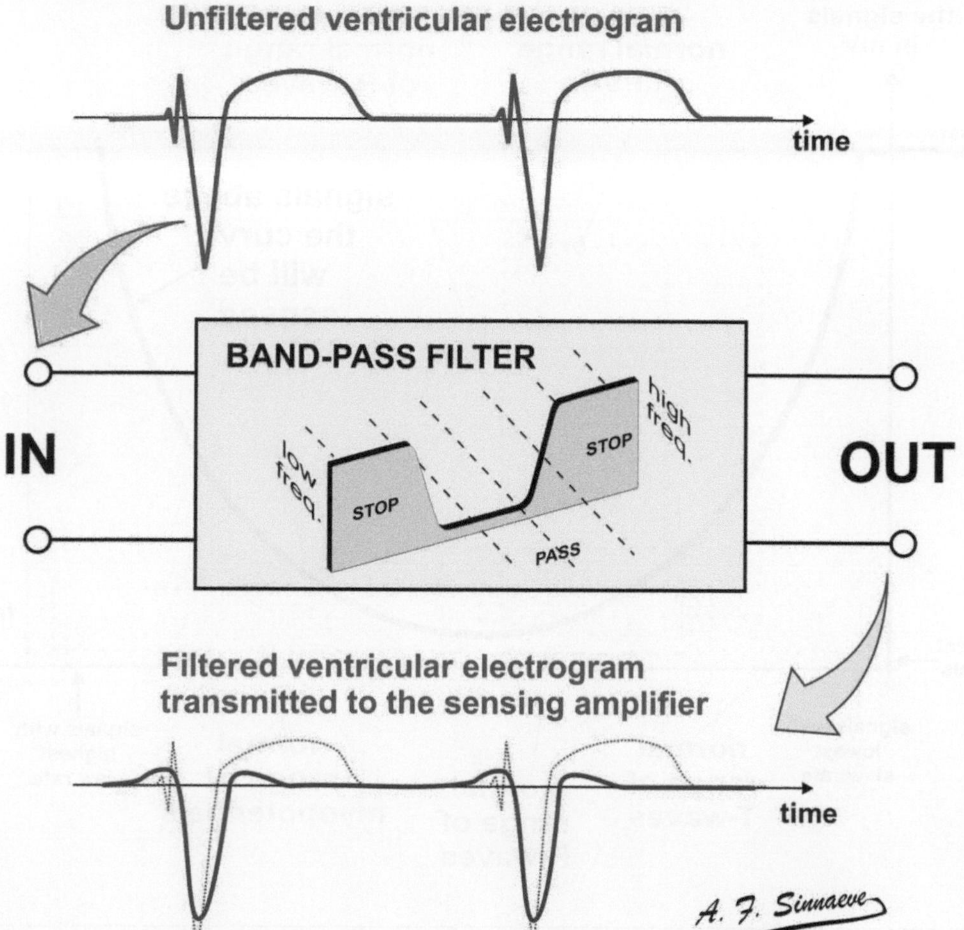

Heart signals with the right slew rate easily pass through the filter without attenuation and can affect the timer of the pacemaker.
Signals with a very high slew rate (i.e. changing very rapidly) probably originate from an external source (myopotentials from skeletal muscles, electromagnetic interference, etc.). They are strongly attenuated so that they no longer can affect the timer. Signals with a very low slew rate corresponding with T waves are also strongly attenuated and unable to affect the timer of the pacemaker.
Only signals with the right slew rate i.e. with the right frequency content, will pass through the filter without attenuation, hence the name "band-pass filter".

THE FILTERING OF SENSED SIGNALS

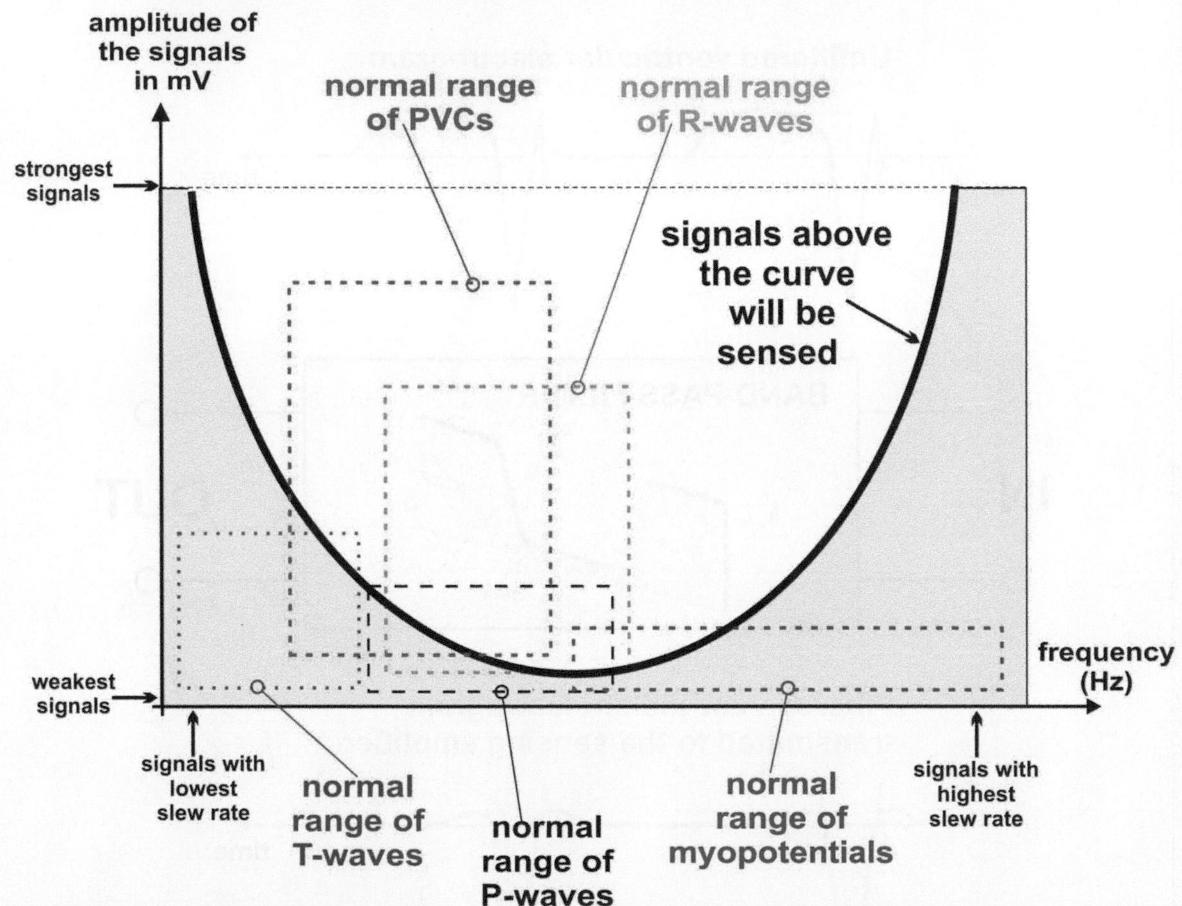

Signals are characterized by their amplitude and their slew rate. Each rectangle is the idealized representation of the set of all possible amplitude & slew rate combinations that are typical for a specific heart signal. Obviously these sets of values overlap each other and discrimination by slew rate only is not possible; a level detector will be necessary.
The shape of the filter characteristic above which detection is guaranteed, is always a technical compromise. Apparently some amplitude & slew rate combinations for T-waves and myopotentials may be above the detection level and can be sensed (over-sensing). Some combinations for PVCs and R- waves are beneath the detection level and cannot be detected (undersensing).

Abbreviations : PVC = premature ventricular complex

THE PACEMAKER REFRACTORY PERIOD TRADITIONAL CONCEPT

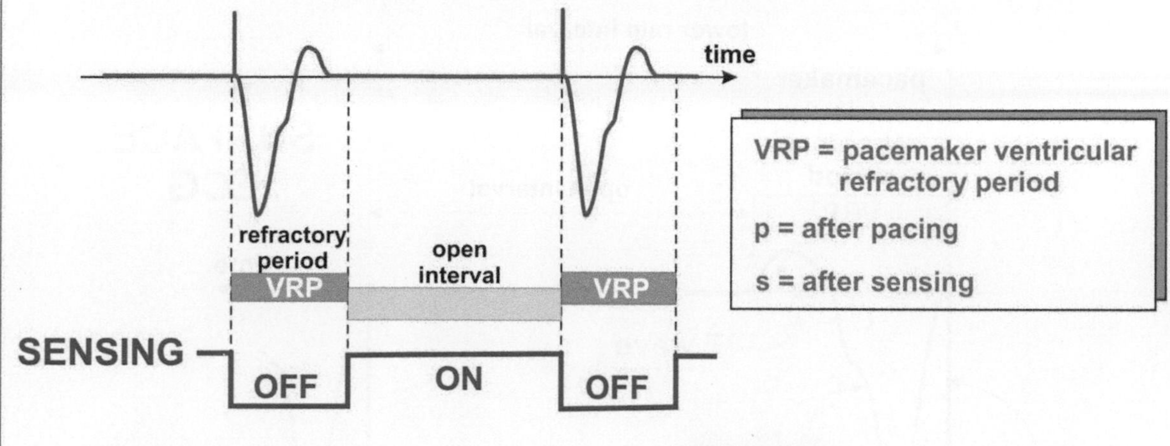

VRP = pacemaker ventricular refractory period

p = after pacing

s = after sensing

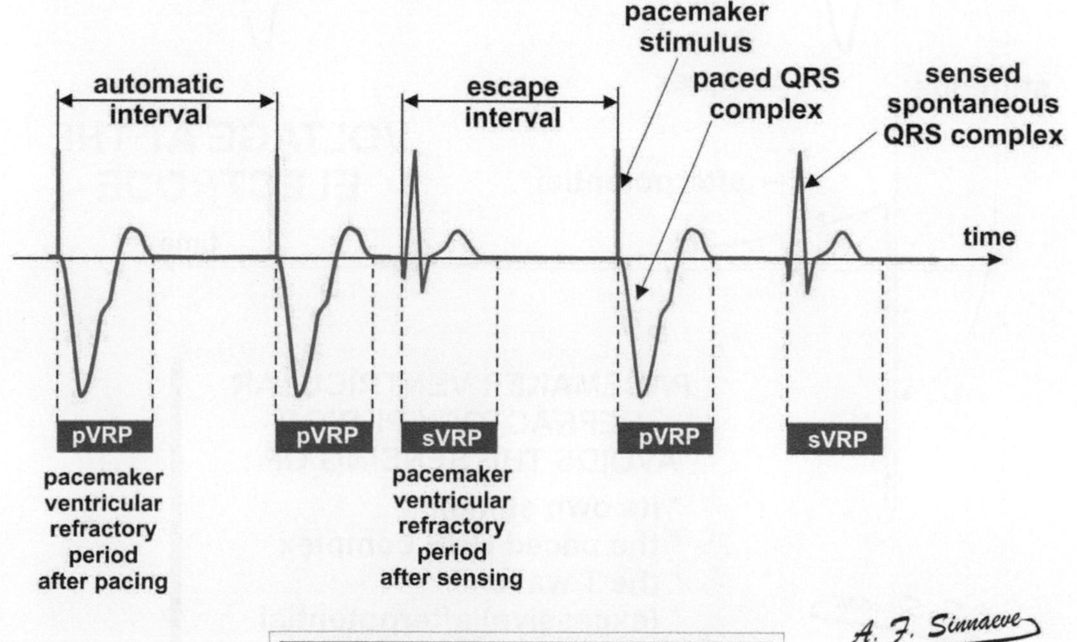

A. F. Sinnaeve

pVRP is often equal to sVRP

FUNCTIONS OF THE PACEMAKER VENTRICULAR REFRACTORY PERIOD

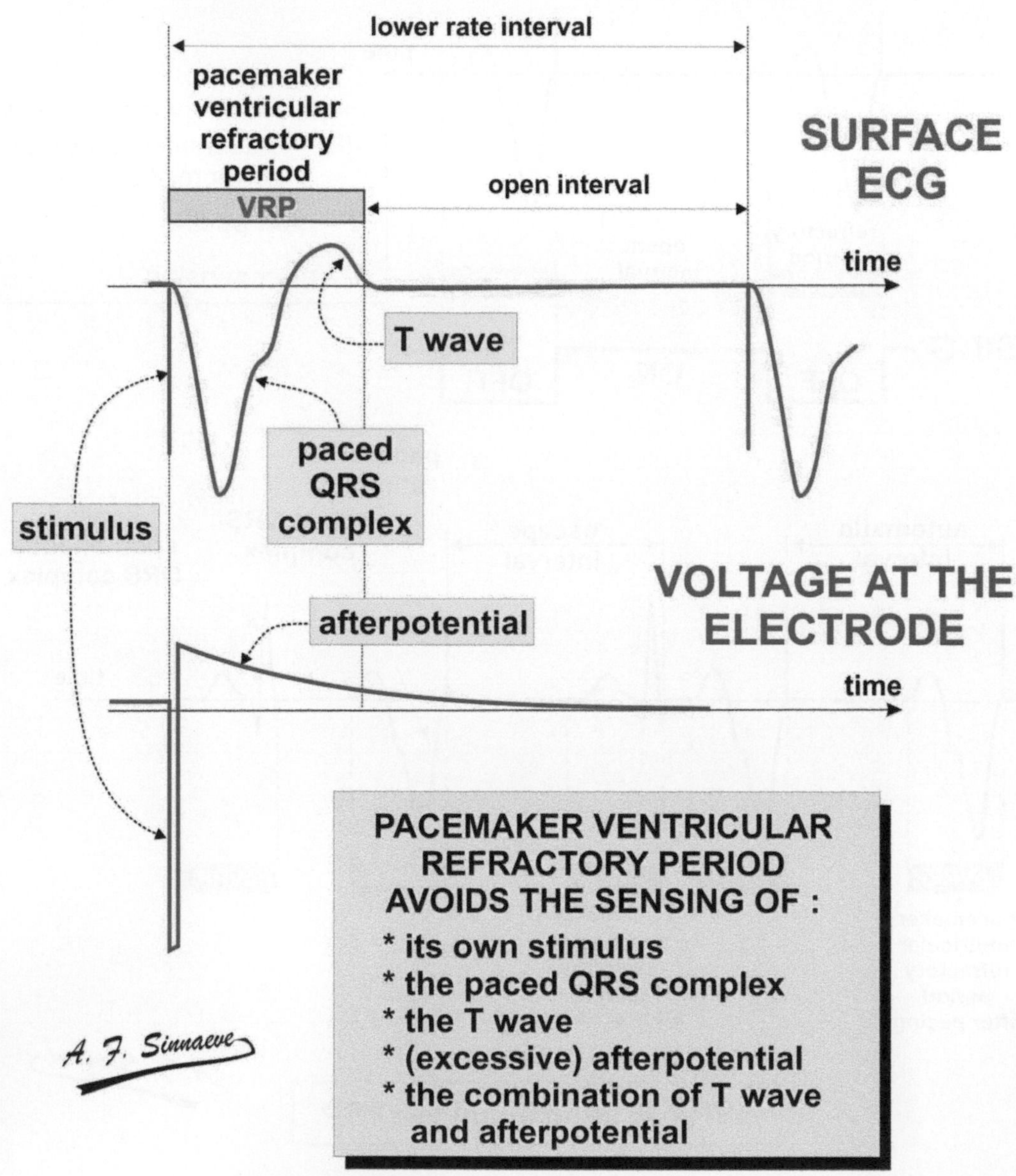

The duration of the pacemaker ventricular refractory period (VRP) is usually 200 - 300 ms

THE PACEMAKER VENTRICULAR REFRACTORY PERIOD

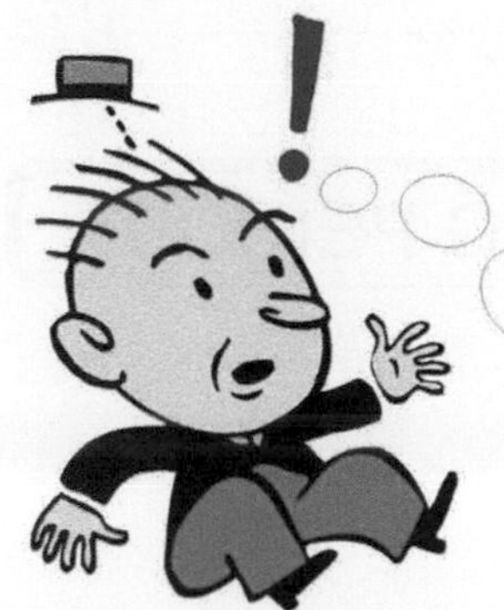

Don't panic ! It is not a malfunction !

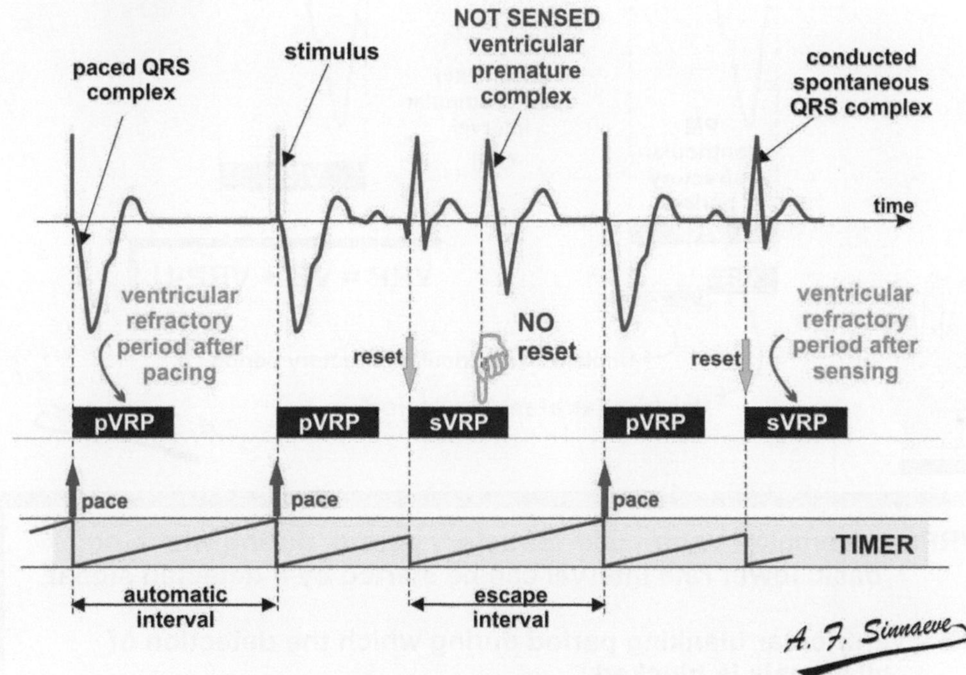

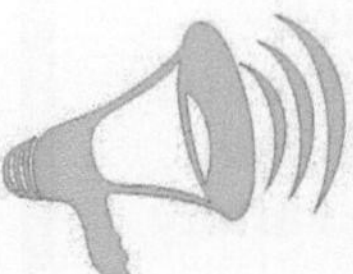

A signal generated during the pacemaker ventricular refractory period can never restart another lower rate interval (corresponding to the lower rate)

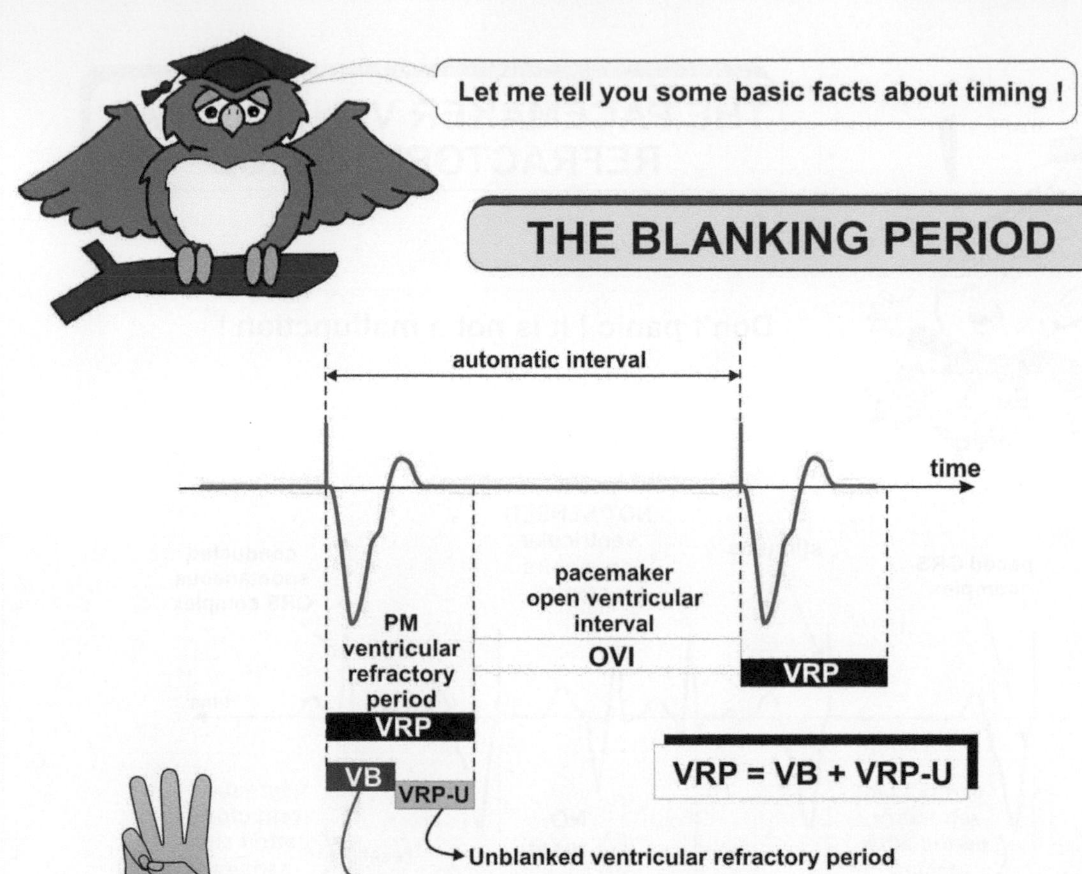

VRP = pacemaker ventricular refractory period, during which no basic lower rate interval can be started by a detected signal

VB = ventricular blanking period during which the detection of all signals is blocked

VRP-U = unblanked ventricular refractory period during which signals can be detected but the lower rate interval cannot be reinitiated. The detected signals in the VRP-U can be used by the pacemaker to control some timing cycles for a variety of functions while the LRI remains unaffected.

RULE

All refractory periods begin with a blanking period. Blanking periods can be free-standing and need not necessarily be followed by an unblanked refractory period such as VPR-U.

PROGRAMMING LOWER SENSITIVITY

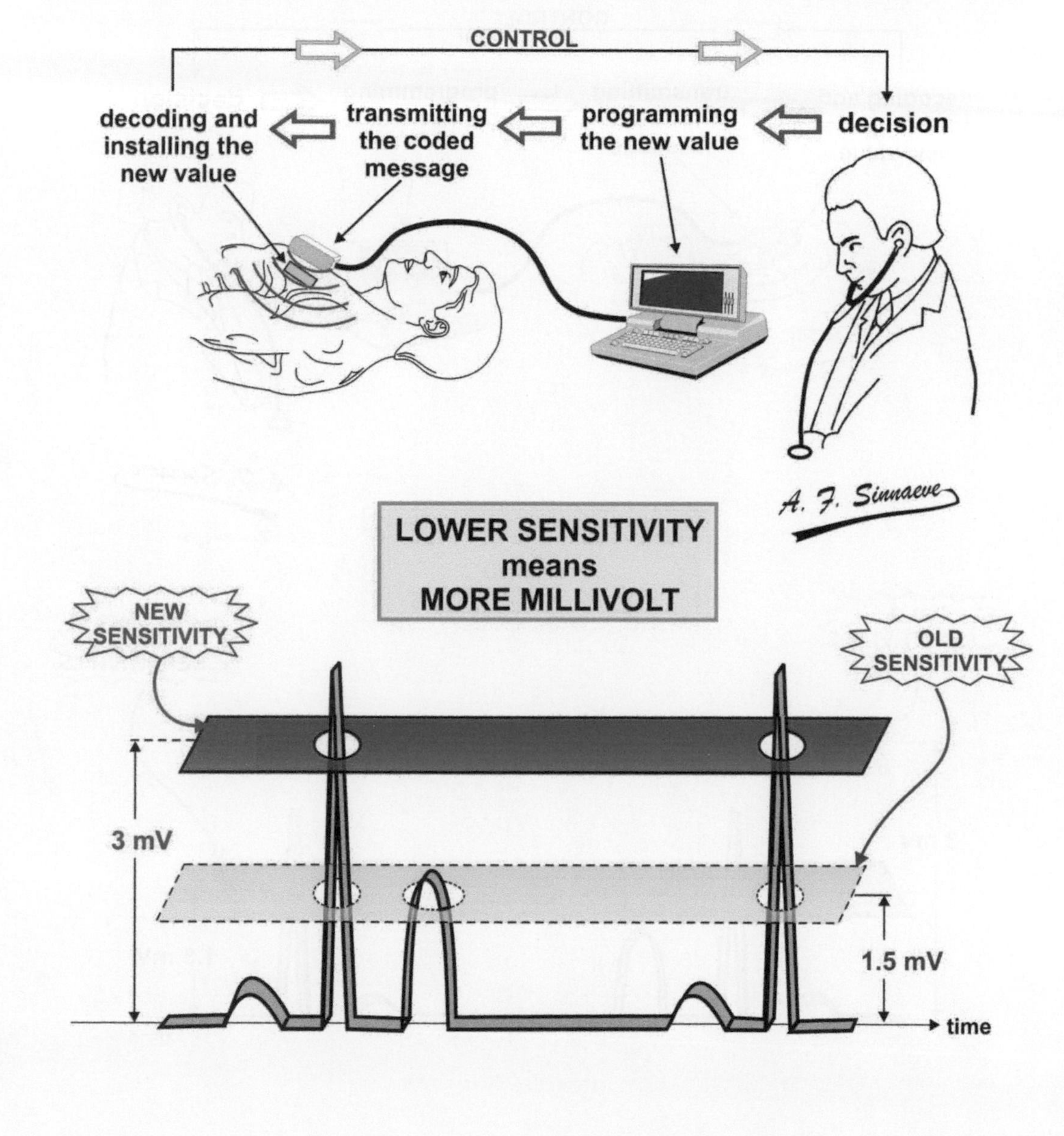

PROGRAMMING HIGHER SENSITIVITY

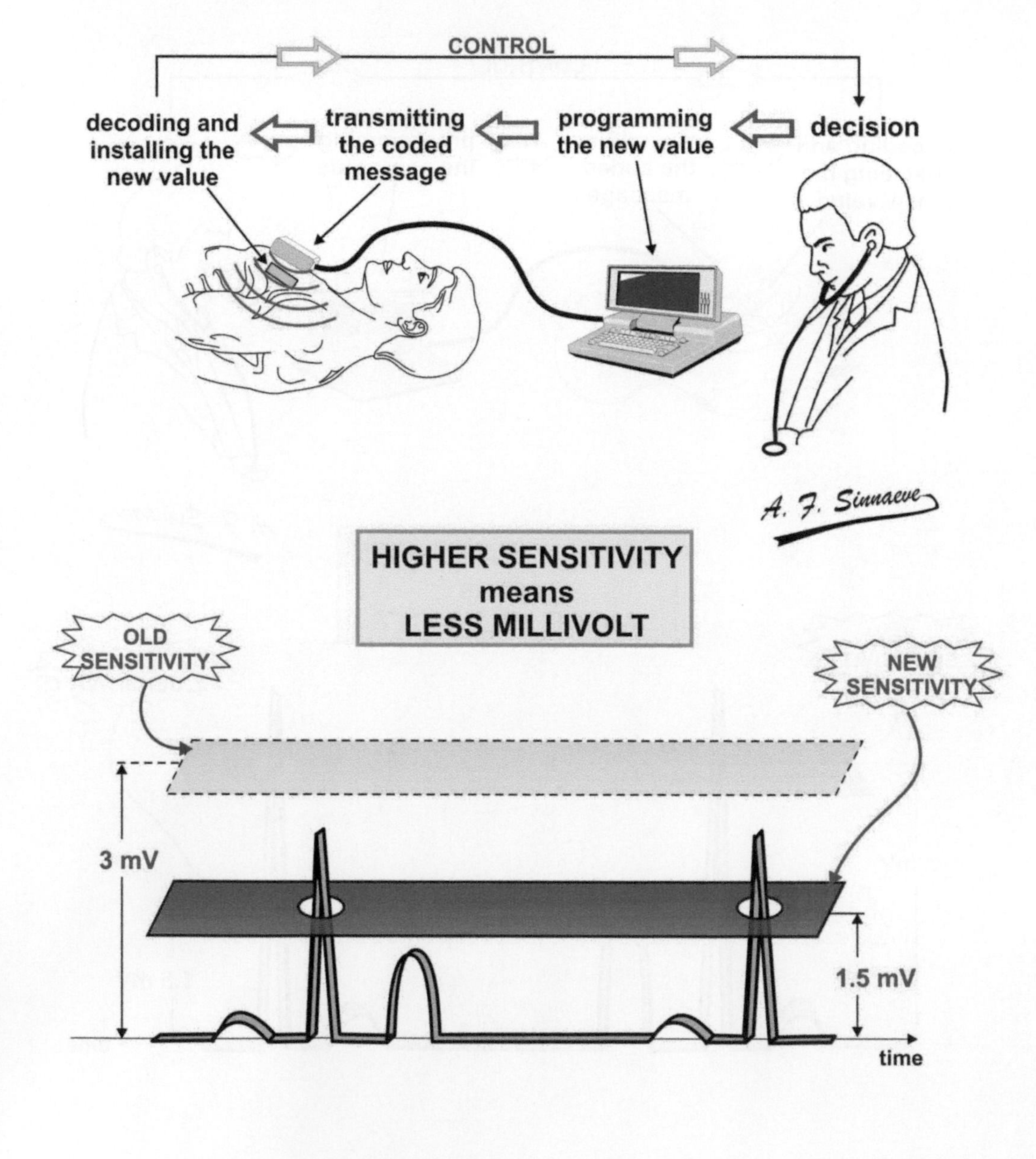

DETERMINATION OF SENSING THRESHOLD

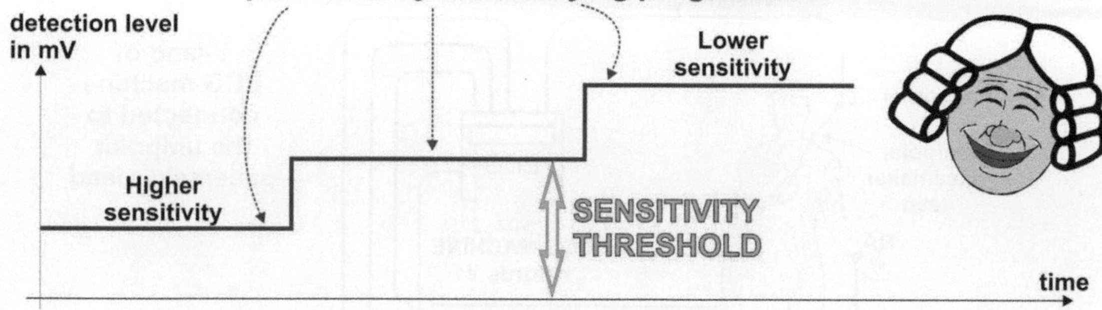

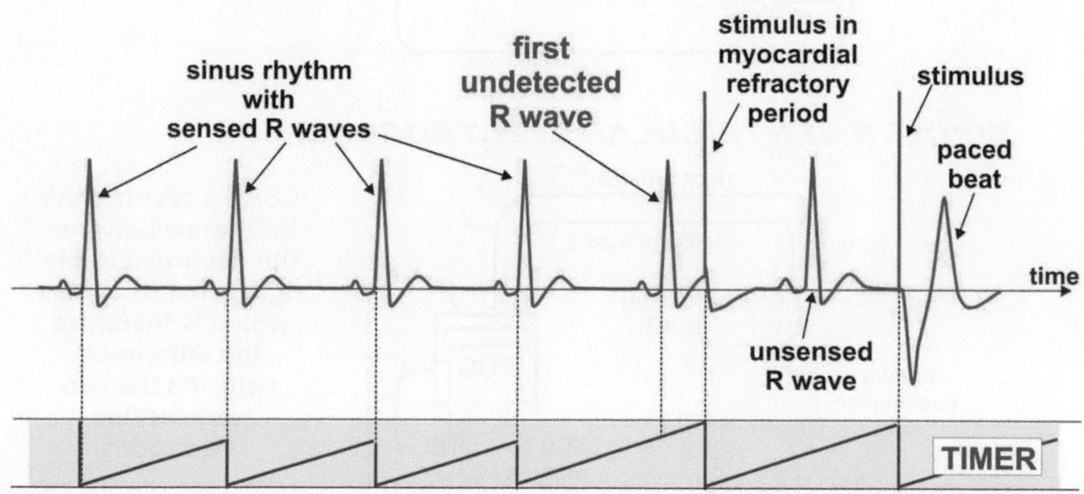

A. F. Sinnaeve

MEASUREMENT OF INTRACARDIAC SIGNALS WITH AN ECG MACHINE AT THE TIME OF IMPLANTATION

UNIPOLAR VENTRICULAR ELECTROGRAM

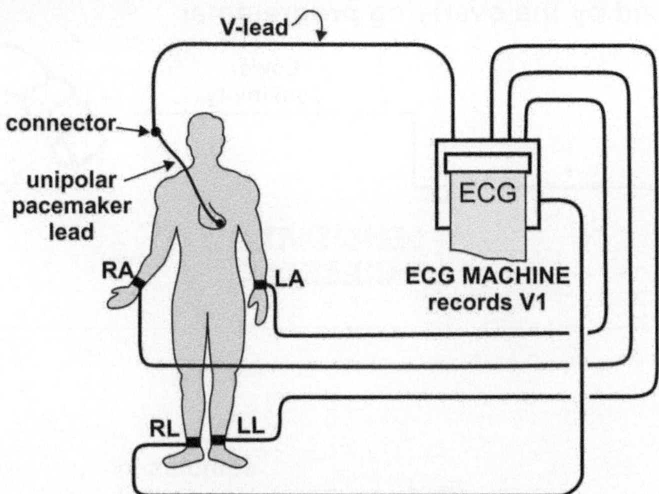

V-lead of ECG machine connected to the unipolar pacemaker lead

BIPOLAR VENTRICULAR ELECTROGRAM

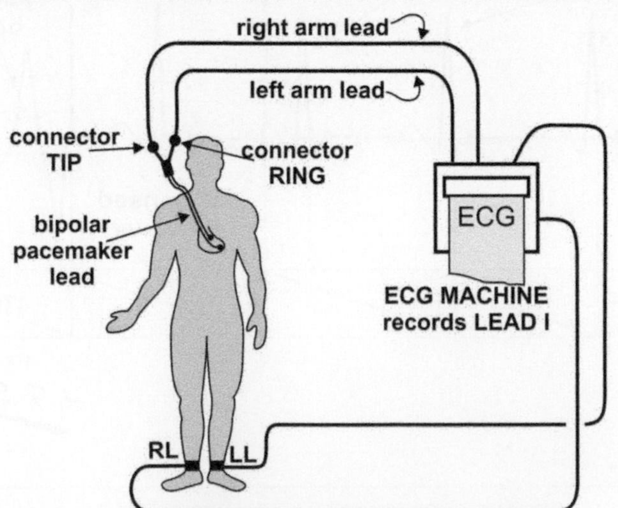

LEAD 1 records the difference between the left arm and the right arm electrodes which is therefore the difference between the two intracardiac electrodes

A. F. Sinnaeve

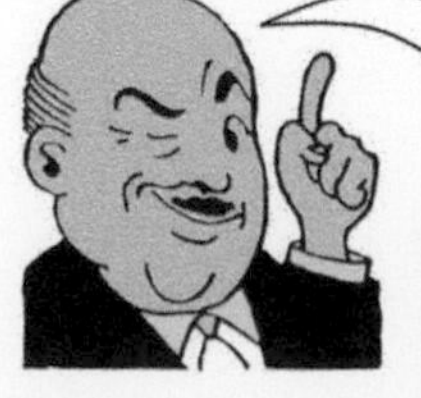

It is important to know that the signal (electrogram) available for sensing by a pacemaker can be easily measured with an ECG machine at the time of implantation. This procedure is sometimes neglected. After implantation, the electrogram can be transmitted noninvasively by telemetry to an appropriate programmer.

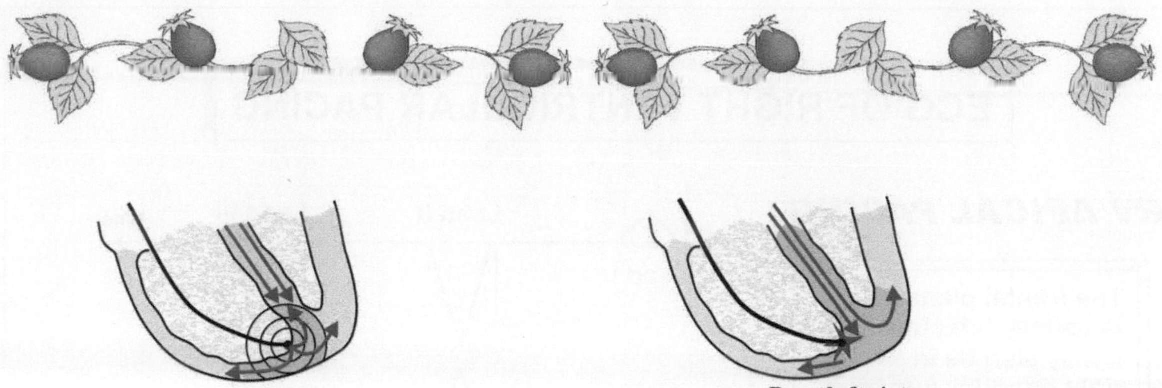

BASIC PACEMAKER ELECTROCARDIOGRAPHY

* ECG of right ventricular pacing : right ventricular apex (RVA) and right ventricular outflow tract (RVOT)
* Axis in the frontal plane with RVA & RVOT pacing
* Myocardial infarct and RV pacing
* Pacing and memory effect
* Patterns of atrial activity with ventricular pacing
* Ventricular fusion
* Ventricular pseudofusion
* Isoelectric ventricular fusion
* Tall R waves in lead V1
* Left ventricular pacing
* Influence of the ECG machine

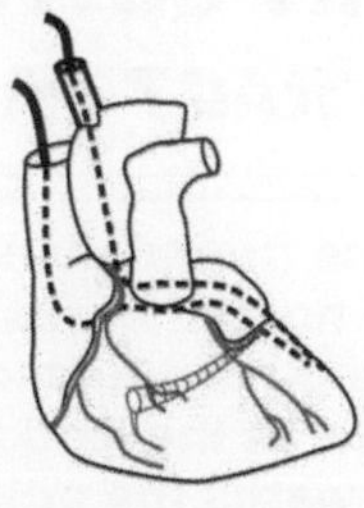

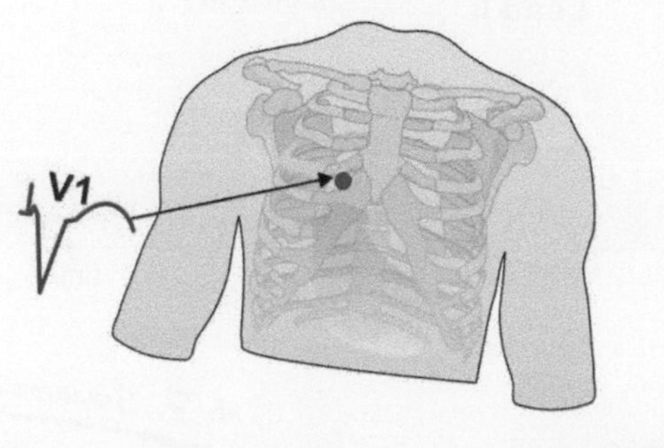

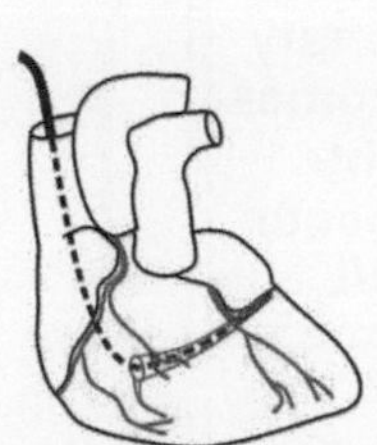

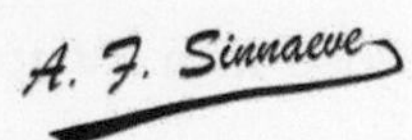

ECG OF RIGHT VENTRICULAR PACING

RV APICAL PACING

The frontal plane axis is usually left superior . It may also be in the right superior quadrant, where it causes leads I, II & III to be negative and lead aVR to show the largest positive deflection.

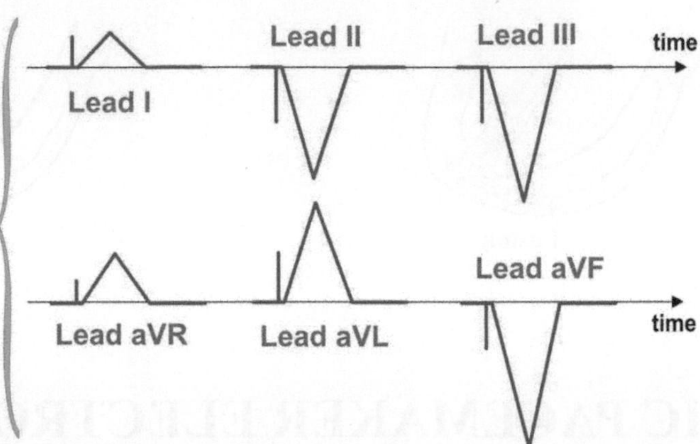

A A typical LBBB pattern in the left precordial leads may not be present and all leads show a QS pattern

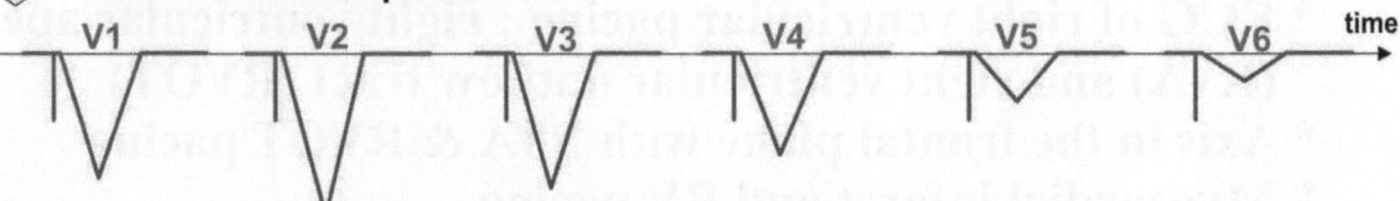

B The left precordial leads may show a dominant R wave

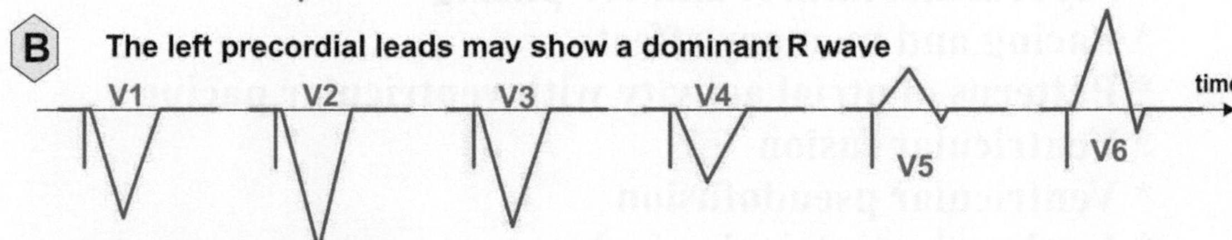

RV OUTFLOW TRACT PACING

The frontal plane axis is normal i.e. as for normally conducted beats. But as the lead moves towards the pulmonary valve, the axis becomes deviated to the right. A qR pattern can occur only in leads I & aVL

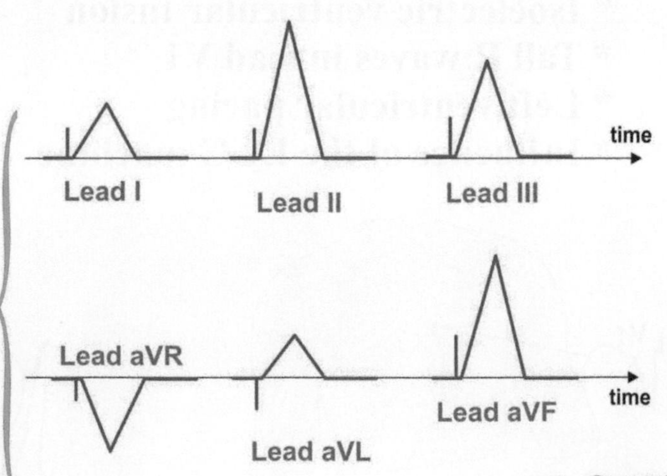

A. F. Sinnaeve

The precordial V leads are similar to those with RV apical pacing !

Abbreviation : LBBB = left bundle branch block

THE MEAN QRS AXIS IN THE FRONTAL PLANE DURING RIGHT VENTRICULAR PACING

During pacing the mean frontal plane QRS axis reflects the site of the pacing !

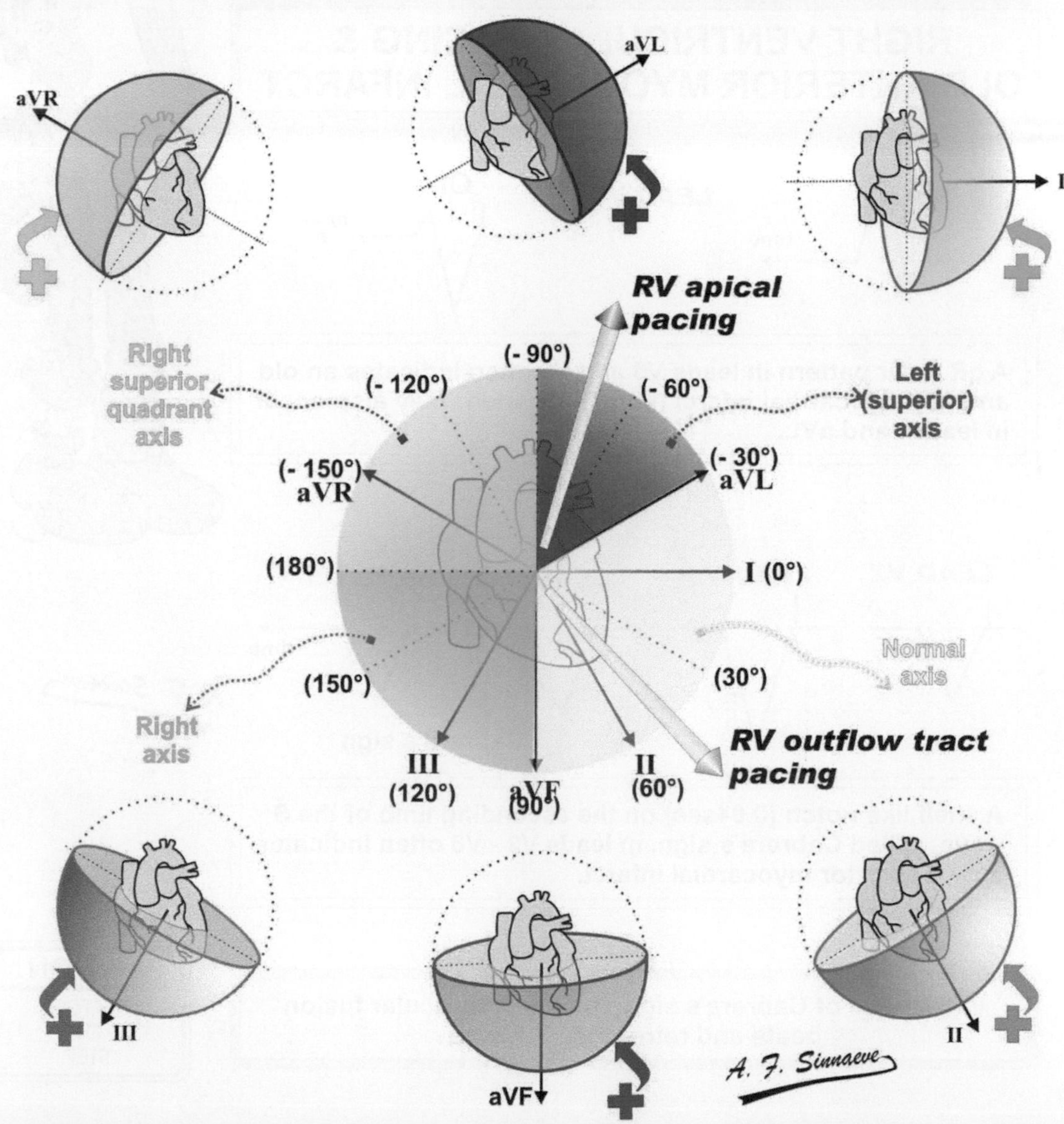

Right ventricular apical pacing activates the inferior part of the heart first. The activation then moves superiorly away from the inferior ECG leads (II, III and aVF) towards the superior leads. The mean frontal plane axis of the paced QRS complex lies superiorly in the left upper quadrant but sometimes in the right superior quadrant. In the latter case, leads I, II and aVF will be negative.
Right ventricular outflow tract pacing, produces a mean frontal plane axis of the paced beat in a direction seen with spontaneous activation of a normal heart: left lower quadrant or "normal" axis. Pacing more superiorly near the pulmonary valve produces right axis deviation: right lower quadrant.

You cannot imagine what little details these cardiologists are looking at ...!

RIGHT VENTRICULAR PACING & OLD ANTERIOR MYOCARDIAL INFARCT

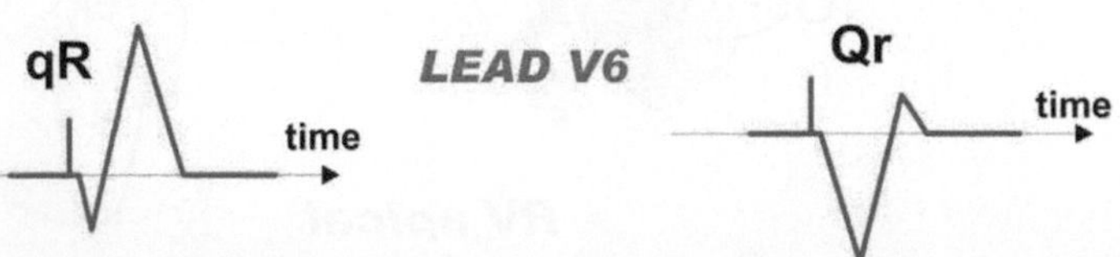

A qR or Qr pattern in leads V5 and V6 often indicates an old anterior myocardial infarct (MI). This pattern may also occur in leads I and aVL.

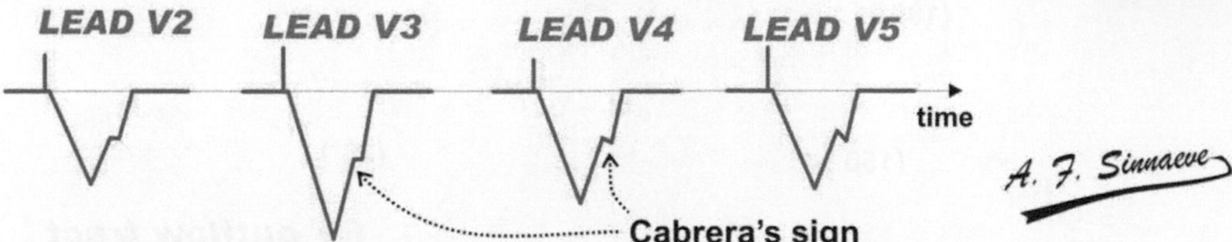

A shelf like notch (0.04sec) on the ascending limb of the S wave, called Cabrera's sign, in leads V2 - V5 often indicates an old anterior myocardial infarct.

In the case of Cabrera's sign, rule out ventricular fusion beats and retrograde P waves

CAUTION
WATCH YOUR STEP

A. F. Sinnaeve

Wow ! The heart has a memory and therefore a brain. I'm flabbergasted !!!

VENTRICULAR PACING & THE MEMORY EFFECT

The underlying ECG cannot be used for the diagnosis of cardiac ischemia because inverted T waves may be due to the memory effect !!!

BEFORE PACING

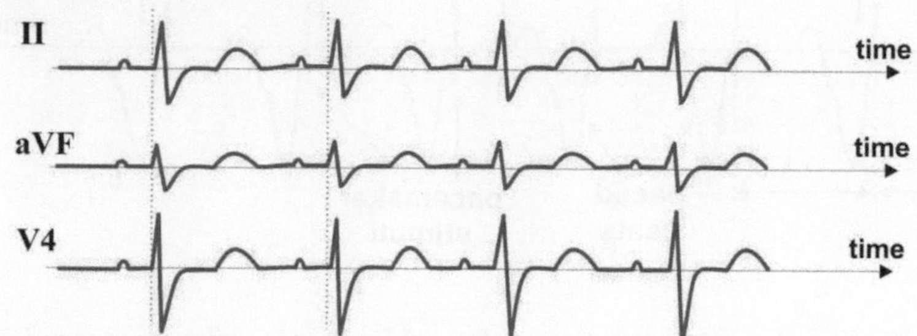

DURING PACING

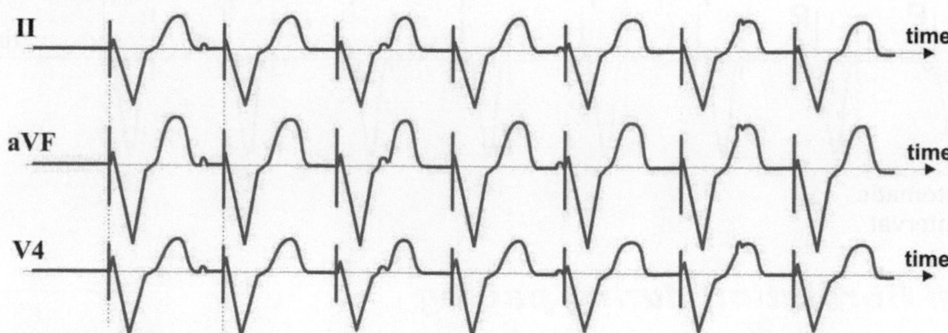

AFTER PACING

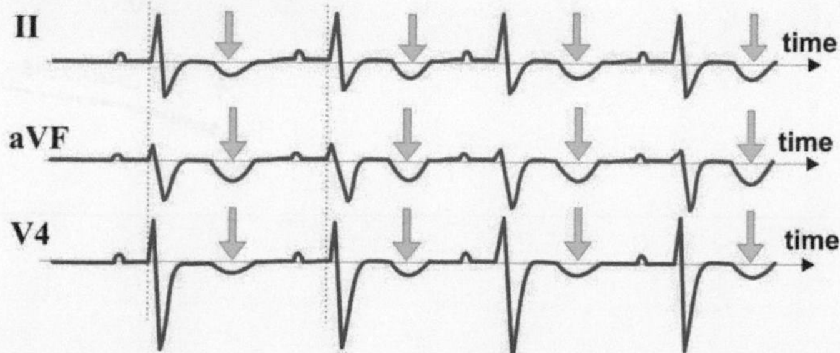

For some time after pacing, the heart seems to remember the abnormal depolarizations.
The duration of the memory effect (negative T waves) depends upon the duration of pacing

A. F. Sinnaeve

PATTERNS OF ATRIAL ACTIVITY DURING VENTRICULAR PACING

AV dissociation during pacing

P waves march through the paced QRS complexes

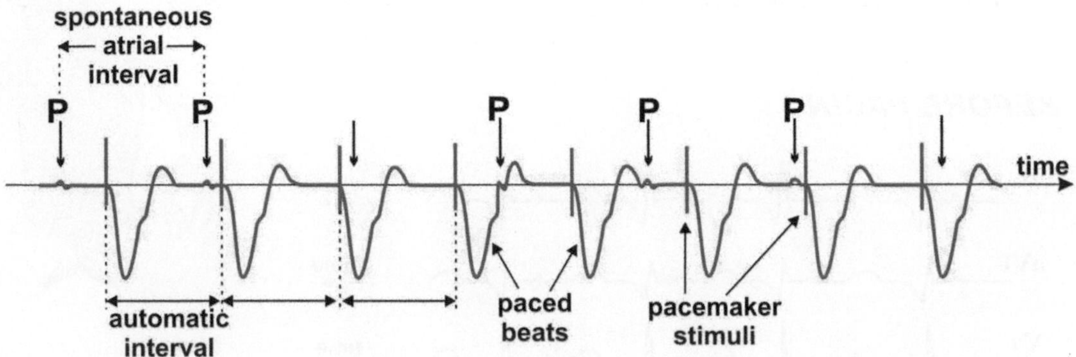

Retrograde ventriculoatrial conduction during pacing

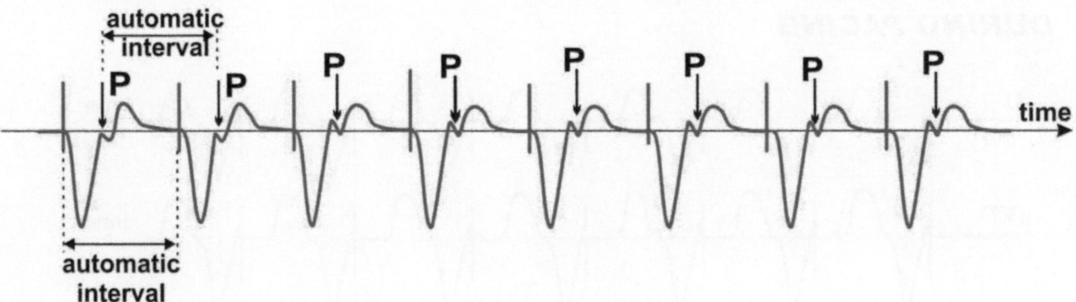

Atrial fibrillation during pacing

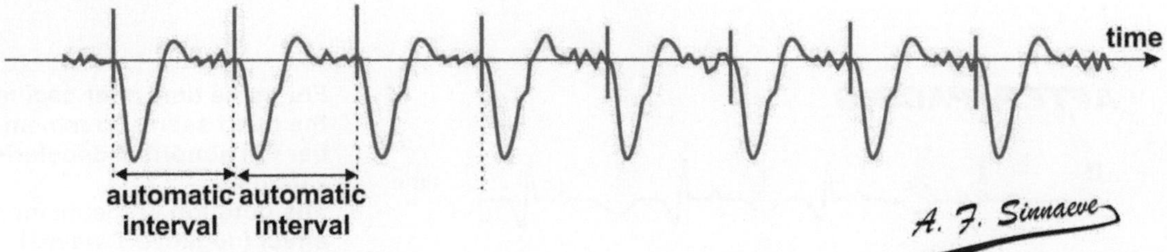

A. F. Sinnaeve

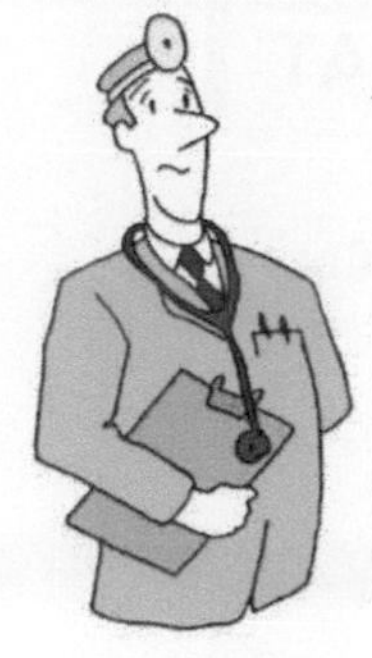

Attention please ! Peculiar QRS complexes may be seen !!!

VENTRICULAR FUSION BEAT

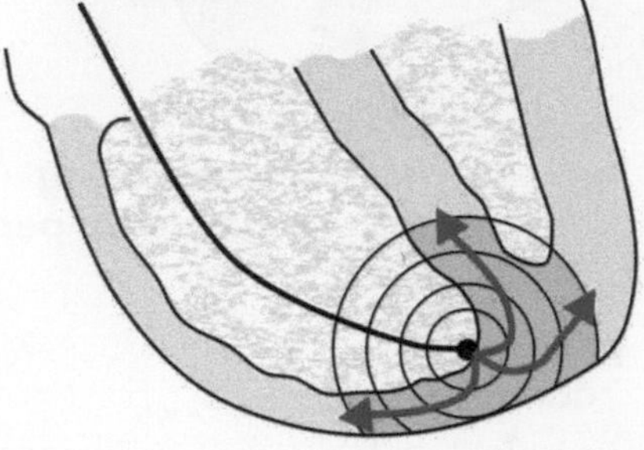

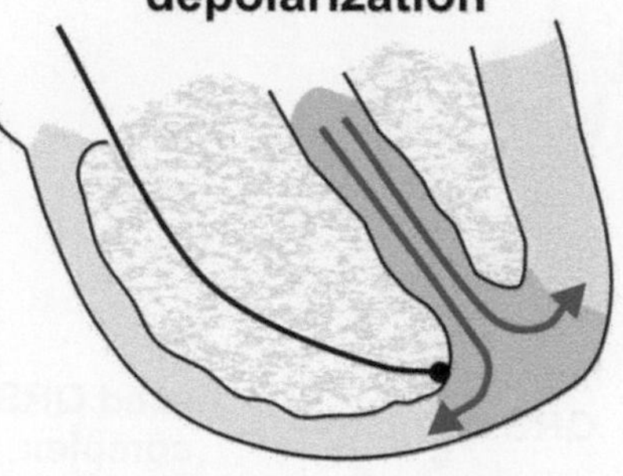

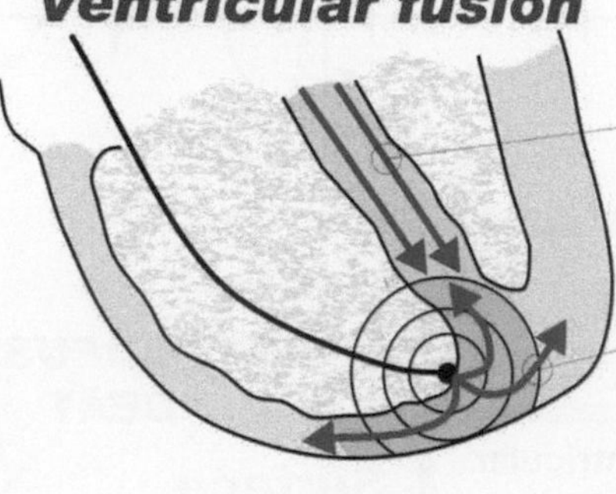

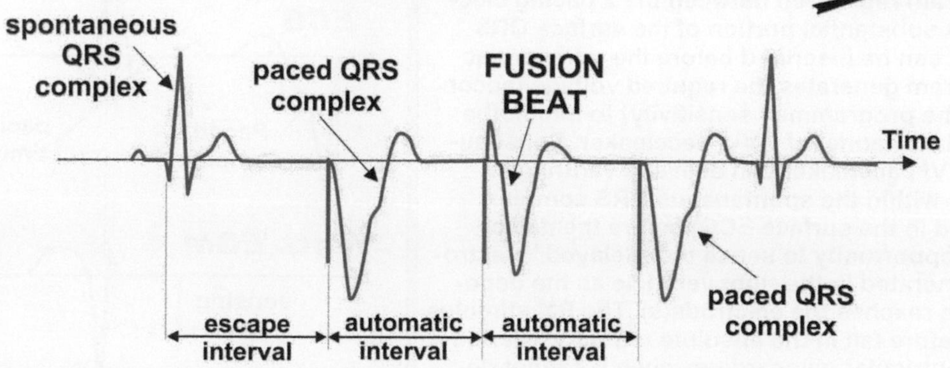

VENTRICULAR PSEUDOFUSION BEAT

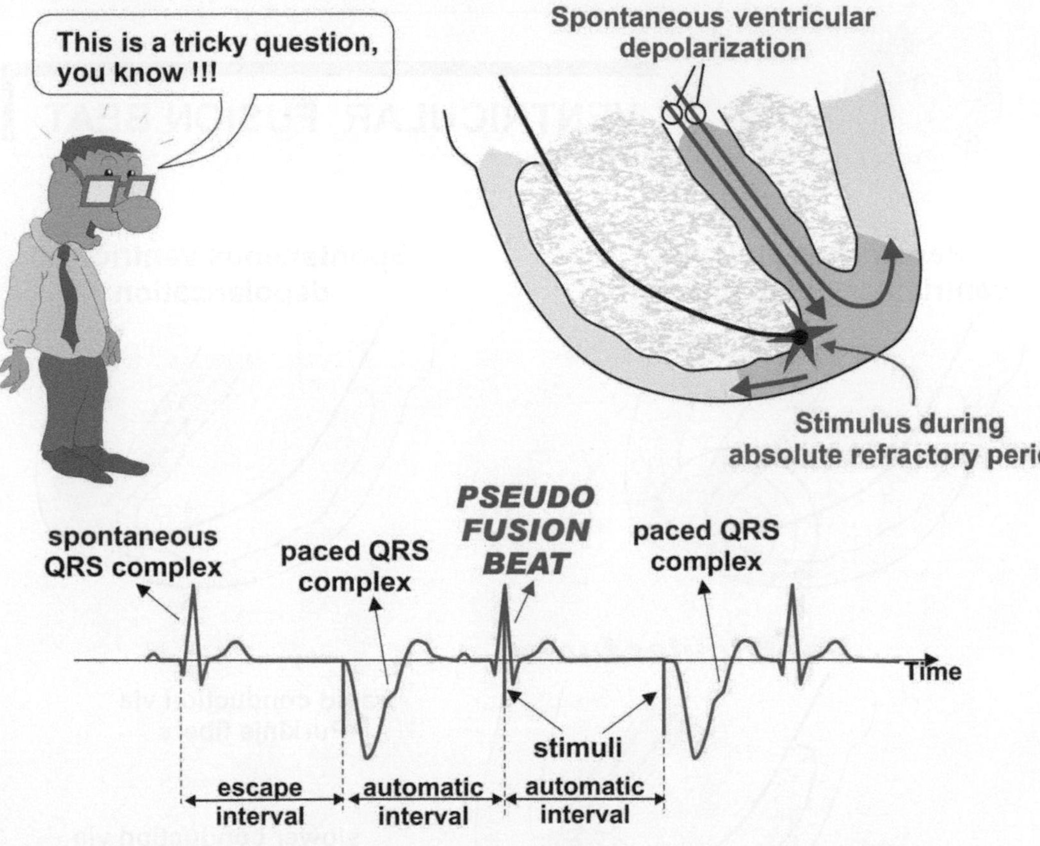

The pacemaker senses the intracardiac ventricular electrogram registered between the 2 pacing electrodes. A substantial portion of the surface QRS complex can be inscribed before the intracardiac electrogram generates the required voltage (according to the programmed sensitivity) to inhibit the ventricular channel of a VVI pacemaker. Consequently a VVI pacemaker can deliver a ventricular stimulus within the spontaneous QRS complex (recorded in the surface ECG) before the device has the opportunity to sense the "delayed" electrogram generated in the right ventricle as the depolarization reaches the electrode(s). The PM stimulus can therefore fall in the absolute refractory period of the ventricular myocardium when it cannot depolarize any portion of the ventricles. True ventricular fusion does not occur. In other words depolarization originates from only one focus !

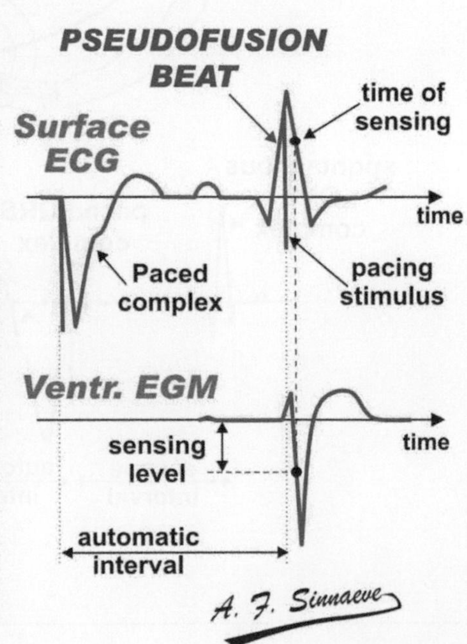

ISOELECTRIC VENTRICULAR FUSION BEATS

Pay attention !!!
The pacemaker may function normally while no QRS complexes are seen on the surface ECG

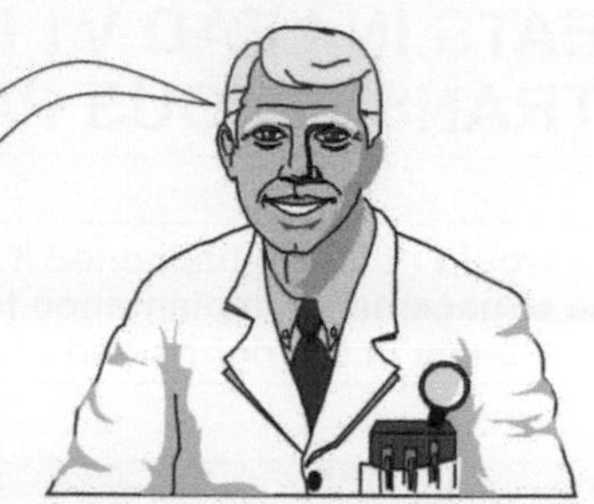

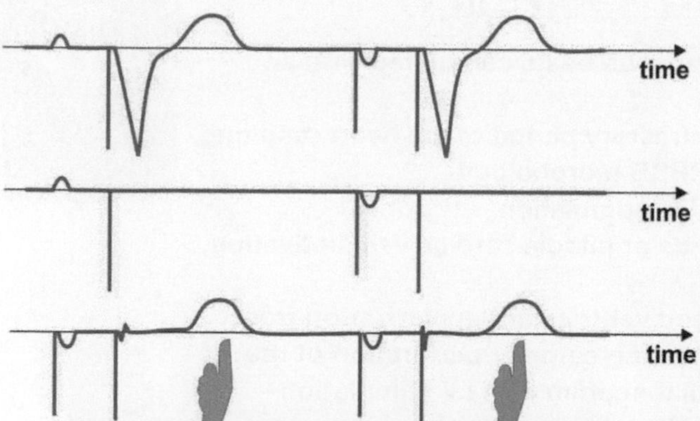

Normal paced ventricular complexes : a depolarization is followed by a repolarization.

There is loss of capture here ! No depolarization is seen.

ISOELECTRIC FUSION BEATS ! The QRS complex may be so narrow as to resemble a stimulus or even zero !!!

Look at the T wave !!! If there is a repolarization, a depolarization has occurred before !

Note that this appearance is seen in only one ECG lead. To confirm the diagnosis, look at different ECG leads where the QRS complex of the ventricular fusion beat will be visible.

A. F. Sinnaeve

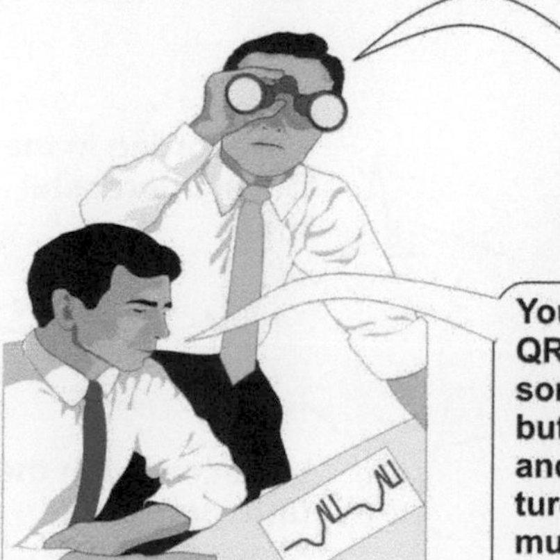

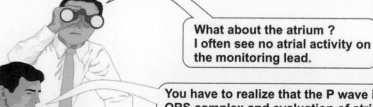

What about the atrium ?
I often see no atrial activity on the monitoring lead.

You have to realize that the P wave is much smaller than the QRS complex and evaluation of atrial activity in the ECG can sometimes be tricky ! Isoelectric atrial fusion beats may occur but are rare. An isoelectric or flat segment between an atrial and ventricular stimulus can be due to successful atrial capture which is not visible in a particular ECG lead. Again, one must examine other ECG leads to determine the presence of a paced P wave and sometimes take an ECG at double standardization to bring out the P wave

SIGNIFICANCE OF A DOMINANT R WAVE OF PACED VENTRICULAR BEATS IN LEAD V1 DURING TRANSVENOUS PACING

A lead in the LV via a foramen ovale !!!

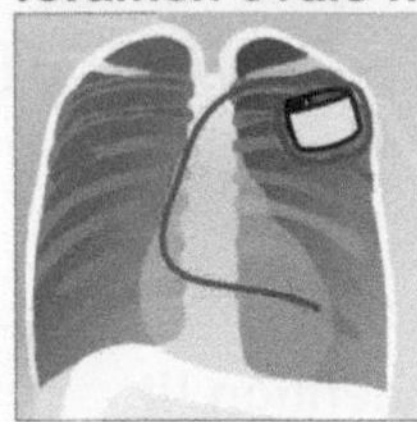

This would not have happened if a 12 lead ECG had been taken at the time of pacemaker implantation to exclude a dominant R wave of the paced beats in the right-sided chest leads !

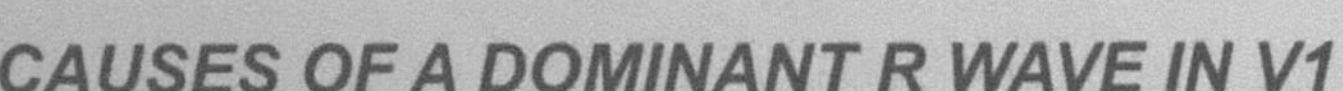

CAUSES OF A DOMINANT R WAVE IN V1

1. Ventricular fusion with spontaneous beats conducted with an RBBB pattern
2. A paced beat in the relative refractory period of the heart resulting in aberrant conduction with RBBB morphology
3. Left ventricular (LV) endocardial stimulation
4. A catheter in the coronary sinus or middle cardiac vein activating the LV epicardial surface
5. A change of electrically induced ventricular depolarization from LBBB to RBBB strongly suggesting catheter perforation of the free wall of RV or the ventricular septum with LV stimulation
6. Uncomplicated RV pacing as shown below

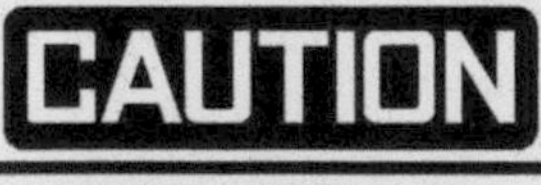

CHECK THE POSITION OF THE LEADS VERY CAREFULLY

* The positivity of V1 depends upon the correct position of the chest (V) electrode

* A dominant R wave may be seen during uncomplicated RV apical pacing

V1 recorded in the third intercostal space

V1 recorded in the fourth intercostal space

V1 recorded in the fourth intercostal space

V1 recorded in the fifth intercostal space

A. F. Sinnaeve

Abbreviations : LBBB = left bundle branch block ; LV = left ventricle ; RBBB = right bundle branch block ; RV = right ventricle ; **Foramen ovale** is a potential communication from the right atrium to the left atrium that may allow passage of a pacemaker lead from the right atrium to the left one and then to the left ventricle. The lead in the left ventricle may appear to be in the right ventricle on standard fluoroscopy.

LEFT VENTRICULAR PACING

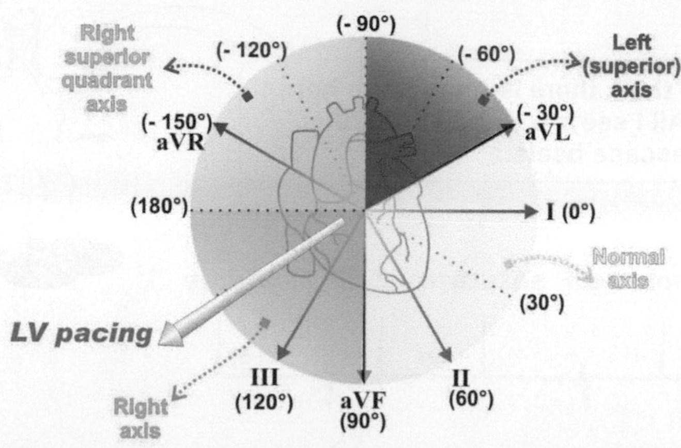

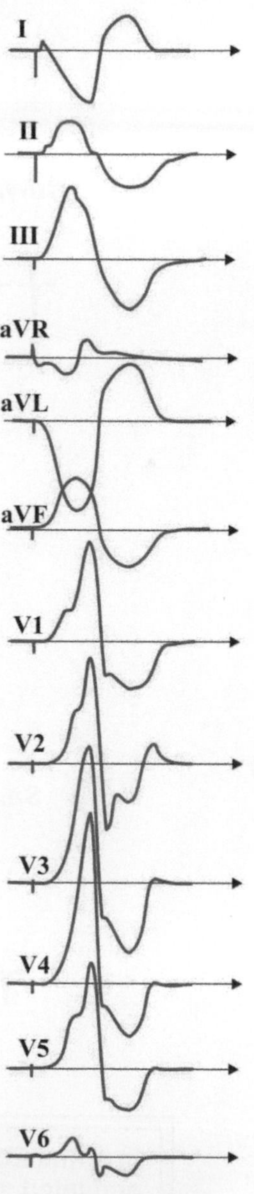

The mean frontal plane axis of the paced beat is directed to the right lower quadrant (right axis deviation). There is a characteristic tall R wave in lead V1 to at least V3 and often further into the left precordial leads.

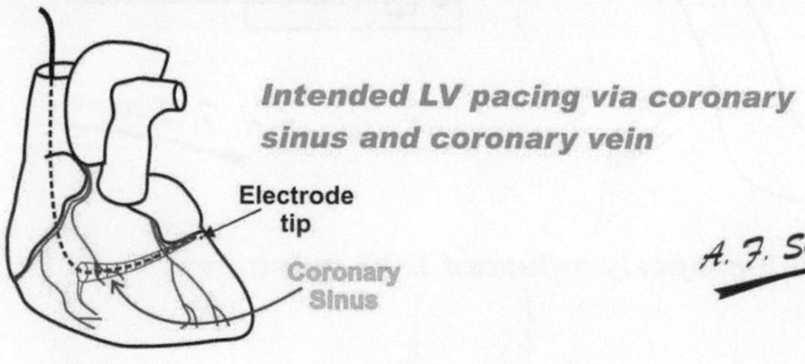

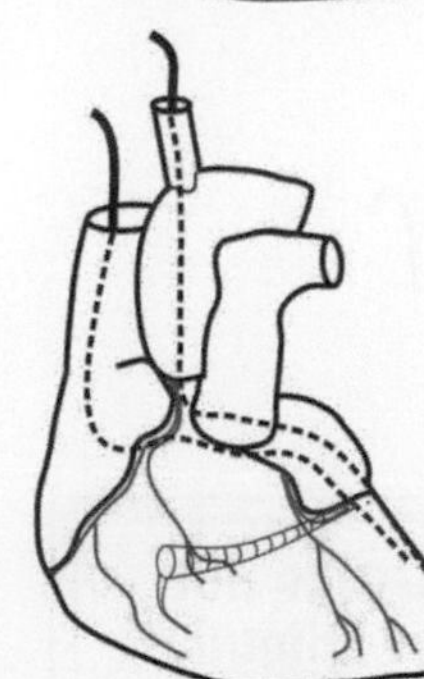

Unintended LV pacing :

- ***Passage of lead into LV via patent foramen ovale (from right atrium to left atrium and LV)***
- ***Via subclavian artery (across the aortic valve) mistaken for the subclavian vein***

A lead within the LV cavity (endocardial site) may cause thrombus formation, cerebral emboli and stroke.
The diagnosis of LV endocardial lead misplacement should be suspected if there is a tall R wave at least in leads V1 to V3 and sometimes further in the left-sided precordial leads. The definitive diagnosis requires echocardiography especially by the transesophageal method.

INFLUENCE OF THE ECG-MACHINE

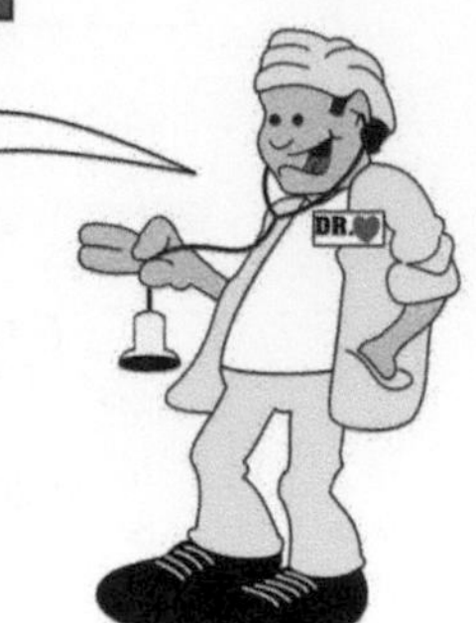

I think there is no capture here ! All I see are some ventricular escape beats...

Surface ECG shown on saturated ECG machine

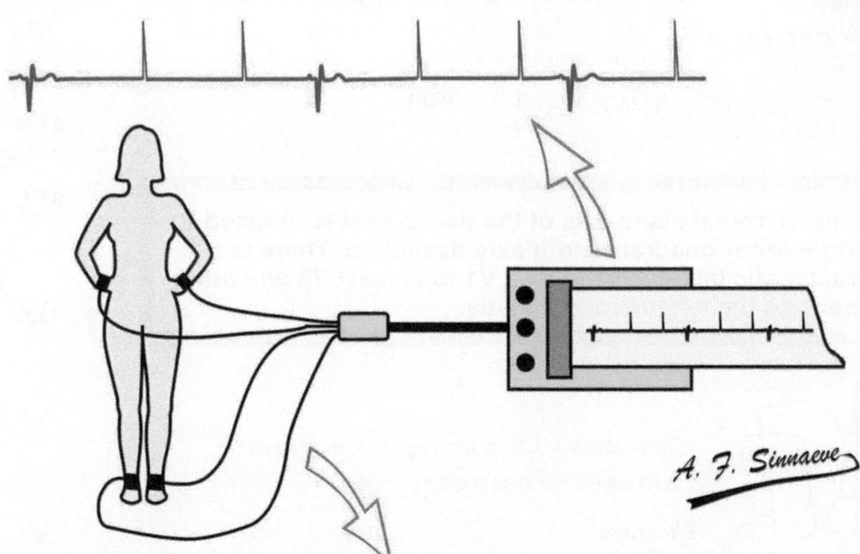

Same ECG with properly adjusted ECG machine

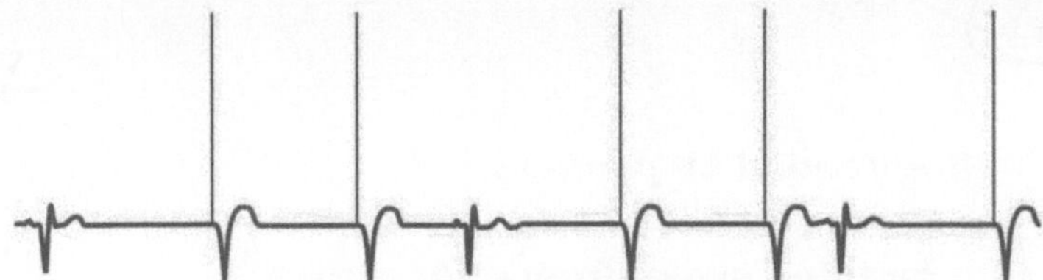

In some ECG machines, when the automatic gain control (AGC) is not activated, the input circuit may be saturated by large unipolar stimuli. During this saturation the machine is unable to detect any small signals and it is impossible to see if the stimuli capture the heart or not.

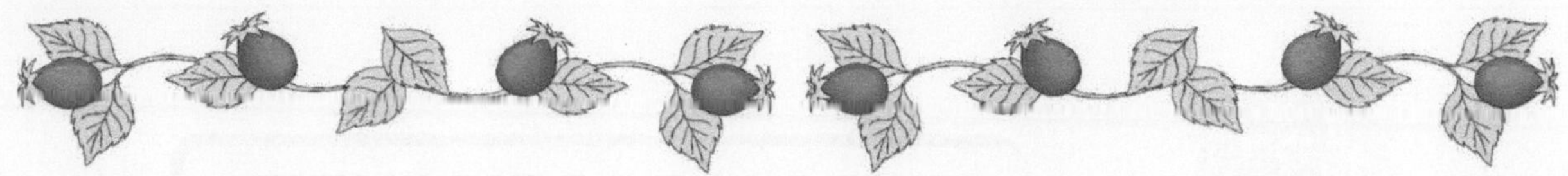

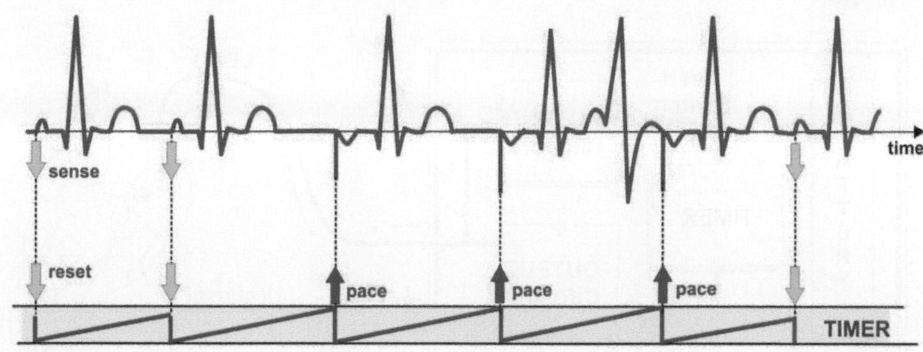

OTHER SINGLE CHAMBER PACEMAKERS

* The AAI pacing mode
* The VVT pacing mode

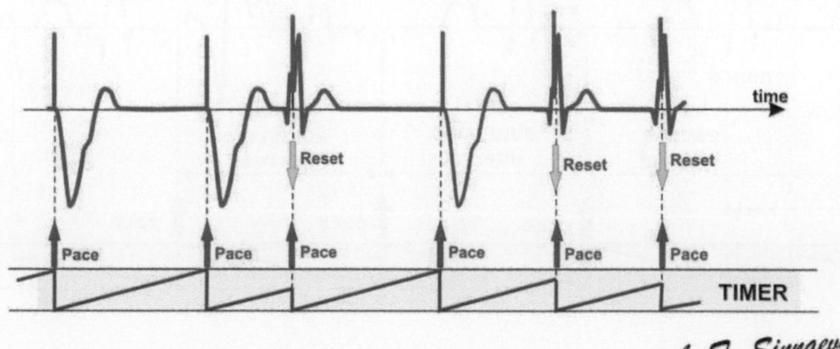

A. F. Sinnaeve

THE AAI PACEMAKER

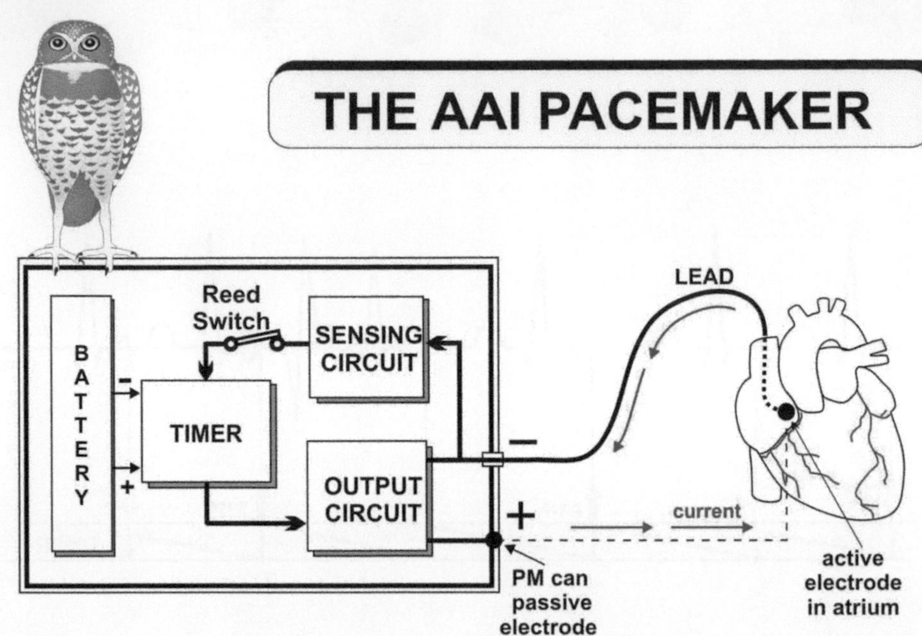

Compared to the VVI pacemaker the SENSITIVITY should be higher (i.e. a lower number in mV) because P waves have lower amplitudes than R waves

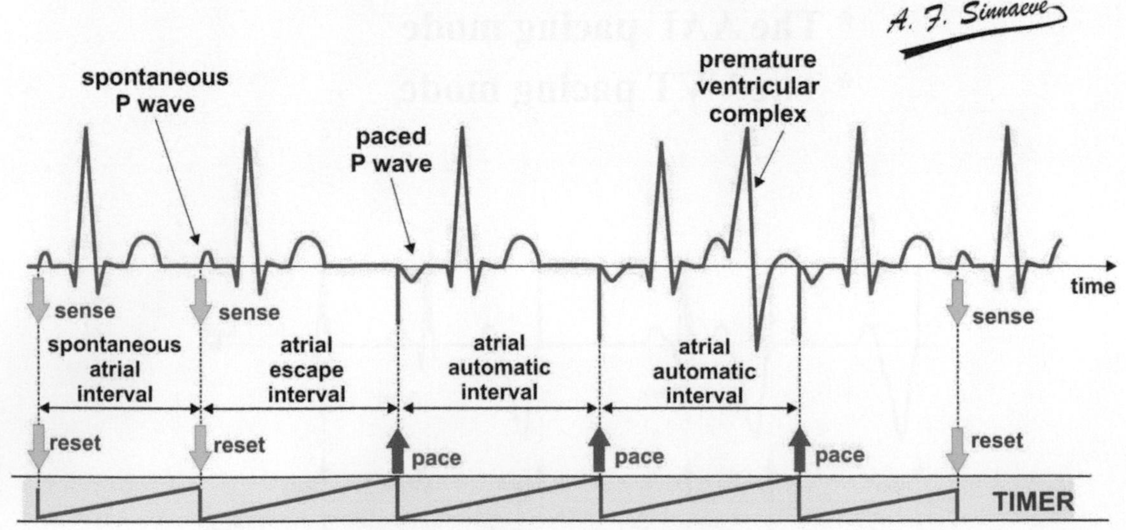

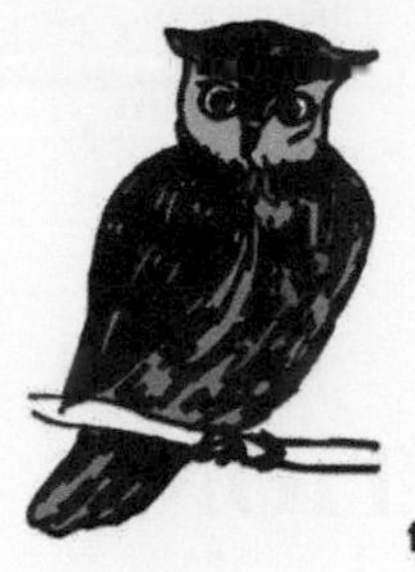

THE VVT MODE

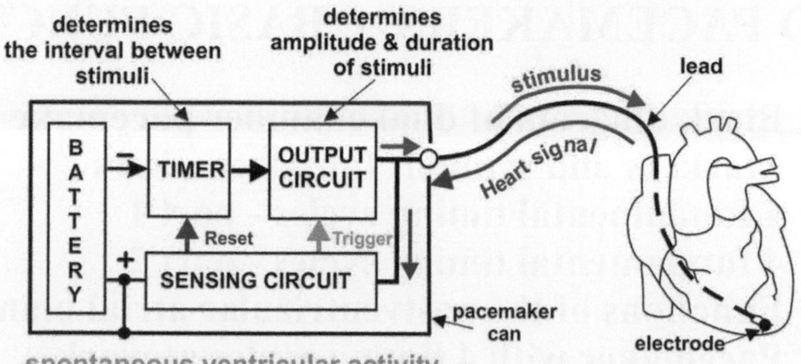
determines
the interval between
stimuli
determines
amplitude & duration
of stimuli
stimulus
lead
B A T T E R Y
TIMER
OUTPUT CIRCUIT
Heart signal
Reset
Trigger
SENSING CIRCUIT
pacemaker can
electrode
spontaneous ventricular activity
triggers the output & resets the timer

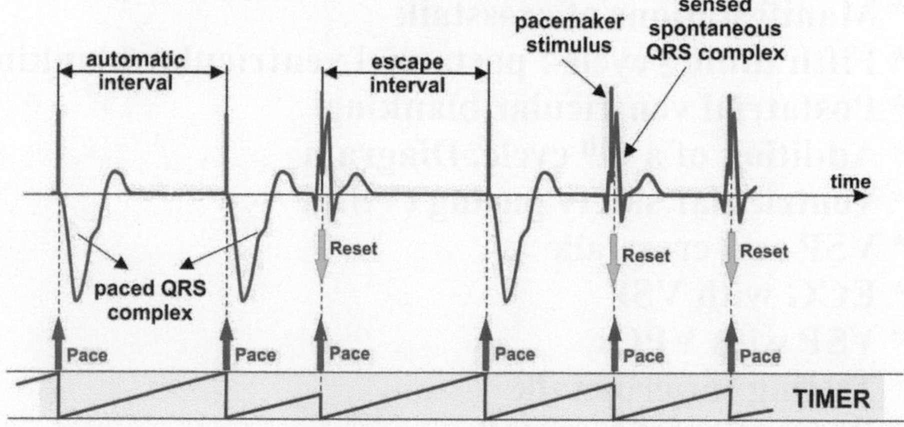
automatic
interval
escape
interval
pacemaker
stimulus
sensed
spontaneous
QRS complex
time
Reset
Reset
Reset
paced QRS
complex
Pace
Pace
Pace
Pace
Pace
Pace
TIMER

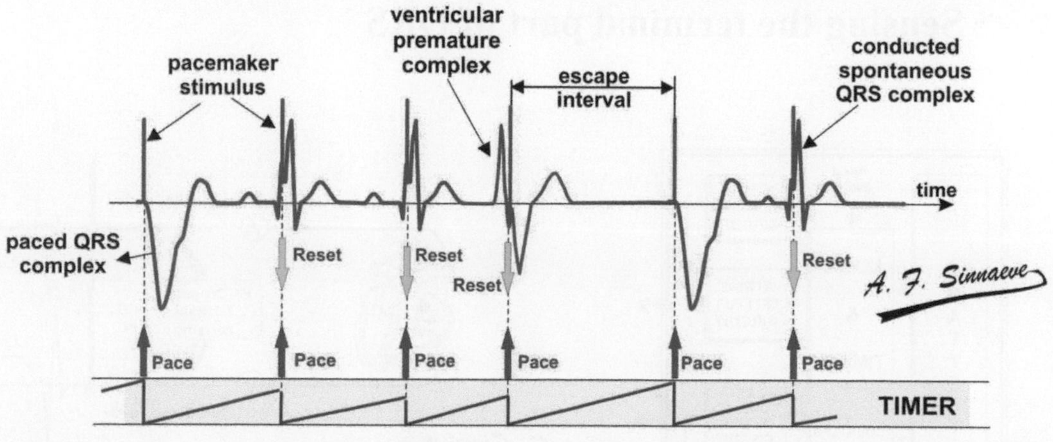
pacemaker
stimulus
ventricular
premature
complex
escape
interval
conducted
spontaneous
QRS complex
time
paced QRS
complex
Reset
Reset
Reset
Reset
Pace
Pace
Pace
Pace
Pace
Pace
TIMER
A. F. Sinnaeve

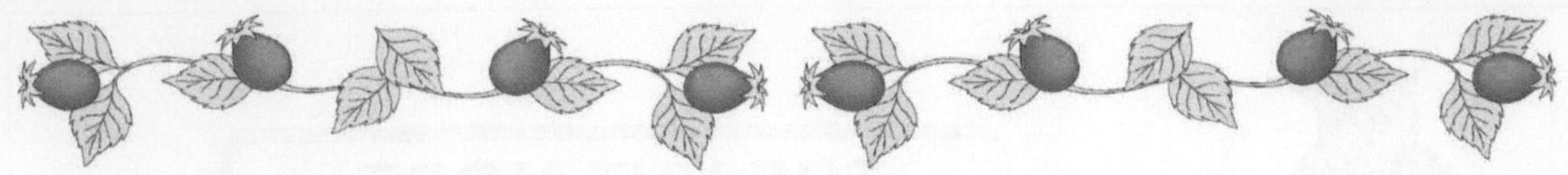

DDD PACEMAKERS - BASIC FUNCTIONS

* Block diagram of dual chamber pacemakers
* Markers and symbols for pacemakers
* 4 fundamental timing cycles - part 1
* 4 fundamental timing cycles - part 2
* Functions of the postventricular atrial blanking period
* Pacemaker with 4 timing cycles at work
* Three-letter-code for dual chamber pacemakers
* Manifestations of crosstalk
* Fifth timing cycle : postatrial ventricular blanking
* Postatrial ventricular blanking
* Addition of a 6th cycle. Diagram
* Ventricular safety pacing (VSP).
* VSP and crosstalk
* ECG with VSP
* VSP with VPCs
* Testing for crosstalk
* Prevention of crosstalk
* Sensing the terminal part of QRS

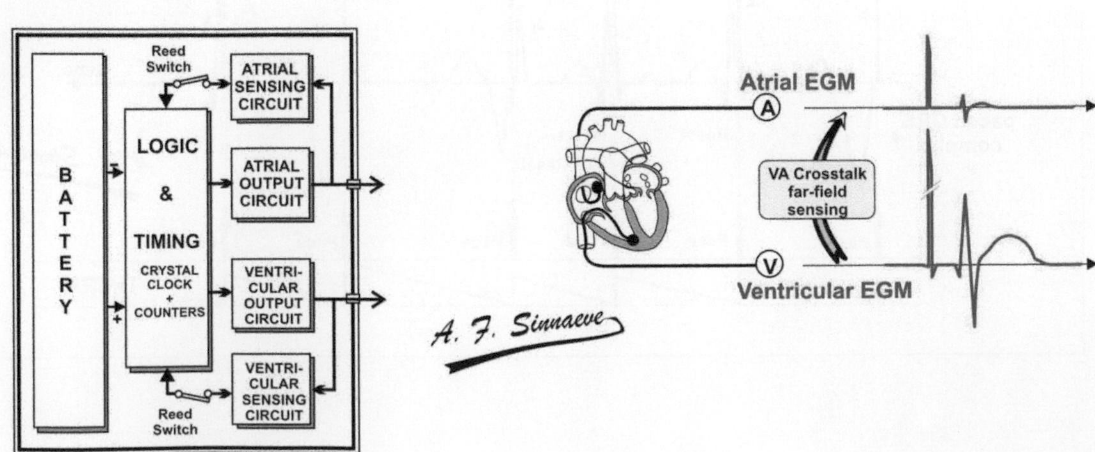

DUAL CHAMBER PACING

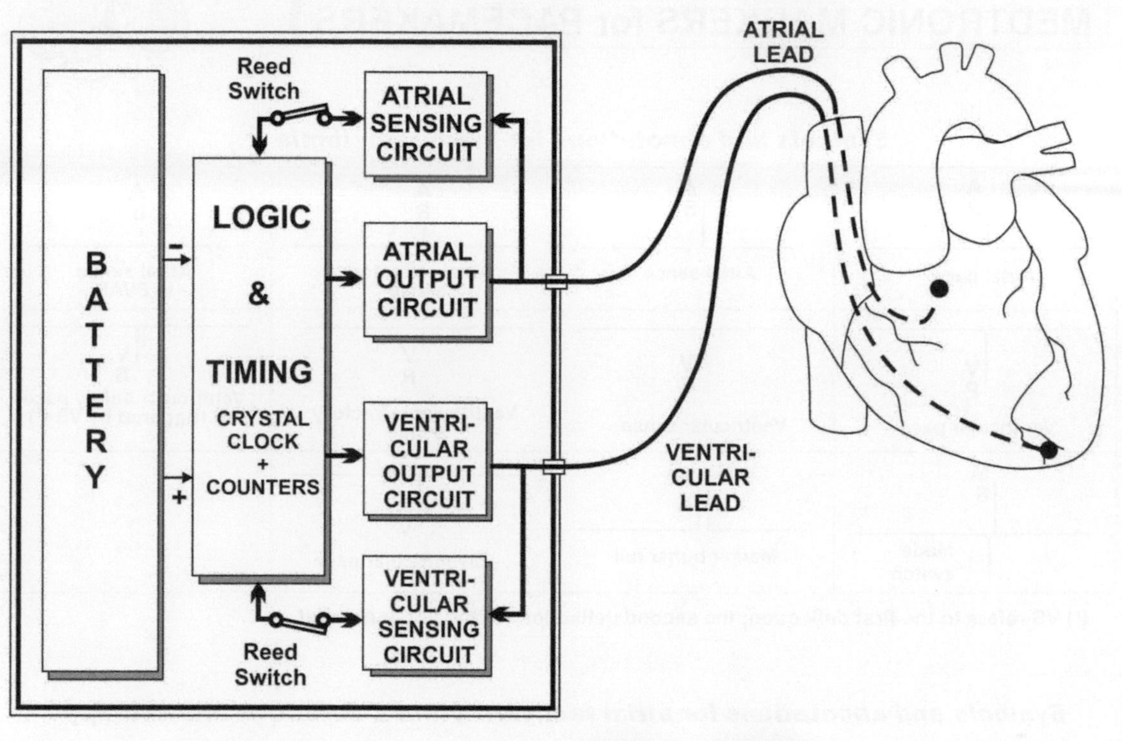

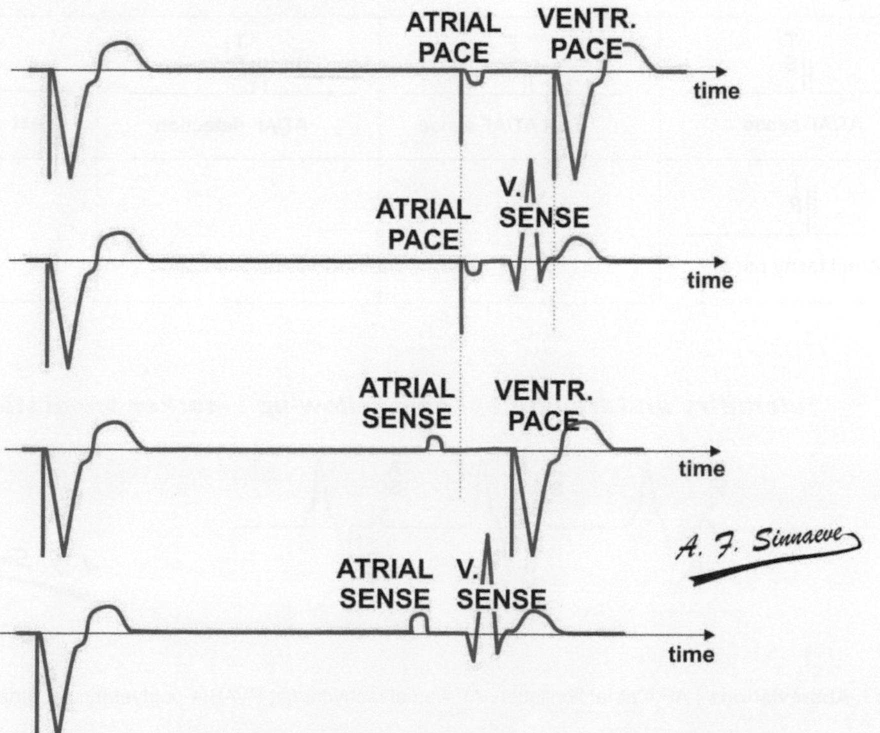

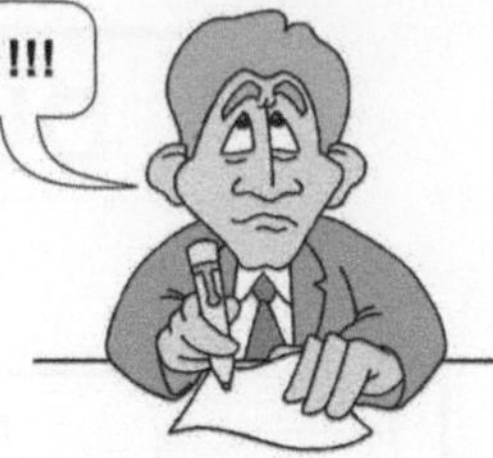

MEDTRONIC MARKERS for PACEMAKERS

Symbols and annotations for bradyarrhythmia

AP — Atrial pace	AS — Atrial sense	AR — Atrial refractory sense	Ab — Atrial sense in PVAB
VP — Ventricular pace	VS — Ventricular sense	VR — Ventricular refractory sense	VS — Ventricular safety pace VP triggered by VS (*)
MS — Mode switch	ER — Marker buffer full	BV — Biventricular pace	

(*) VS refers to the first deflection; the second deflection (VP) is not annotated

Symbols and annotations for atrial tachyarrhythmia detection and therapy

TS — AT/AF sense	FS — Fast AT/AF sense	TD — AT/AF detection	FD — Fast AT/AF detection
TP — Atrial tachy pace			

Telemetry and transtelephonic follow-up : marker annotations

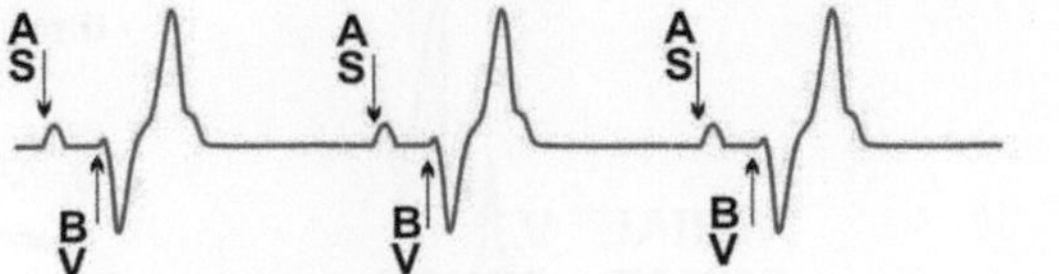

A. F. Sinnaeve

Abbreviations : AF = atrial fibrillation; AT = atrial tachycardia; PVAB = postventricular atrial blanking;

BOSTON SCIENTIFIC MARKER CHANNEL for PACEMAKERS

The markers in bold red are included in the subset available when real-time EGMs are selected.

Marker Description	Annotations	
	Printed	Screen
PVARP extension end	PVP->	–
Atrial tachy fallback end	ATR-End	–
PMT detection and PVARP extension	PMT-B	–
Atrial tachycardia sense-count up	ATR↑	AS
Atrial tachycardia sense-count down	ATR↓	AS
Atrial tachy response - duration started	ATR-Dur	–
Atrial tachy response - fallback started	ATR-FB	–
A. Sense after refractory and AFR window	**AS**	AS
A. Sense-rate hysteresis active	AS-Hy	AS
A. Sense during PVARP	**(AS)**	–
A. Sense in atrial flutter response (AFR window)	AS-Fl	AS
A. Pace - rate hysteresis active	AP-Hy	AP
A. Pace - lower rate	**AP**	AP
A. Pace - rate smoothing down	AP↓	AP
A. Pace - rate smoothing up	AP↑	AP
A. Pace - trigger mode	AP-Tr	AP
A. Pace at sensor rate	AP-Sr	AP
A. Pace inserted after flutter protection (AFR)	AP→	AP
A. Pace - noise (asynchronous pacing)	AP-Ns	AP
A. Pace - fallback (in ATR)	AP-FB	AP
A. Pace - atrial pacing preference	AP-PP	AP
A. Pace - sudden brady response	AP-SBR	AP

Marker Description	Annotations	
	Printed	Screen
Ventricular sense afer refractory	**VS**	VS
V. Sense - AV hysteresis active	VS-Hy	VS
V. Sense - rate hysteresis active	VS-Hy	VS
PVC after refractory	PVC	VS
V. Sense during refractory	**(VS)**	–
V. Pace at hysteresis rate	VP-Hy	VP
V. Pace at lower rate	**VP↓**	VP
V. Pace - down rate smoothing	VP↑	VP
V. Pace - up rate smoothing	VP	VP
V. Pace - trigger mode	VP-Tr	VP
V. Pace - in atrial tachy response	VP-FB	VP
V. Pace - at sensor rate	VP-Sr	VP
V. Pace - atrial tracked	**VP**	VP
V. Pace - atrial tracked, MTR	VP-MT	VP
V. Pace - sense amp noise	VP-Ns	VP
V. Pace - ventricular rate regulation	VP-VR	VP
V. Pace - sudden brady response	VP-SBR	VP
V. Pace after A-pace during atrial pacing preference	VP-PP	VP

TN : noise indication, telemetry noise
#.# V : amplitude in V during voltage threshold test
#.## ms : pulse width in ms during threshold test

A. F. Sinnaeve

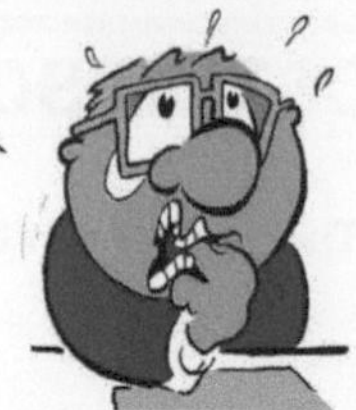
All manufacturers say their system is very logical and self-explanatory. But they are all different and I cannot afford any mistakes when I am using different systems. So I have to study them very carefully !

St JUDE MEDICAL MARKERS for PMs

Brady Basic Event Markers

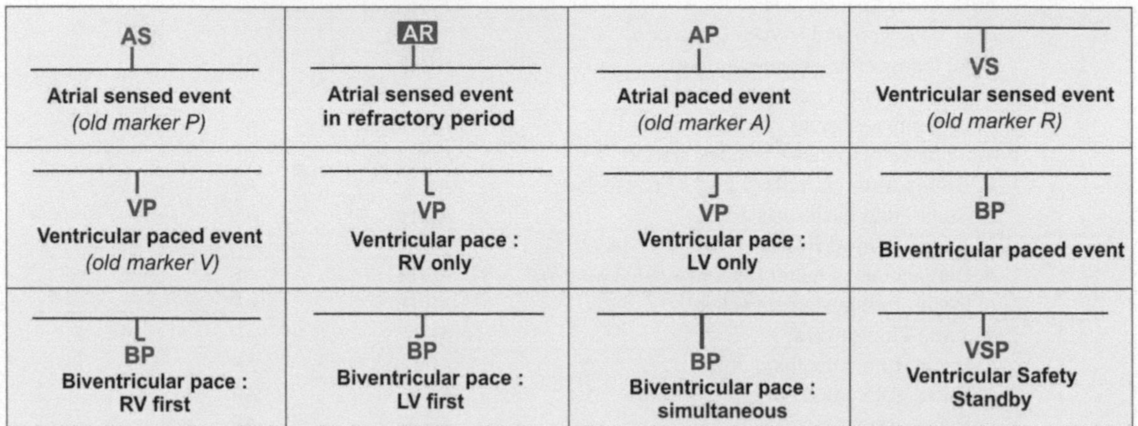

Bradyarrhythmia : special events markers

AMS .... Automatic mode switching (ongoing)
->AMS......... AMS entry
AFx .... AF suppression algorithm operation
SIR .... Activity sensor-indicated rate
HYS .... Rate hysteresis started by search timer or sensed event
Neg-HYS..... Negative AV-hysteresis search started
VIP............... VIP search started
(VIP = Ventricular Intrinsic Preference : an algorithm which allows the pacemaker to search for intrinsic conduction).
LOC............. Loss of capture
PVC............. PVC detection

Episode trigger event markers

If an event triggers EGM storage, a vertical bar with a 'Trigger' flag appears at the trigger point

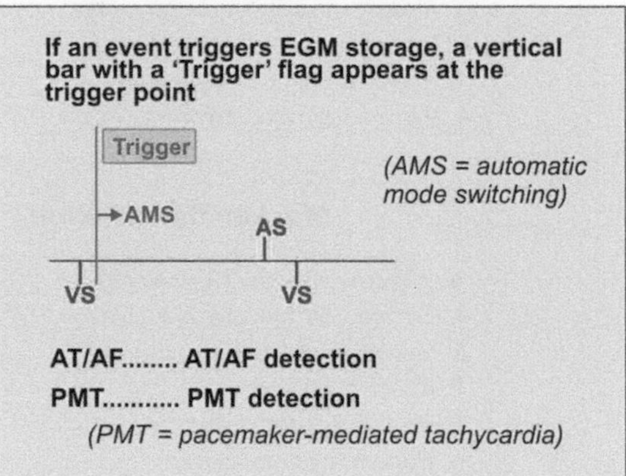

AT/AF........ AT/AF detection
PMT........... PMT detection
(PMT = pacemaker-mediated tachycardia)

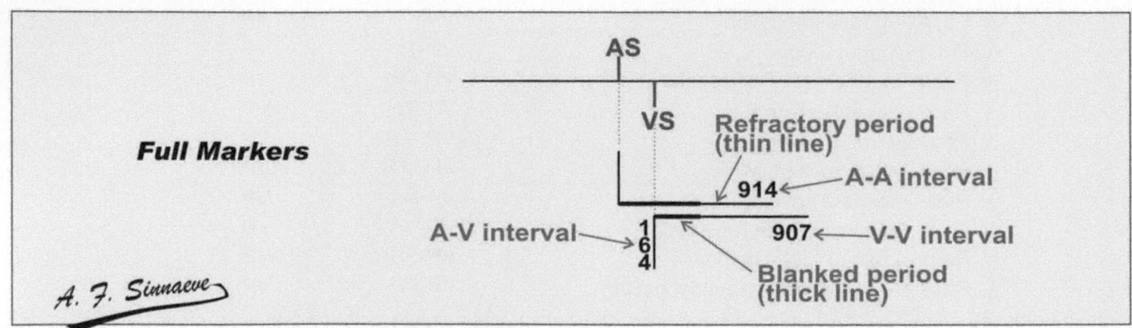

Full Markers

A. F. Sinnaeve

Abbreviations : AF = atrial fibrillation; AT = atrial tachycardia; AMS = auto mode switching; PMT = pacemaker mediated tachycardia;

THE 4 FUNDAMENTAL TIMING CYCLES OF A DDD PACEMAKER

PART 1 : THE VENTRICULAR CHANNEL

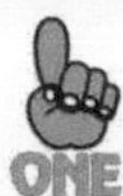

FUNDAMENTAL TIMING CYCLE 1
LRI = LOWER RATE INTERVAL

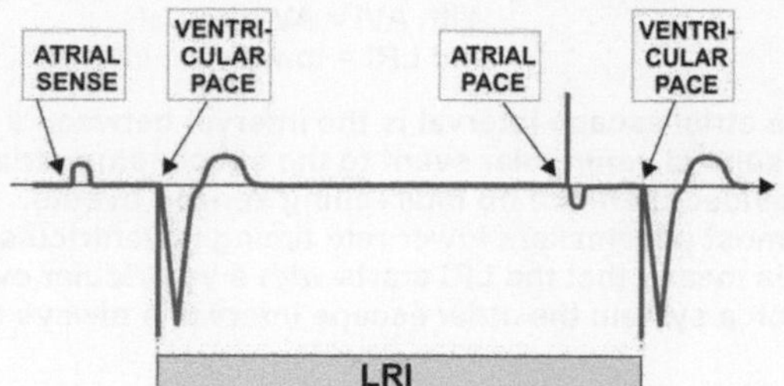

Longest interval between a paced or sensed ventricular event and the succeeding ventricular paced event without intervening sensed events

FUNDAMENTAL TIMING CYCLE 2
VRP = VENTRICULAR REFRACTORY PERIOD

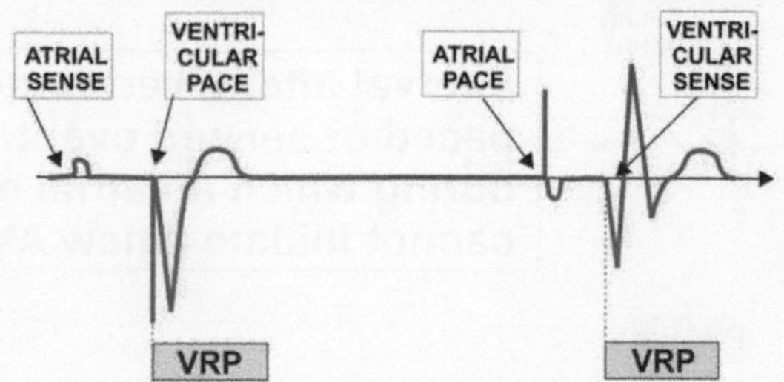

Interval initiated by a ventricular event during which a new lower rate interval (LRI) cannot be initiated

A. F. Sinnaeve

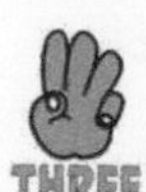

FUNDAMENTAL TIMING CYCLE 3
AVI = ATRIOVENTRICULAR INTERVAL

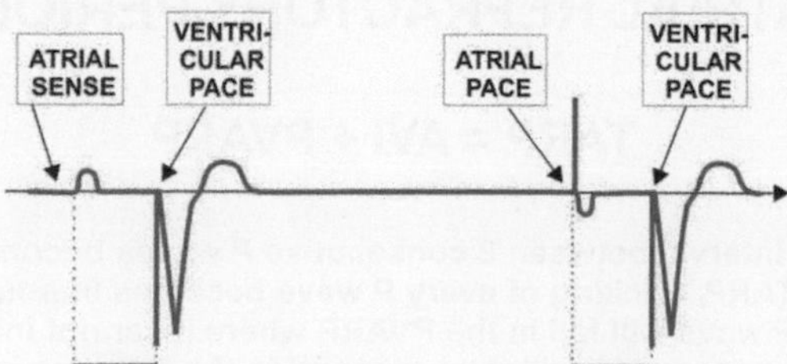

Interval between an atrial event and the sheduled delivery of a ventricular stimulus

sAVI = after a sensed atrial event
pAVI = after a paced atrial event

* the electronic analog of the P-R interval
* the atrial channel is refractory during the AV interval (a new AV delay cannot be initiated when one is already in progress)

THE 4 FUNDAMENTAL TIMING CYCLES OF A DDD PACEMAKER

PART 2 : THE ATRIAL CHANNEL

DERIVED : AEI = ATRIAL ESCAPE INTERVAL

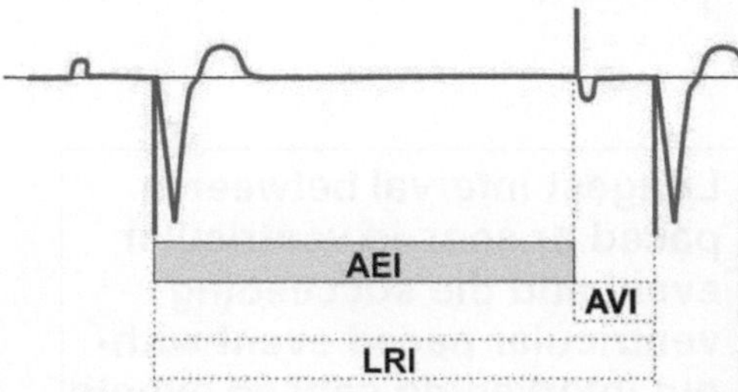

AEI = LRI - AVI

With AVI = AV interval and LRI = lower rate interval

The atrial escape interval is the interval between a paced or sensed ventricular event to the succeeding atrial stimulus provided there are no intervening sensed events. In most pacemakers lower rate timing is ventricular-based. This means that the LRI starts with a ventricular event. In such a system the atrial escape interval is always constant.

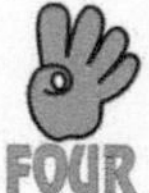

FUNDAMENTAL TIMING CYCLE 4
PVARP = POSTVENTRICULAR REFRACTORY PERIOD

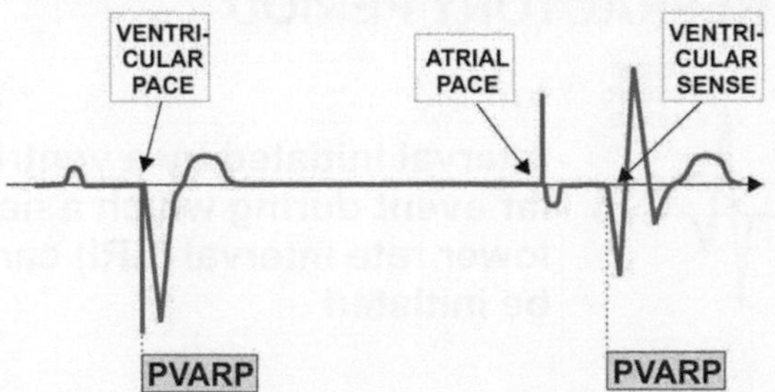

Interval after a ventricular paced or sensed event during which an atrial event cannot initiate a new AVI

*** avoids inappropriate atrial sensing of ventricular events**
*** eliminates sensing of retrograde P waves from ventriculoatrial conduction**

DERIVED : TARP = TOTAL ATRIAL REFRACTORY PERIOD

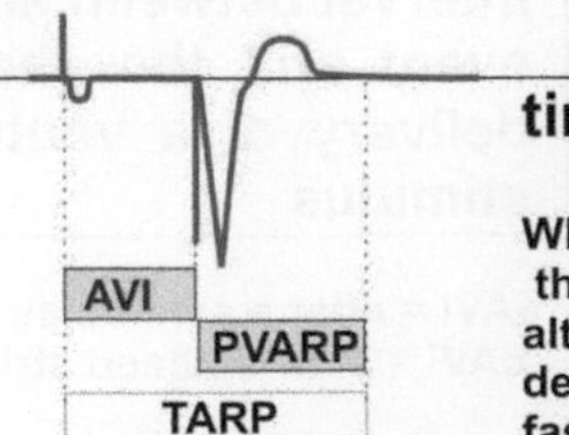

TARP = AVI + PVARP

When the interval between 2 consecutive P waves becomes shorter than the TARP, tracking of every P wave becomes impossible. Every alternate P wave will fall in the PVARP where it cannot initiate an AV delay. The pacemaker will thus respond to the P waves in a 2 : 1 fashion. This form of upper rate response is called 2 : 1 block and the TARP effectively becomes the upper rate interval.

A. F. Sinnaeve

All examples of pacemaker timing in this book involve ventricular-based lower rate timing, unless otherwise specified.

FUNCTIONS OF THE POSTVENTRICULAR ATRIAL REFRACTORY PERIOD (PVARP)

PVARP Interval after a ventricular paced or sensed event during which the atrial channel is refractory !!!

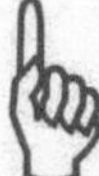

1. Avoids the inappropriate atrial sensing of ventricular events (ventricular stimuli, QRS complexes, aberrant T waves)

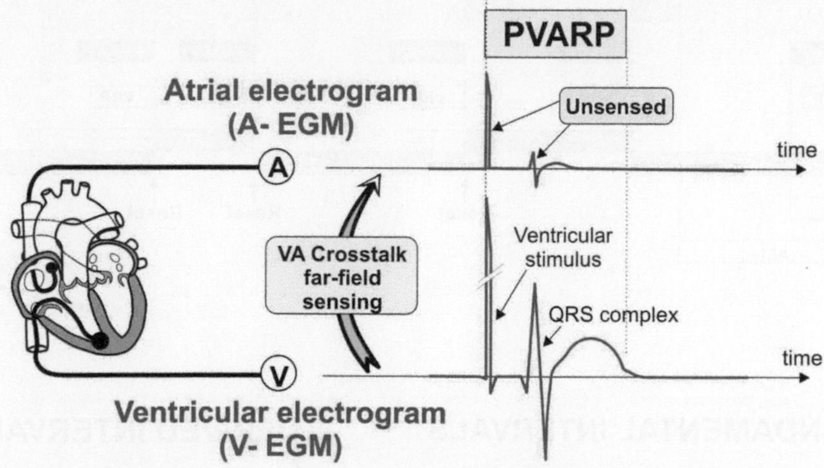

2. Avoids sensing of retrogradely conducted P waves

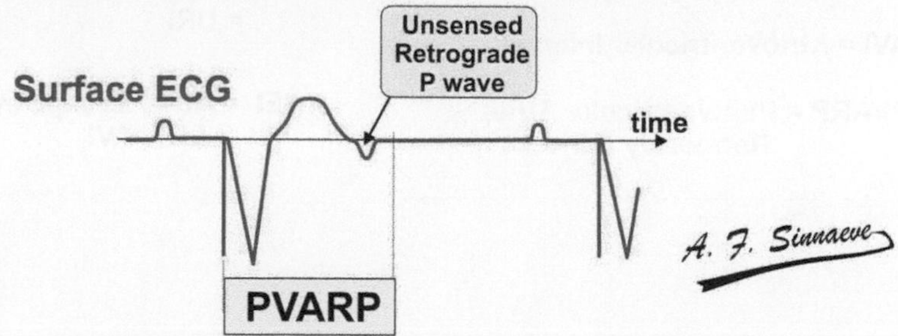

A. F. Sinnaeve

DDD PACEMAKER WITH 4 TIMING CYCLES AT WORK

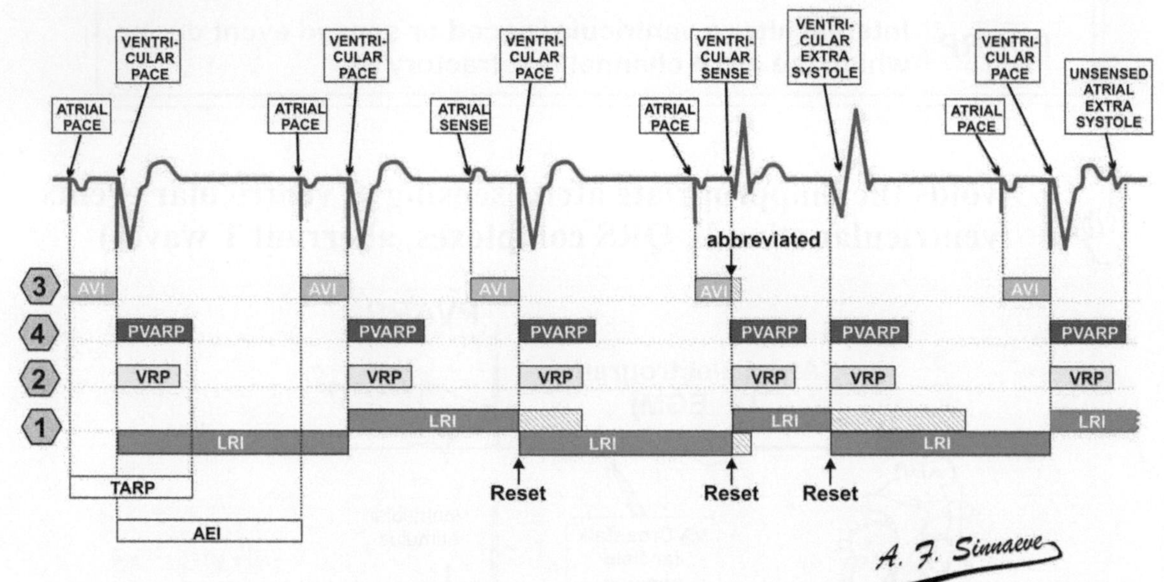

FUNDAMENTAL INTERVALS

1. LRI = Lower Rate Interval
2. VRP = Ventricular Refractory Period
3. AVI = Atrioventricular Interval
4. PVARP = Postventricular Atrial Refractory Period

DERIVED INTERVALS

TARP = Total Atrial Refractory Period
= AVI + PVARP
= Upper Rate Interval
= URI

AEI = Atrial Escape Interval
= LRI - AVI

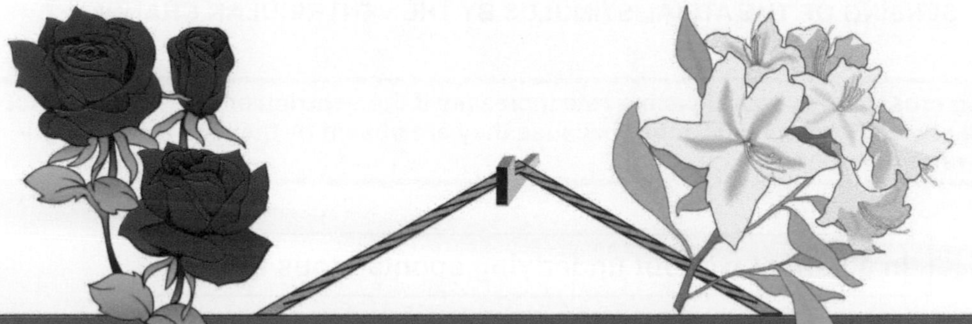

THREE-LETTER PACEMAKER CODE (ICHD)

POSITION	1st	2nd	3rd
CATEGORY	CHAMBER(S) PACED	CHAMBER(S) SENSED	MODE OF RESPONSE
LETTERS	V = VENTRICLE A = ATRIUM S = SINGLE D = DOUBLE (V & A)	V = VENTRICLE A = ATRIUM S = SINGLE O = NONE D = DOUBLE (V & A)	T = TRIGGERED I = INHIBITED O = NONE D = DOUBLE inhibited & triggered

EXAMPLE :

DDD = a pacemaker pacing and sensing in both the atrium and the ventricle; pacing is inhibited in the atrial channel by sensed ventricular or atrial activity and is inhibited in the ventricular channel by ventricular activity but triggered by sensing atrial activity.

A. F. Sinnaeve

MANIFESTATIONS of AV CROSSTALK

SENSING OF THE ATRIAL STIMULUS BY THE VENTRICULAR CHANNEL

During crosstalk, the atrial pacing rate increases if the ventricular channel does not sense any QRS complexes either because they are absent or they fall in the ventricular refractory period

In a patient without underlying spontaneous rhythm

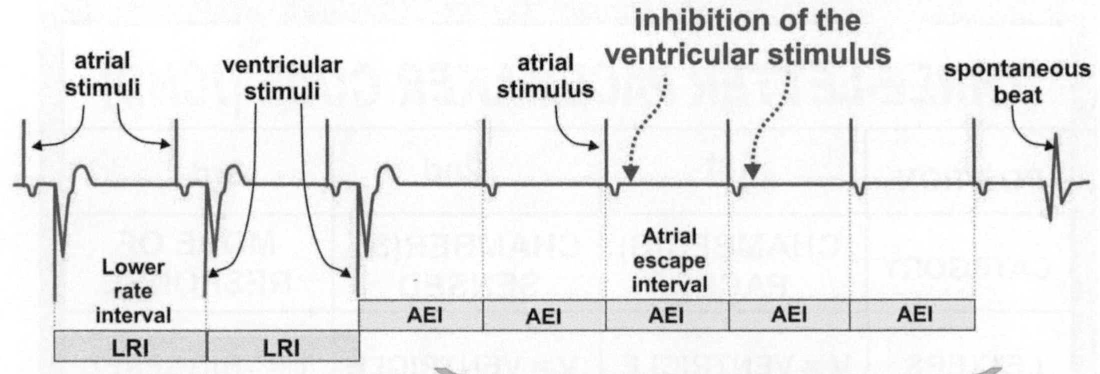

In a patient with first-degree AV block

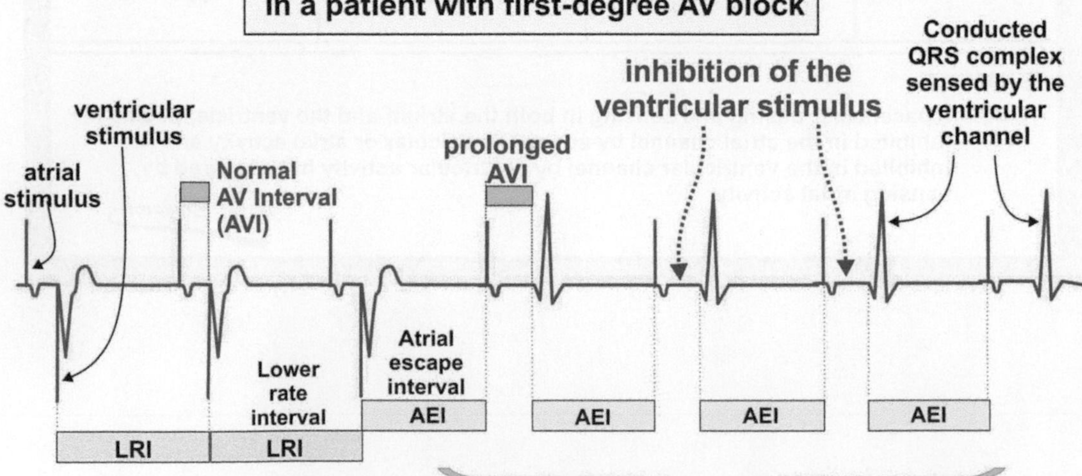

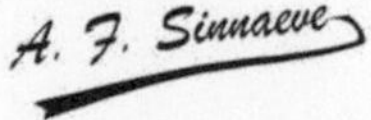

ADDITION OF A FIFTH TIMING CYCLE TO A SIMPLE DDD PACEMAKER TO PREVENT AV CROSSTALK

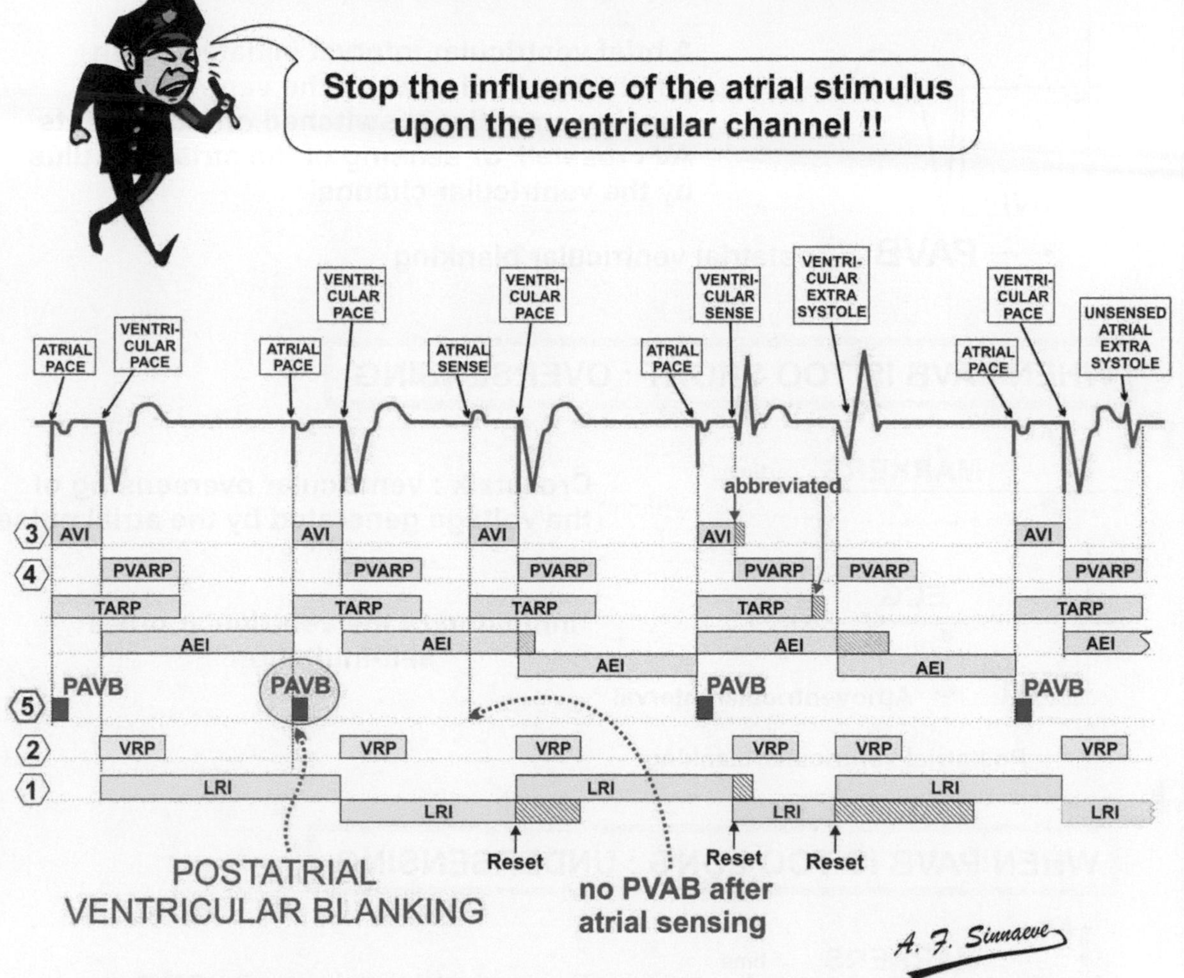

PAVB = a brief interval (10 to 60 ms) initiated by an atrial output pulse when the ventricular channel is switched off and cannot sense.
PVAB is often programmable

Abbreviations : AEI = atrial escape interval ; AVI = atrioventricular interval ; LRI = lower rate interval ; PAVB = postatrial ventricular blanking ; PVARP = postventricular atrial refractory period ; TARP = total atrial refractory period ; VRP = ventricular refractory period ;

THE POSTATRIAL VENTRICULAR BLANKING PERIOD

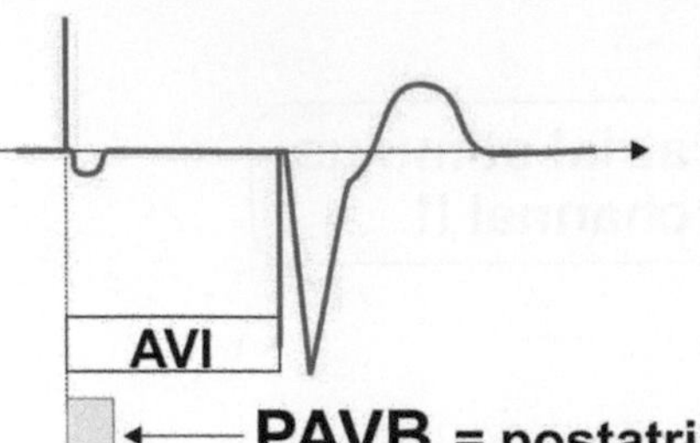

A brief ventricular interval initiated by an atrial output pulse when the ventricular sensing amplifier is switched off. It prevents AV crosstalk or sensing of the atrial stimulus by the ventricular channel

PAVB = postatrial ventricular blanking

WHEN PAVB IS TOO SHORT : OVERSENSING

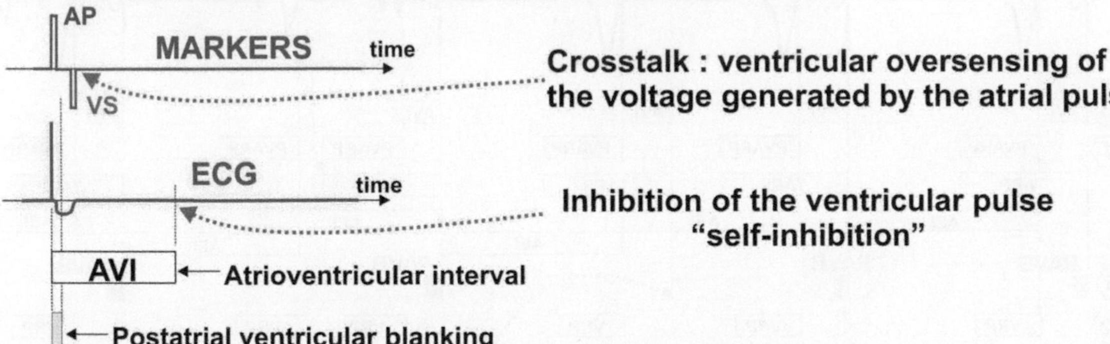

WHEN PAVB IS TOO LONG : UNDERSENSING

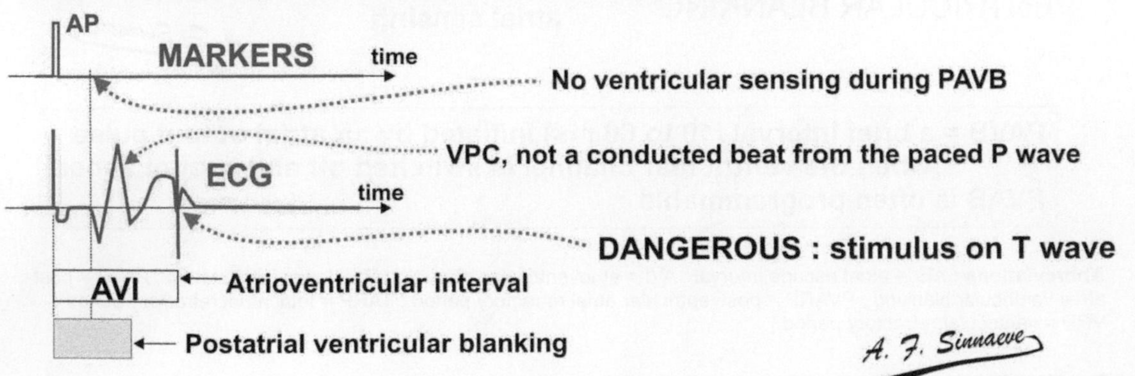

A. F. Sinnaeve

Abbreviations : AVI = atrioventricular interval ; AP = atrial pace ; VS = ventricular sense ;

THE ADDITION OF THE 6th CYCLE : VSP or VENTRICULAR SAFETY PACING

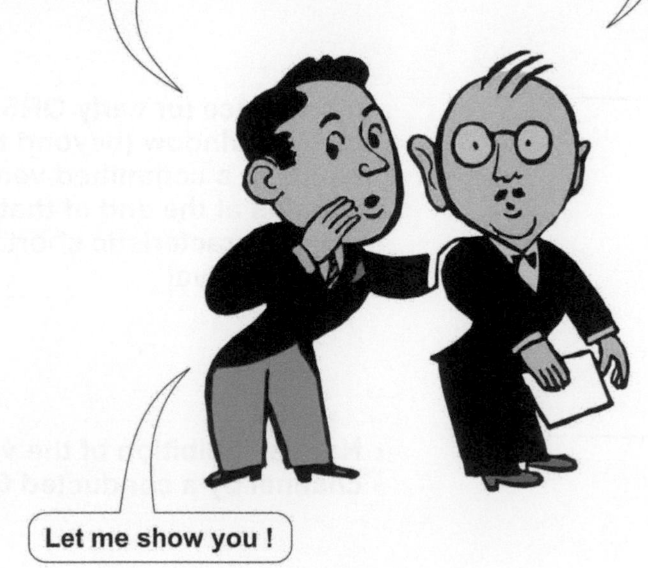
The postatrial ventricular blanking period does not always prevent crosstalk !?
If this happens, the consequences of crosstalk can be prevented by adding a 6th timing cycle often called the VSP period in the first part of the AV delay. A signal sensed in the VSP will trigger a premature stimulus at the end of the VSP. In this way ventricular inhibition by crosstalk cannot occur....
Let me show you !

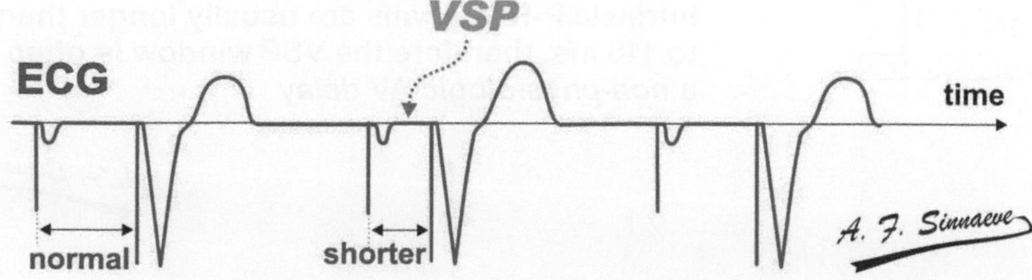

VSP does not prevent crosstalk.
It simply prevents its consequences !

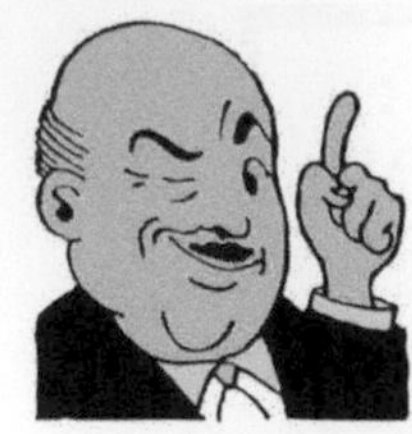

VENTRICULAR SAFETY PACING

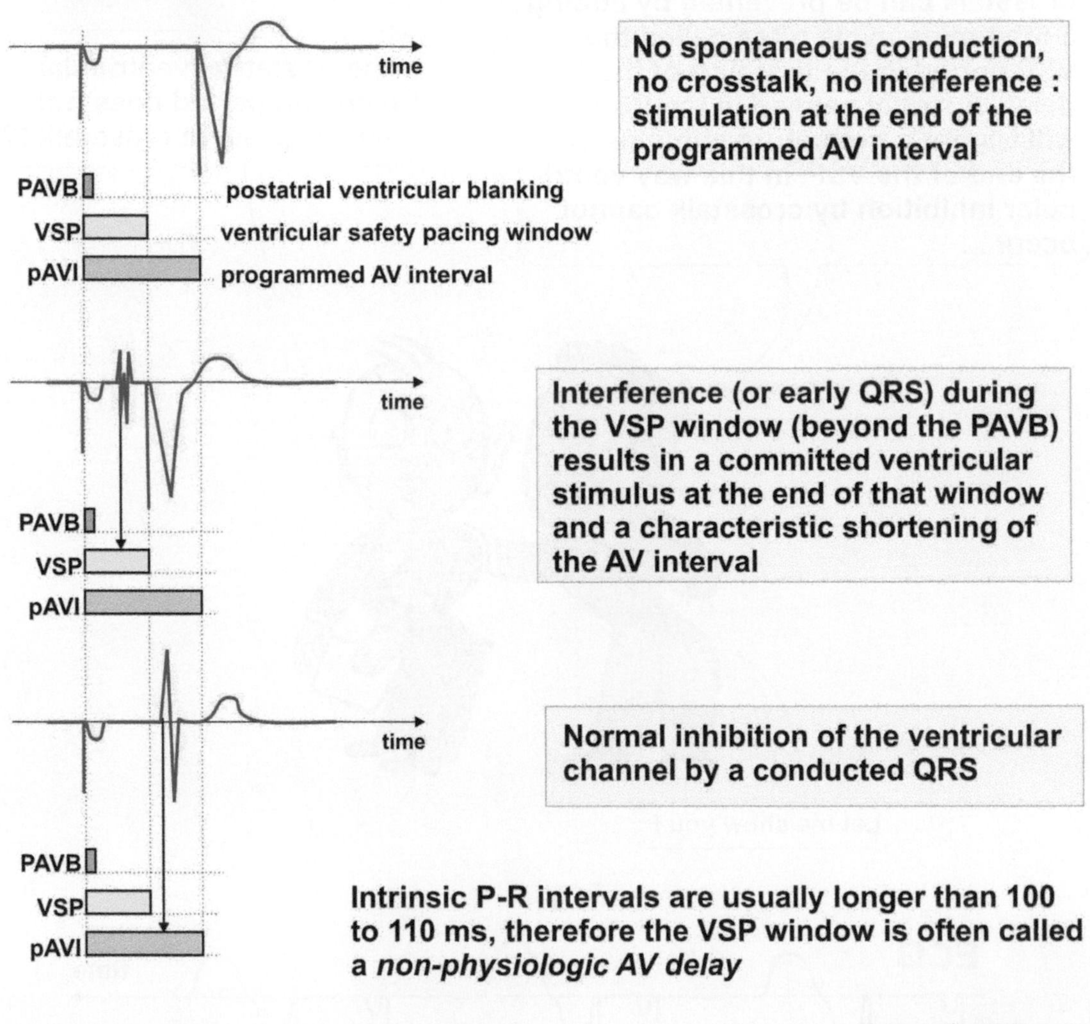

No spontaneous conduction, no crosstalk, no interference : stimulation at the end of the programmed AV interval

Interference (or early QRS) during the VSP window (beyond the PAVB) results in a committed ventricular stimulus at the end of that window and a characteristic shortening of the AV interval

Normal inhibition of the ventricular channel by a conducted QRS

Intrinsic P-R intervals are usually longer than 100 to 110 ms, therefore the VSP window is often called a *non-physiologic AV delay*

A. F. Sinnaeve

ADDITION OF A SIXTH TIMING CYCLE TO A SIMPLE DDD PACEMAKER TO PREVENT THE CONSEQUENCES AV CROSSTALK

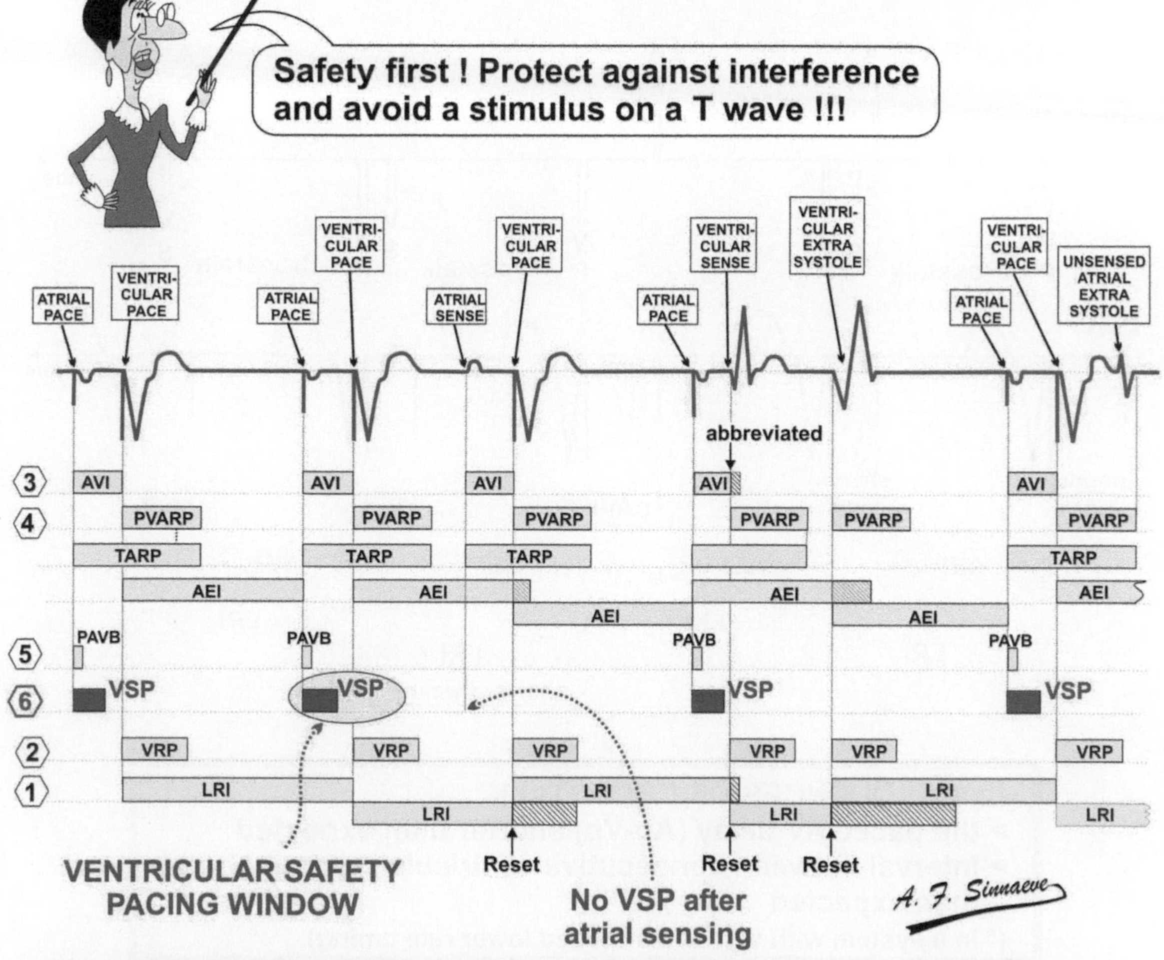

Ventricular Safety Pacing Window : by convention the VSP starts at the time of the atrial stimulus and its duration is usually 100 to 110 ms. The PAVB period, also activated by the atrial stimulus, occupies the initial portion of the VSP. Ventricular sensing cannot occur during this blanking period. Therefore ventricular sensing can occur in the VSP only after completion of the relatively short PAVB period.

ABBREVIATIONS : AVI = AV interval; PVARP = postventricular atrial refractory period; TARP = total atrial refractory period; AEI = atrial escape interval; PAVB = postatrial ventricular blanking; VSP = ventricular safety pacing window; VRP = ventricular refractory period; LRI = lower rate interval

ECG PATTERNS of VENTRICULAR SAFETY PACING

Intermittent crosstalk during DDD pacing

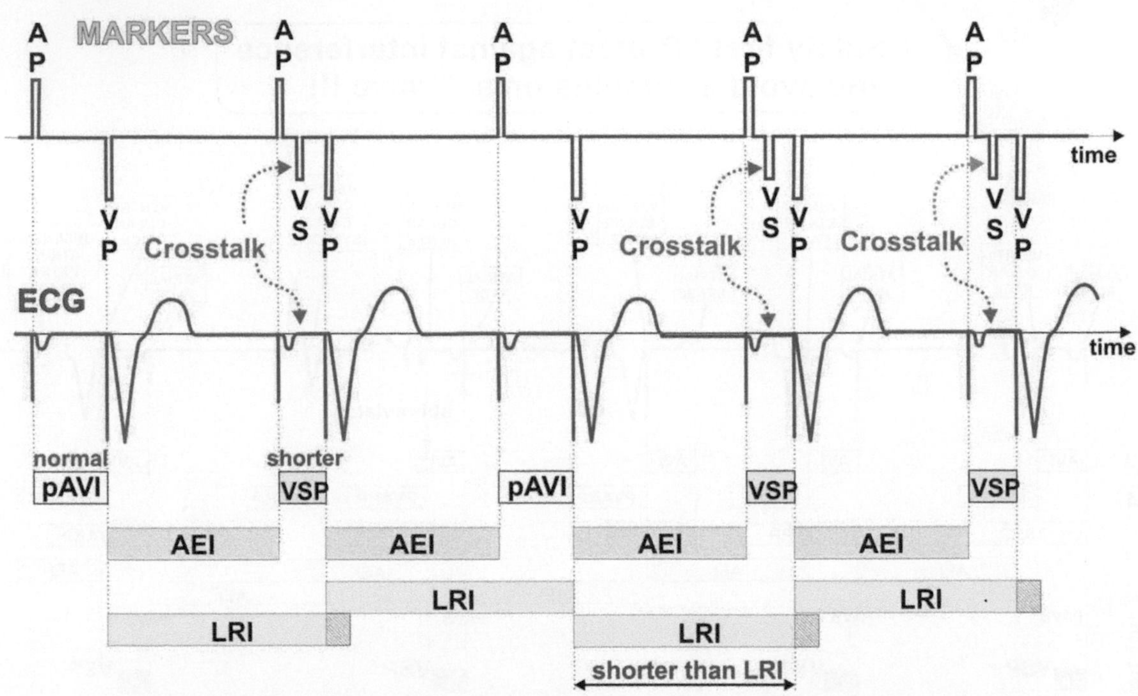

CONSEQUENCES OF CROSSTALK* :

> the paced AV delay (Ap-Vp) shorter than expected

> interval between consecutive ventricular stimuli shorter than expected

(* In a system with ventricular-based lower rate timing)

ABBREVIATIONS : Ap = atrial paced event; Vp = ventricular paced event; Vs = ventricular sensed event; pAVI = paced atrioventricular interval; VSP = ventricular safety pacing window; AEI = atrial escape interval; LRI = lower rate interval

A. F. Sinnaeve

MANIFESTATIONS of VENTRICULAR SAFETY PACING with VENTRICULAR PREMATURE COMPLEXES

UNSENSED QRS COMPLEX

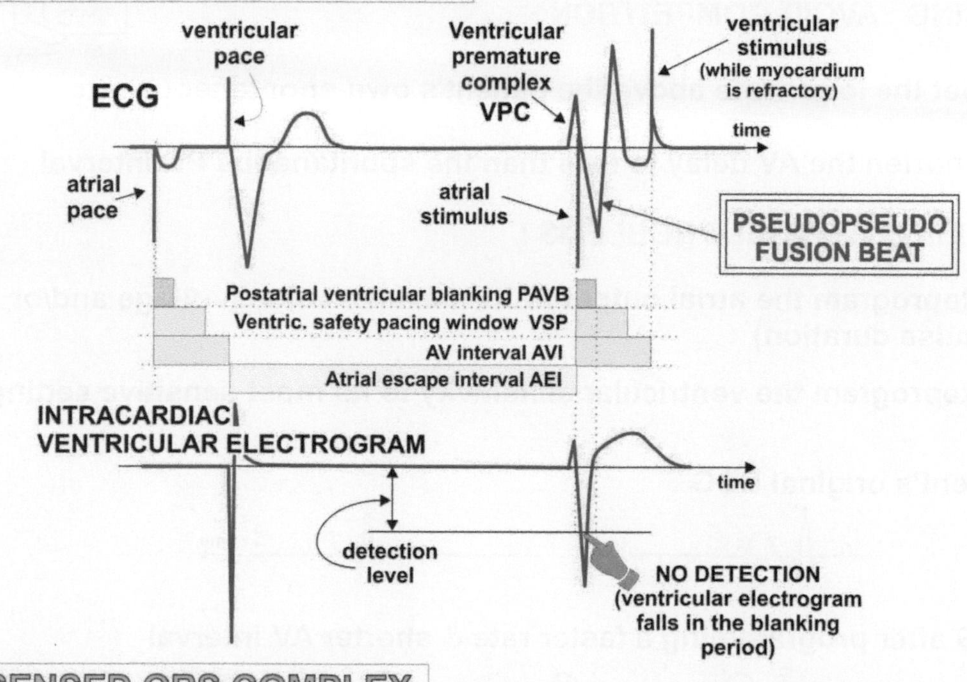

SENSED QRS COMPLEX

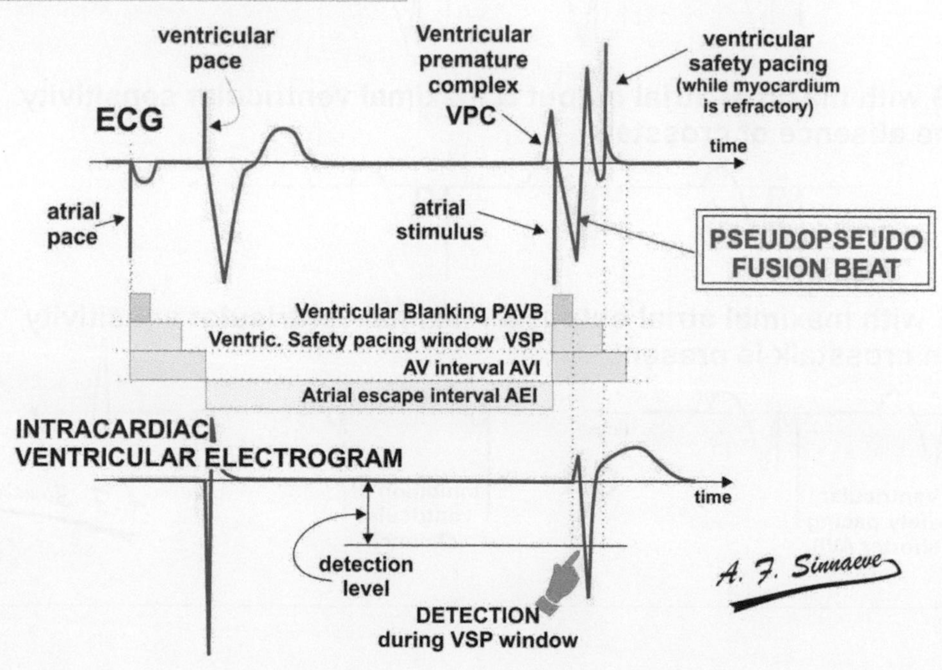

TESTING FOR AV CROSSTALK

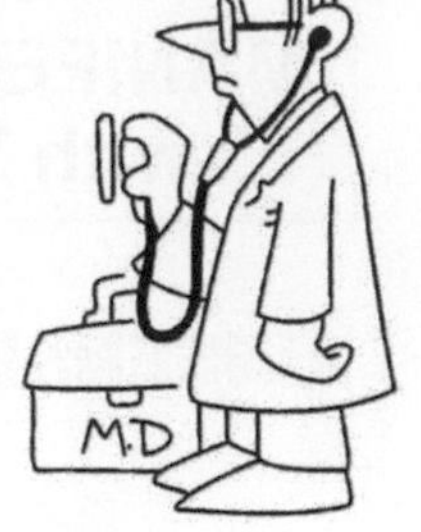

ESTABLISH CONTINUAL ATRIAL AND VENTRICULAR PACING : AVOID COMPETITION

♣ **Set the lower rate above the patient's own spontaneous rate**

♠ **Shorten the AV delay to less than the spontaneous PR interval**

UNVEIL POTENTIAL PROBLEMS :

♦ **Reprogram the atrial output to its maximal value (voltage and/or pulse duration)**

♥ **Reprogram the ventricular sensitivity to its most sensitive setting**

Patient's original ECG

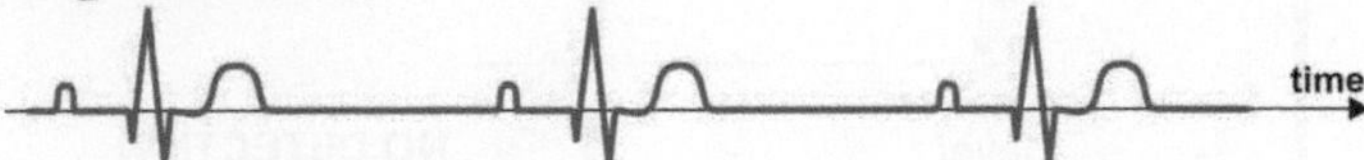

ECG after programming a faster rate & shorter AV interval

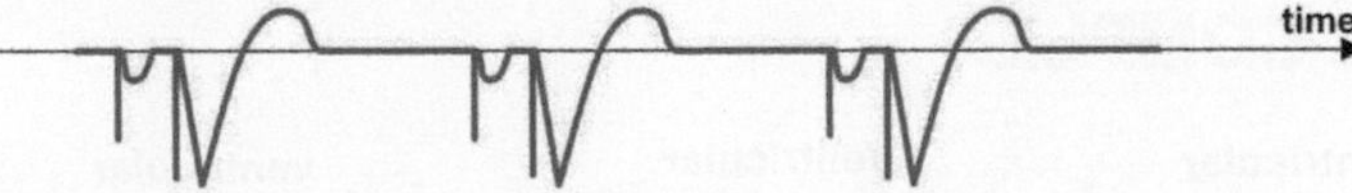

ECG with maximal atrial output & maximal ventricular sensitivity in the absence of crosstalk

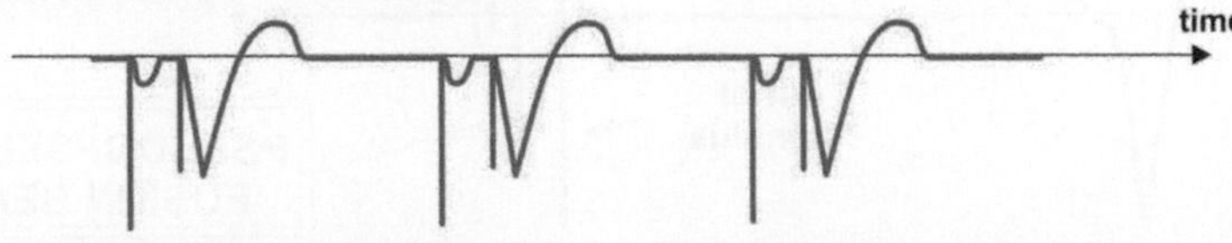

ECG with maximal atrial output & maximal ventricular sensitivity when crosstalk is present

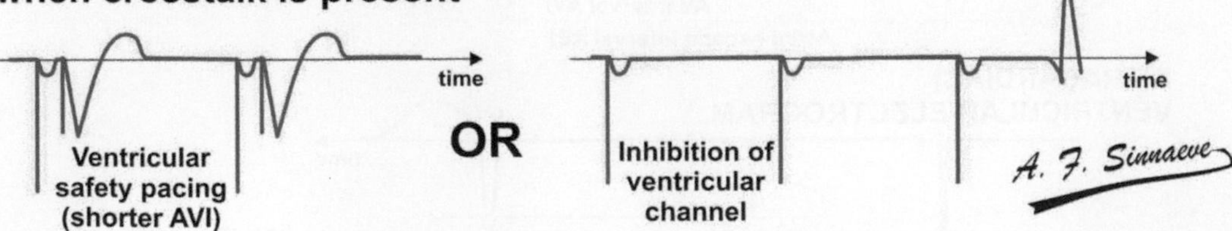

A. F. Sinnaeve

PREVENTION of AV CROSSTALK

(or SELF- INHIBITION)

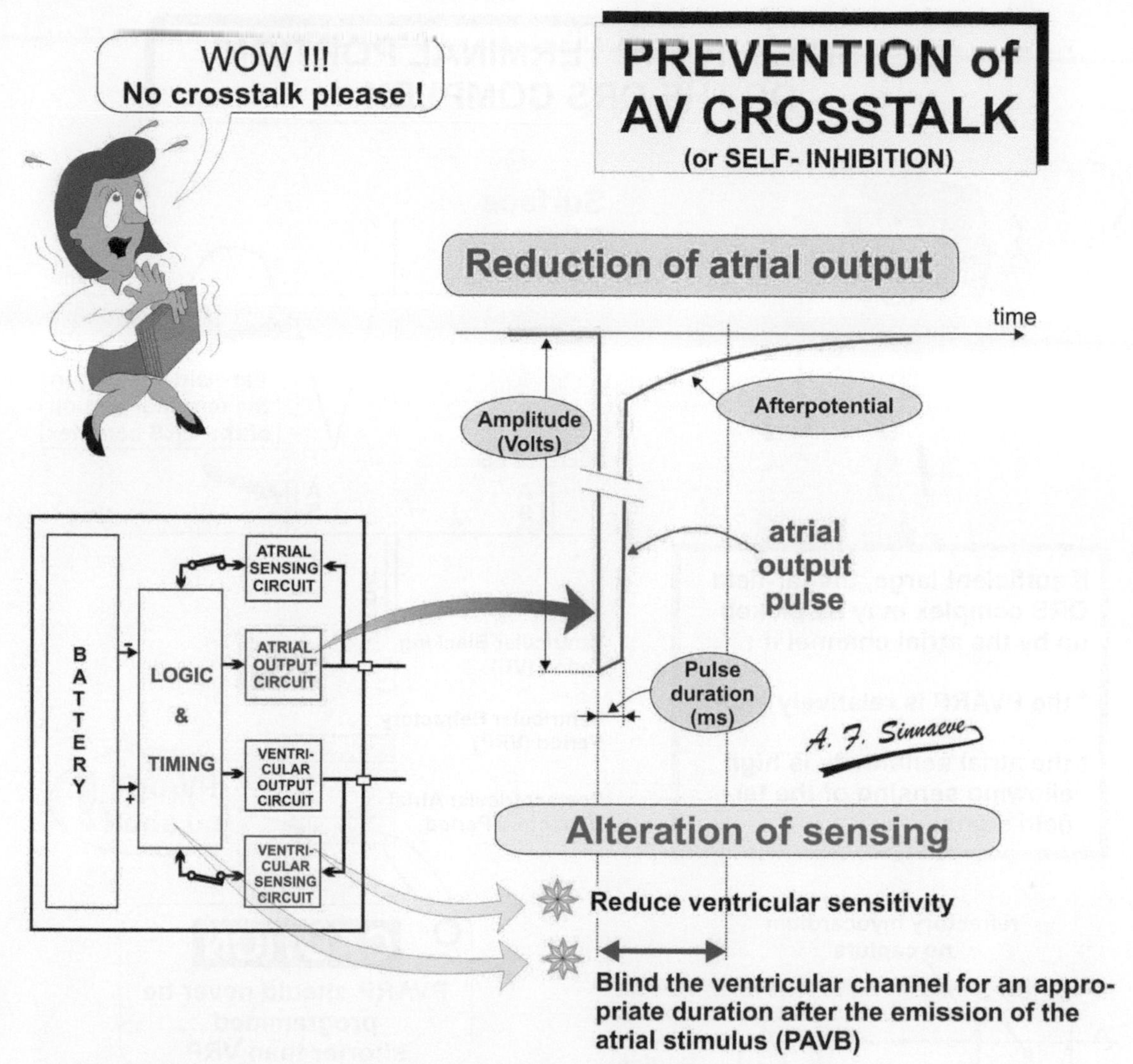

MANAGEMENT OF CROSSTALK

1. Crosstalk is best prevented by using bipolar dual-chamber devices.
2. If crosstalk is observed, decrease the atrial output (voltage and/or pulse duration).
3. Decrease the sensitivity of the ventricular channel (the numerical value - mV - of the sensitivity on the programmer will therefore increase).
4. Prolong the postatrial ventricular blanking period (PAVB). The PAVB lasts 10 to 60 ms and is programmable in most pacemakers !
5. Program ventricular safety pacing ON (if VSP is available).

SENSING OF THE TERMINAL PORTION OF THE QRS COMPLEX

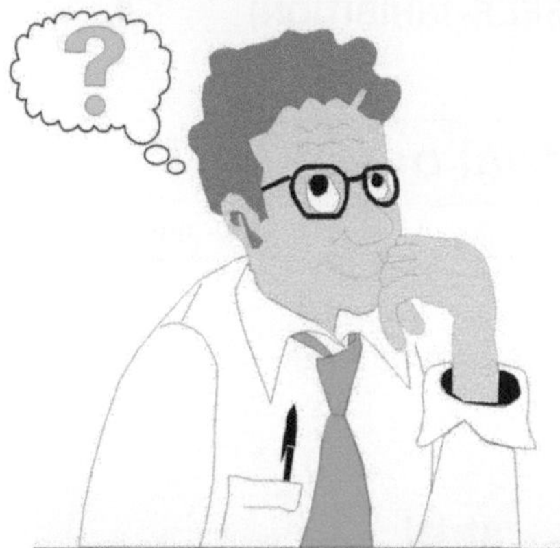

If sufficient large, the far-field QRS complex may be picked up by the atrial channel if :

* the PVARP is relatively short

* the atrial sensitivity is high allowing sensing of the far-field signal

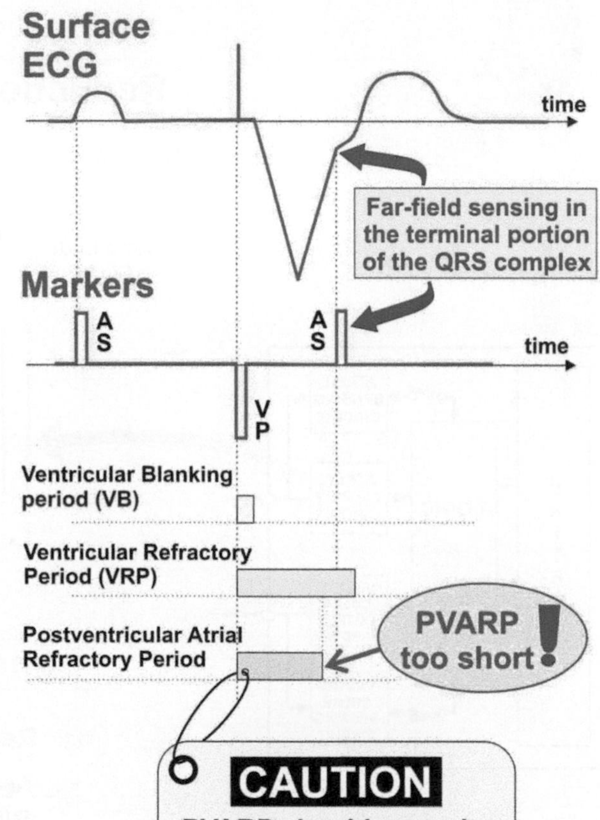

CAUTION

PVARP should never be programmed shorter than VRP

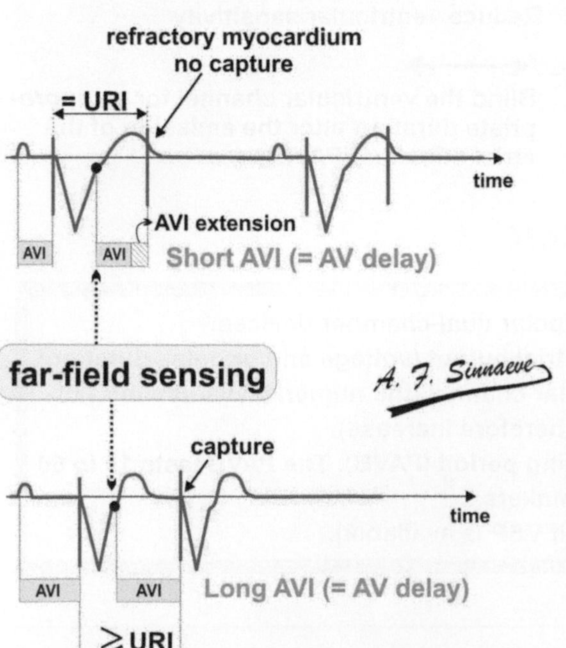

If the far-field QRS is sensed by the atrial channel, the pacemaker interprets it as a P wave, initiates an AV delay and triggers a ventricular stimulus at the completion of this AV delay (AVI). The ventricular stimulus may or may not capture the ventricle according to its timing relative to the ventricular myocardial refractory period.

Abbreviations : AS = atrial sense ; VP = ventricular pace ; URI = upper rate interval ; PVARP = postventricular atrial refractory period ; VRP = ventricular refractory period ; VB =ventricular blanking ; AVI = AV delay

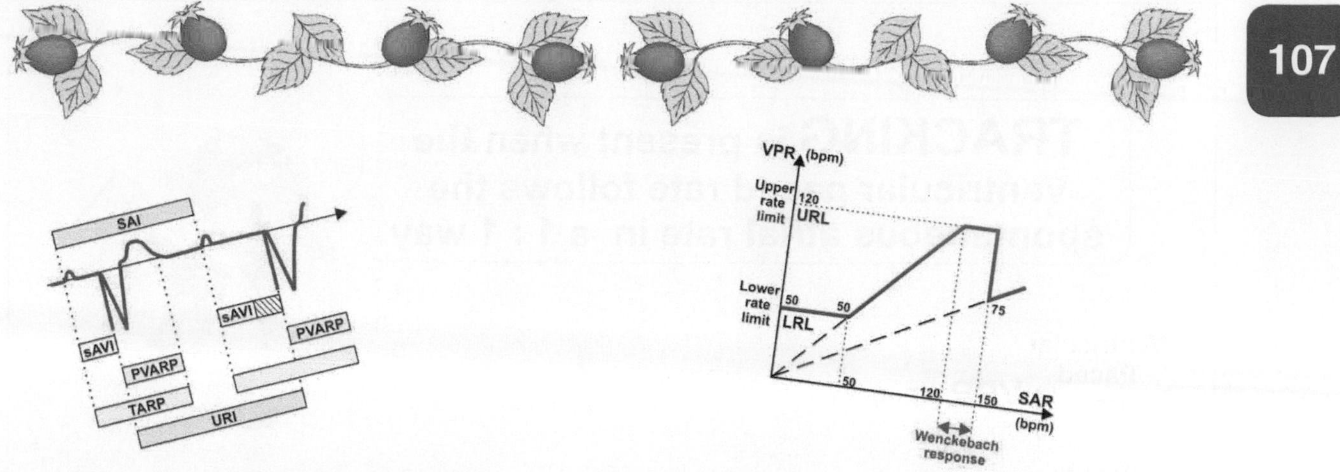

DDD PACEMAKERS - UPPER RATE RESPONSE

- Tracking
- Fixed-ratio block 2 : 1
- Fixed-ratio block - Stress test
- Addition of 7th timing cycle to obtain upper rate response with Wenckebach block
- Wenckebach upper rate limitation
- How to ensure Wenckebach block
- Wenckebach upper rate response - part 1
- Wenckebach upper rate response - part 2
- Management of upper rate
- Rate smoothing
- Atrial premature complexes (APCs)
- APCs - More difficult
- Premature ventricular events - Definitions
- Functional atrial undersensing
- Apparent lack of atrial tracking

A. F. Sinnaeve

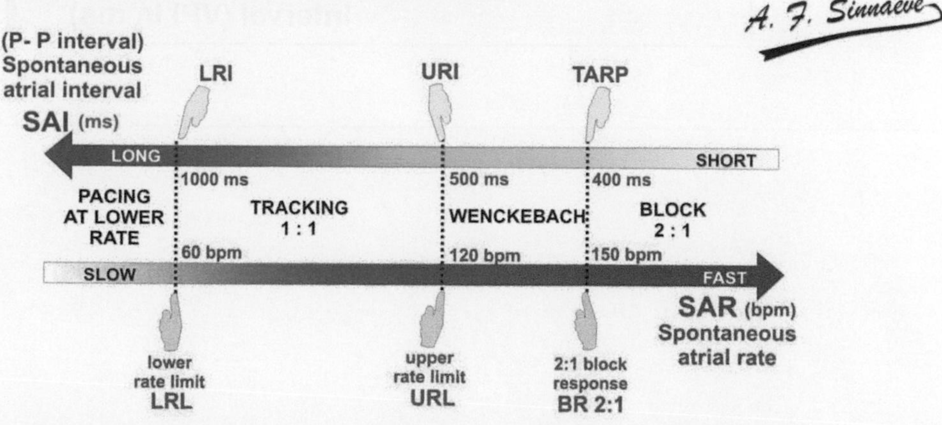

TRACKING is present when the ventricular paced rate follows the spontaneous atrial rate in a 1 : 1 way

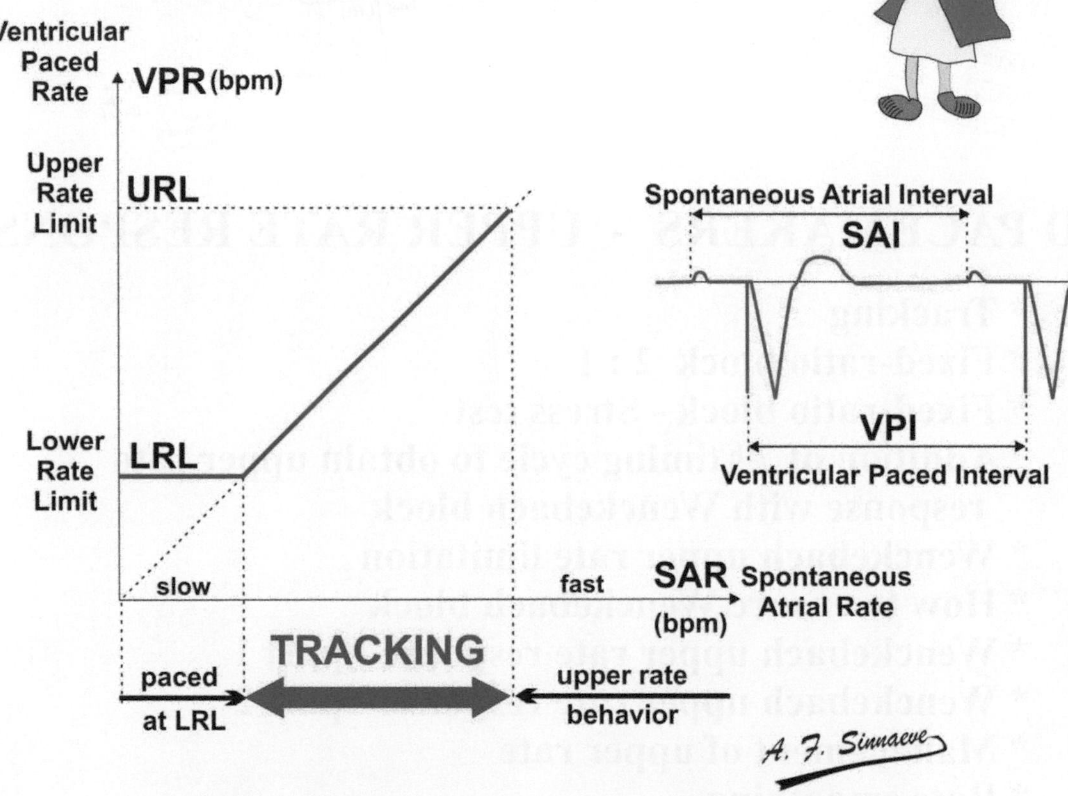

$$\text{Spontaneous Atrial Rate (SAR in bpm)} = \frac{60{,}000}{\text{Spontaneous Atrial Interval (SAI in ms)}}$$

$$\text{Ventricular paced Rate (VPR in bpm)} = \frac{60{,}000}{\text{Ventricular Paced Interval (VPI in ms)}}$$

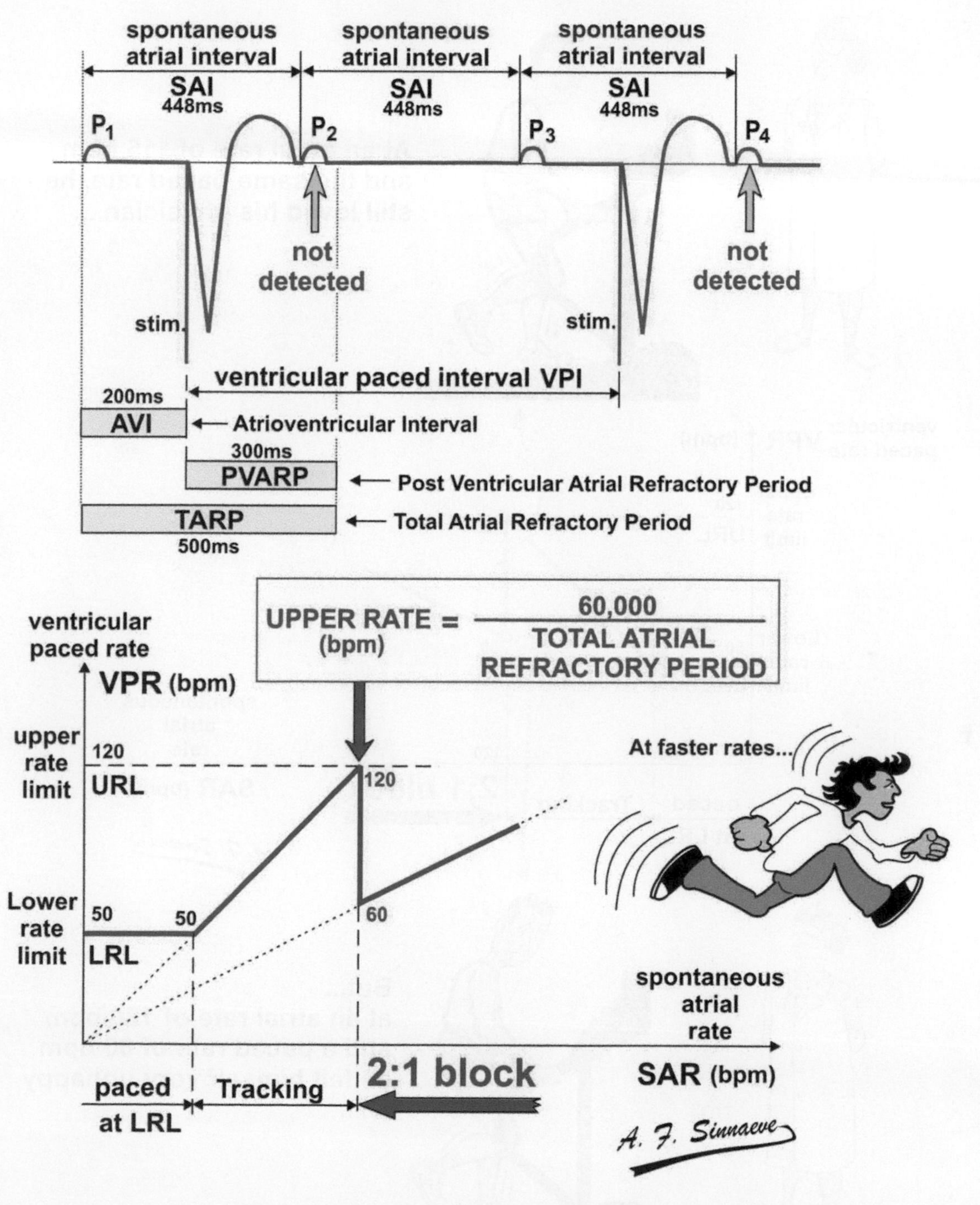
FIXED RATIO BLOCK 2 :1
spontaneous atrial interval
SAI
448ms
spontaneous atrial interval
SAI
448ms
spontaneous atrial interval
SAI
448ms
P1
P2
P3
P4
not detected
not detected
stim.
stim.
ventricular paced interval VPI
200ms
AVI
Atrioventricular Interval
300ms
PVARP
Post Ventricular Atrial Refractory Period
TARP
Total Atrial Refractory Period
500ms
UPPER RATE (bpm) = 60,000 / TOTAL ATRIAL REFRACTORY PERIOD
ventricular paced rate
VPR (bpm)
upper rate limit
120
URL
120
Lower rate limit
50
LRL
50
60
At faster rates...
spontaneous atrial rate
SAR (bpm)
paced at LRL
Tracking
2:1 block
A. F. Sinnaeve

THE TREADMILL STRESS TEST

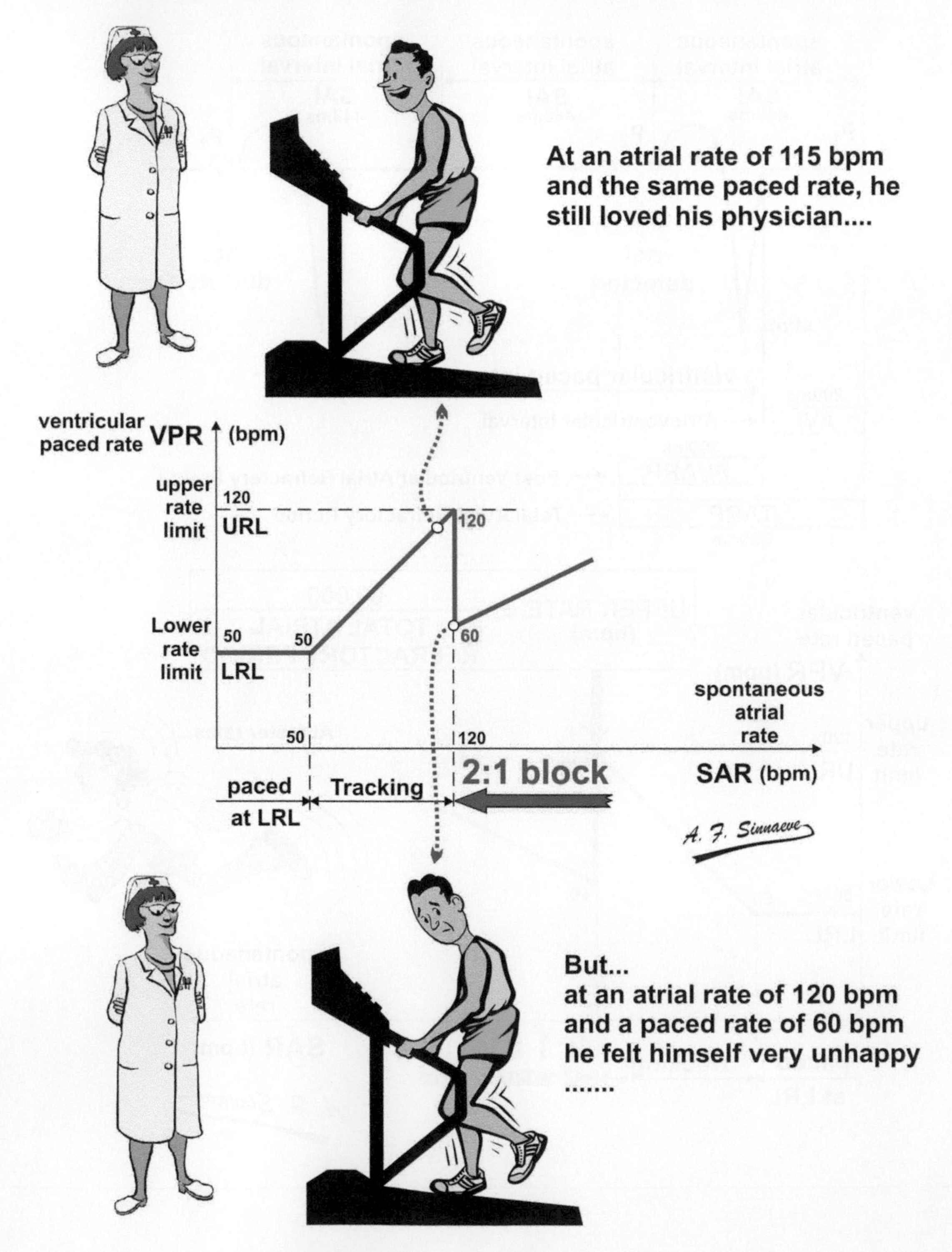

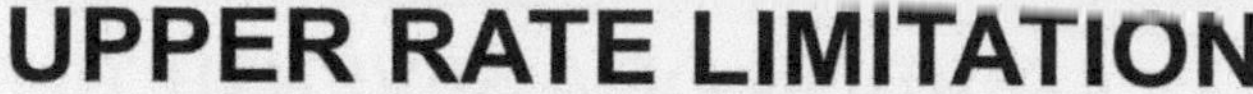

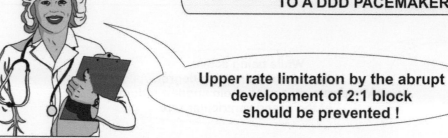

UPPER RATE LIMITATION

ADDITION OF A SEVENTH TIMING CYCLE TO A DDD PACEMAKER

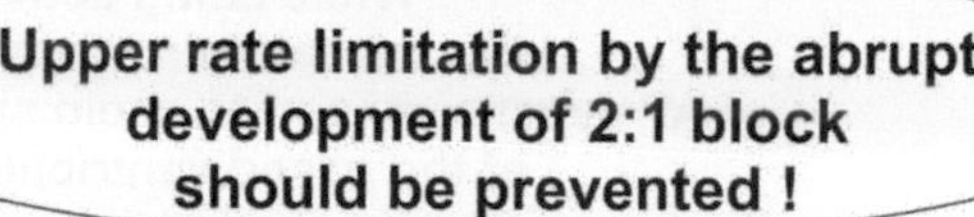

Upper rate limitation by the abrupt development of 2:1 block should be prevented !

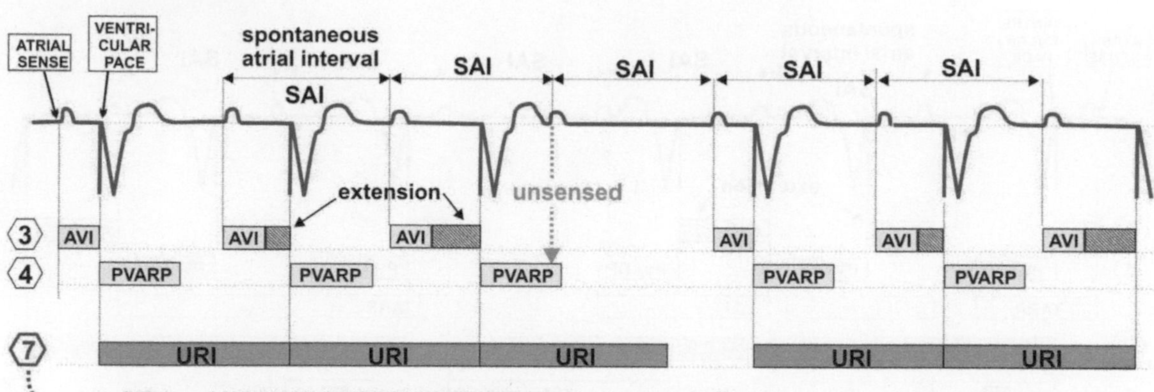

A Wenckebach upper rate response can only occur when the upper rate interval (URI) is programmed longer than the total atrial refractory period (TARP). The latter is the sum of the atrioventricular interval (AVI) and the postventricular atrial refractory period (PVARP) i.e. TARP = AVI + PVARP

If the upper rate interval (URI) equals the total atrial refractory period (TARP), no Wenckebach upper rate behavior is possible and the upper rate response will consist of 2:1 block.

ADDITION OF A SEVENTH TIMING CYCLE TO A DDD PACEMAKER TO AVOID ABRUPT 2:1 BLOCK

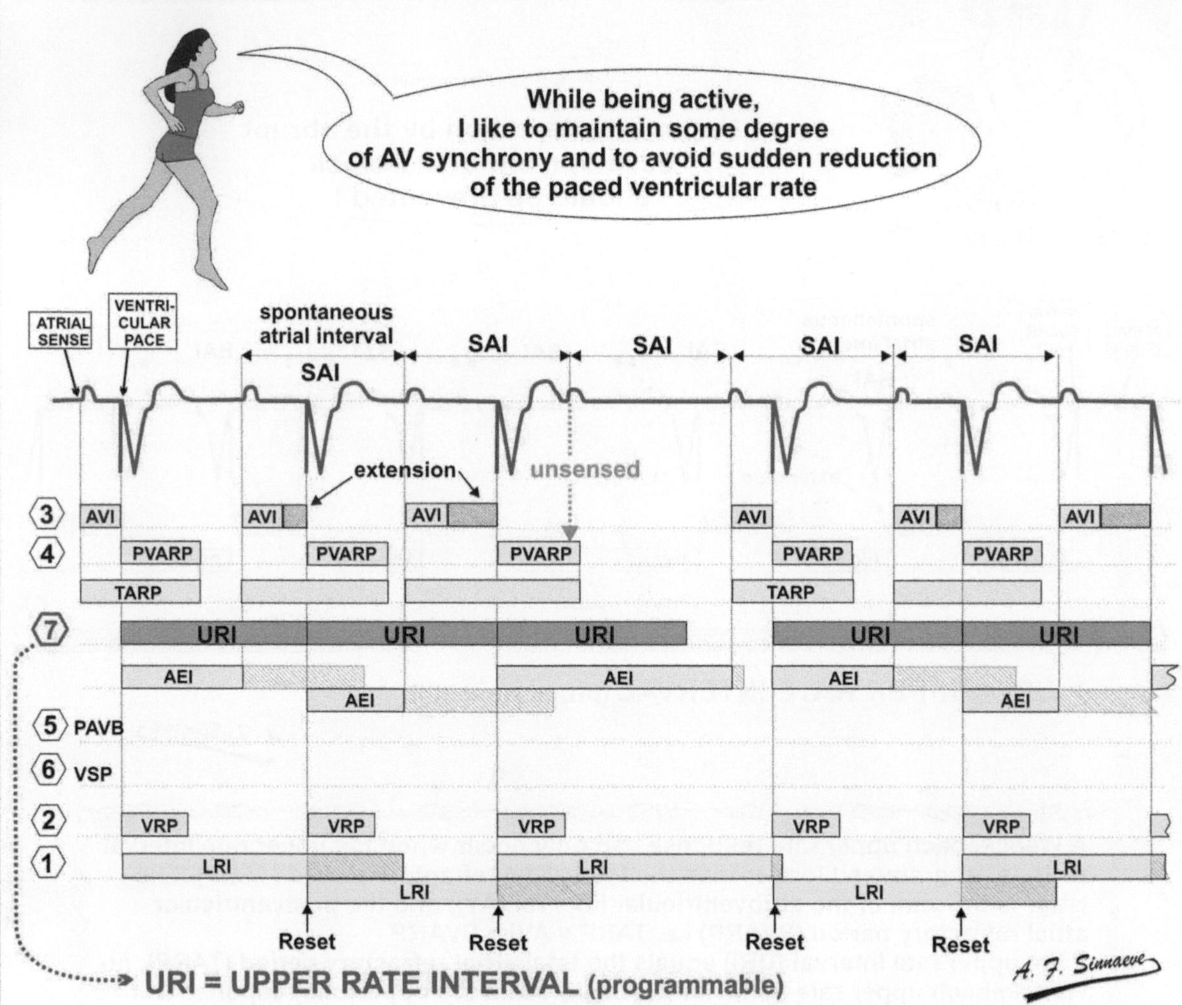

A pacemaker Wenckebach upper rate response can only occur if the pacemaker permits an upper rate interval (URI) longer than the pacemaker total atrial refractory period (TARP)

ABBREVIATIONS : AVI = AV interval; PVARP = postventricular atrial refractory period; TARP = total atrial refractory period; AEI = atrial escape interval; PAVB = postatrial ventricular blanking; VSP = ventricular safety pacing window; VRP = ventricular refractory period; LRI = lower rate interval

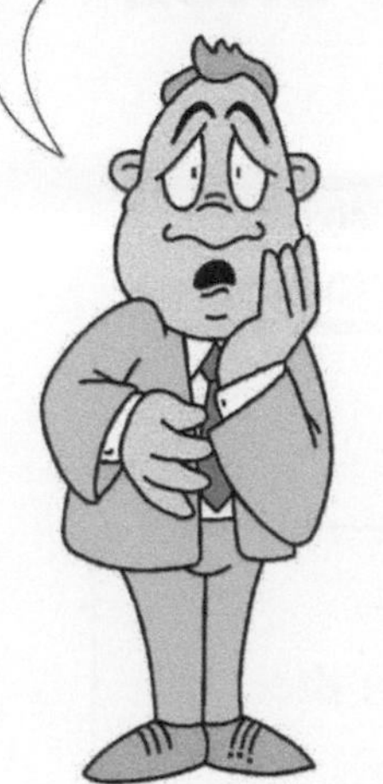

HOW TO ENSURE A WENCKEBACH UPPER RATE BEHAVIOR OF A PACEMAKER

A pacemaker Wenckebach upper rate response can only occur if the pacemaker permits an upper rate interval longer than the pacemaker total atrial refractory period

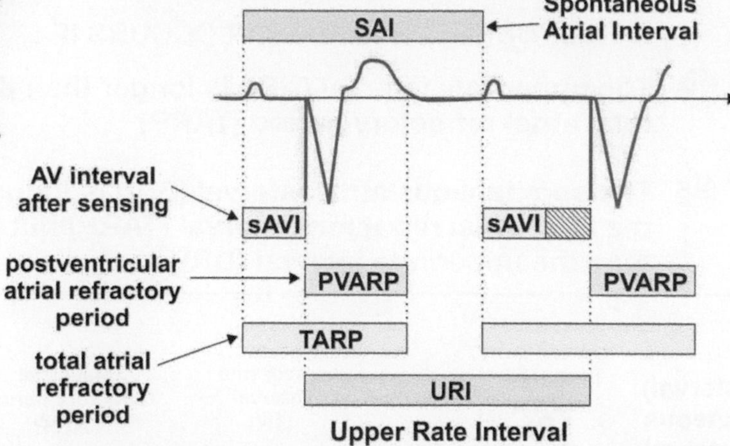

A shorter Total Atrial Refractory Period (TARP) pushes the 2 : 1 block rate to a higher level, thereby allowing the programming of a faster rate at which the Wenckebach response begins.
Manipulation of the sAVI and/or the PVARP allows the establishment of a faster upper rate by :

 **Programming a shorter basic AV Interval after sensing (sAVI)**

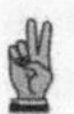 **Shortening the sAVI with an increase in atrial rate**

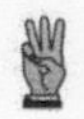 **Programming a shorter Postventricular Atrial Refractory Interval (PVARP)**

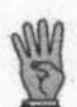 **An adaptive PVARP shortening on exercise**

A. F. Sinnaeve

WENCKEBACH UPPER RATE RESPONSE

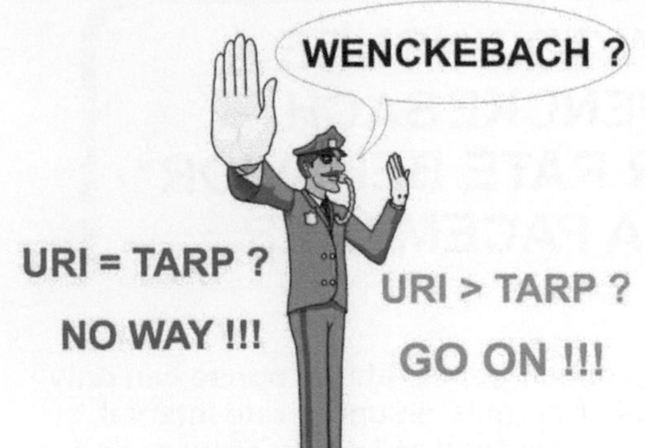

$$\text{RATE (bpm)} = \frac{60{,}000}{\text{INTERVAL (ms)}}$$

WENCKEBACH BEHAVIOR OCCURS IF :

1. The upper rate interval (URI) is longer than the total atrial refractory period (TARP)
2. The spontaneous atrial interval (SAI) is longer than the total atrial refractory interval (TARP) but shorter than the upper rate interval (URI)

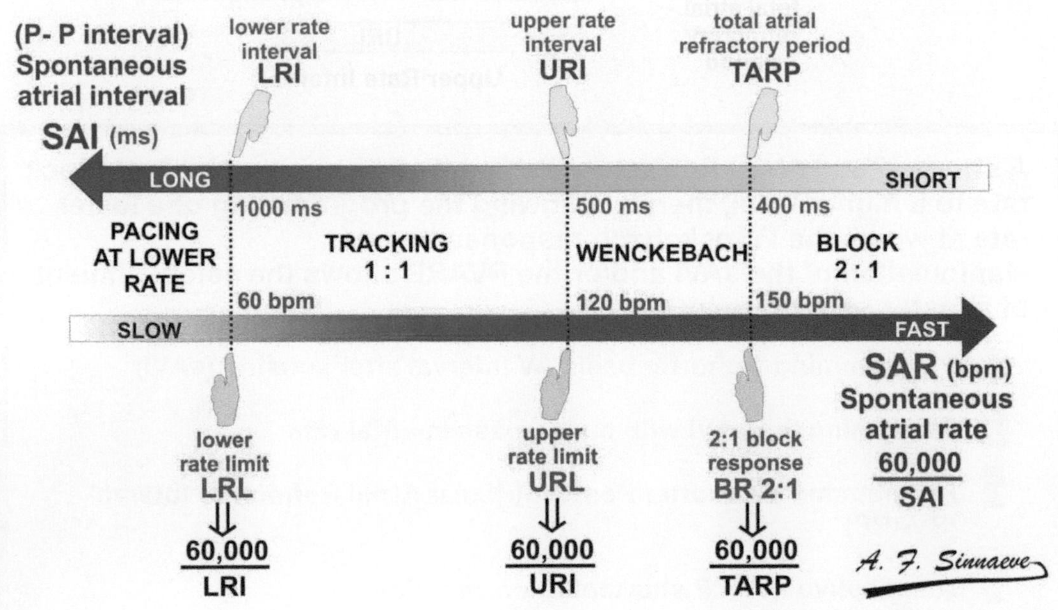

WENCKEBACH UPPER RATE RESPONSE

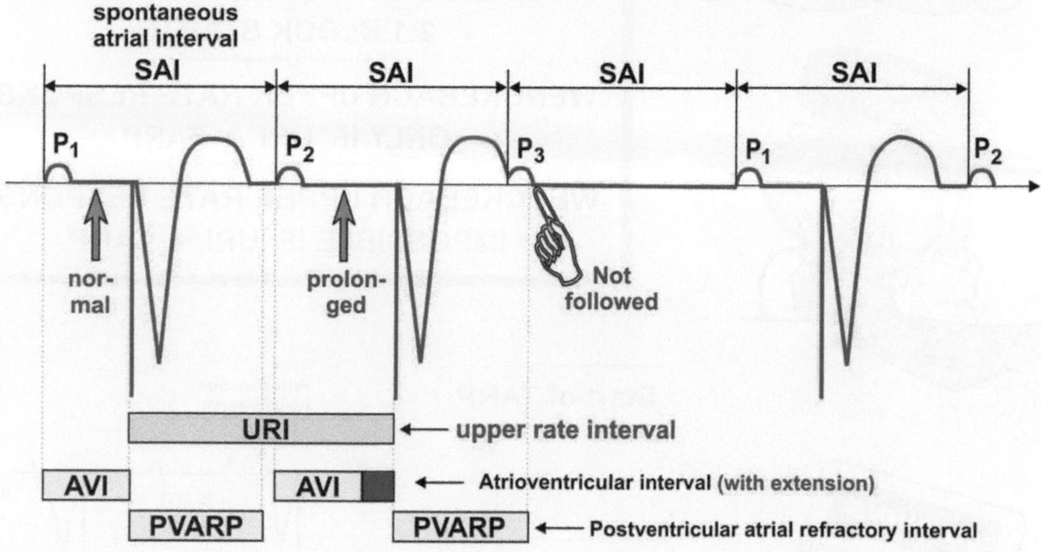

spontaneous
atrial interval
SAI
SAI
SAI
SAI
P1
P2
P3
P1
P2
nor-
mal
prolon-
ged
Not
followed
URI
upper rate interval
AVI
AVI
Atrioventricular interval (with extension)
PVARP
PVARP
Postventricular atrial refractory interval

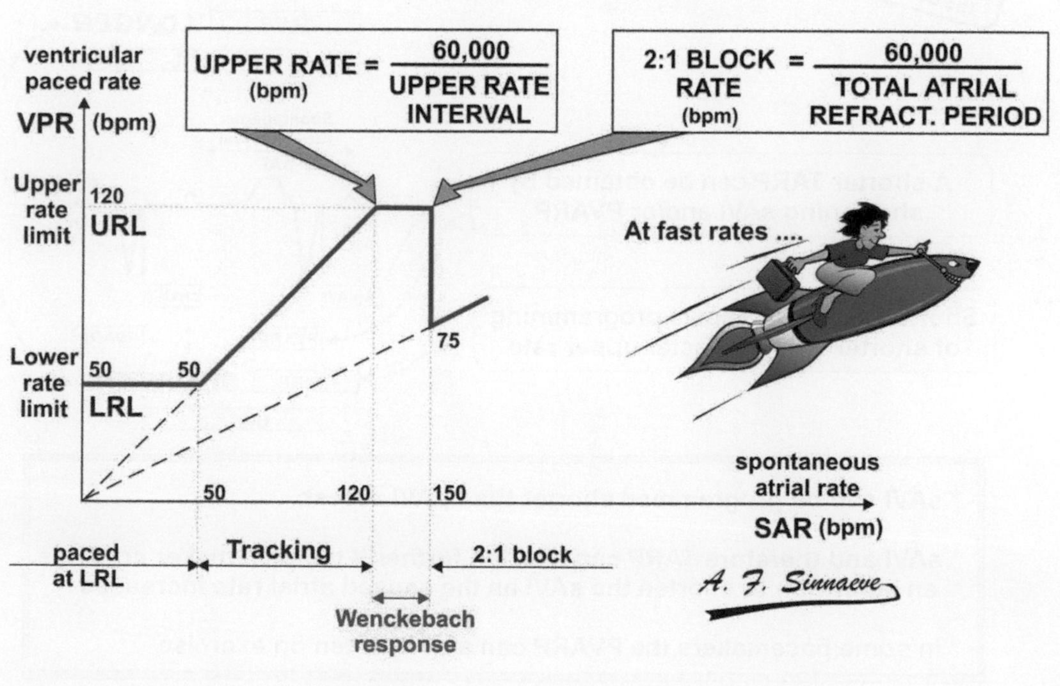

ventricular
paced rate
VPR (bpm)
UPPER RATE (bpm) = 60,000 / UPPER RATE INTERVAL
2:1 BLOCK RATE (bpm) = 60,000 / TOTAL ATRIAL REFRACT. PERIOD
Upper
rate
limit
120
URL
Lower
rate
limit
50
50
LRL
75
At fast rates ....
50
120
150
spontaneous
atrial rate
SAR (bpm)
paced
at LRL
Tracking
2:1 block
Wenckebach
response
A. F. Sinnaeve

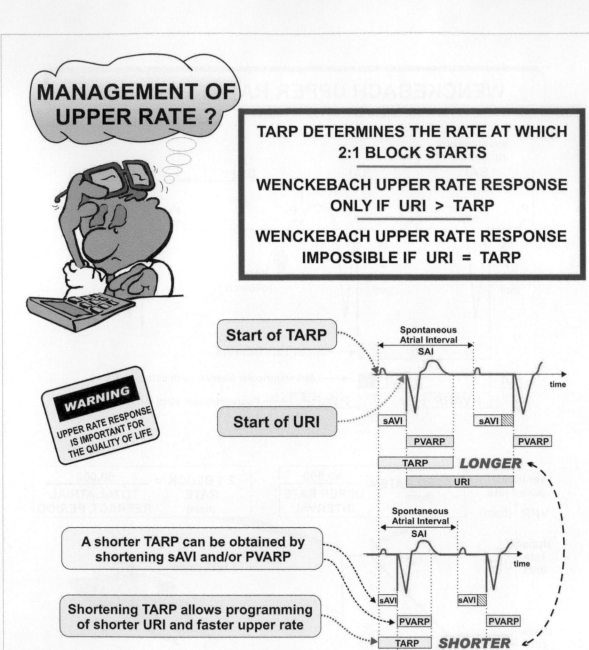

MANAGEMENT OF UPPER RATE ?

TARP DETERMINES THE RATE AT WHICH 2:1 BLOCK STARTS

WENCKEBACH UPPER RATE RESPONSE ONLY IF URI > TARP

WENCKEBACH UPPER RATE RESPONSE IMPOSSIBLE IF URI = TARP

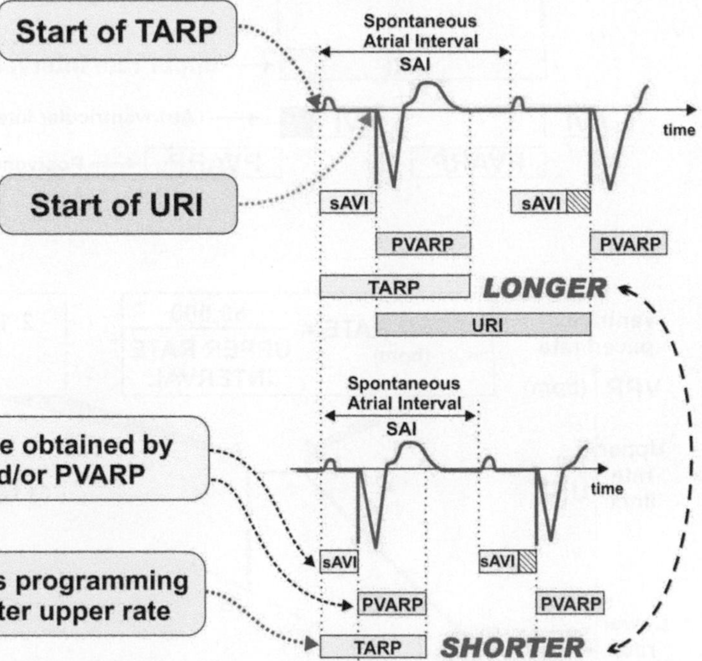

*** sAVI can be programmed shorter than pAVI at rest**

*** sAVI and therefore TARP can shorten further if the pacemaker contains an algorithm to shorten the sAVI as the sensed atrial rate increases**

*** in some pacemakers the PVARP can also shorten on exercise**

Abbreviations : sAVI = AV interval after sensing; SAI = spontaneous atrial interval; PVARP = postventricular atrial refractory period; TARP = total atrial refractory period; URI = upper rate interval;

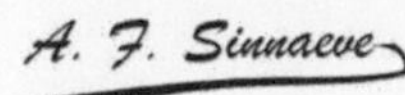

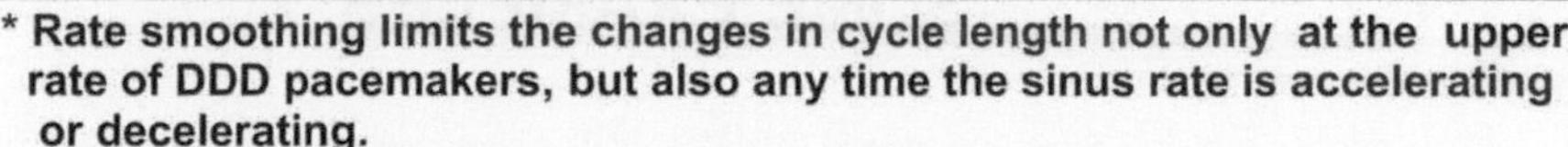

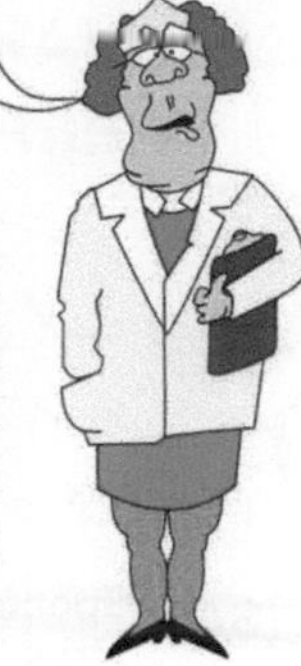
I hate sudden changes !!!

* Rate smoothing limits the changes in cycle length not only at the upper rate of DDD pacemakers, but also any time the sinus rate is accelerating or decelerating.
* The permitted maximum change in the pacing cycle length is programmable (3%,6%, 9%, 12%)

Wenckebach upper rate response without rate smoothing

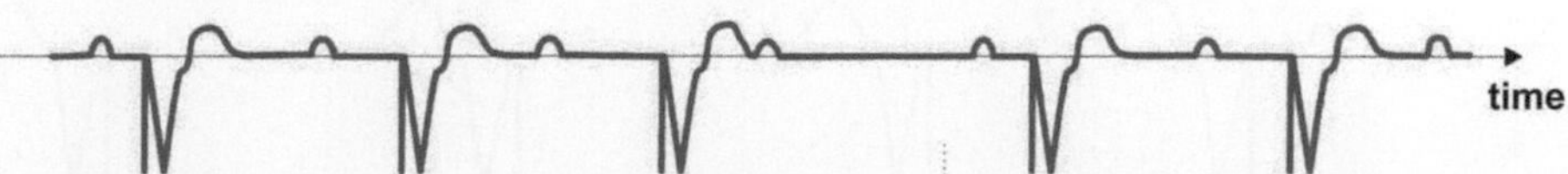

Same upper rate response, but with true rate smoothing (9%)

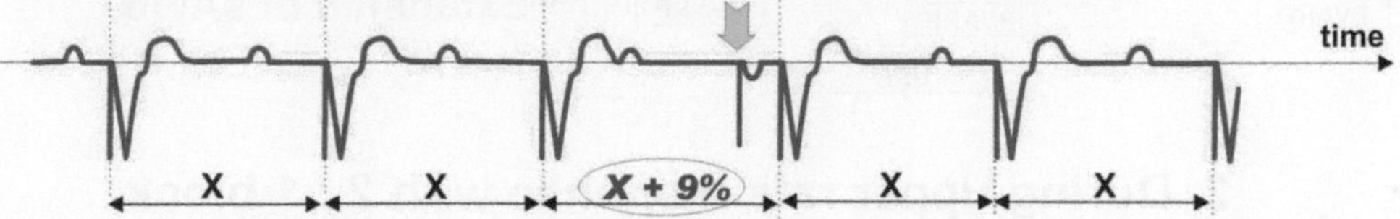

Note : A response similar to rate smoothing can also occur during rate-responsive DDDR pacing. With increased sensor input generated by exercise or activity, the pause at the end of a Wenckebach upper rate response can be attenuated or eliminated according to the prevailing sensor-driven interval. This response is potentially important in patients who do not tolerate the pauses in the Wenckebach upper rate response of DDD pacemakers

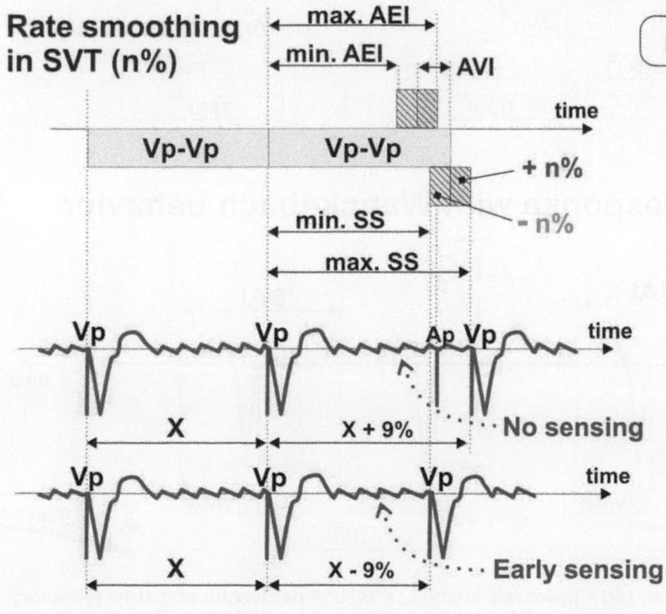

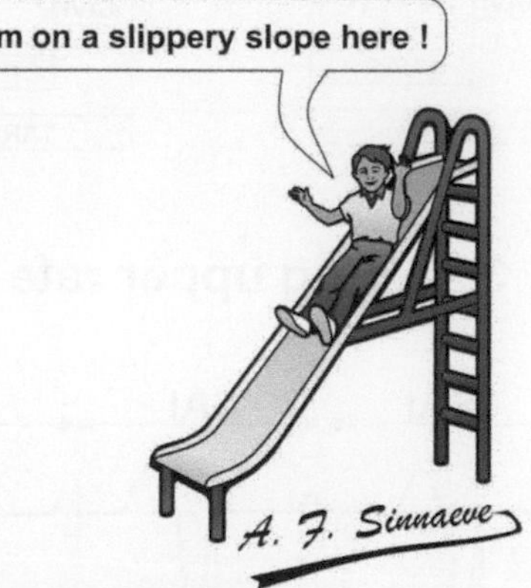
I'm on a slippery slope here !
A. F. Sinnaeve

Abbreviations :
AEI = atrial escape interval ; AVI = AV delay
Ap = atrial pace ; Vp = ventricular pace ;
SS = interstimulus interval ; SVT = supraventriclar tachycardia

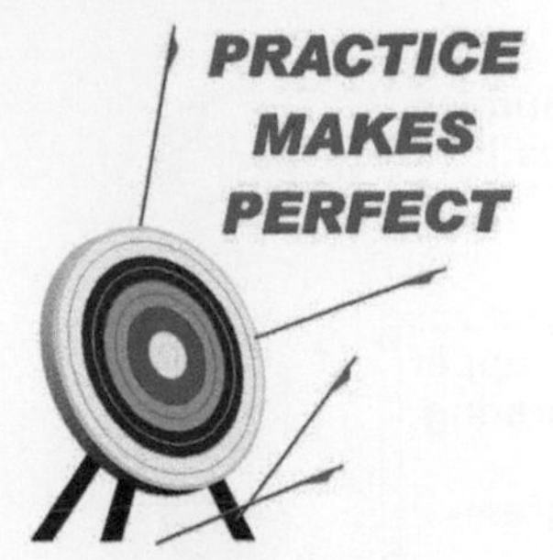

ATRIAL PREMATURE COMPLEXES AND UPPER RATE LIMITATION * SOME EXAMPLES *

1. While tracking (LRI > SAI > URI)

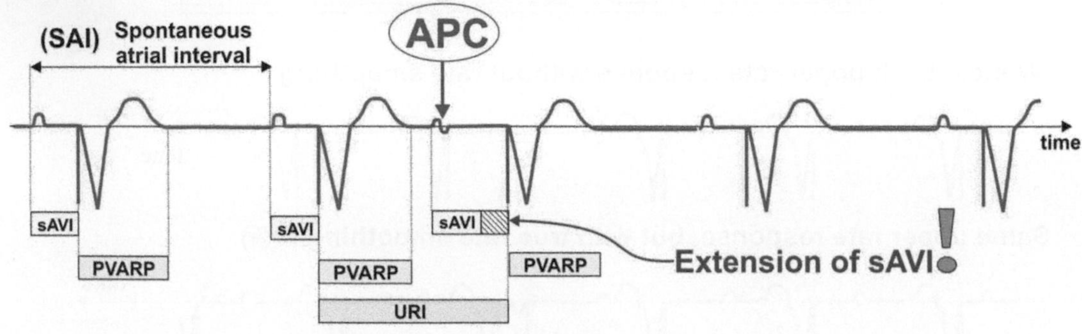

2. During upper rate response with 2 : 1 block

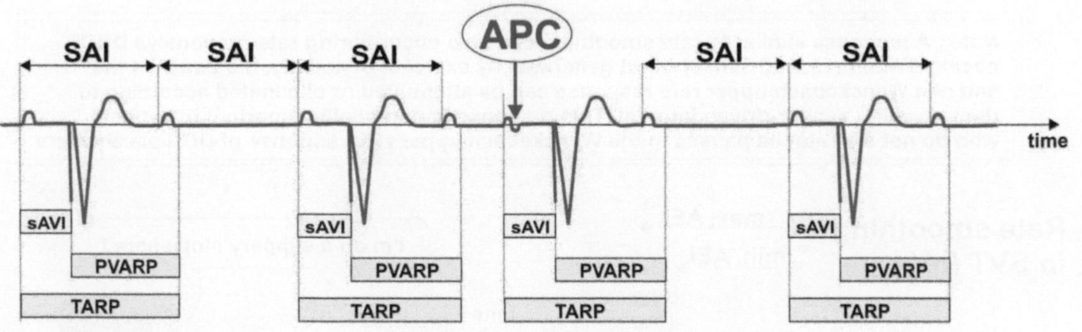

3. During upper rate response with Wenckebach behavior

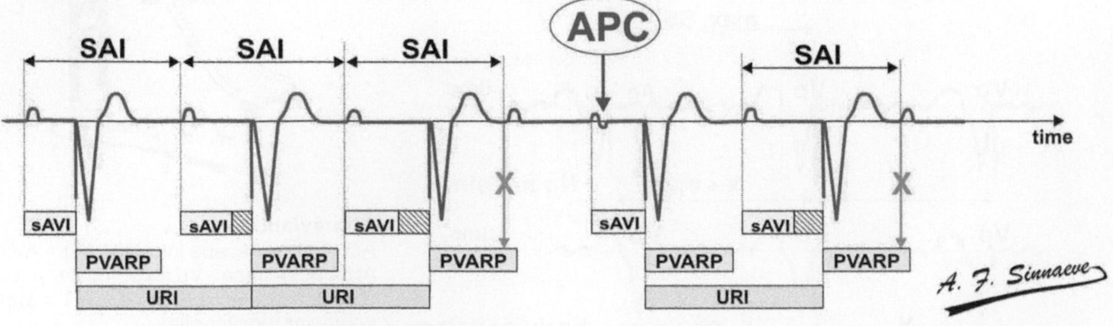

Abbreviations : APC = atrial premature complex ; LRI = lower rate interval ; PVARP = postventricular atrial refractory period ; SAI = spontaneous atrial interval ; sAVI = AV delay after sensing ; TARP = total atrial refractory period ; URI = upper rate interval

ATRIAL PREMATURE COMPLEXES AND UPPER RATE LIMITATION DDD pacemaker with URI > TARP

The AV delay initiated by an APC depends on its timing in the pacemaker cycle ! Unexplained upper rate limitation is often due to an APC !!!

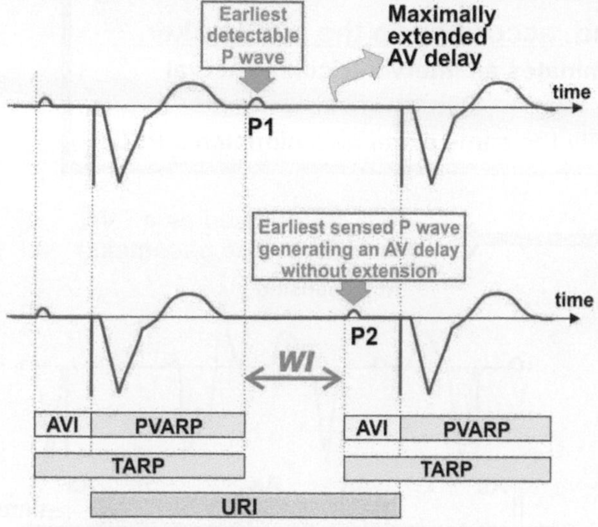

The Wenckebach interval (WI) is equal to the longest prolongation of the AV delay. It is therefore equal to :

WI = URI - (AVI + PVARP)

WI = URI - TARP

A P wave (P1) immediately after PVARP termination will exhibit the longest interval (AVI +WI) to conform to the constancy of the URI. A P wave (P2) just beyond the WI will initiate an AV interval equal to the programmed value. P waves in the WI will exhibit varying degrees of AV prolongation to conform to the URI.

Use your calipers and measure the suspected interval !

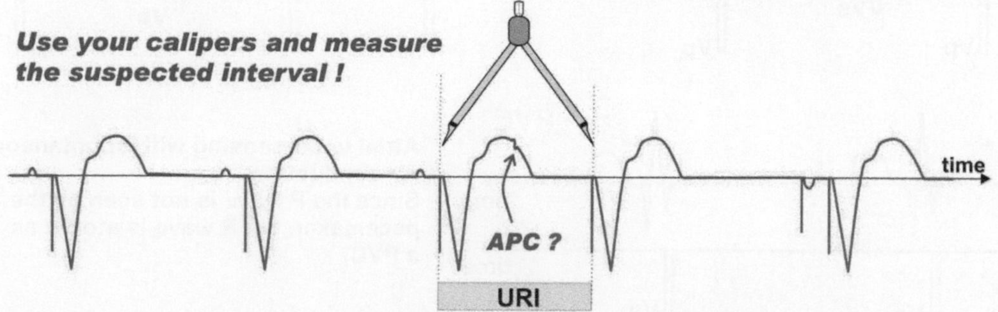

The URI can be identified on the ECG by moving calipers from the early ventricular stimulus back to the previous ventricular event. If this measured interval equals URI, it provides proof that an atrial sensed event occurred between the two ventricular events bracketing the URI. By far the most likely cause is an APC or less commonly a retrograde P wave as an isolated event. Far-field T wave sensing by the atrial channel is very rare, even at very high atrial sensitivity.

Abbreviations : APC = atrial premature complex; AVI = AV interval or AV delay; PVARP = postventricular atrial refractory period; TARP = total atrial refractory period; URI = upper rate interval; WI = Wenckebach interval

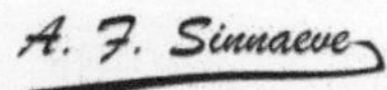

ABOUT PREMATURE VENTRICULAR EVENTS (PVE)

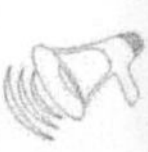

DEFINITION **: a PVE is a sensed R wave that is not preceded by an atrial event, paced or sensed, <u>according to the pacemaker.</u>**

Thus a pacemaker-defined PVE terminates an interventricular interval without an intervening atrial event.

A pacemaker's PVE is not necessarily the same event as a clinician's PVC !

Recognized as a PVC (or PVE) by the pacemaker ⟷ **NOT recognized as a PVC (or PVE) by the pacemaker**

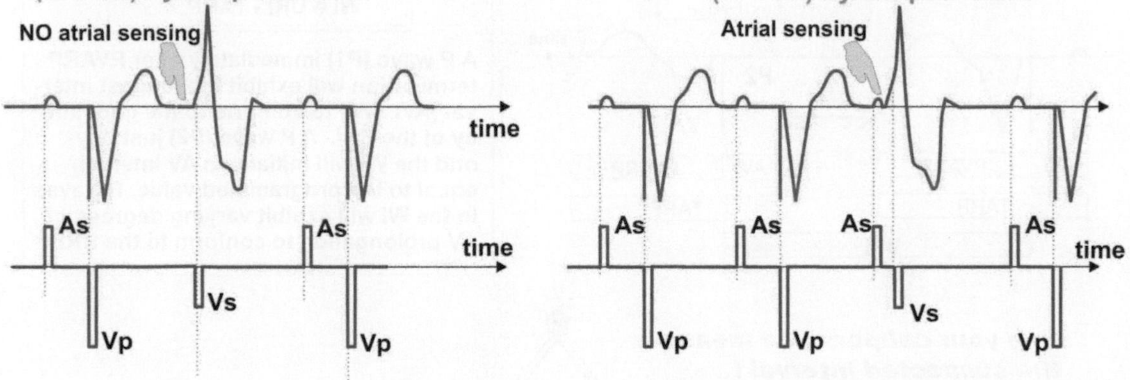

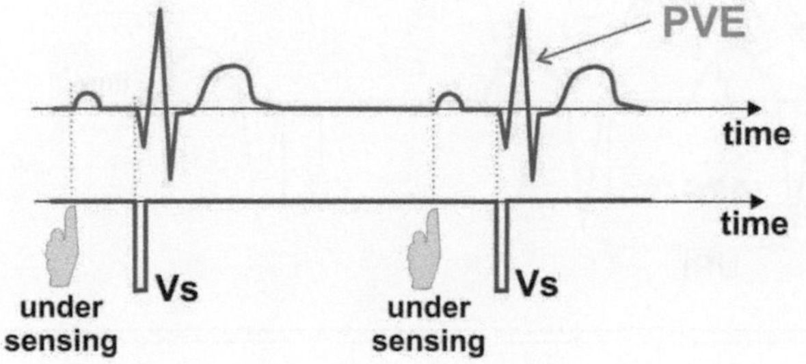

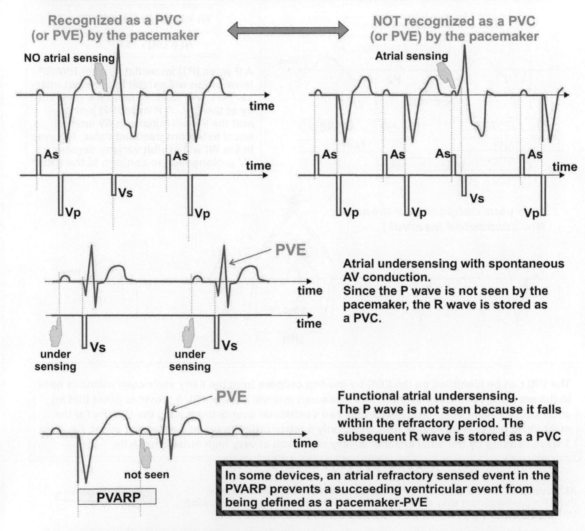

Atrial undersensing with spontaneous AV conduction.
Since the P wave is not seen by the pacemaker, the R wave is stored as a PVC.

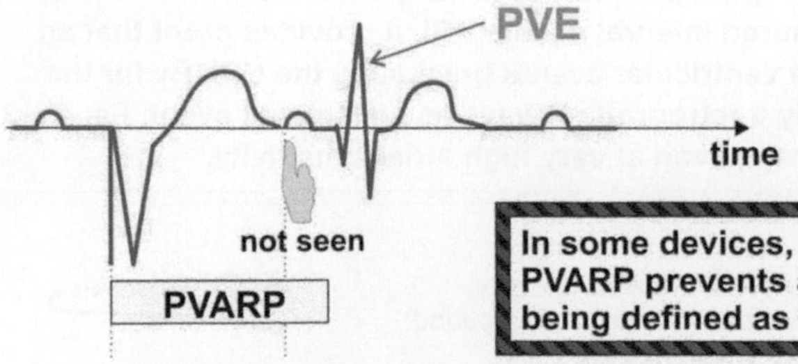

Functional atrial undersensing.
The P wave is not seen because it falls within the refractory period. The subsequent R wave is stored as a PVC

In some devices, an atrial refractory sensed event in the PVARP prevents a succeeding ventricular event from being defined as a pacemaker-PVE

Abbreviations : PVARP = postventricular atrial refractory period; PVE = premature ventricular event; PVC = premature ventricular complex ; As = atrial sensed event; Ap = atrial paced event; Vp = ventricular paced event; Vs = ventricular sensed event

A. F. Sinnaeve

FUNCTIONAL ATRIAL UNDERSENSING

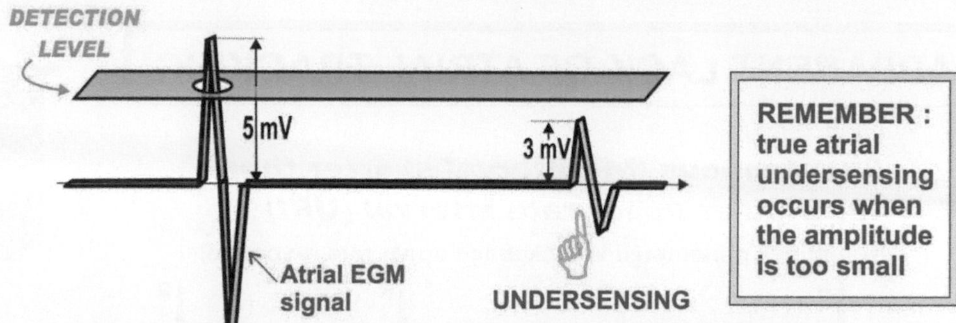

REMEMBER : true atrial undersensing occurs when the amplitude is too small

Functional atrial undersensing with a long PVARP

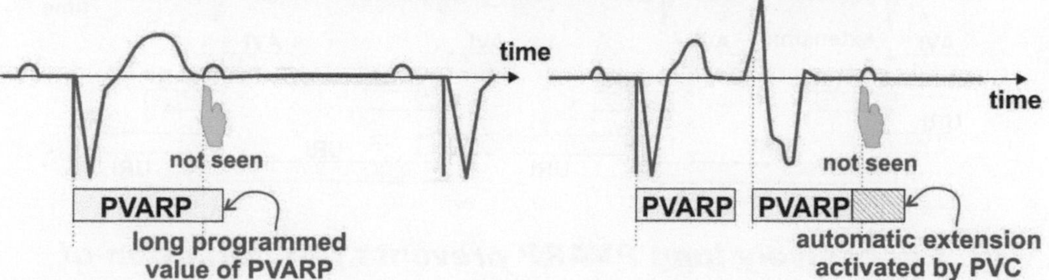

Apparent or functional atrial undersensing due to upper rate limitation (displacement of the P wave in the PVARP as a function of the atrial rate).

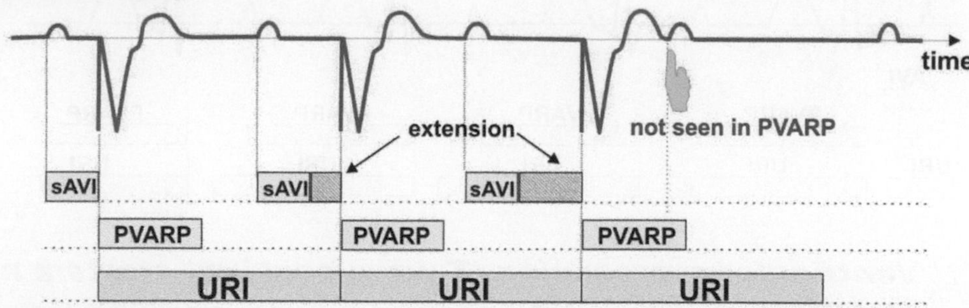

A. F. Sinnaeve

CAUTION

Remember that automatic PVARP extension after a pacemaker-defined PVC may cause functional atrial undersensing even when the basic PVARP is relatively short.

Abbreviations : EGM = electrogram; mV = millivolt; PVC = premature ventricular complex; PVARP = postventricular atrial refractory period; sAVI = AV delay after a sensed atrial event; URI = upper rate interval

Sometimes we see a prolongation of the interval between atrial-sensed and ventricular-sensed events beyond the programmed AV interval, while there is no true atrial undersensing because the amplitude of the atrial electrogram is adequate for atrial sensing !!!

APPARENT LACK OF ATRIAL TRACKING

1 *Spontaneous R-R interval shorter than ventricular upper rate interval (URI)*

(Repetitive pre-empted Wenckebach upper rate response)

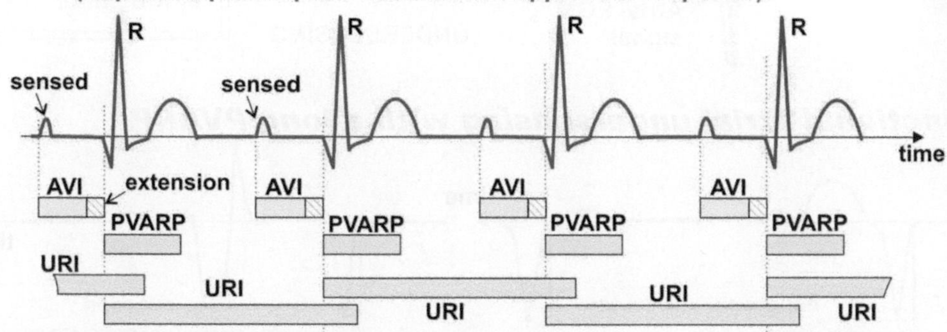

2 *Excessively long PVARP prevents the detection of P waves (at relatively fast spontaneous atrial rate)*

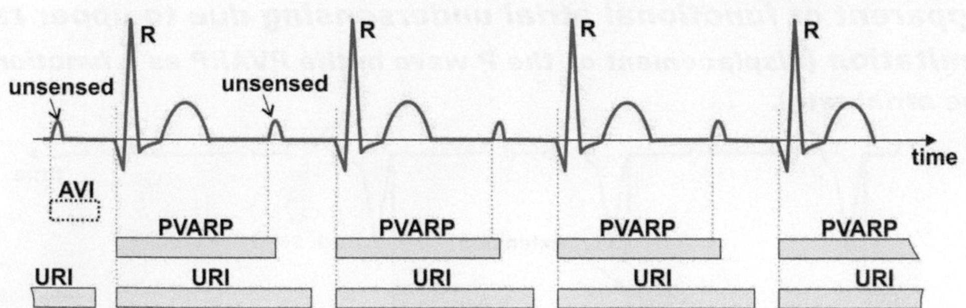

3 *Ventricular oversensing (T wave sensing) starts a new PVARP thus preventing normal P wave sensing*

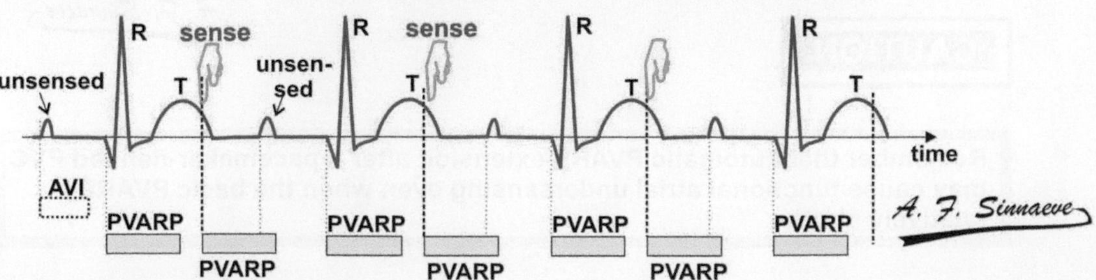

Abbreviations : AVI = programmed AV delay; PVARP = postventricular atrial refractory period; URI = upper rate interval

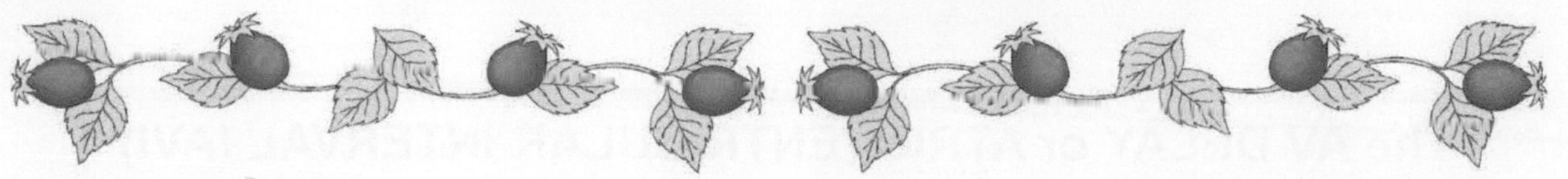

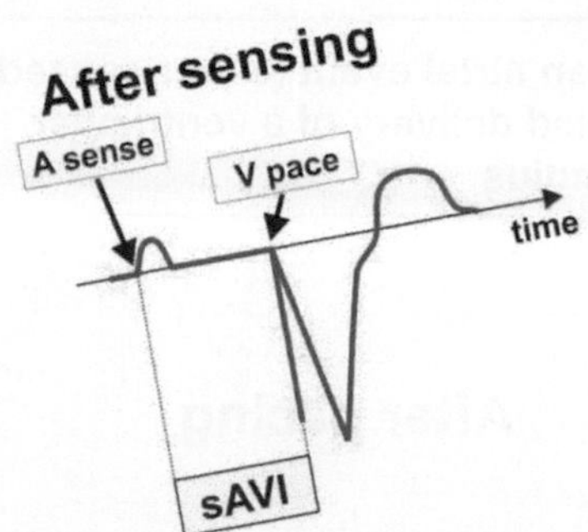

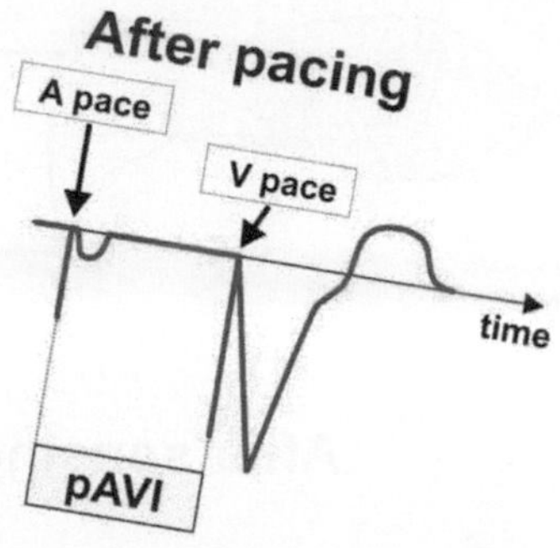

ATRIOVENTRICULAR INTERVAL (AVI)

* AV delay - paced and sensed
* Rate-adaptive AV delay
* How to program the AV delay ?
* AV search hysteresis

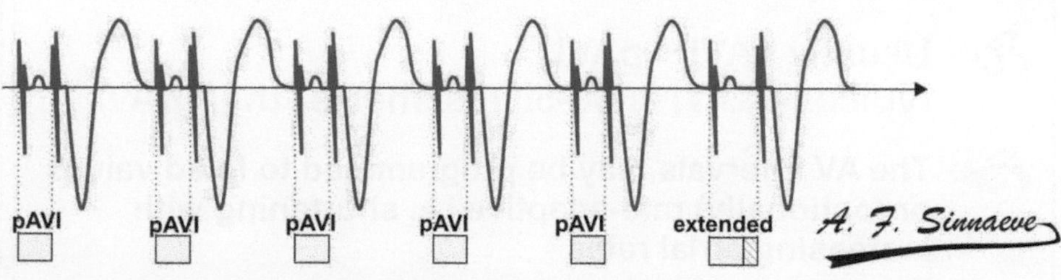

A. F. Sinnaeve

The AV DELAY or ATRIOVENTRICULAR INTERVAL (AVI)

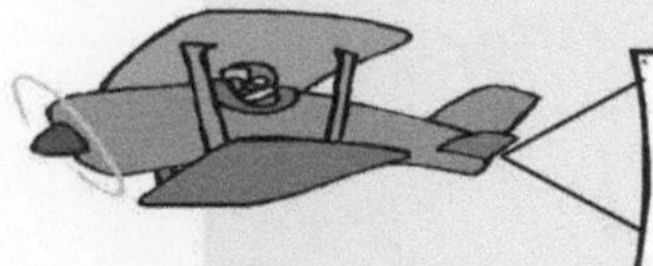

AVI is the interval between an atrial event (either sensed or paced) and the scheduled delivery of a ventricular stimulus

After sensing

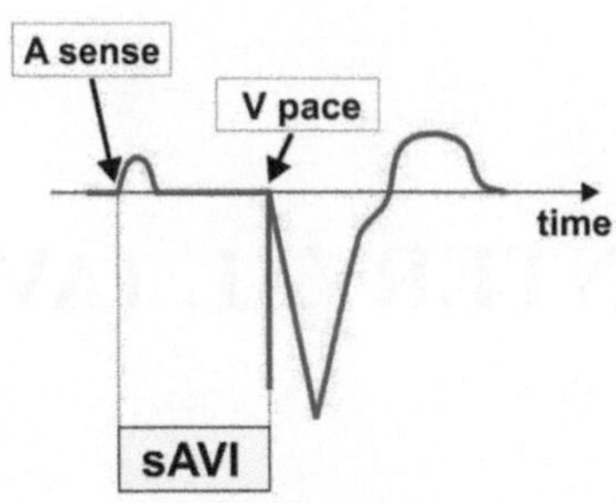

sAVI starts with an atrial sensed event

After pacing

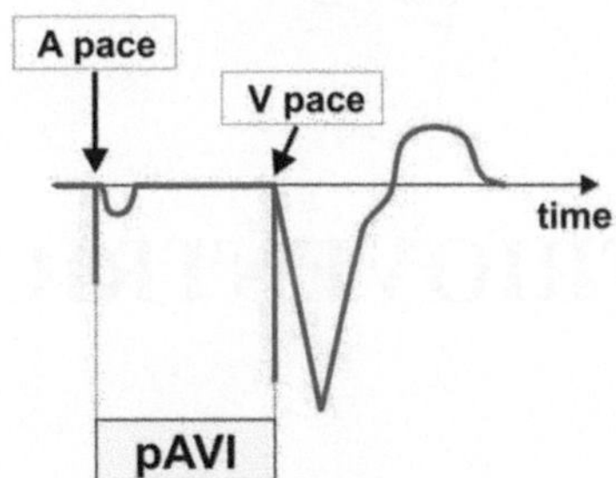

pAVI starts with an atrial stimulus

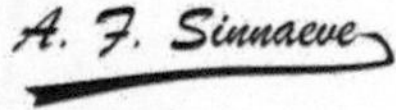

 Separate AV intervals for paced and sensed atrial events are available

 Usually sAVI < pAVI
typically sAVI is 30-50 ms shorter than pAVI

 The AV intervals may be programmed to fixed values or (optionally) rate-adaptive i.e. shortening with increasing atrial rates

THE RATE-ADAPTIVE AV INTERVAL

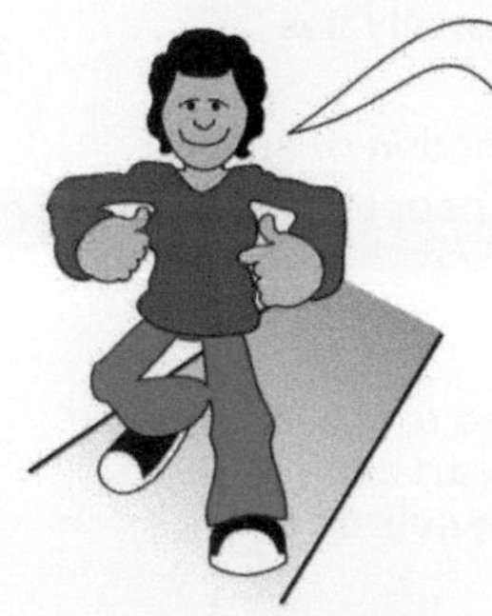
My AV delay is normal or physiologic.
It shortens whenever I exercise !

The rate-adaptive AV interval mimics the physiologic response of the heart

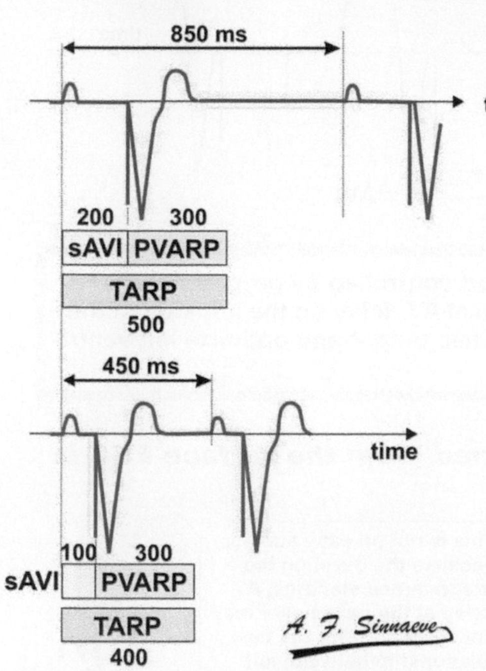

RELATIVELY SLOW ATRIAL RATE
→ **LONGER AV DELAY**

Spontaneous atrial interval SAI = 850 ms

Spontaneous atrial rate SAR = 71 bpm

Sensed atrioventricular interval sAVI = 200 ms

FASTER ATRIAL RATE
→ **SHORTER AV DELAY**

Spontaneous atrial interval SAI = 450 ms

Spontaneous atrial rate SAR = 133 bpm

Sensed atrioventricular interval sAVI = 100 ms

THE PROGRAMMER MAY CHANGE

- **the maximum value of sAVI**
- **the minimum value of sAVI**
- **the value of the gradual decrement of sAVI between this 2 rates**
- **the range of rates where the change in the sAVI occurs**

pAVI can also shorten according to the input of a nonatrial sensor that reflects increased activity

HOW TO OBTAIN AN OPTIMAL AV DELAY ?

* In healthy individuals at rest, the optimal basic PR or AV interval normally lies between 120 and 210 ms
* The optimal value varies greatly from one patient to another as a function of several physiologic and pathologic factors including age (shorter in young people)
* Optimization of the AV delay (AVI) is needed at rest and exercise

Normal

time

AVI

The P wave is too close to the ventricular complex so that the heart cannot derive the full benefit of AV synchrony

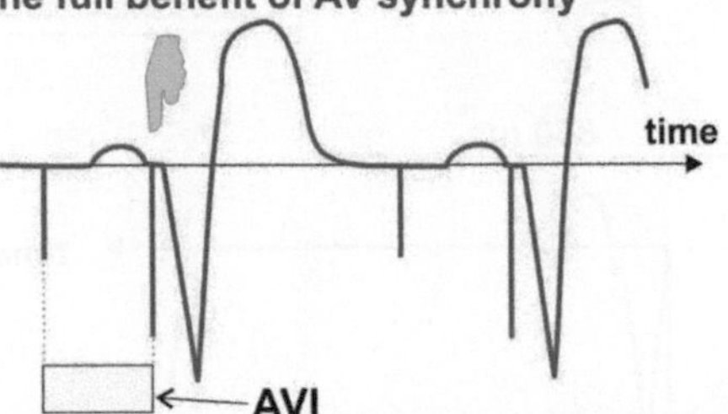

The electrical AV delay on the right side of the heart controlled by programming the pacemaker must produce an appropriate mechanical AV delay on the left side of the heart to preserve the atrial contribution to the cardiac output and optimize left ventricular function !!!

The optimal AV delay cannot be determined from the surface ECG !!!

Doppler echocardiography is required to determine the optimal AV delay that produces the best stroke volume and cardiac output for each individual

This is not an easy subject because the duration the programmed electrical AV delay of the pacemaker may not correlate with the best relationship between left atrial systole and left ventricular systole. What is important, is the optimal mechanical AV delay on the left side of the heart

Echo - Doppler equipment

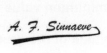

Echocardiogram

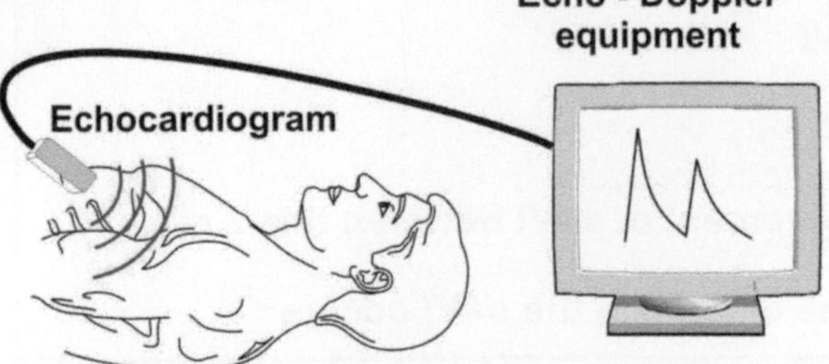

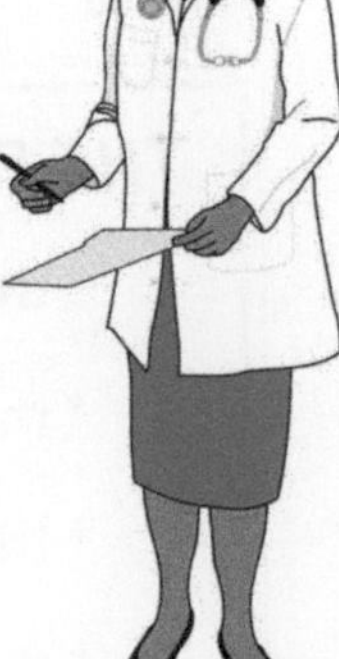

A. F. Sinnaeve

AV DELAY HYSTERESIS

Facilitation of normal AV conduction to promote normal ventricular depolarization

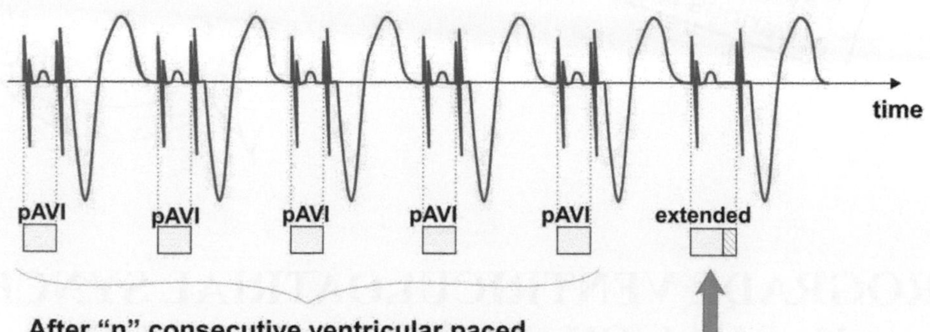

After "n" consecutive ventricular paced complexes, the AV delay is prolonged for "1" cycle

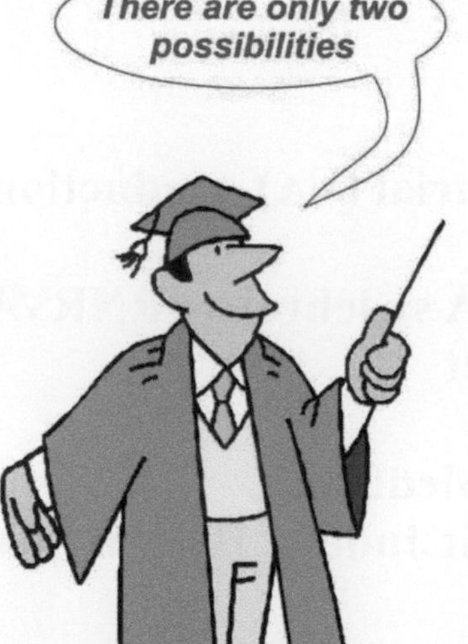

1 **If an intrinsic ventricular event is sensed, the AV delay remains prolonged**

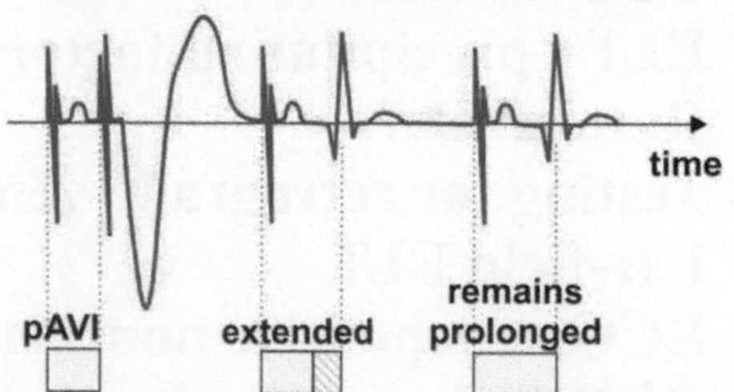

2 **If no intrinsic ventricular event is sensed, the AV delay returns to the programmed value**

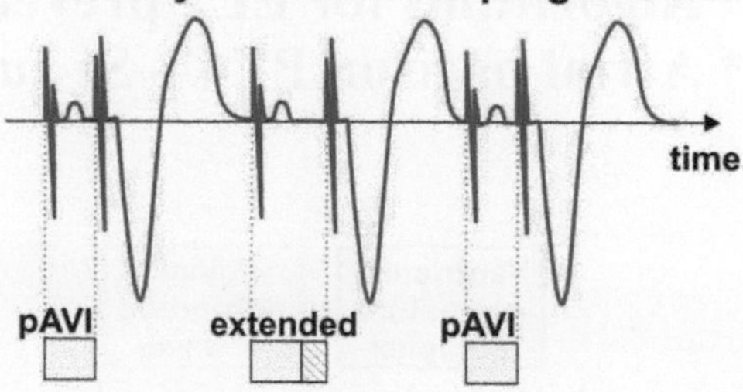

Abbreviations : AV = atrio-ventricular ; pAVI = paced atrioventricular interval ;

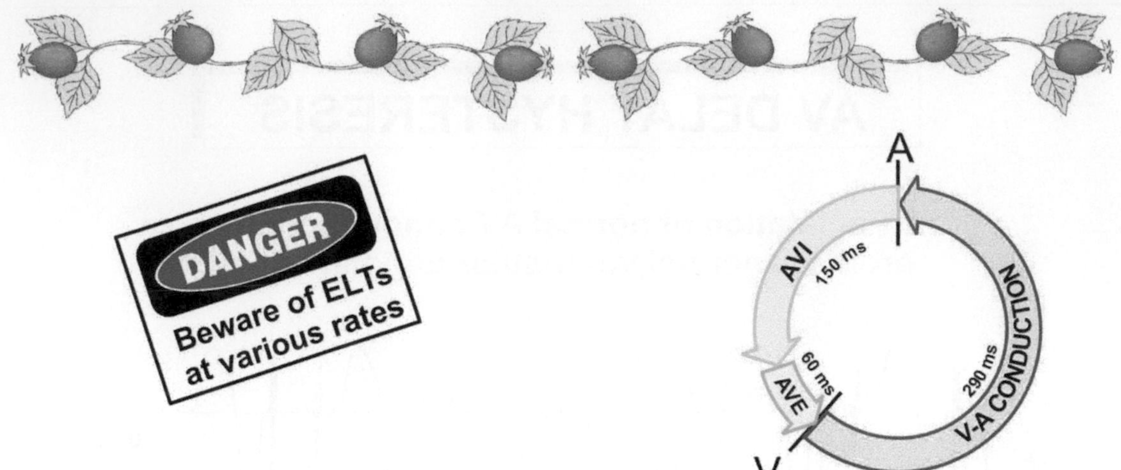

RETROGRADE VENTRICULOATRIAL SYNCHRONY IN DUAL CHAMBER PACEMAKERS

- **Mechanism of endless loop tachycardia (ELT)**
- **ECG of ELT**
- **ELT : precipitating factors**
- **Rate of ELTs**
- **Testing for retrograde ventriculoatrial (VA) conduction**
- **Far-field ELT**
- **ECG of repetitive nonreentrant VA synchrony (RNRVAS)**
- **RNRVAS : prevention & treatment**
- **The cousins : ELT and RNRVAS**
- **Algorithms for ELT prevention - Medtronic**
- **Algorithms for ELT prevention - St Jude & Boston Scientific**
- **Atrial pace on PVC - St Jude**

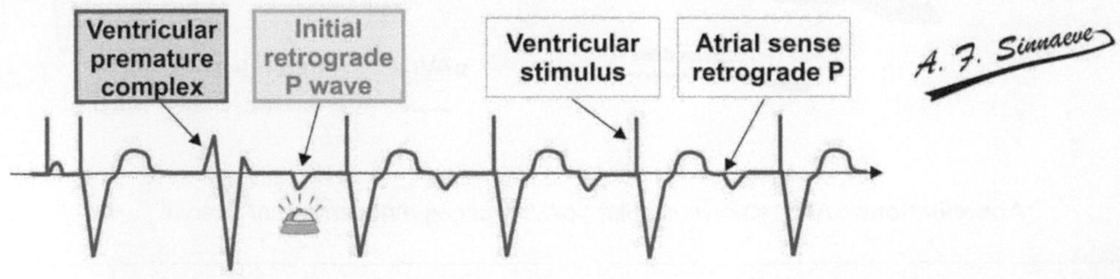

ENDLESS LOOP TACHYCARDIA (ELT)

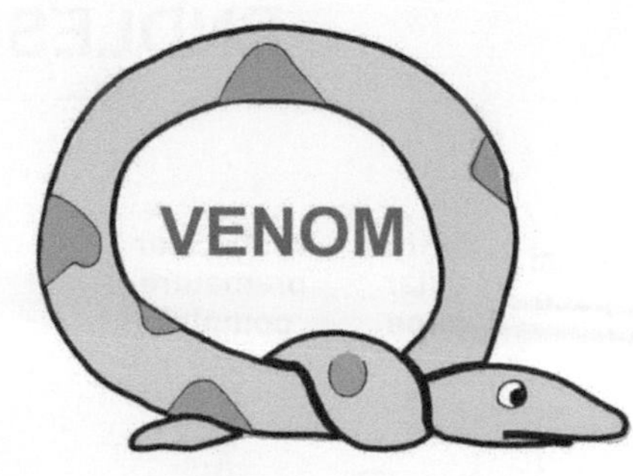

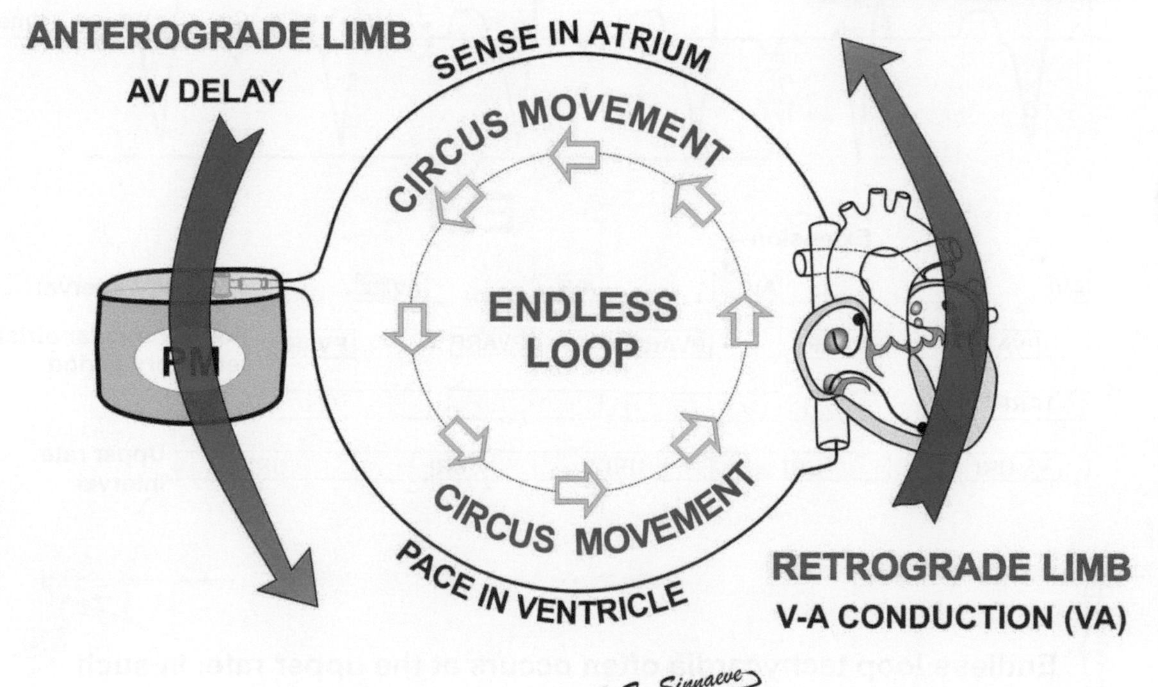

A. F. Sinnaeve

DDD PACEMAKER & ENDLESS LOOP TACHYCARDIA

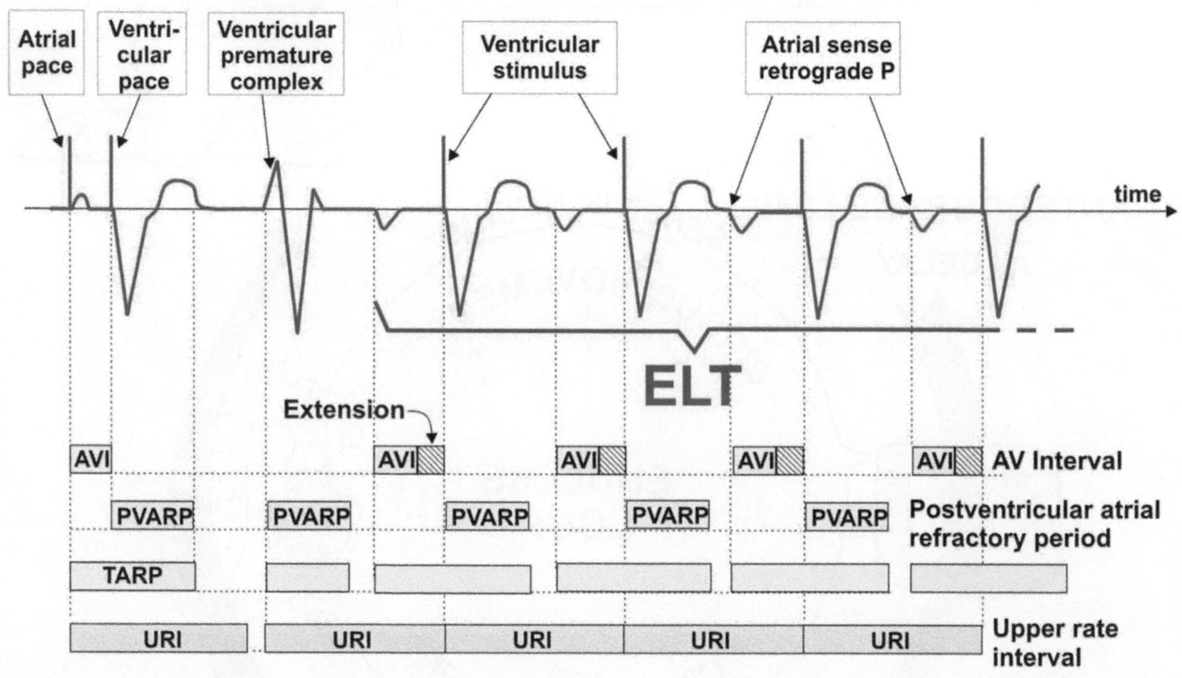

Endless loop tachycardia often occurs at the upper rate. In such a case as the programmed upper rate interval (URI) is longer than the total atrial refractory interval (TARP), the AV delay is extended to conform to the upper rate interval (URI)

Abbreviations : AVI = atrioventricular interval ; AVE = extension of AVI ; ELT = endless loop tachycardia ; PVARP = postventricular atrial refractory period ; TARP = total atrial refractory period ; URI = upper rate interval

A. F. Sinnaeve

ENDLESS LOOP TACHYCARDIA PRECIPITATING FACTORS

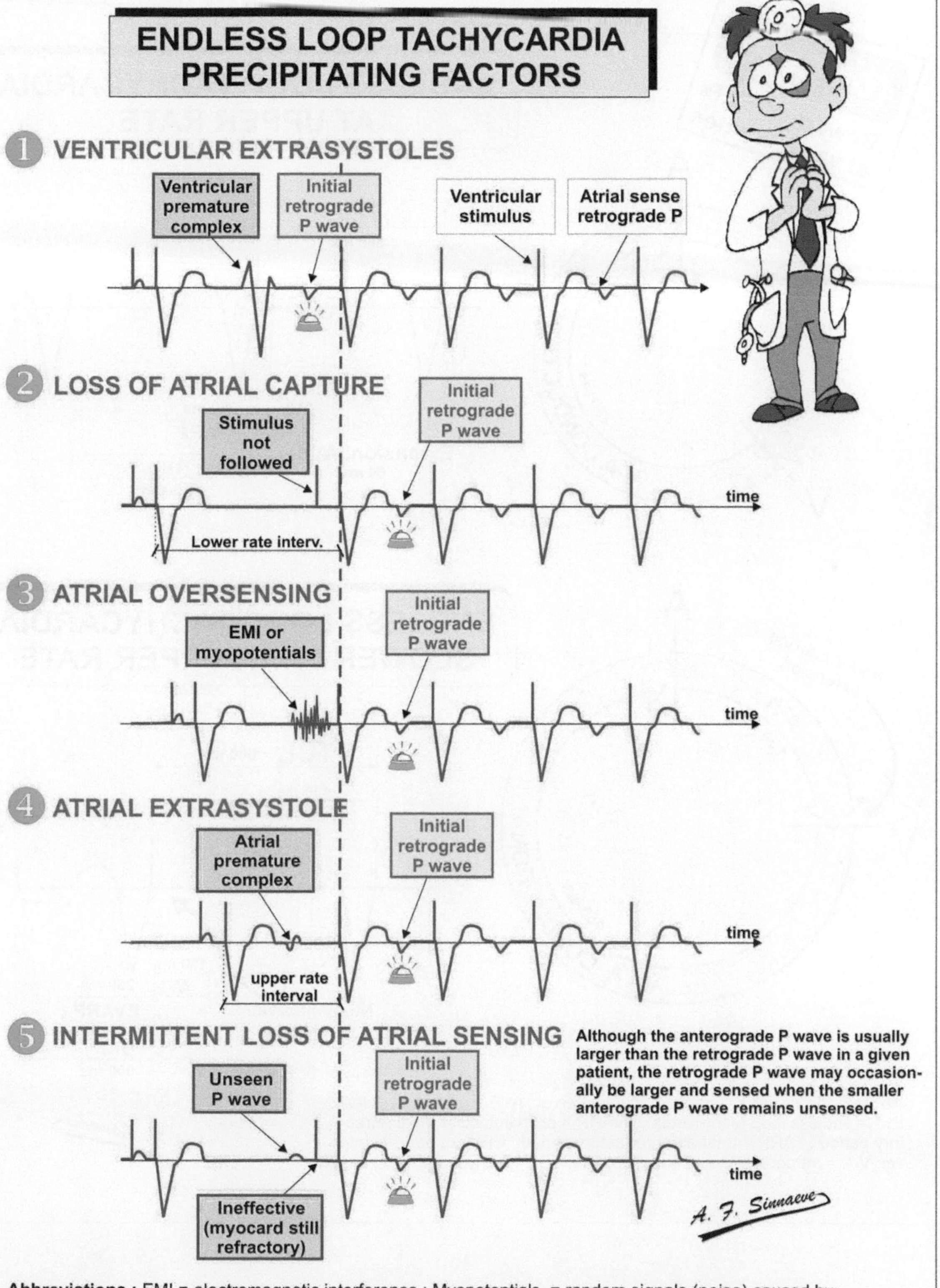

1 VENTRICULAR EXTRASYSTOLES

2 LOSS OF ATRIAL CAPTURE

3 ATRIAL OVERSENSING

4 ATRIAL EXTRASYSTOLE

5 INTERMITTENT LOSS OF ATRIAL SENSING

Although the anterograde P wave is usually larger than the retrograde P wave in a given patient, the retrograde P wave may occasionally be larger and sensed when the smaller anterograde P wave remains unsensed.

Abbreviations : EMI = electromagnetic interference ; Myopotentials = random signals (noise) caused by the action of some muscles ; myocard = myocardium or cardiac muscle

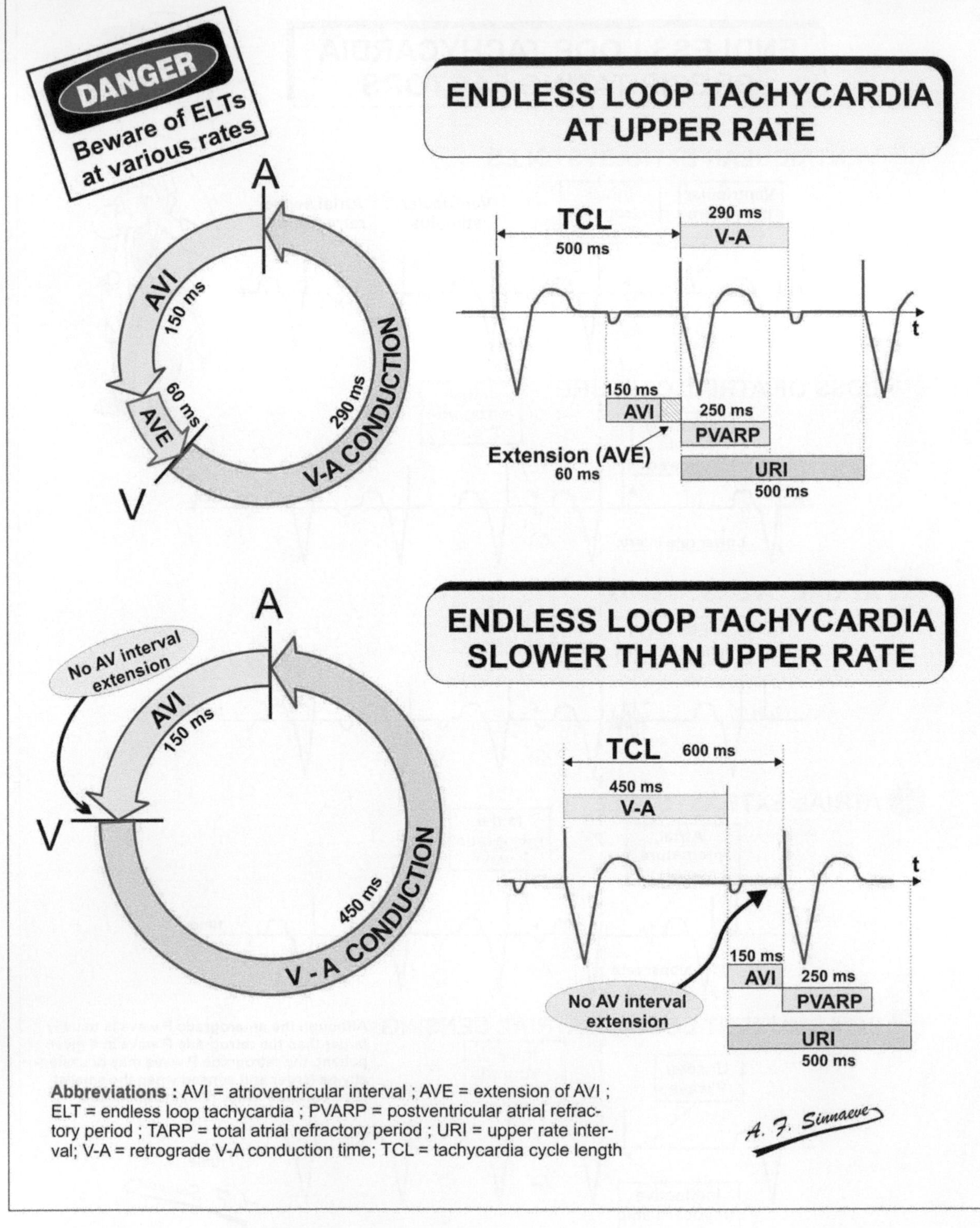

Abbreviations : AVI = atrioventricular interval ; AVE = extension of AVI ; ELT = endless loop tachycardia ; PVARP = postventricular atrial refractory period ; TARP = total atrial refractory period ; URI = upper rate interval; V-A = retrograde V-A conduction time; TCL = tachycardia cycle length

EVALUATION OF RETROGRADE VA CONDUCTION

Reprogram the pacemaker to the VVI mode at a rate faster than the spontaneous rhythm

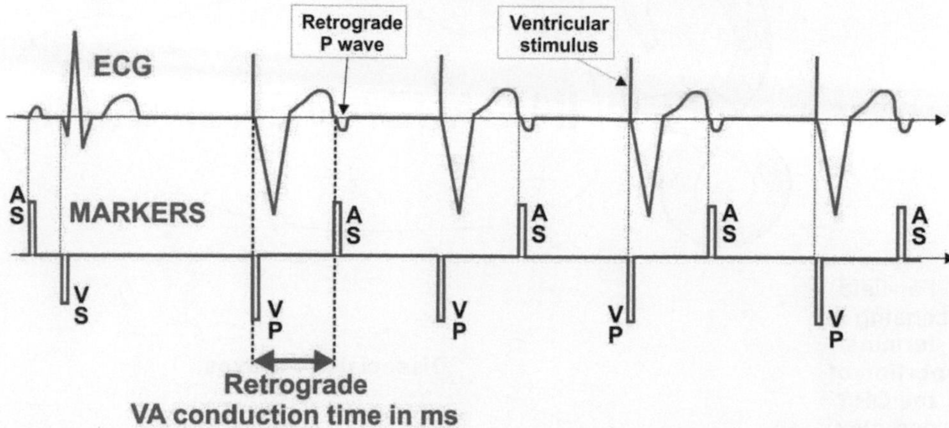

TEST FOR PROPENSITY TO ENDLESS LOOP TACHYCARDIA

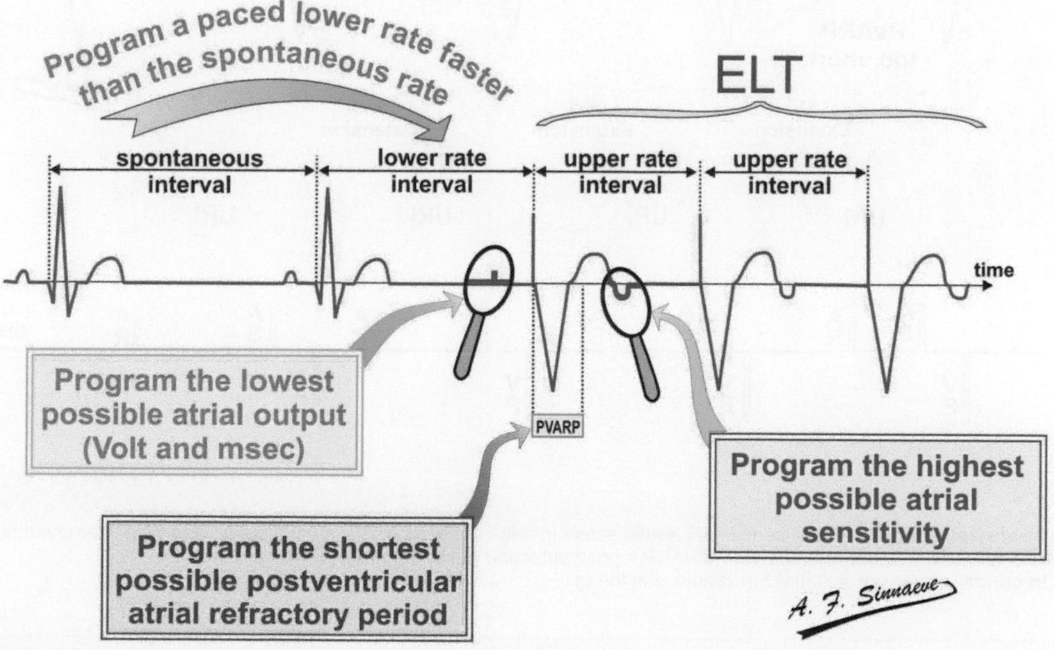

Abbreviations : AS = atrial sense ; ELT = endless loop tachycardia ; ms = millisecond ; PVARP = postventricular atrial refractory period ; VA = ventriculoatrial ; VP = ventricular pace ; VS = ventricular sense

FAR-FIELD ENDLESS LOOP TACHYCARDIA

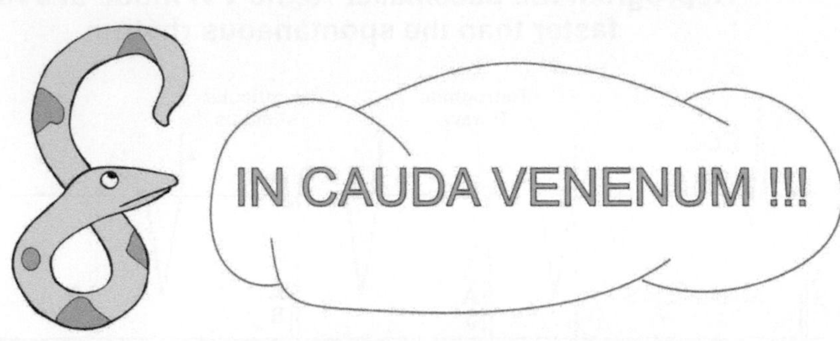

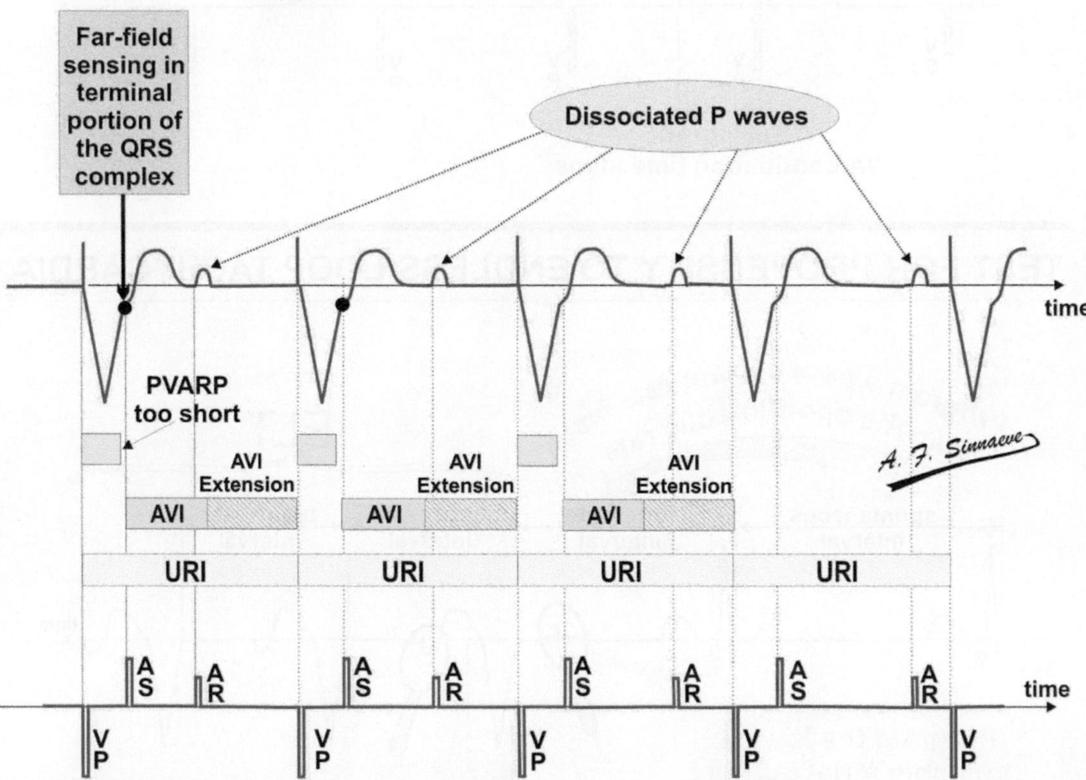

Abbreviations : AS = atrial sense ; AR =atrial sense in refractory period ; VP = ventricular pace ; AVI = atrioventricular interval ; URI = upper rate interval ; PVARP = postventricular atrial refractory period ;
In cauda venenum = (latin) the venom is in the tail !

REPETITIVE NONREENTRANT VA SYNCHRONY (RNRVAS)

A self-perpetuating process ? Another pacemaker mediated rhythm resulting from AV dyssynchrony? And the pacemaker is functioning properly? I'm stunned !!!

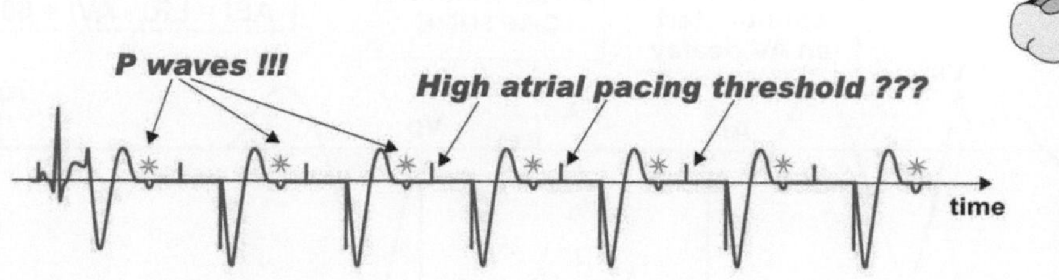

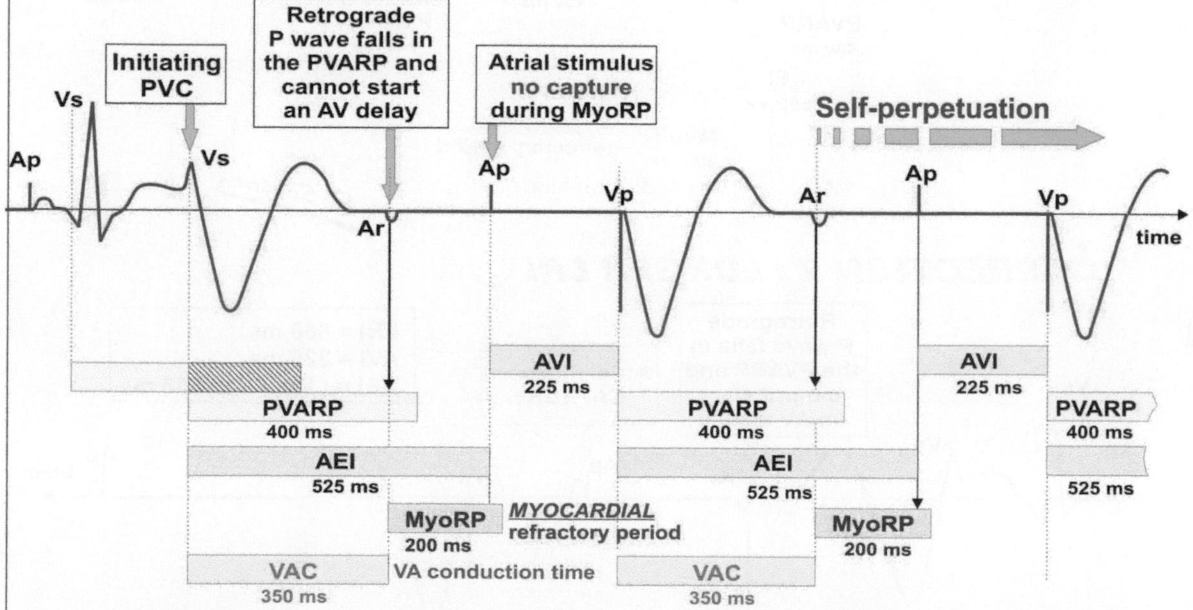

PREDISPOSING FACTORS
- Long VA conduction time
- Long PVARP
- Short LRI (lower rate interval)
- Long AVI

Abbreviations : Ap = atrial pace ; Ar = atrial sense during refractory period ; Vp = ventricular pace ; Vs = ventricular sense ; AVI = pacemaker AV delay ; PVARP = postventricular atrial refractory period ; PVC = ventricular premature complex ; AEI = atrial escape interval

A. F. Sinnaeve

RNRVAS - PREVENTION AND TREATMENT

PROLONGATION OF THE ATRIAL ESCAPE INTERVAL TO DISPLACE THE ATRIAL STIMULUS FROM THE RETROGRADE P WAVE

CORRECTION 1 : SHORTER AVI

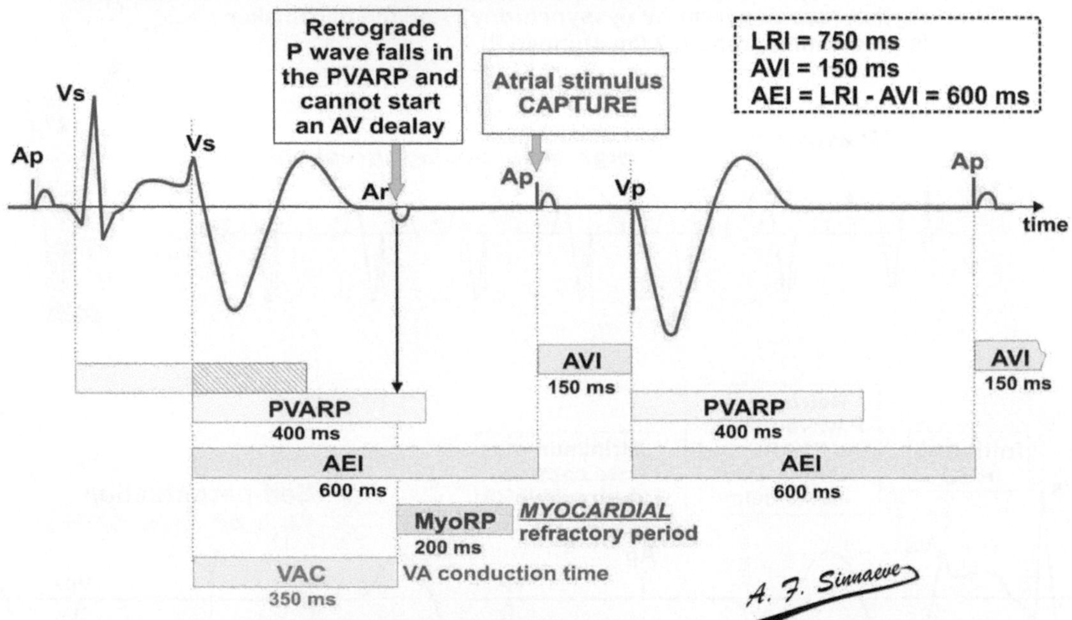

CORRECTION 2 : LONGER LRI

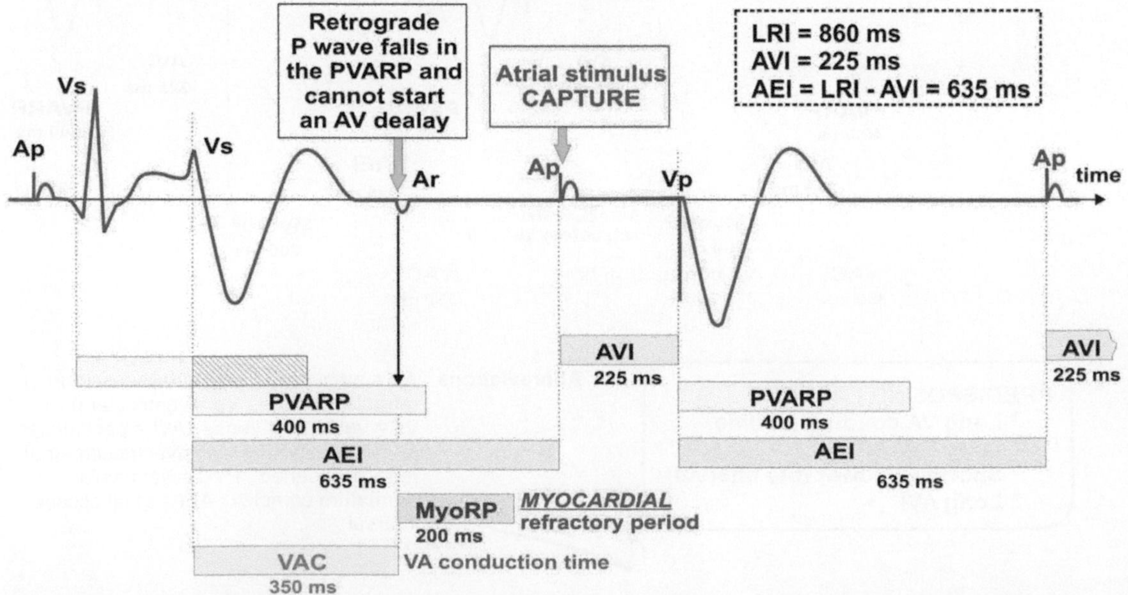

Abbreviations : AEI = atrial escape interval ; Ap = atrial pace ; Ar = atrial sense during refractory period ; Vp = ventricular pace ; Vs = ventricular sense ; AVI = pacemaker AV delay ; PVARP = postventricular atrial refractory period PVC = ventricular premature complex ; LRI = lower rate interval ; RNRVAS = repetitive nonreentrant VA synchrony

SUSTAINED PACEMAKER MEDIATED RHYTHMS RELATED TO VENTRICULOATRIAL (VA) SYNCHRONY

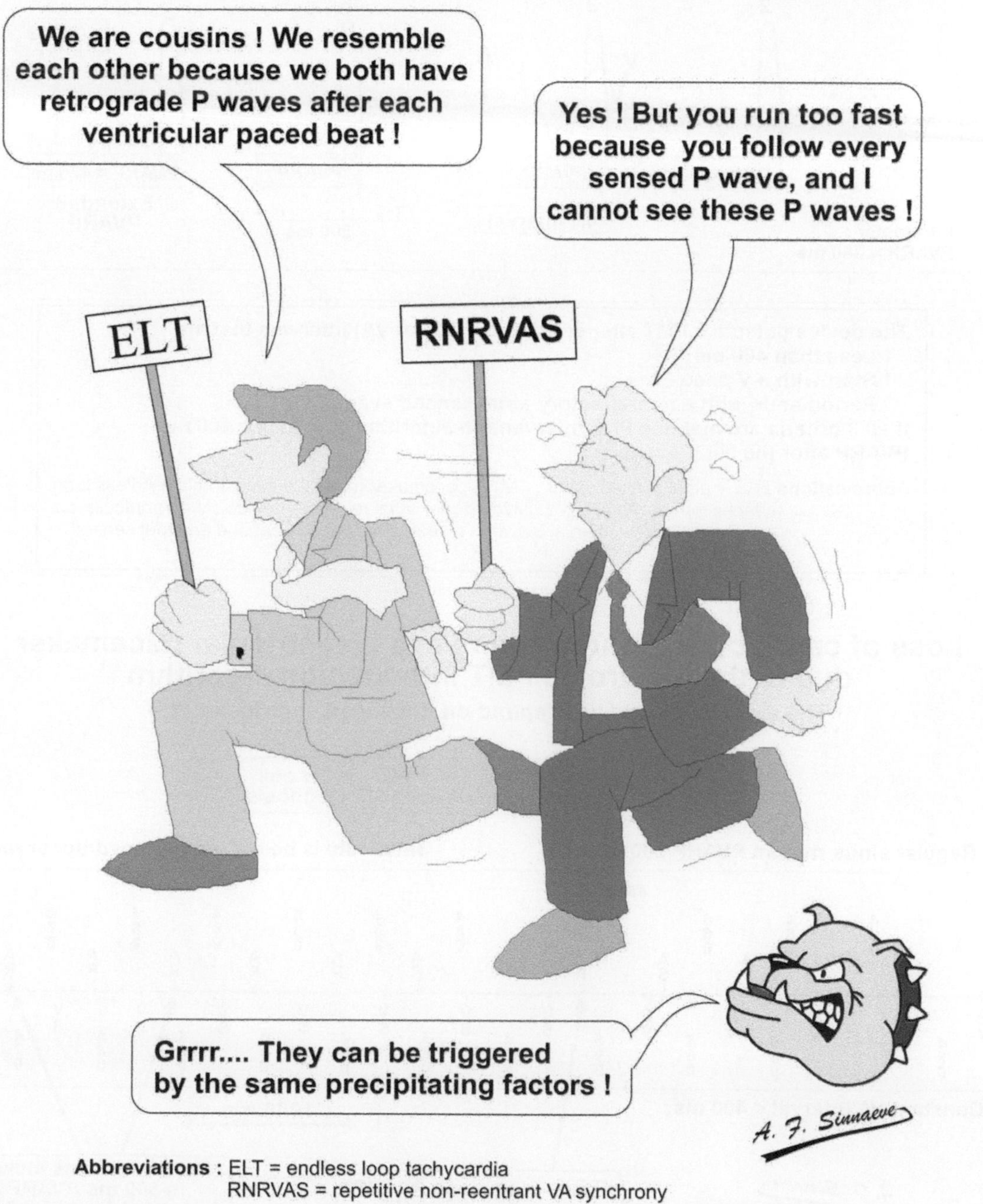

We are cousins ! We resemble each other because we both have retrograde P waves after each ventricular paced beat !
Yes ! But you run too fast because you follow every sensed P wave, and I cannot see these P waves !
ELT
RNRVAS
Grrrr.... They can be triggered by the same precipitating factors !
A. F. Sinnaeve

Abbreviations : ELT = endless loop tachycardia
RNRVAS = repetitive non-reentrant VA synchrony

MEDTRONIC PMT INTERVENTION ALGORITHM

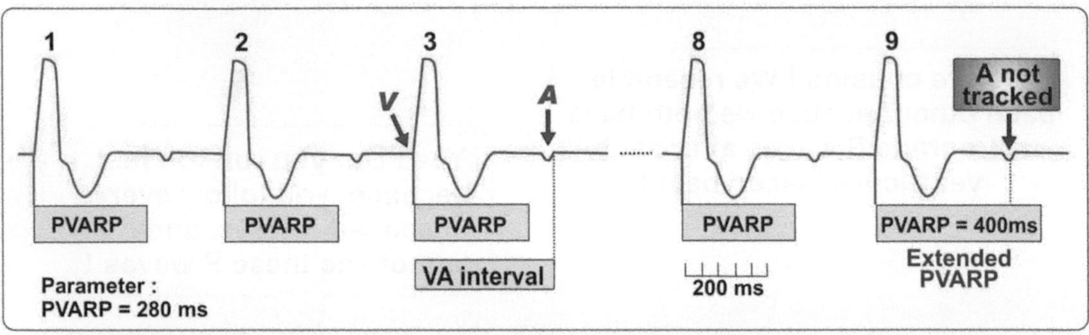

The device detects a PMT after sensing 8 V-AS (or VA) intervals that are :
*** Less than 400 ms**
*** Start with a V pace**
*** Period ends with a nonrefractory atrial sensed event**
If all 3 criteria are met, the PMT intervention algorithm activates a 400 ms PVARP after the 9th V event.

Abbreviations : AS = atrial sensed event ; PMT = pacemaker-mediated tachycardia (endless loop tachycardia) ; PVARP = postventricular atrial refractory period ; V = ventricular paced event ; VA = interval between a ventricular paced beat and an atrial sensed event ;

Loss of cardiac resynchronization in a biventricular pacemaker due to the Medtronic PMT intervention algorithm

The algorithm does not depend on the paced ventricular rate

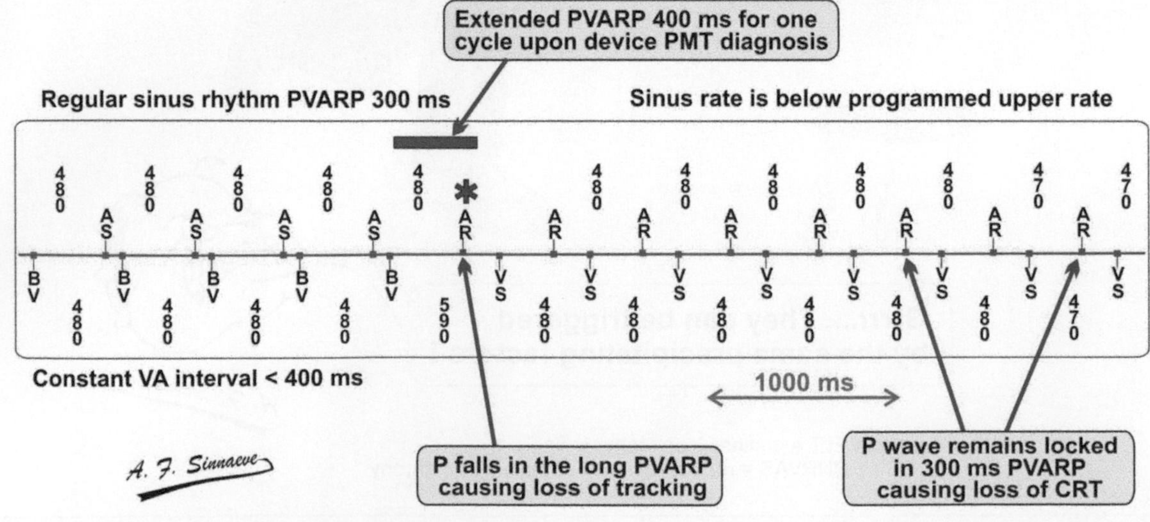

Abbreviations : AR = atrial event sensed in the atrial refractory period ; AS = atrial sensed event ; BV = BiV pacing ; CRT = cardiac resynchronization therapy ; PVARP = postventricular atrial refractory period ; VS = ventricular sensed event ;

PMT TERMINATION ALGORITHMS

St JUDE Algorithm :

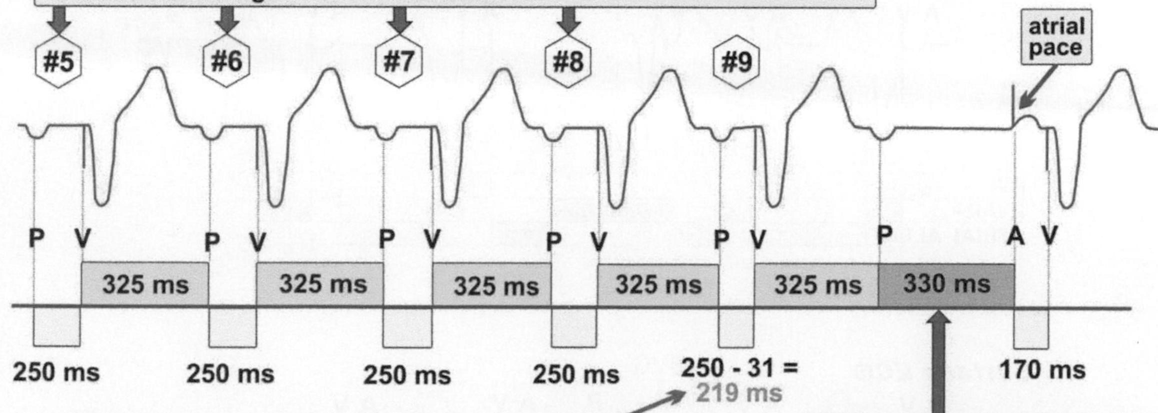

Abbreviations : AS = atrial sensed event ; A = atrial stimulus ; P = sensed P wave ; PMT = pacemaker mediated tachycardia ; V = ventricular stimulus ;

BOSTON SCIENTIFIC Algorithm :

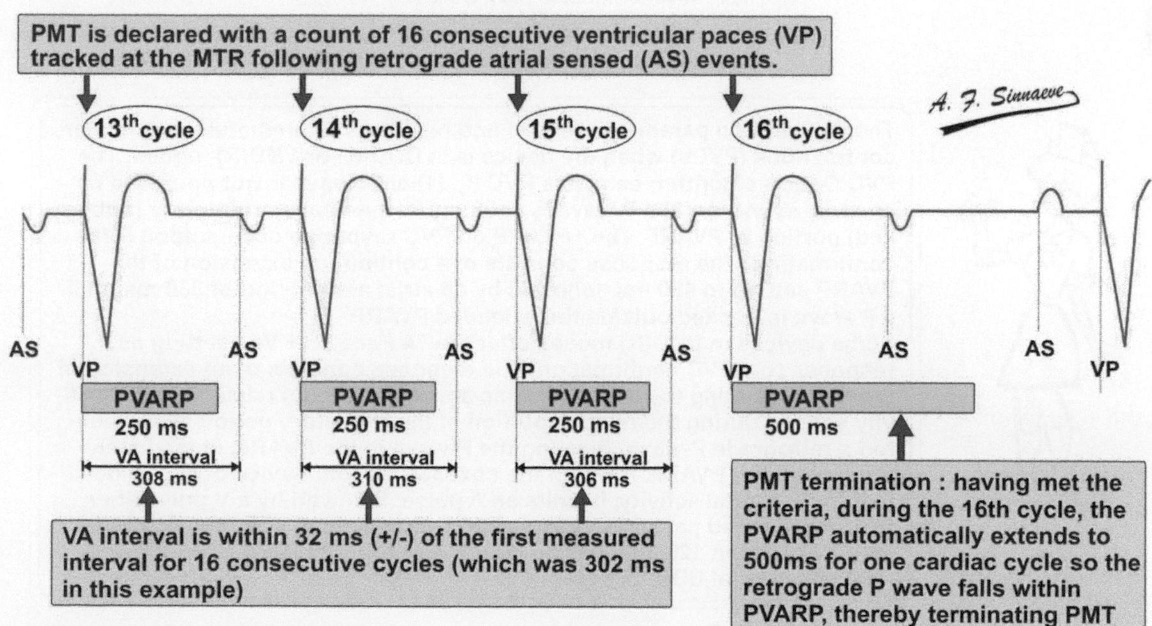

Abbreviations : AS = Atrial sensed event ; MTR = maximum tracking rate ; PMT = pacemaker mediated tachycardia ; PVARP = postventricular atrial refractory period ; VP = ventricular paced event ;

ATRIAL PACE ON PVC (St JUDE)

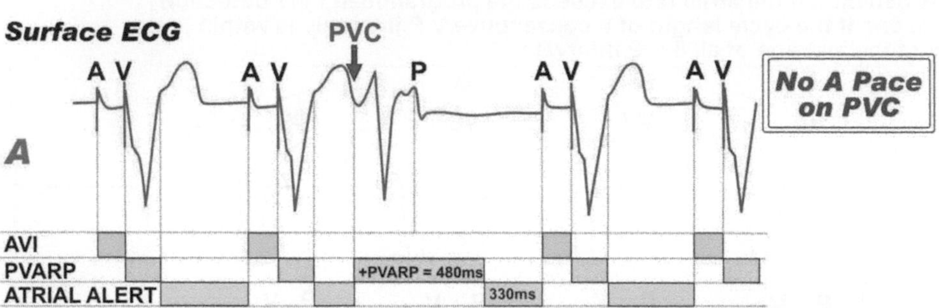

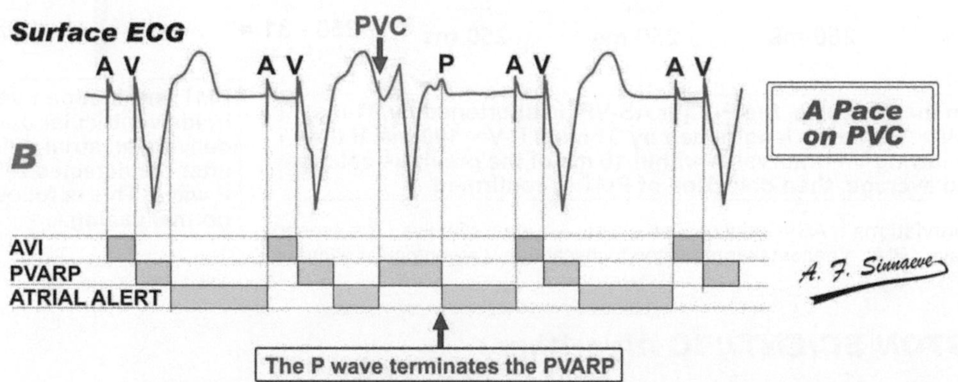

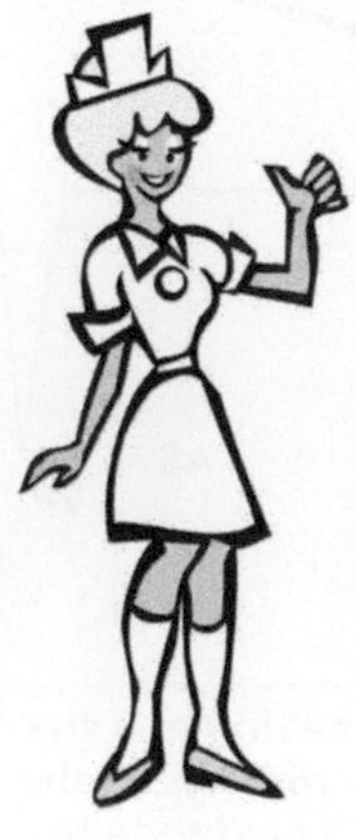

The PVC Option parameter detects and responds to premature ventricular contractions (PVCs) when the device is in DDD(R) or VDD(R) modes. The PVC Option algorithm detects a PVC if : (1) an R wave is not preceded by an atrial event; or (2) a P wave is detected in the relative refractory (unblanked) portion of PVARP. The +PVARP on PVC response occurs upon PVC confirmation. The response consists of a continuous extension of the PVARP setting to 480 ms, followed by an atrial alert period of 330 ms until a P-wave is tracked outside the extended PVARP.
Some devices in DDD(R) modes offer the *"A Pace on PVC"* setting as a response to a PVC confirmation. The response consists of an extension of the PVARP setting to 480 ms (150 ms absolute, 330 ms relative). Atrial activity sensed during the relative portion of the refractory period is considered a retrograde P-wave. Sensing the P-wave in the PVARP, immediately terminates the PVARP. If within the next 330 ms, the device does not detect further atrial activity, it emits an A pulse, followed by a V pulse after the programmed paced AV delay setting. If the device does sense atrial activity between 120 and 330 ms after the retrograde P-wave, the device resumes normal DDD timing.

Abbreviations : AVI = atrioventricular interval or AV delay ; PVARP = postventricular atrial refractory period ; PVC = premature ventricular complex ;

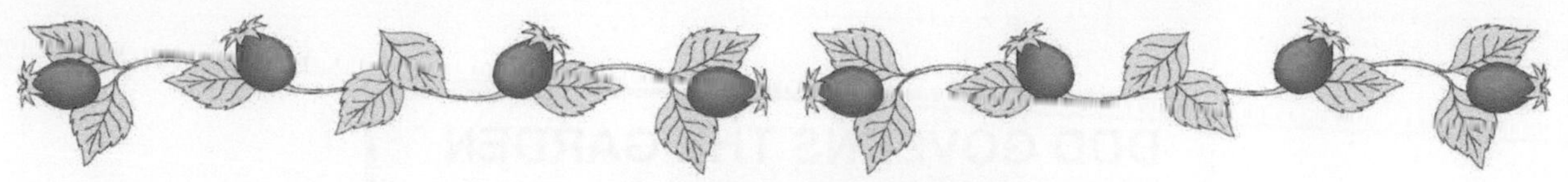

DDD

DVI ? VDD ? DOO ? DDI ?

ALL DUAL CHAMBER PACEMAKERS FUNCTION IN THE DDD MODE

* The garden of dual chamber pacemakers
* The DVI mode
* The DDI mode
* The VDD mode
* Two types of VDD timing cycles
* Single lead VDD pacing
* Selection of pacing mode - 1 & 2
* Choice of the pacing site
* RV apical pacing and risk of LV dysfunction
* Alternative RV pacing sites
* RV outflow tract & septal pacing
* His bundle pacing
* Importance of the atrial pacing site
* Selection of a pacing site

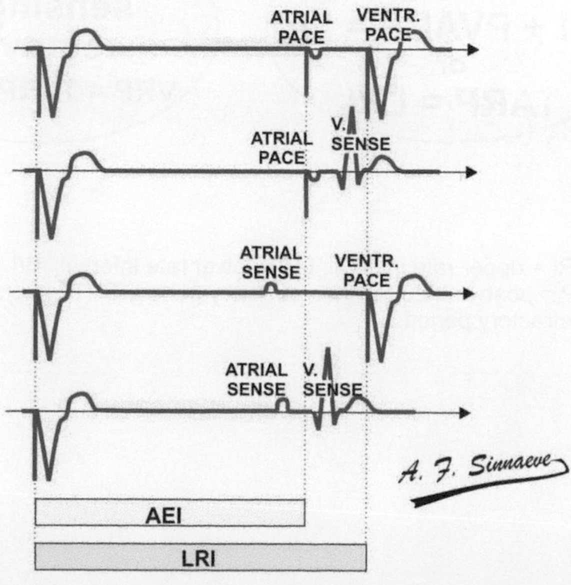

DDD GOVERNS THE GARDEN OF DUAL CHAMBER PACING

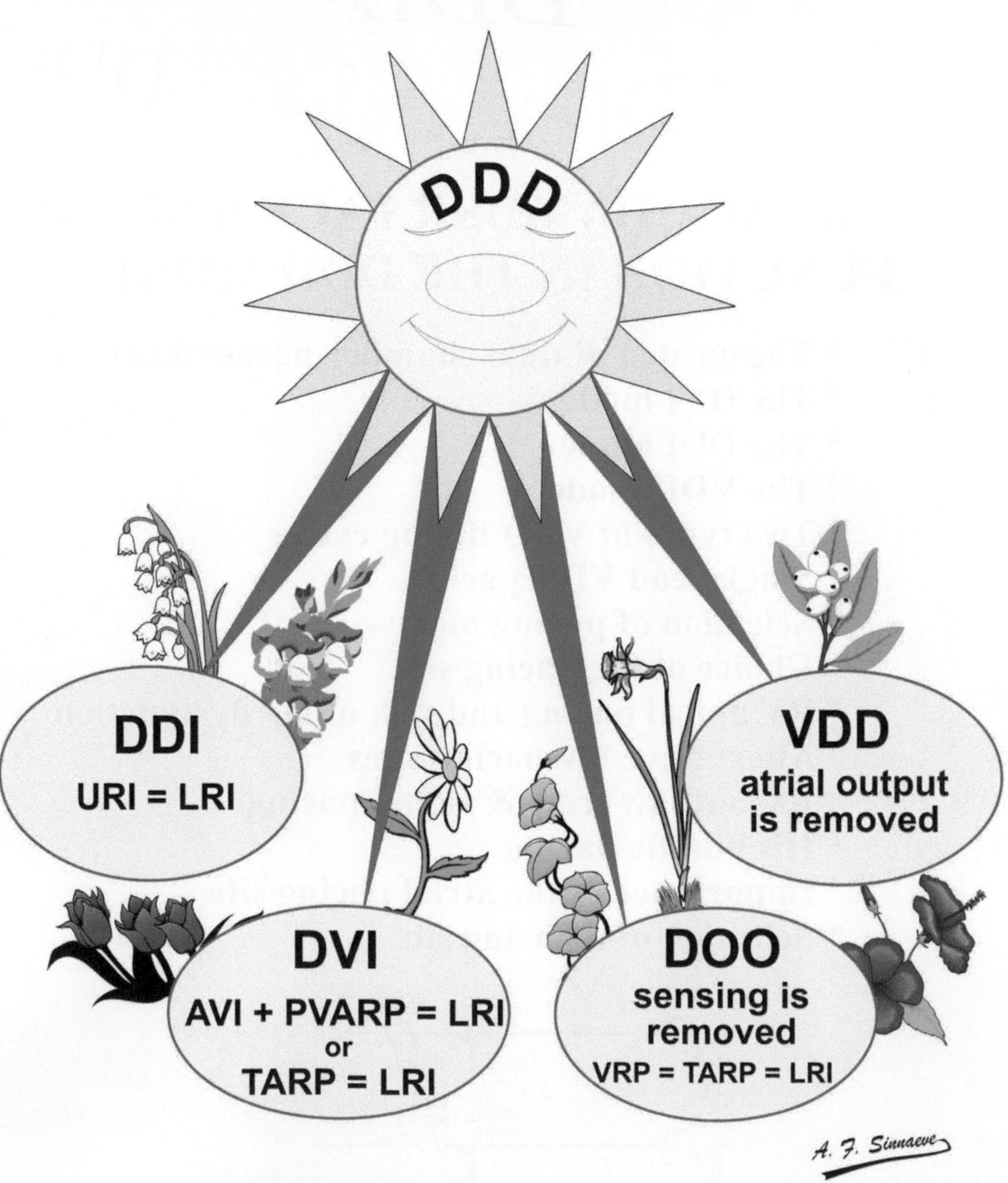

Abbreviations : URI = upper rate interval; LRI = lower rate interval; AVI = atrioventricular interval or AV delay; PVARP = postventricular atrial refractory period; TARP = total atrial refractory period; VRP = ventricular refractory period.

DUAL CHAMBER PACING in DVI MODE

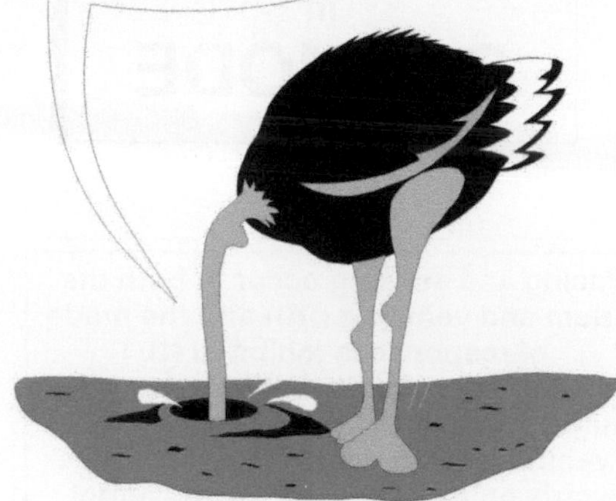

Pacing occurs in both the atrium and ventricle (D) but there is only sensing in the ventricle (V). The mode of response is inhibition (I). No sensing of the atrial electrogram and lack of tracking results in asynchronous atrial pacing (competitive atrial pacing may precipitate atrial fibrillation).

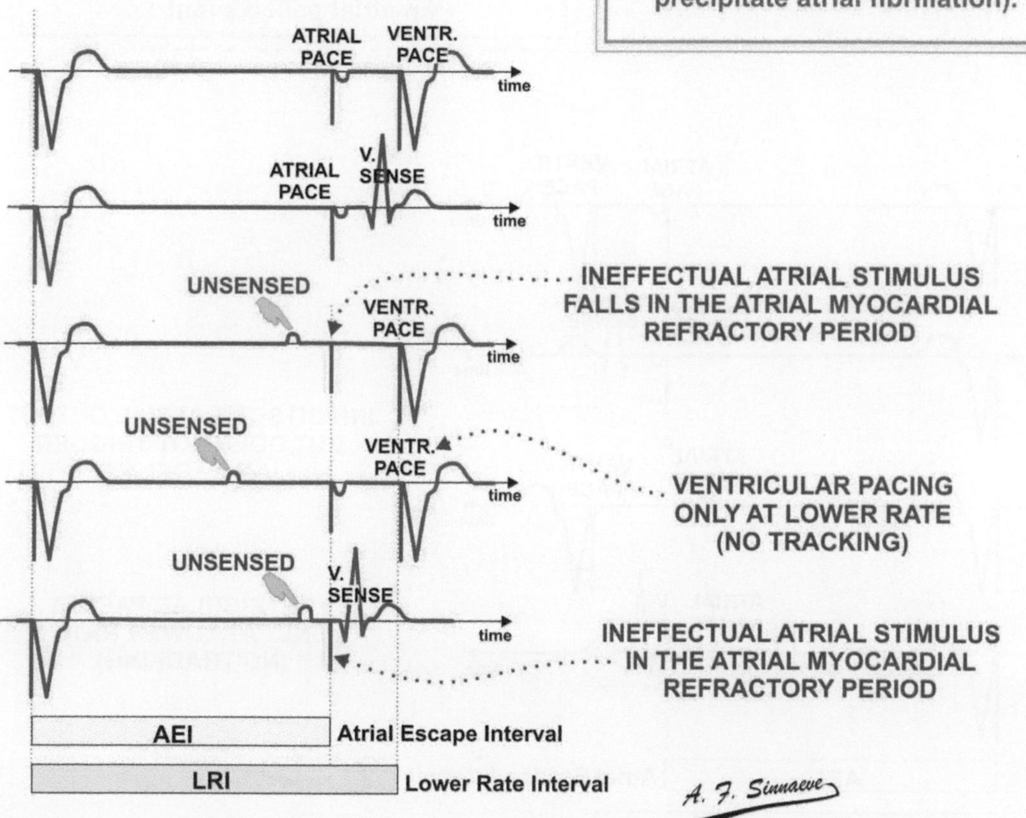

A. F. Sinnaeve

DUAL CHAMBER PACING in DDI MODE

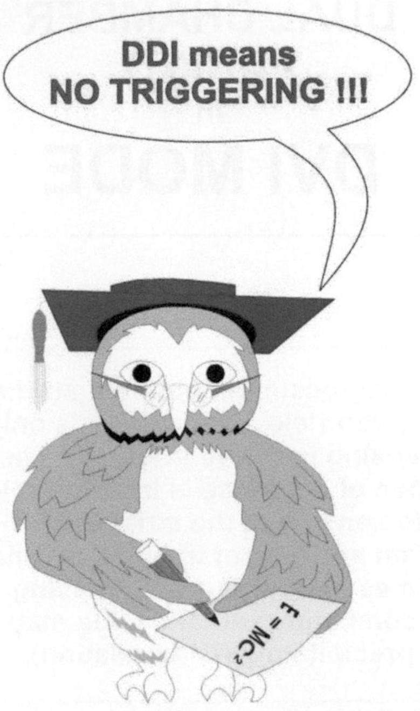

Pacing and sensing occur in both the atrium and ventricle (DD) and the mode of response is inhibited (I).
Sensed atrial activity inhibits the atrial output impulse, but does not trigger a ventricular output impulse. In other words an atrial sensed event cannot produce a physiologic AV delay equal or shorter to the AV delay initiated by an atrial paced event .

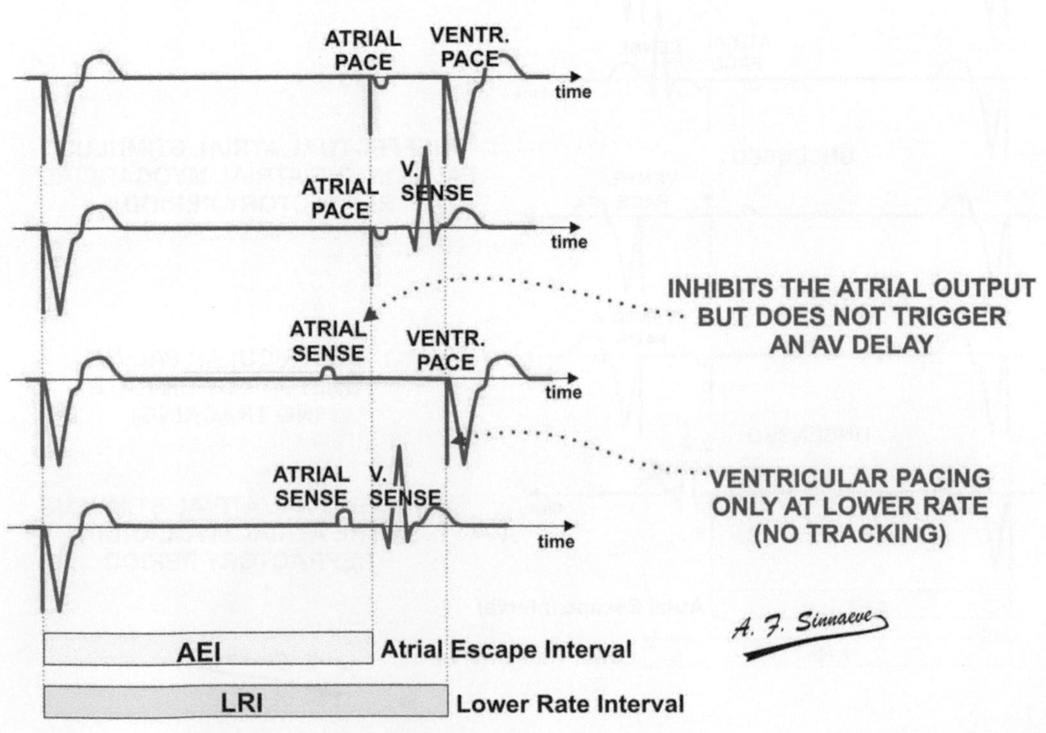

DUAL CHAMBER PACING in VDD MODE

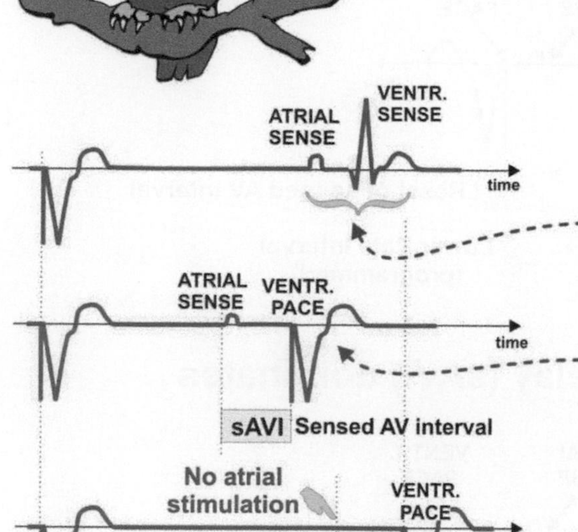

In the VDD mode there is no atrial stimulus and therefore no AV crosstalk. There are no crosstalk timing cycles : postatrial ventricular blanking period and ventricular safety pacing function.
But, this is not for me... This is for young people and they can have fast upper rates!!!

Pacing occurs in the ventricle only (V) but there is sensing in both the atrium and ventricle (D). The mode of response is inhibition and triggering (D).
A sensed atrial event triggers (T) a ventricular stimulus after completion of the AVI. A sensed ventricular event inhibits the ventricular output (I). Hence the response is T + I = D.

ATRIAL SENSE
VENTR. SENSE
time
Atrial sensing. Conducted QRS occurs before completion of the AV delay and therefore inhibits the ventricular stimulus
ATRIAL SENSE
VENTR. PACE
time
sAVI Sensed AV interval
Atrial tracking : atrial sensing followed by ventricular pacing after the programmed AV delay
No atrial stimulation
VENTR. PACE
time
VVI pacing at the lower rate during sinus bradycardia slower than the programmed pacemaker lower rate
As there is no atrial stimulation, there is no need for an atrial escape interval
VENTR. SENSE
time
Resets the lower rate interval
ATRIAL SENSE
VENTR. PACE
time
The P wave is sensed but not tracked, i.e. it does not trigger a ventricular stimulus after the programmed AV delay. The P wave is not tracked because it falls in the implied AV delay which terminates with the emission of a ventricular stimulus at the completion of the lower rate interval.
Reset of sensed AV interval
LRI
Lower Rate Interval (programmed)
A. F. Sinnaeve

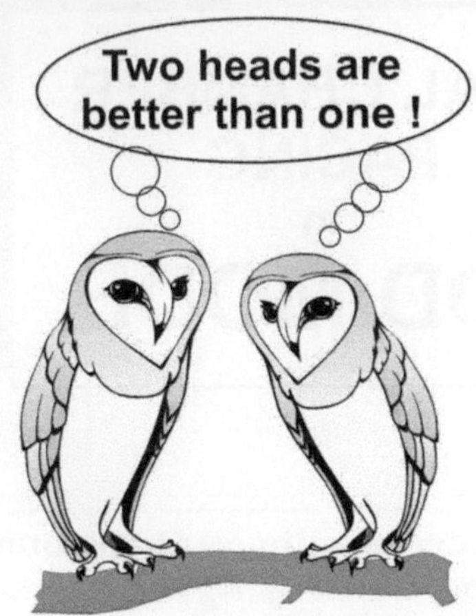

2 TYPES OF VDD TIMING CYCLES

TYPE 1 : The lower rate interval dominates

TYPE 2 : The AV delay (sAVI) dominates

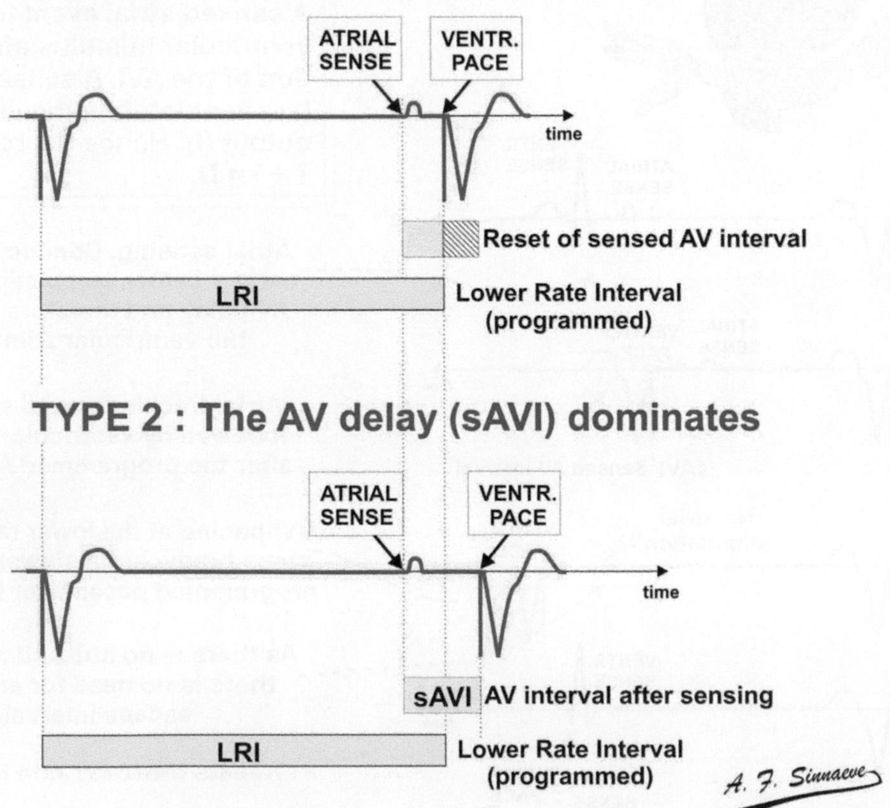

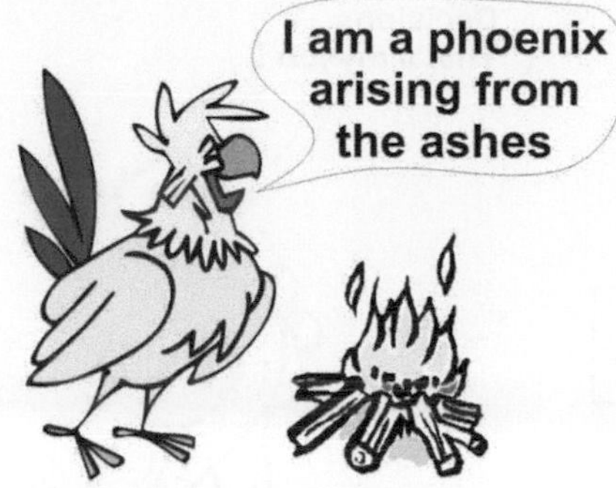

SINGLE LEAD VDD PACING

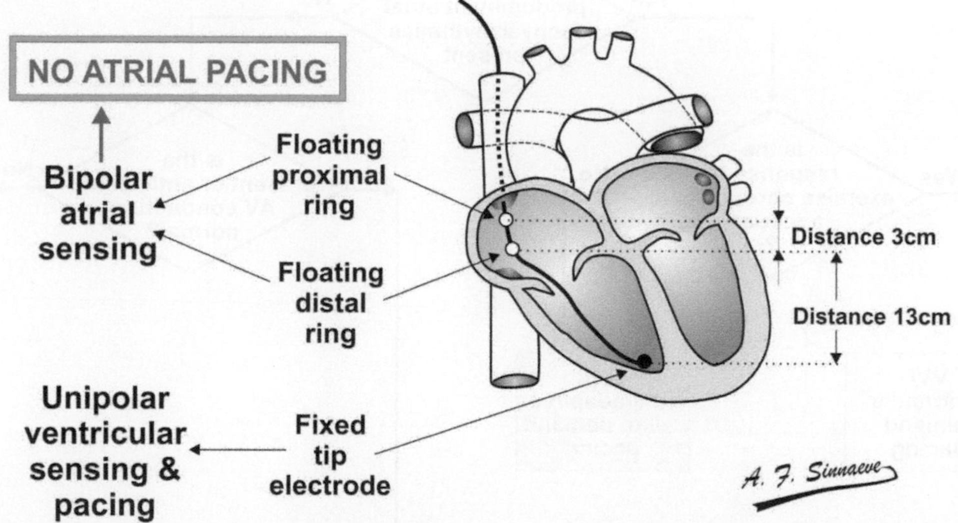

Atrial signals from floating (non-contact) electrodes tend to be small and therefore high atrial sensitivity is required for sensing

This system should not be used in patients with sick sinus syndrome (sinus bradycardia) or atrial chronotropic incompetence (abnormal response of atrial rate on exercise)

WHICH PACING MODE SHOULD BE CHOSEN? A DECISION TREE

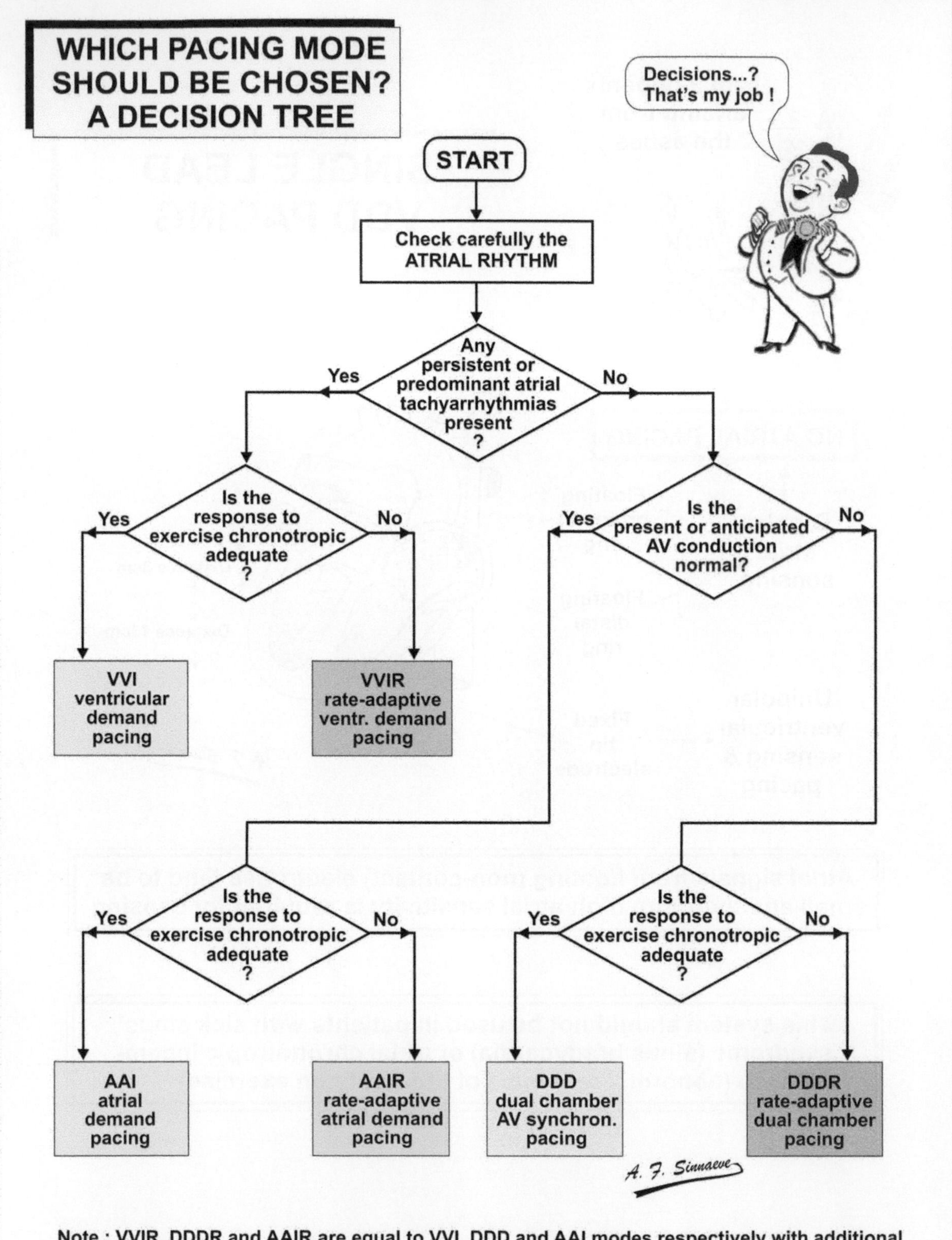

Decisions...?
That's my job !
START
Check carefully the ATRIAL RHYTHM
Any persistent or predominant atrial tachyarrhythmias present ?
Yes
No
Is the response to exercise chronotropic adequate ?
Yes
No
VVI ventricular demand pacing
VVIR rate-adaptive ventr. demand pacing
Is the present or anticipated AV conduction normal?
Yes
No
Is the response to exercise chronotropic adequate ?
Yes
No
AAI atrial demand pacing
AAIR rate-adaptive atrial demand pacing
Is the response to exercise chronotropic adequate ?
Yes
No
DDD dual chamber AV synchron. pacing
DDDR rate-adaptive dual chamber pacing
A. F. Sinnaeve

Note : VVIR, DDDR and AAIR are equal to VVI, DDD and AAI modes respectively with additional rate-adaptive function provided by an artificial sensor for rate increase on activity.

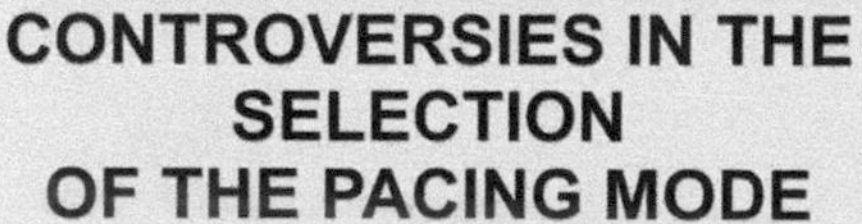

JOGGING PATH

Well, in Europe we believe that they can be used in patients with sick sinus syndrome if there is no AV block or bundle branch block.
AAI and AAIR allow normal ventricular depolarization which promotes better left ventricular function.

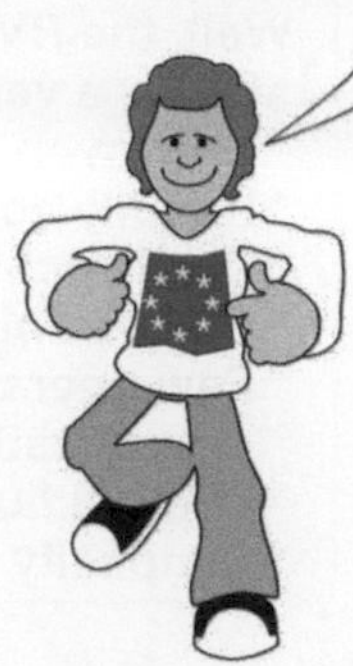

We, in America believe that AAI and AAIR are obsolete ! They are rarely used in the USA

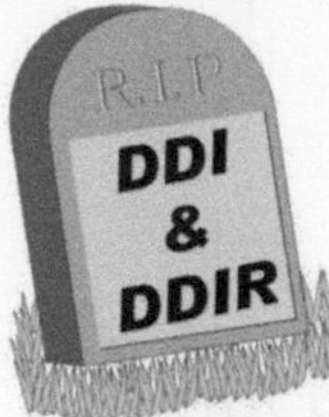

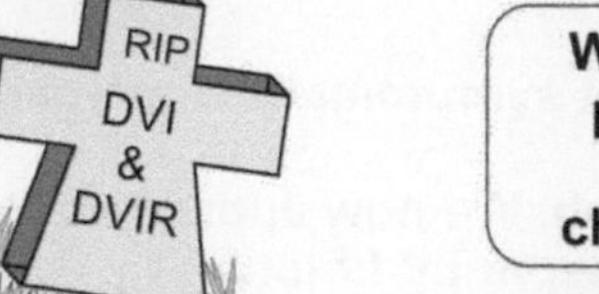

We, in the USA, prefer 2 leads for dual chamber pacing

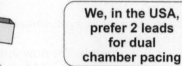

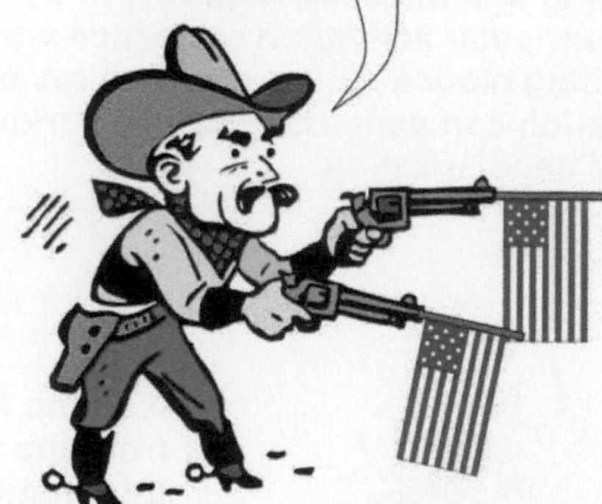

We Europeans believe that VDD is useful in patients with AV block and no atrial chronotropic incompetence in whom the sinus rate increases normally with exercise

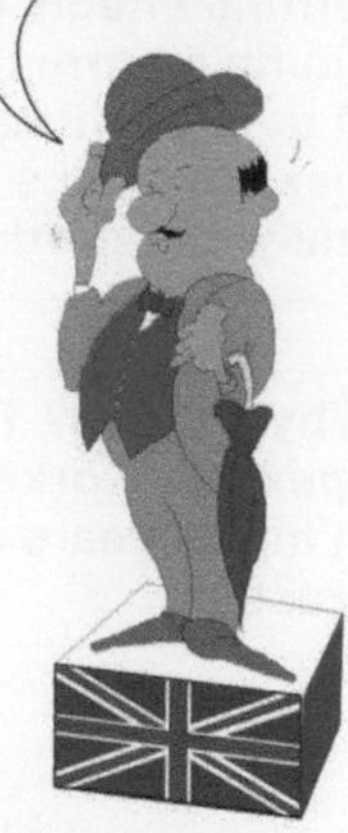

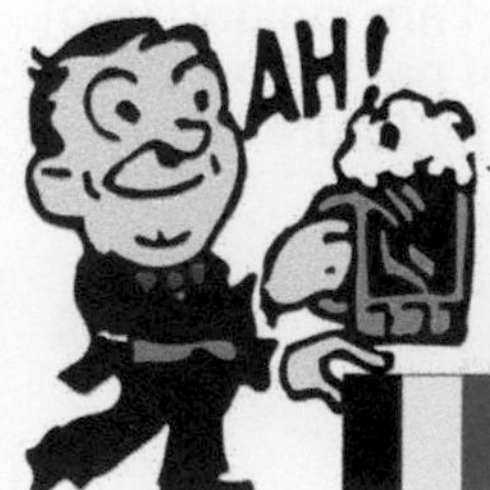

OK, you are all right there... But the Belgian beer is the best there is !!!

A. F. Sinnaeve

IS THE RV APEX STILL THE RIGHT PLACE TO PACE ?

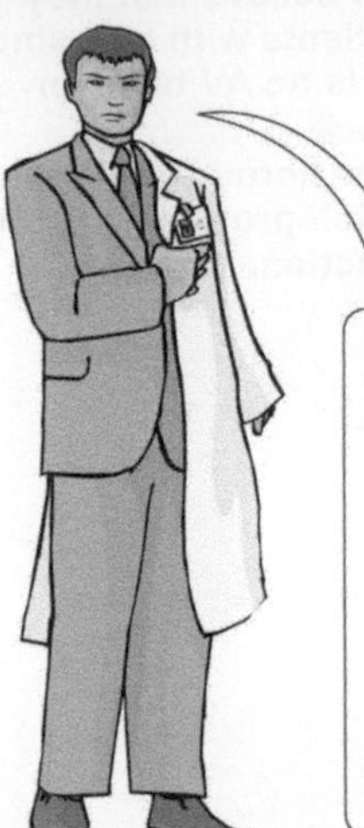

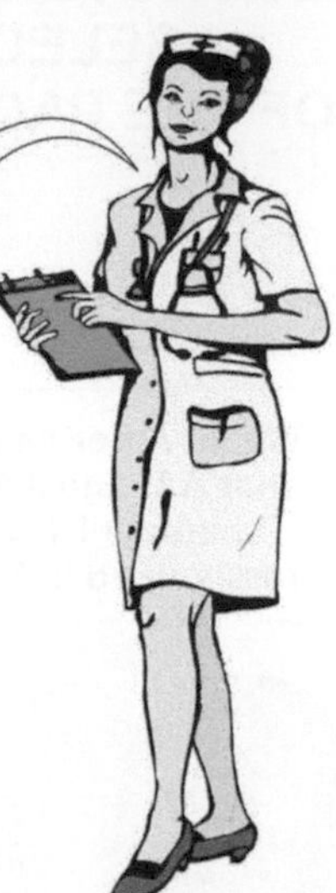

Doctor, why has RV apical pacing been so popular for such a long time ?
Well, the RV apex has been an attractive site for a variety of reasons :
* Unproven and unscientific tradition
* Readily accessible
* Easily achieved
* Lead stability
* Few operative and postoperative complications
* Limited fluoroscopy
* Simplicity and reliability

There are new developments in the area of pacing for bradycardia (as well as for ICD patients).

The traditional use of pacing has always been to prevent symptomatic bradycardia and provide chronotropic competence when necessary.
In the last decade we have learned that this is not enough. We now appreciate the harmful effects of RV apical pacing and the need to preserve LV function by maintaining a normal or improved ventricular activation sequence whenever possible by using minimal ventricular pacing modes and/or pacing sites away from the RV apex. One aims where the activation can penetrate the His-Purkinje system more easily and produce improved LV depolarization.

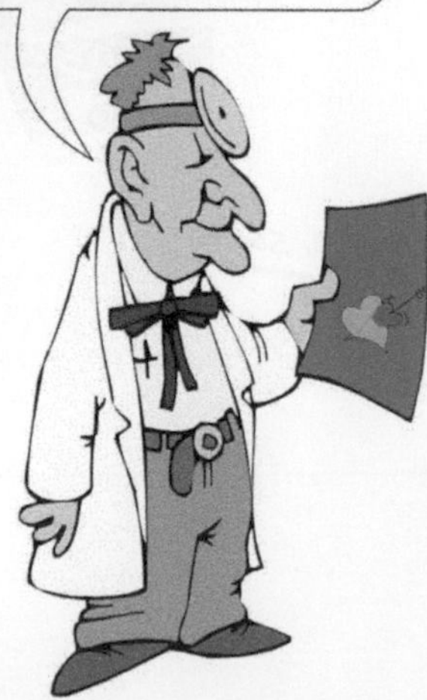

Why change? The RV apex has worked fine in my 40 years of practice.

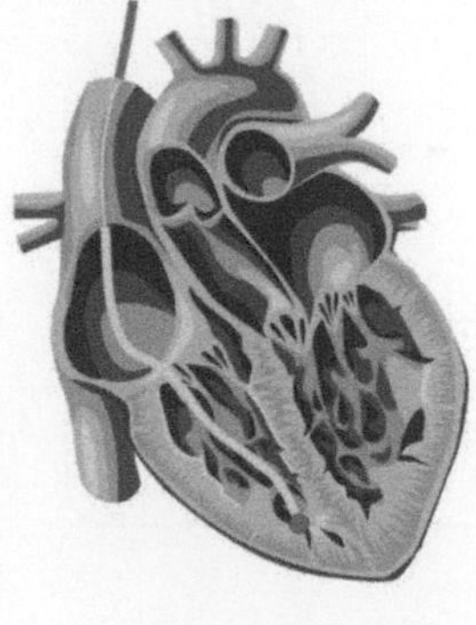

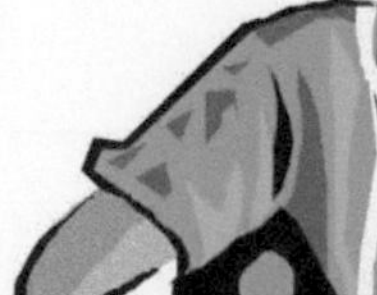

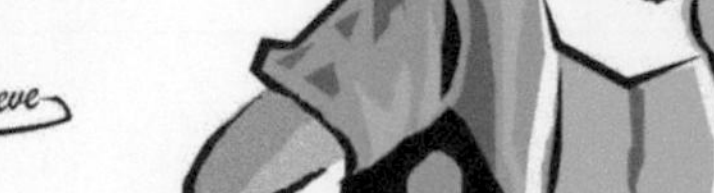

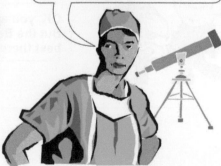

Abbreviations : ICD = implantable cardioverter-defibrillator ; LV = left ventricle ; RV = right ventricle

LONG-TERM RISK OF LV DYSFUNCTION AND HEART FAILURE WITH RV APICAL PACING

Deleterious effects of right ventricular apical pacing

* Intra-LV conduction delay
* LV mechanical dyssynchrony
* Heterogeneous myocardial perfusion and metabolism
* Heterogeneous contraction and relaxation within the LV
* Molecular : Regional disparities in protein expression
* Abnormalities in myocardial histopathology : Cellular disarray
* LV remodeling with asymmetric hypertrophy
* Heart failure
* Mitral regurgitation
* Atrial fibrillation, increased LA size

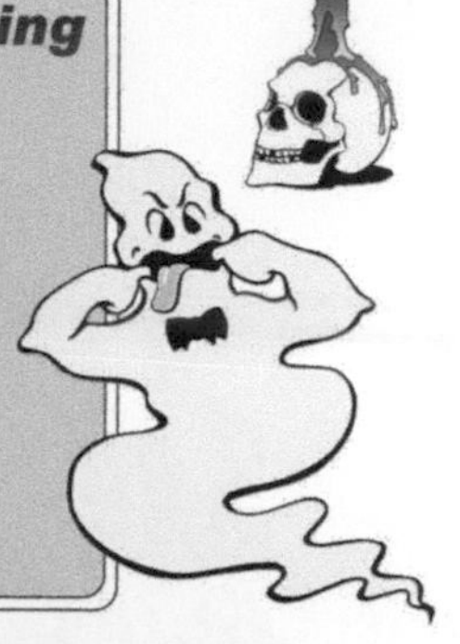

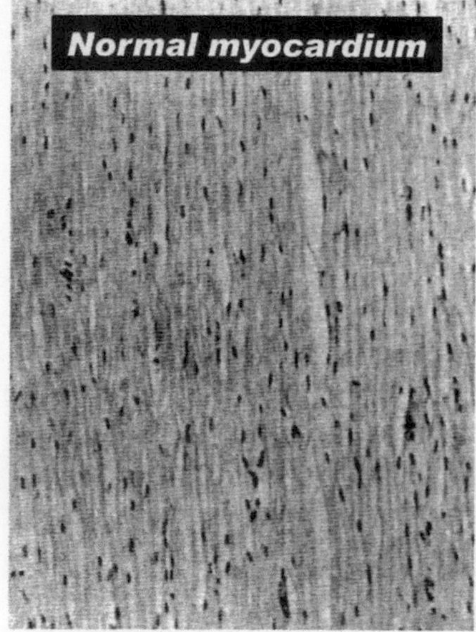

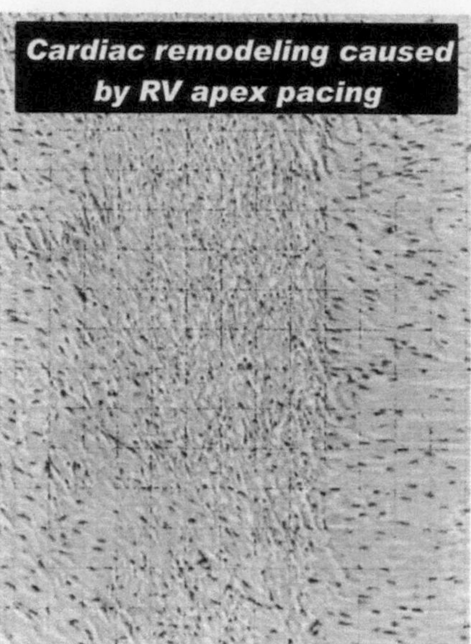

Profound myocardial disarray following 6 months of RV apical pacing

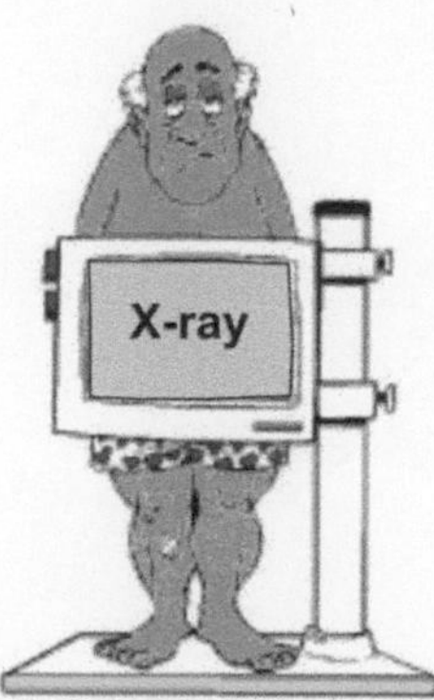
X-ray

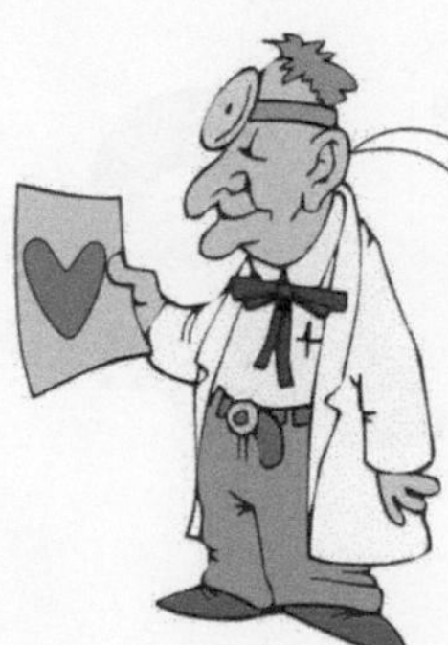
The RV pacemaker is OK 3 years after implantation but the previously normal LV is now dysfunctional !

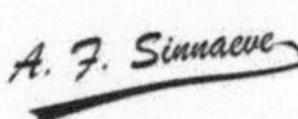

LONG-TERM RISK of LV DYSFUNCTION and HEART FAILURE with RV APICAL PACING

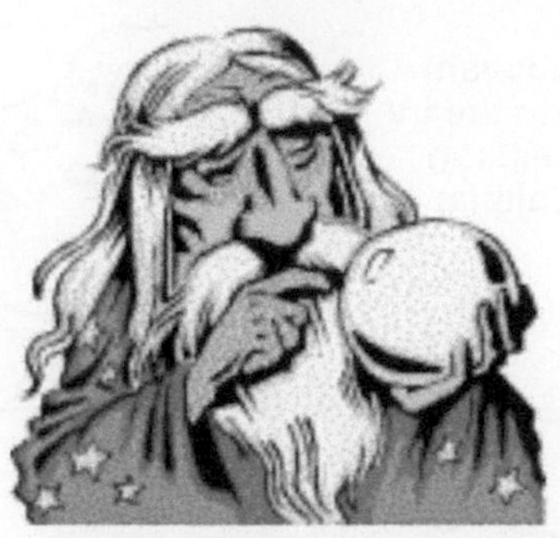

We cannot predict the risk of HF in patients with RV apical pacing but we know some of the risk factors (excluding Cum% VP) for the development of new LV dysfunction (or aggravation of pre-existing LV dysfunction) and new HF (or aggravation of HF documented before implantation) :

* **Older age**
* **Coronary artery disease**
* **Pre-existing LV dysfunction**
* **Wide QRS complex**

- **With long-term RV apical pacing (> 90% ventricular pacing) for acquired AV block in patients with normal LVEF without a prior history of HF, new-onset HF develops in about 25% in about 8 years or earlier.**
- **7% of chronically paced children develop heart failure after an average of 8 years of RV pacing.**

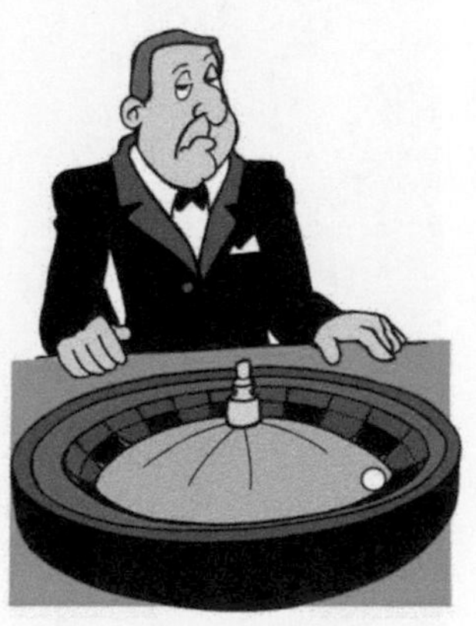

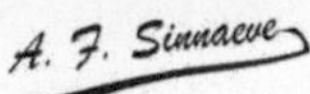

The prediction of HF due to RV apical pacing is extremely difficult !

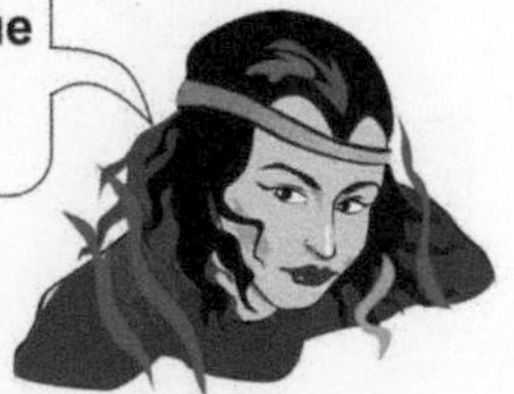

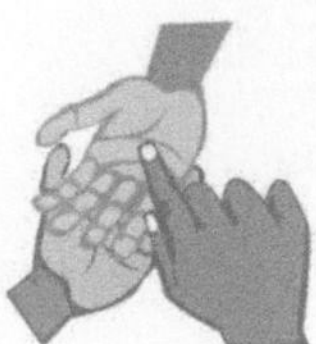

Abbreviations : Cum% VP = cumulative % ventricular pacing ; CAD = coronary artery disease ; HF heart failure ; LV = left ventricle ; RV = right ventricle ; LVEF = left ventricular ejection fraction ;

ALTERNATIVE RV PACING SITES

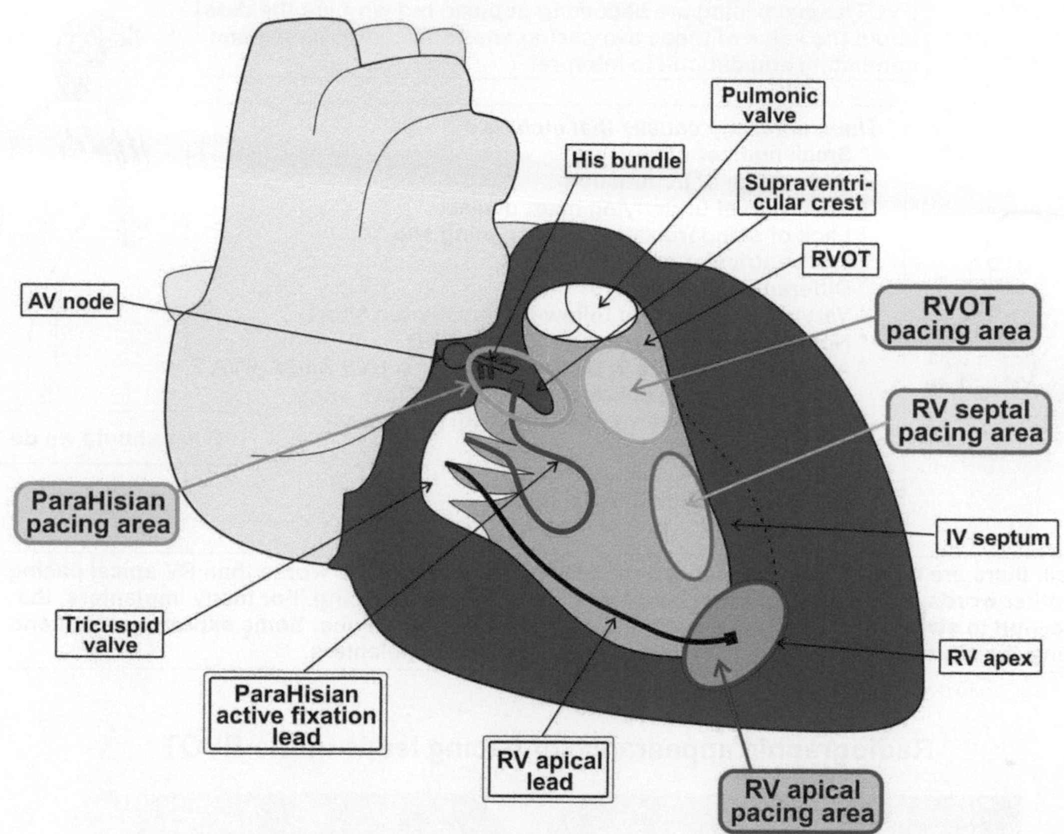

BASIC ANATOMY OF THE RV OUTFLOW TRACT

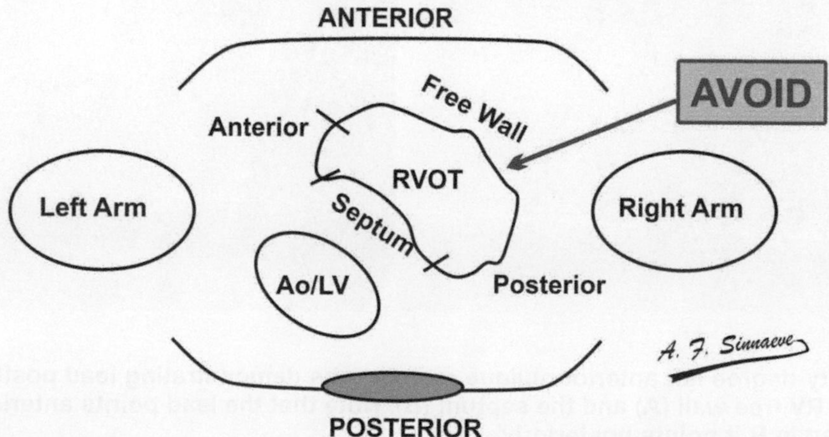

Abbreviations : Ao = aorta ; AV = atrioventricular ; IV = interventricular ; LV = left ventricle ; RV = right ventricle ; RVOT = RV outflow tract

RIGHT VENTRICULAR OUTFLOW TRACT / SEPTAL PACING

RVOT/septal pacing are becoming popular, but why are the data about the value of these two pacing sites still controversial and conflicting and difficult to interpret ?

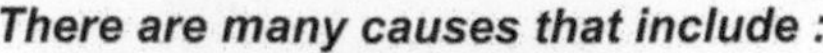

There are many causes that include :

* Small number of patients
* Wide range of LV function
* Spectrum of underlying heart disease
* Lack of standardization of RV pacing site
* ? % ventricular pacing
* Different endpoints
* Varying durations of follow-up (mostly too short)
* Non-physiological pacing : VVI not DDD
* Arbitrary AV delays in DDD : similar for A-RVS and A-RVA ? 30-50 ms delay in conduction between these sites
* Many studies involved patients with permanent atrial fibrillation
* QRS duration ?
* Long-term studies are needed !

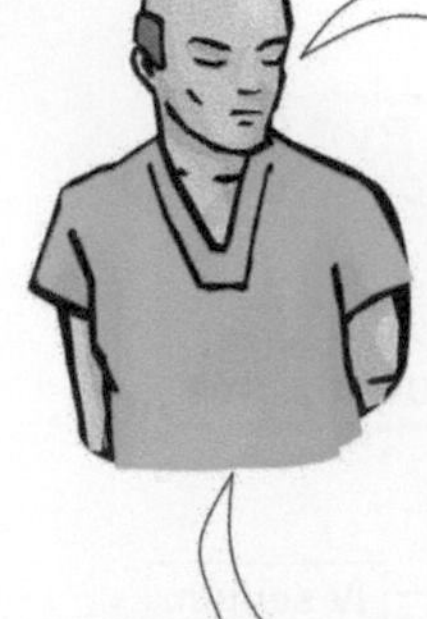

What should we do ?

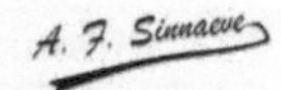

Well, there are no data to cause concern that RVOT/septal pacing is worse than RV apical pacing. In other words, RVOT/septal pacing is not inferior to RV apical pacing. For many implanters, the decision to switch to RVOT/septal sites is basically an emotional one. Some experts recommend using the sites in all patients and train a new generation of implanters.

Radiographic appearance of pacing leads in the RVOT

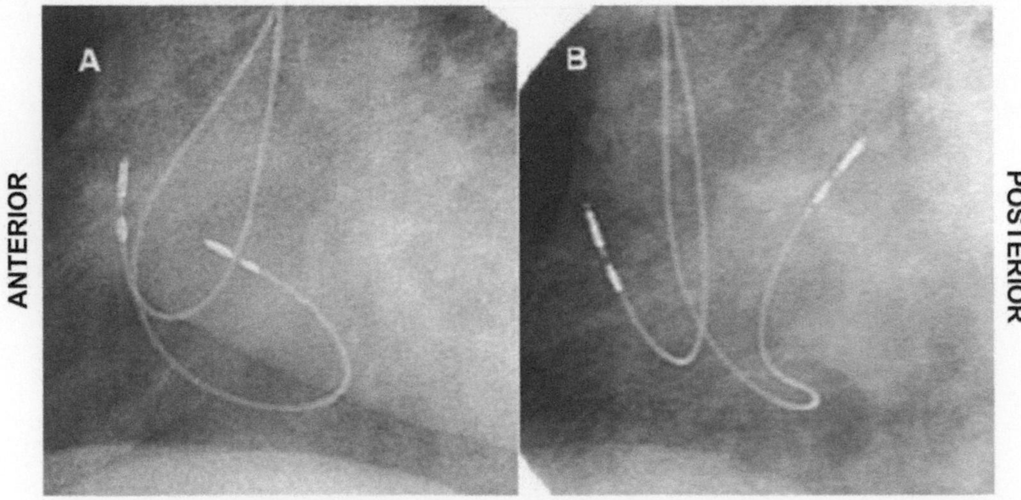

Forty-degree left anterior oblique radiographs demonstrating lead position on the RV free wall (A) and the septum (B). Note that the lead points anteriorly in A but in B it points posteriorly.

Abbreviations : RVA = right ventricular apex ; RVOT = right ventricular outflow tract ; RVS = right ventricular septum

RIGHT VENTRICULAR OUTFLOW TRACT / SEPTAL PACING
continued

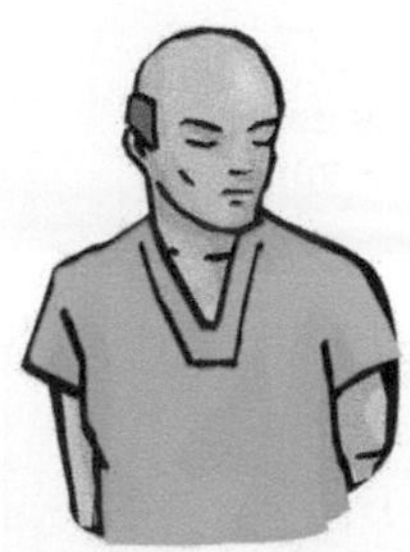

RVOT pacing generates a LBBB pattern with an inferior axis. Pacing from the septal and free wall aspects of the RVOT are associated with different ECG patterns which is a function of their relative anatomical relationship, with the septum being a more posterior and leftward structure than the free wall. As such, a negative vector in lead I is a highly specific feature of septal lead placement. Septal pacing may also cause an isoelectric complex in lead I. These two ECG patterns are not sensitive. Septal pacing is also associated with a shorter QRS duration than RV free wall pacing. Notching in the inferior leads is a function of prolonged total activation time during pacing from the free wall, which may reflect late activation of the left ventricular lateral wall.

A. F. Sinnaeve

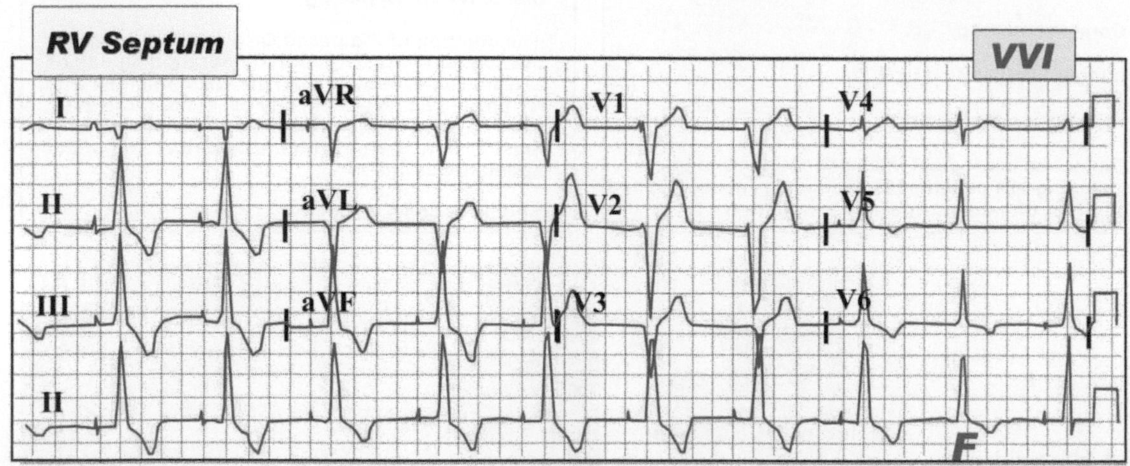

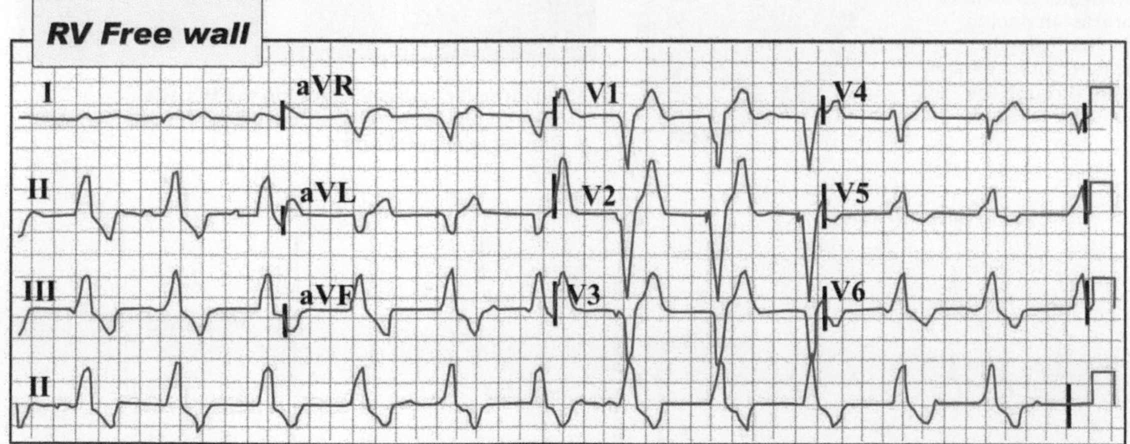

Typical ECG appearance of pacing from the free wall and septal aspects of the RV outflow tract. QRS duration is shorter with septal pacing and is often associated with a negative vector in lead I. Notching of the inferior leads is more often seen in free wall pacing.

Abbreviations : F = fusion ; LBBB = left bundle branch block ; RVOT = right ventricular outflow tract

HIS BUNDLE PACING

There is a lot of interest recently about His bundle pacing. Do you think it is a viable technique ?

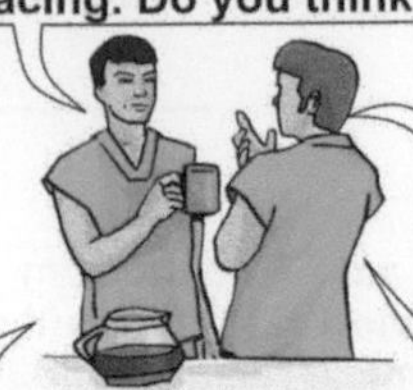

The recent developments are based on the concept that one must pace as close as possible to the His-Purkinje system to promote its participation in the LV depolarization process. In this way you seem to provide a better opportunity to preserve LV function.

But His bundle pacing is difficult ?

Yes. ParaHisian pacing (very close to the His bundle) is easier to perform and may give similar results. I believe that this approach will become popular.

DIRECT HIS BUNDLE PACING

* Spike-QRS is equal to HV (His to ventricle) interval during spontaneous AV junctional escape interval. Paced QRS identical to spontaneous QRS
* Not applicable to patients with bundle branch block
* Complex method
* Longer implantation time
* High pacing thresholds
* Cannot be carried out in all patients. In 5 studies including 126 patients HB pacing was accomplished in < 70% of patients in whom it was tried

PARAHISIAN PACING

* Easy to perform and reliable
* Limited data and follow-up
* Acute hemodynamic response is superior to that of RV apical pacing
* The duration of the paced QRS can be larger than the spontaneous QRS, but the duration should be at least 50 ms shorter than the QRS obtained with RV apical pacing and, in any case, not more than 120-130 ms. The electrical axis of the paced QRS must be concordant with the electrical axis of the spontaneous QRS
* Should become popular

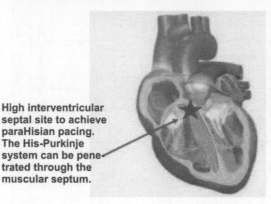

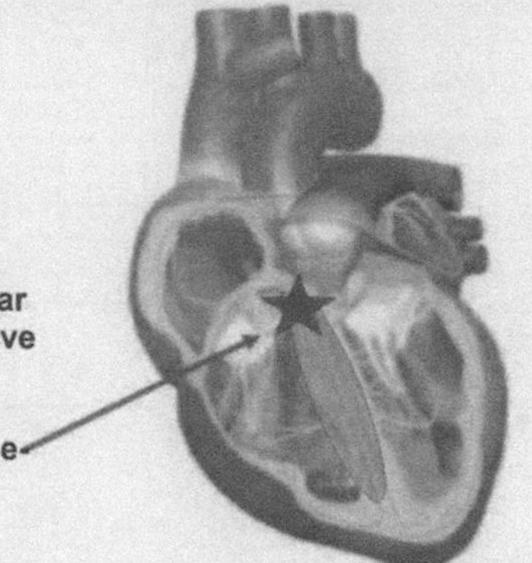

High interventricular septal site to achieve paraHisian pacing. The His-Purkinje system can be penetrated through the muscular septum.

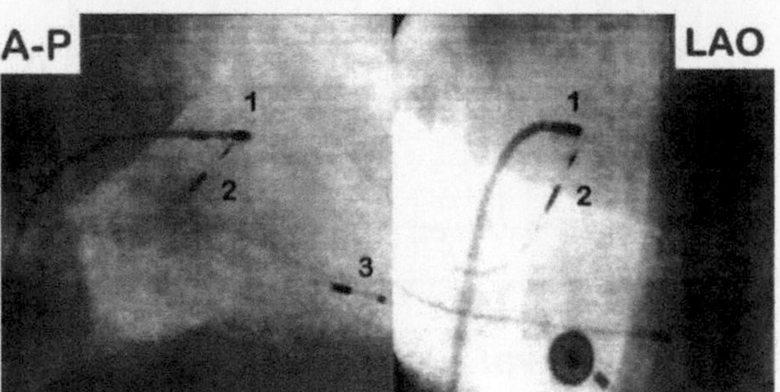

1. Quadripolar catheter mapping the His site
2. Srew-in bipolar lead positioned near the His bundle
3. Bipolar lead at RV apex

5 volts paraHisian pacing

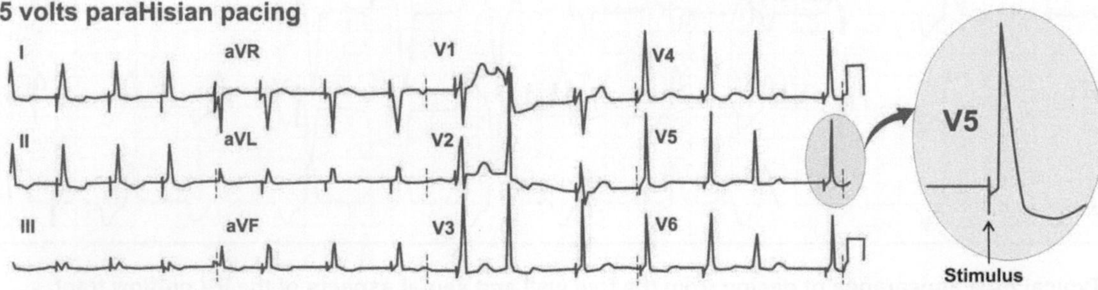

Post radiofrequency AV ablation for chronic atrial fibrillation. QRS = 120ms and a normal axis which is concordant with the non-paced spontaneous QRS. Note the pre-excitation-like pattern at the onset of the QRS.

A. F. Sinnaeve

WHY IS THE ATRIAL PACING SITE IMPORTANT ?

* Interatrial septal (IAS) pacing may be useful in the prevention of paroxysmal atrial fibrillation
* IAS pacing is important for the treatment of interatrial conduction delay requiring optimization of mechanical left-sided AV delay
* Enhanced atrial contractile function ?

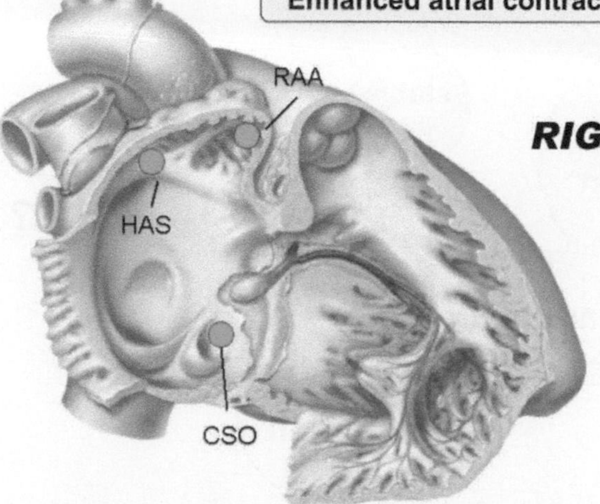

RIGHT ATRIAL PACING SITES

RAA = right atrial appendage

HAS = high atrial septum

CSO = coronary sinus os (triangle of Koch)

In IACD, consider placing the atrial lead in the interatrial septum where pacing produces a more homogeneous activation of both atria and abbreviates total atrial conduction time !

ALTERNATE SITE ATRIAL PACING

* high right atrium (Bachmann's bundle)
* mid-septal
* proximal coronary sinus or site near it
* dual site right atrial
* bi-atrial with one site in the proximal coronary sinus (pacing the left atrium)

INTERATRIAL CONDUCTION DELAY (IACD)

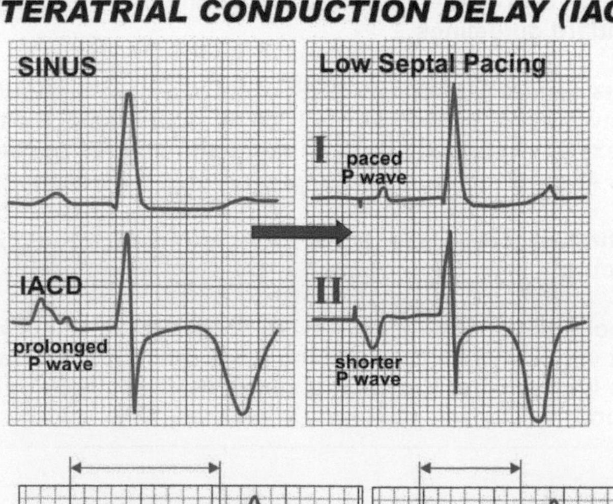

Pacing low atrial septum (LAS) vs right atrial appendage (RAA)

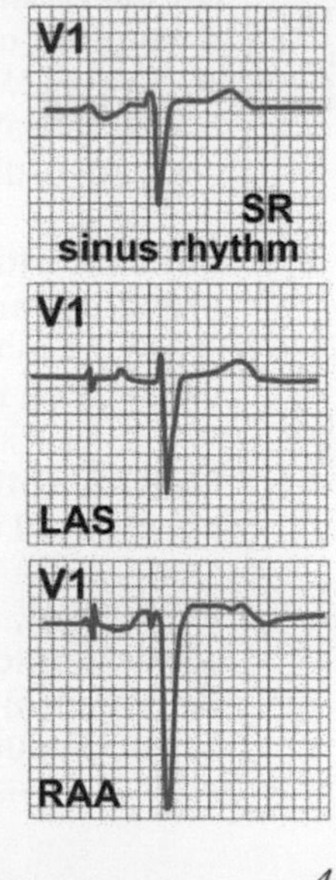

IACD

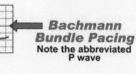

intrinsic P wave (120 ms)

paced P wave (80 ms)

Bachmann Bundle Pacing
Note the abbreviated P wave

A. F. Sinnaeve

WHAT FACTORS NEED TO BE CONSIDERED IN SELECTING THE PACING SITE ?

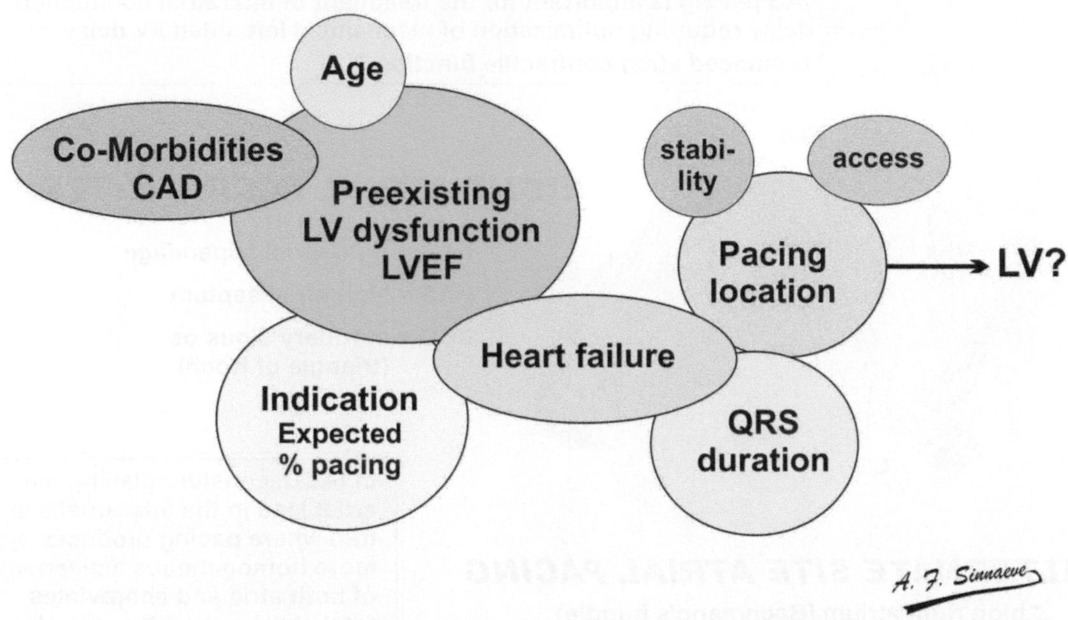

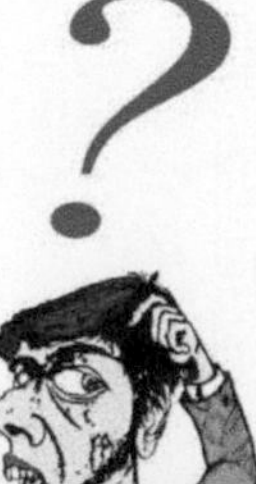

WHAT TO DO IN THE PRESENCE OF LV DYSFUNCTION ?

On the basis of little data it would seem reasonable to consider BiV pacing if frequent or continuous RV pacing is anticipated (high Cum% VP) for bradycardia (AV block) in the setting of LVEF < 35% especially if there is associated mitral regurgitation even if the patient is not a candidate for BiV pacing according to standard guidelines.

Patients with sick sinus syndrome, narrow QRS, and LVEF ≤ 35% should probably receive a conventional pacemaker (+ ICD) at an optimal RV site (away from the RV apex) if the clinical situation suggests that RV pacing is likely to be infrequent. Algorithms to minimize pacing may be important.

Patients with marked first-degree AV block and LV dysfunction should be considered for BiV pacing.

In children, acute hemodynamic effects have been shown to correlate well with chronic effects at various ventricular pacing sites, and thus permanent lead(s) should be implanted at the pacing site(s) that results in optimal acute LV pump function.

Abbreviations : BiV : biventricular ; CAD : coronary artery disease ; Cum% VP : cumulative % ventricular pacing ; LV : left ventricle ; LVEF : left ventricular ejection fracture

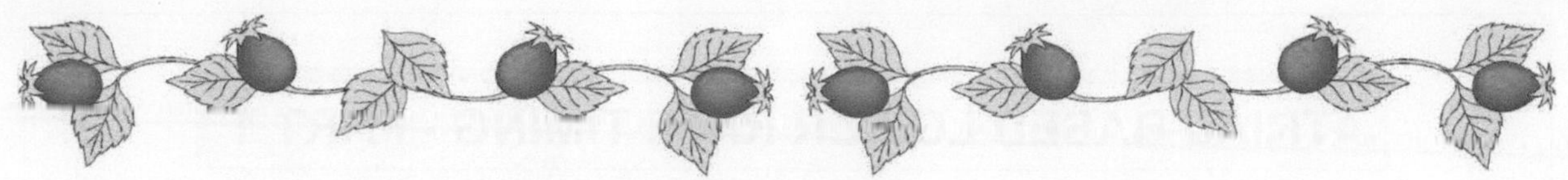

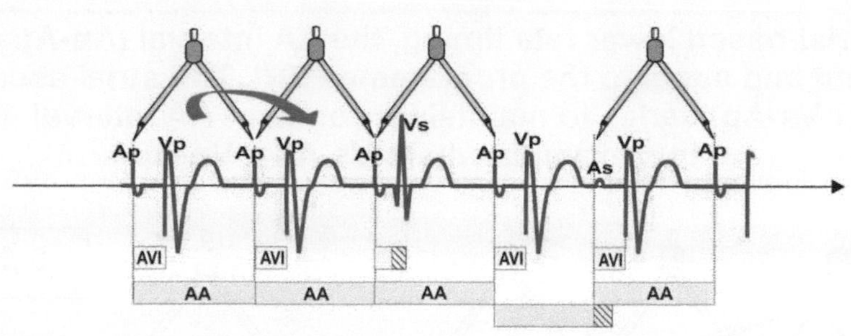

TYPES OF LOWER RATE TIMING

* Atrial-based lower rate timing - part 1.
* Atrial-based lower rate timing - part 2.
* Atrial-based lower rate timing - part 3 (AV delay).
* Faster atrial pacing rate with ventricular-based lower rate timing.
* What is the pacing mode during inhibition ?
* Spike in QRS complex.

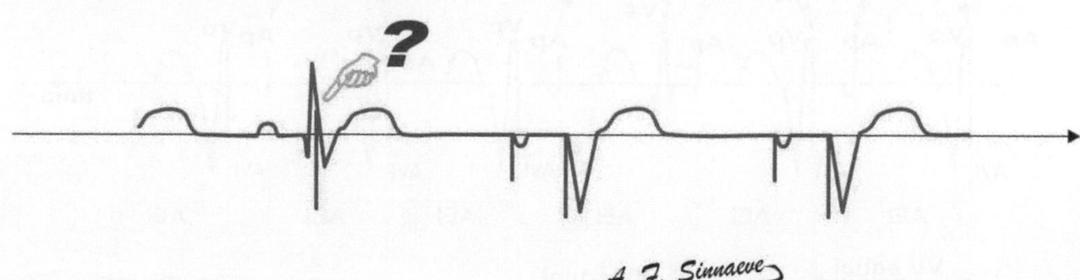

A. F. Sinnaeve

ATRIAL-BASED LOWER RATE TIMING - PART 1

With atrial-based lower rate timing, the AA interval (Ap-Ap or As-Ap) is constant and equal to the programmed LRI. The atrial escape interval (Vp-Ap or Vs-Ap) varies to maintain a constant AA interval as shown in this example where Vs-Ap > Vp-Ap .

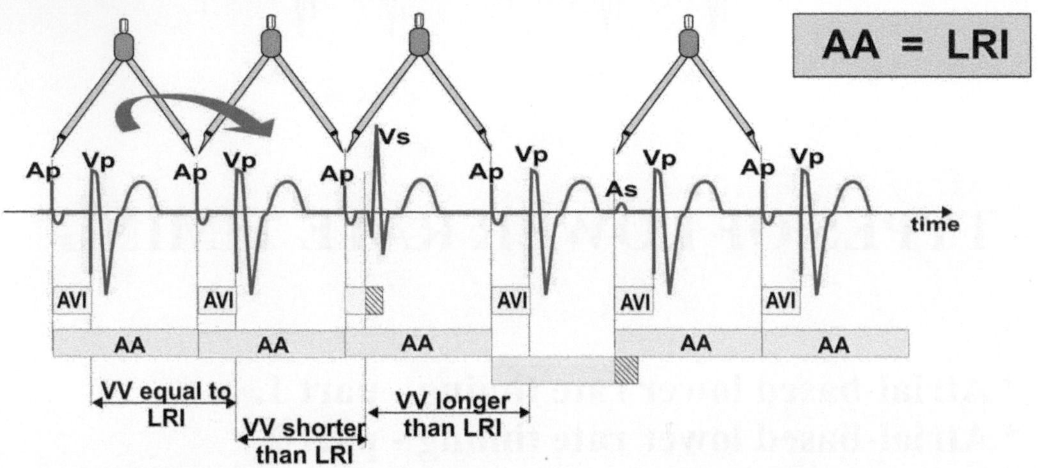

With ventricular-based lower rate timing the AEI or atrial escape interval (Vp-Ap or Vs-Ap) is constant

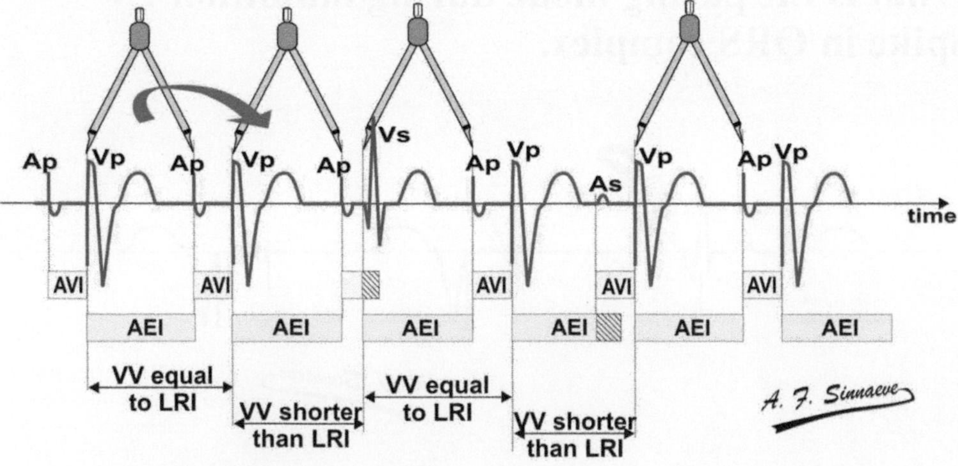

Abbreviations : Ap = atrial pace ; As = atrial sense ; AEI = atrial escape interval ; AVI = AV delay ; AA = programmed atrial lower rate interval = Ap-Ap or As-Ap ; LRI = lower rate interval ; VV = interval between two consecutive ventricular events

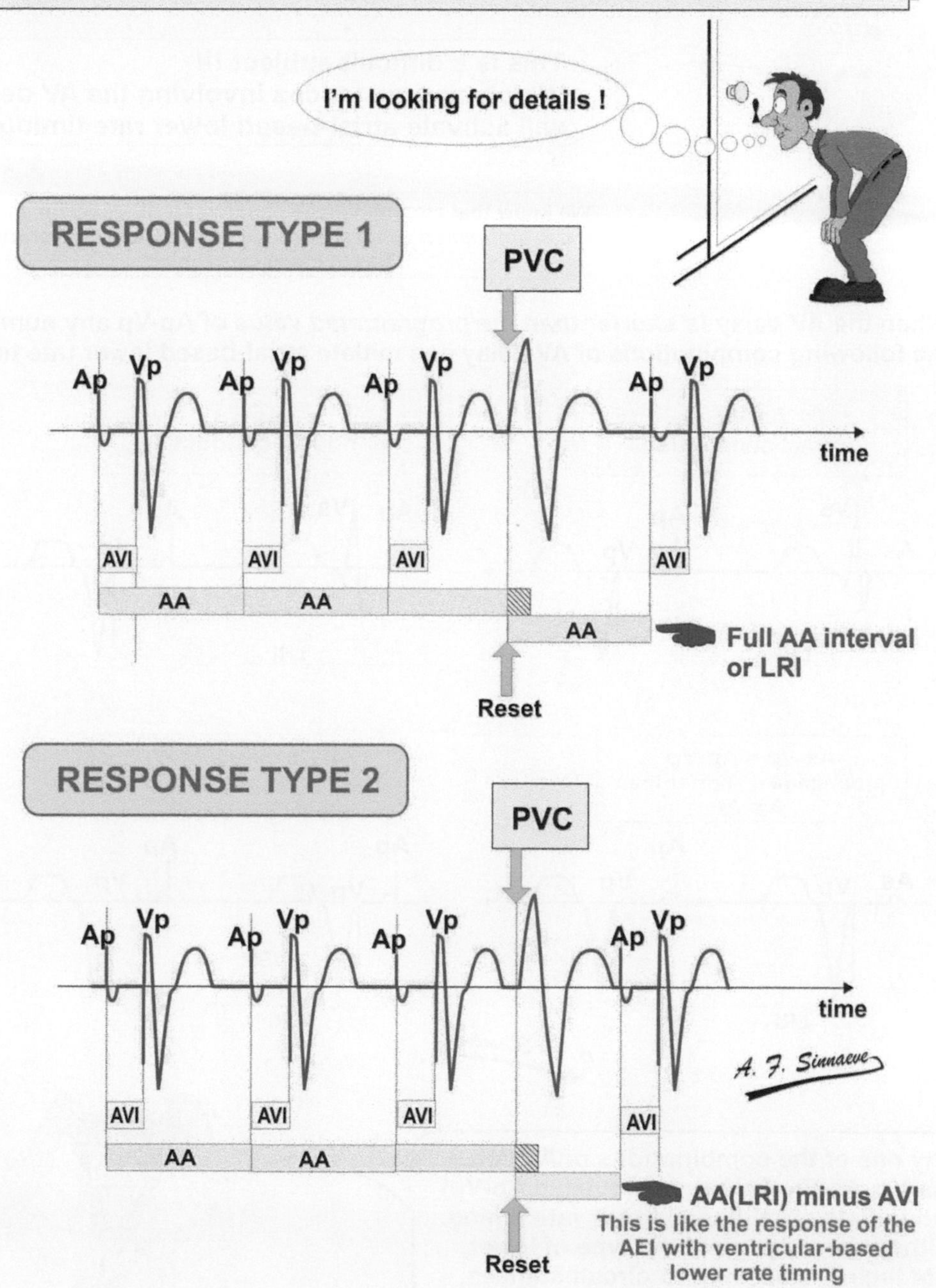

Abbreviations : Ap = atrial pace ; As = atrial sense ; AEI = atrial escape interval ; AVI = AV delay ; AA = programmed atria-based lower rate interval = Ap-Ap or As-Ap interval ; LRI = lower rate interval ; PVC = premature ventricular complex

ATRIAL-BASED LOWER RATE TIMING - PART 3

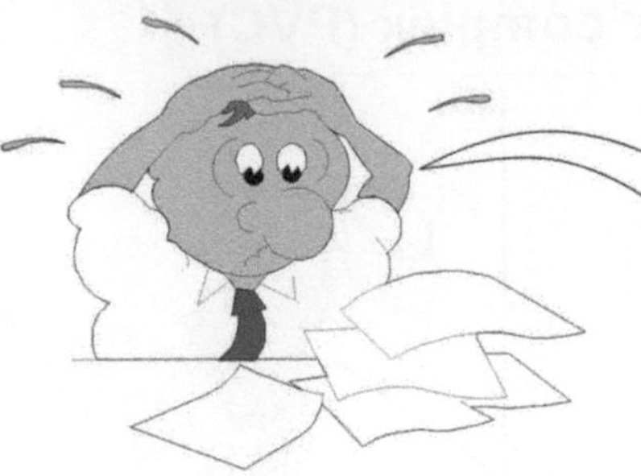

This is a difficult subject !!!
Which circumstances involving the AV delay will activate atrial-based lower rate timing ??

We know that circumstances causing an *AV delay longer than the programmed value* are always associated with ventricular-based lower rate timing

When the *AV delay is shorter than the programmed value* of Ap-Vp any number of the following combinations of AV delay can initiate atrial-based lower rate timing

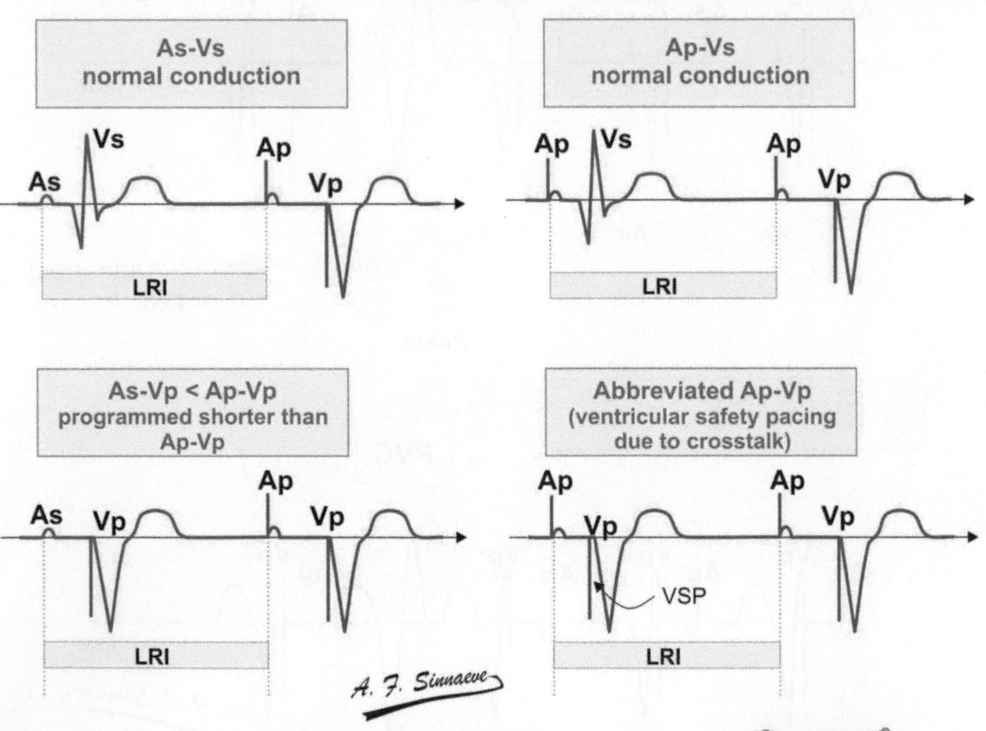

Any one of the combinations of AV delay (As-Vp, As-Vs, Ap-Vs, abbreviated Ap-Vp) can initiate atrial-based lower rate timing. Without knowledge of the type of lower rate timing according to circumstances, one cannot interpret the ECG !!!!

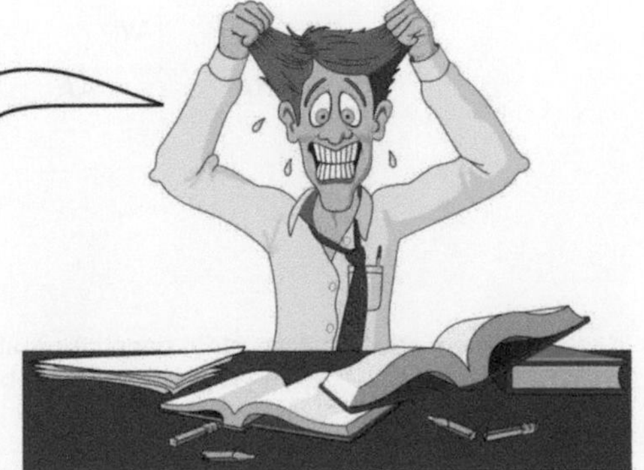

Abbreviations : AVI = AV delay ; AEI = atrial escape interval ; AVE = extension of AVI ; LRI = lower rate interval ;Ap = atrial pacing ; As = atrial sensing ; Vp = ventricular pacing ; Vs = ventricular sensing ; VSP = ventricular safety pacing

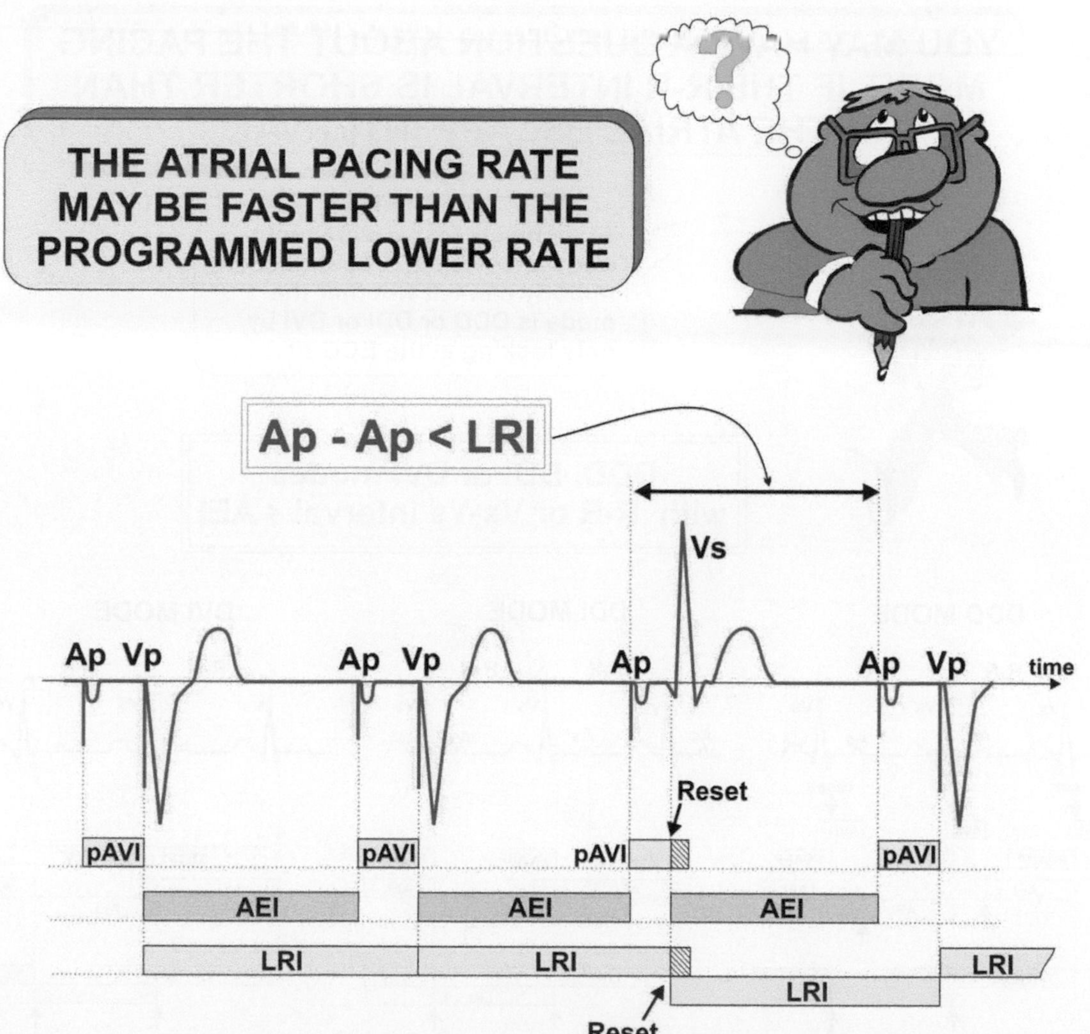

With ventricular-based lower rate timing, the atrial escape interval (AEI) and the lower rate interval (LRI) start from a sensed or paced ventricular event. The hallmark of ventricular-based lower rate timing is constancy of the AEI

Abbreviations : Ap = atrial pace ; Vp = ventricular pace ; Vs = ventricular sense ; pAVI = AV delay after pacing ; AEI = atrial escape interval ; LRI = lower rate interval

A. F. Sinnaeve

YOU MAY HAVE A QUESTION ABOUT THE PACING MODE IF THE R-R INTERVAL IS SHORTER THAN THE ATRIAL ESCAPE INTERVAL

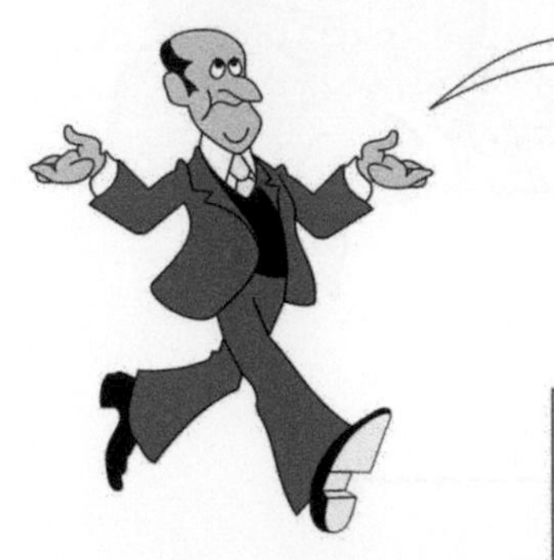

At relatively fast spontaneous rates and normal AV conduction, nobody can tell whether the mode is DDD or DDI or DVI by only looking at the ECG !!!

DDD, DDI or DVI modes with R-R or Vs-Vs interval < AEI

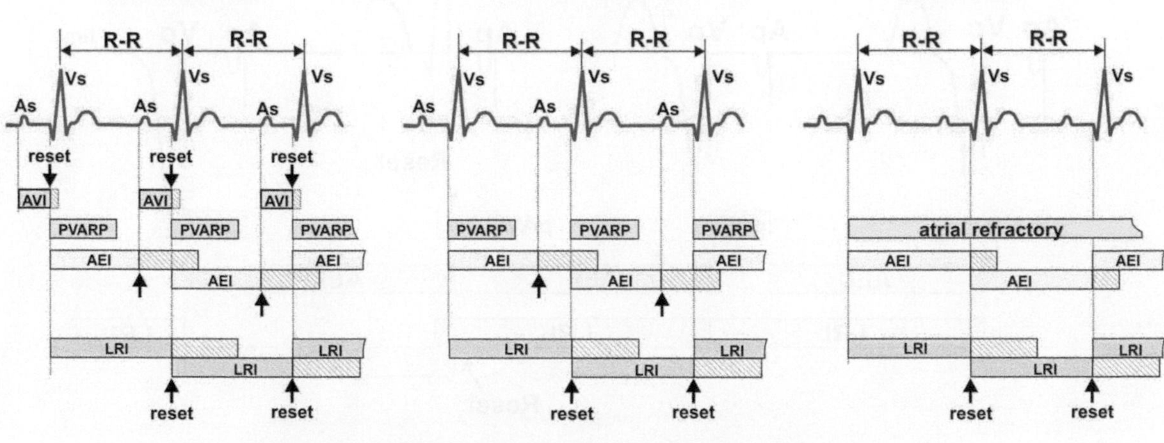

The same ECG may also represent the VDD mode if As-Vs < programmed As-Vp and the spontaneous atrial rate is faster than the programmed lower rate

A. F. Sinnaeve

Abbreviations : As = atrial sense ; Vs = ventricular sense ; AVI = AV delay ; AEI = atrial escape interval ; LRI = lower rate interval ; PVARP = postventricular atrial refractory period

It took some time and a lot of exercise to become an expert in marching backwards, but at the end it isn't difficult at all......

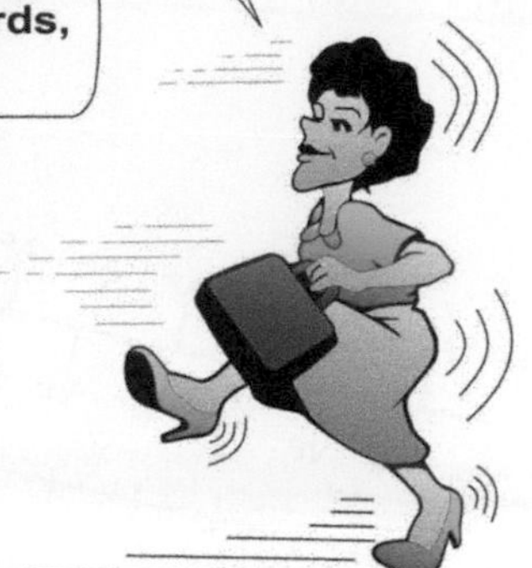

A SPIKE WITHIN A QRS COMPLEX ! IS IT AN ATRIAL OR A VENTRICULAR STIMULUS ?

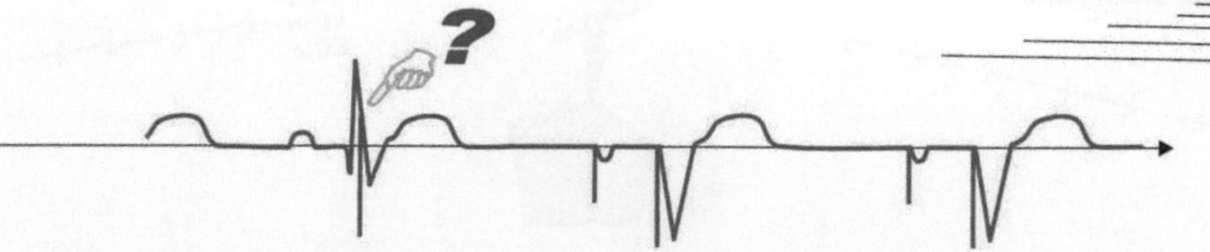

① **Establish the duration of the AEI, starting with any VP**
(alternatively the duration of AEI can be determined from the onset of a sensed QRS complex to the succeeding atrial stimulus)

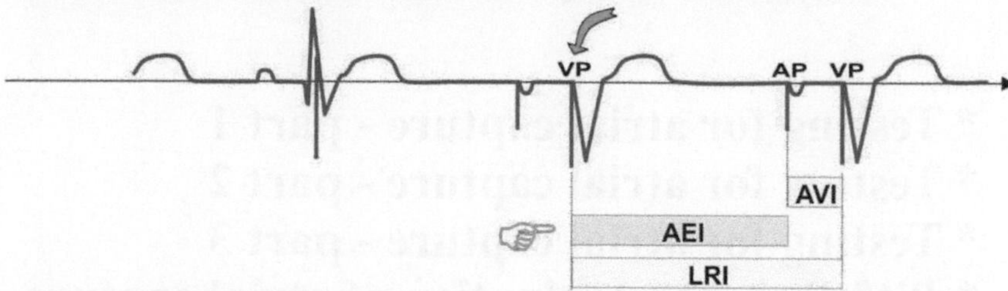

② **Measure the interval from the stimulus in question back to the preceding ventricular event ......**

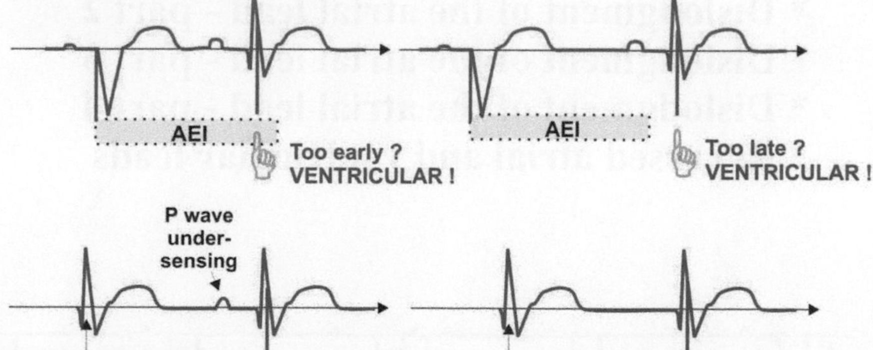

In all probability ATRIAL ! **In all probability ATRIAL !**

This rule is only valid for DDD pacemakers with ventricular-based lower rate timing

A. F. Sinnaeve

Abbreviations : Ap = atrial pace; Vp = ventricular pace; AEI = atrial escape interval; AVI = AV delay; LRI = lower rate interval

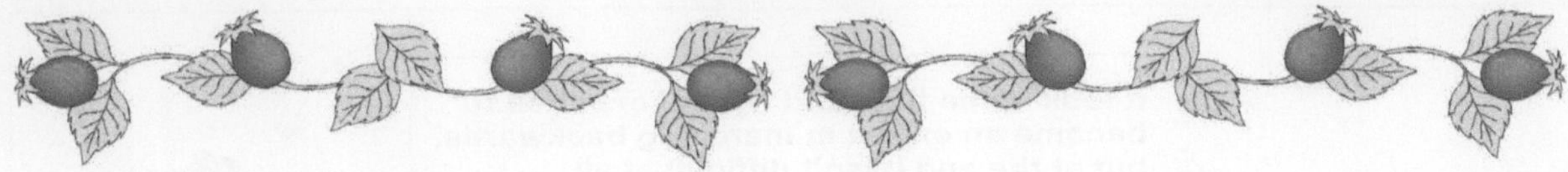

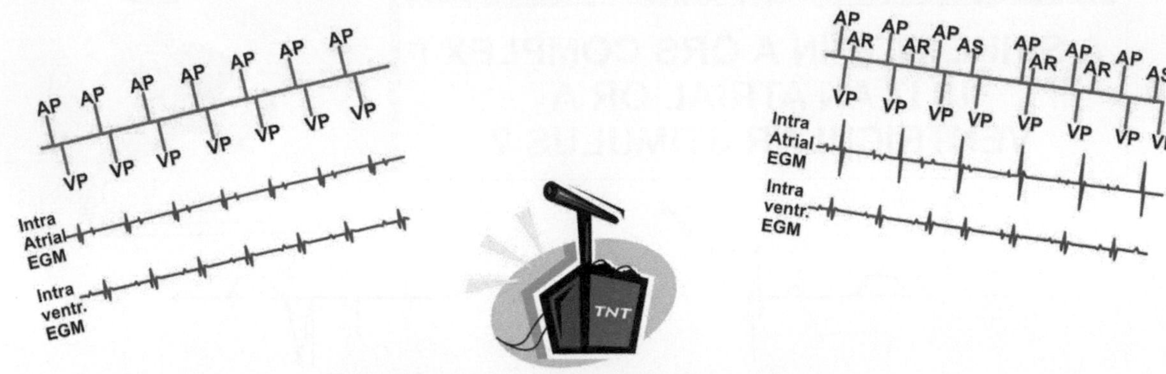

ATRIAL CAPTURE

* Testing for atrial capture - part 1
* Testing for atrial capture - part 2
* Testing for atrial capture - part 3
* Pitfalls in the evaluation of atrial capture
* Dislodgment of the atrial lead - part 1
* Dislodgment of the atrial lead - part 2
* Dislodgment of the atrial lead - part 3
* Dislodgment of the atrial lead - part 4
* Reversed atrial and ventricular leads

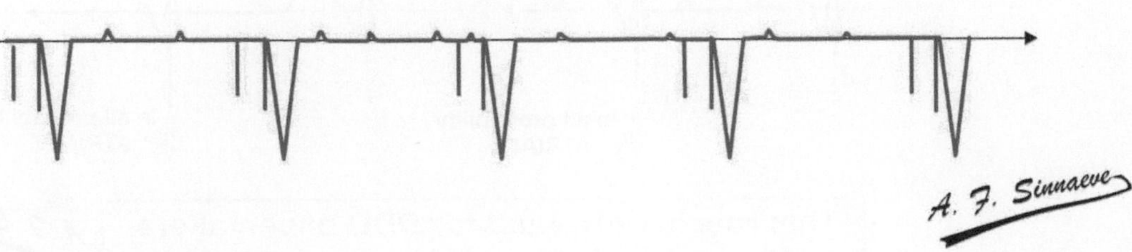

A. F. Sinnaeve

HOW TO TEST FOR ATRIAL CAPTURE - PART1

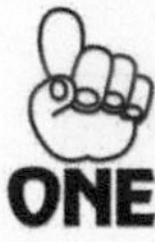

ONE

Take a 12-lead ECG recorded at double standardization to bring out paced P waves and/or tiny bipolar stimuli

NORMAL

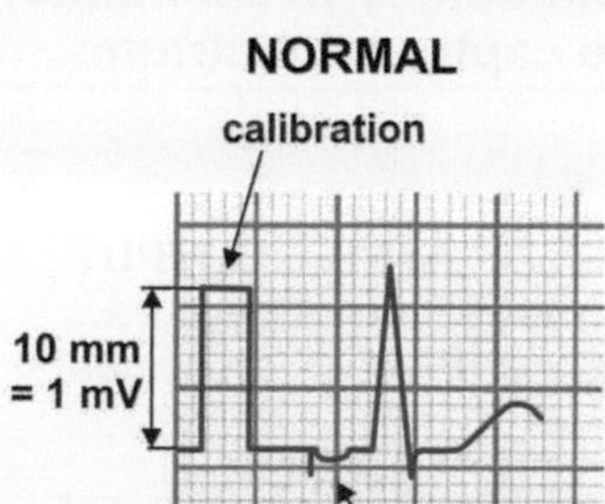

DOUBLE STANDARD

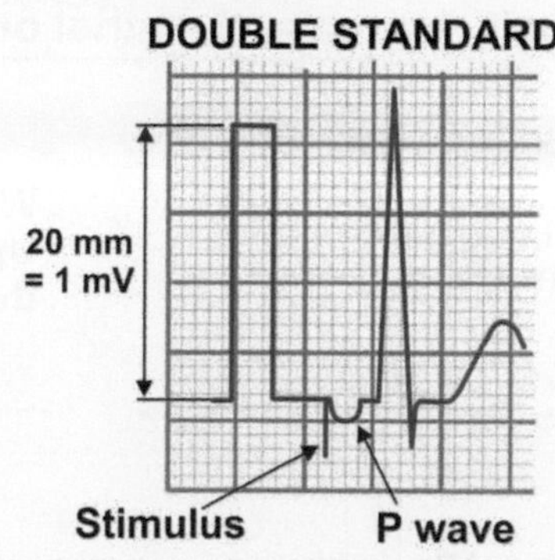

TWO

Reprogram to the AAI or AOO mode (at several pacing rates)

AAI mode in patient with intact AV conduction

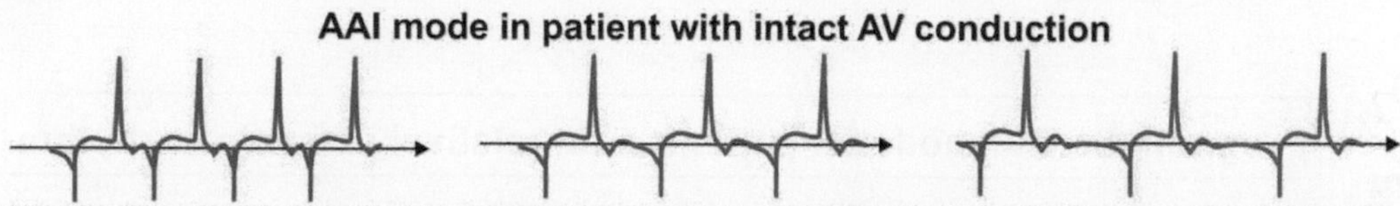

Atrial capture is present when the rate of the conducted QRS complexes (ventricular rate) always remains equal to the changing atrial pacing rates used during testing

AAI mode in patient with complete AV block and idioventricular rhythm

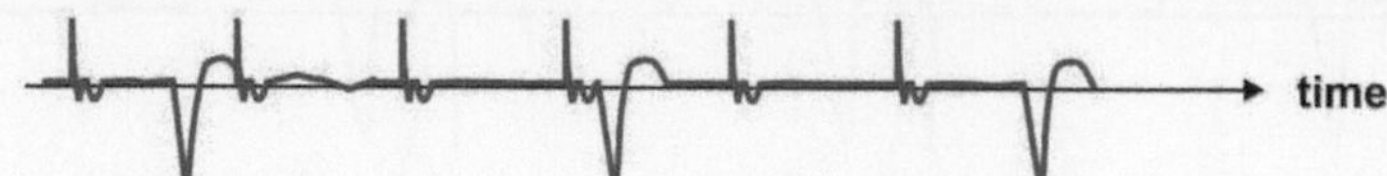

This maneuver can only be performed if there is an underlying ventricular rhythm during AAI pacing. A spontaneous ventricular rhythm is often present when the pacing rate in the VVI mode is slowly decreased to allow the emergence of a slow spontaneous idioventricular rhythm. If this rate is satisfactory, testing is done in the AAI mode.

THREE

Unmask P waves by programming a long AV delay (250-300 ms) e.g. with latency or considerable delay in interatrial conduction

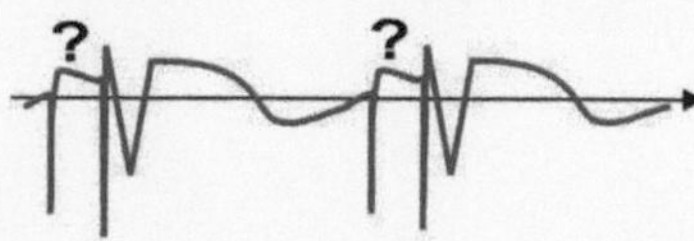

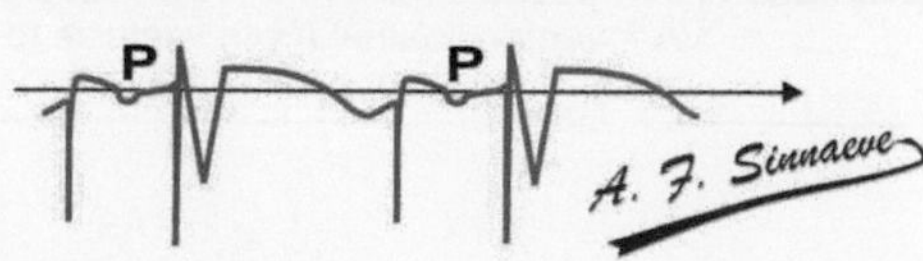

A. F. Sinnaeve

HOW TO TEST FOR ATRIAL CAPTURE - PART2

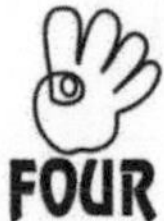

Retrograde VA conduction suggests lack of capture by the preceding atrial stimulus. Verify retrograde conduction by event markers and eventually increase the atrial output to capture the atrium

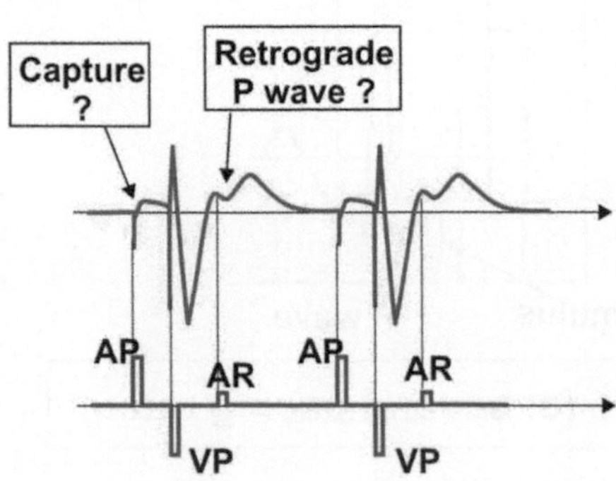

WITH LARGER ATRIAL OUTPUT
Upon successful atrial capture, the retrograde P wave disappears

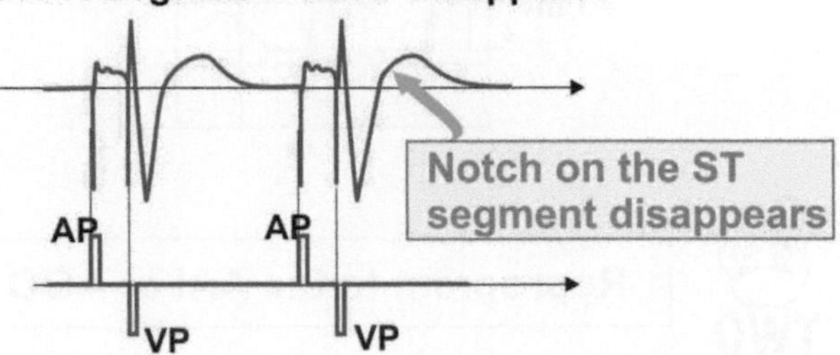

Program the DVI mode for patients with relatively fast sinus rhythm

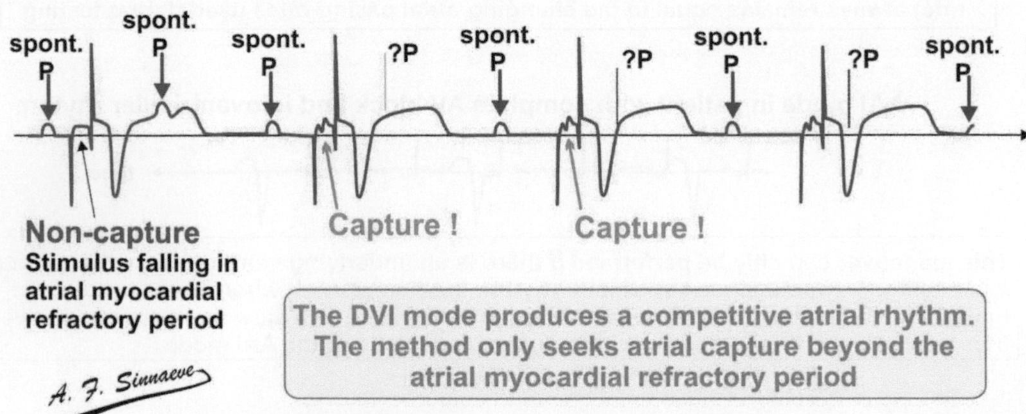

The DVI mode produces a competitive atrial rhythm. The method only seeks atrial capture beyond the atrial myocardial refractory period

A. F. Sinnaeve

Abbreviations : AP = paced atrial event ; AR = atrial sensing in atrial refractory period ; VP = ventricular paced event ; VA = ventriculoatrial (from ventricle to atrium)

HOW TO TEST FOR ATRIAL CAPTURE - PART 3

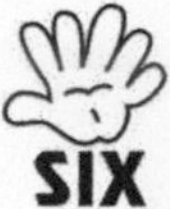

Using only the programmer, program the DDD mode and increase the atrial pacing rate above the spontaneous rate, then increase or decrease the atrial output and look at the markers

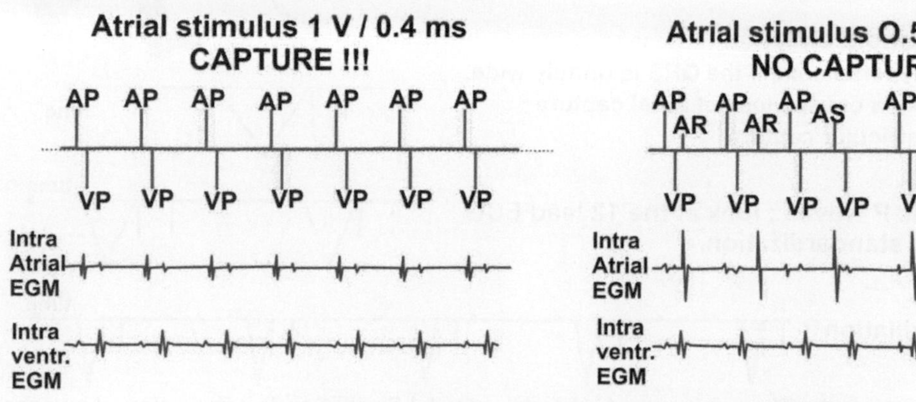

CLARIFICATION OF THE MARKERS

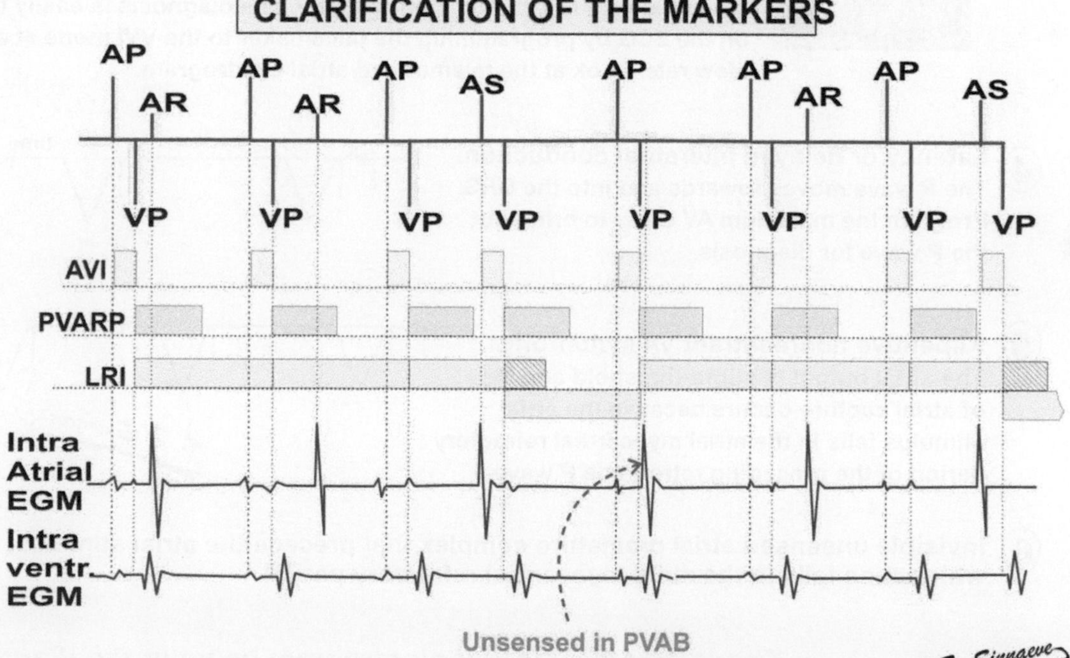

Abbreviations : AVI = AV delay ; PVARP = postventricular atrial refractory period ; LRI = lower rate interval ; AP =atrial pacing ; AS = atrial sensing ; AR = atrial sensing during refractory period ; VP = ventricular pacing ; EGM = electrogram ; PVAB = postventricular atrial blanking period ;

PITFALLS IN THE EVALUATION OF ATRIAL CAPTURE

This is like a mine field !!!

1. **High threshold situation**
   Suspect hyperkalemia if the QRS is unduly wide. Hyperkalemia causes loss of atrial capture before ventricular capture.

2. **Isoelectric P waves : look at the 12 lead ECG at double standardization.**

3. **Atrial fibrillation**

WARNING **The presence of underlying atrial fibrillation is often missed and the patient is denied anticoagulant therapy. The diagnosis is easily made on the ECG by programming the pacemaker to the VVI mode at a slow rate. Look at the telemetered atrial electrogram.**

4. **Latency or delayed interatrial conduction.**
   The P wave moves towards and into the QRS. Program the maximum AV delay to bring out the P wave for diagnosis

5. **Repetitive nonreentrant VA synchrony.**
   The atrial output is supra-threshold and loss of atrial capture occurs because the atrial stimulus falls in the atrial myocardial refractory period of the preceding retrograde P wave

A. F. Sinnaeve

6. **Invisible unsensed atrial premature complex that precede the atrial stimulus which then falls in the atrial myocardial refractory period.**

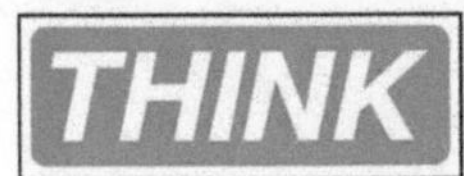

The telemetered atrial electrogram helps in the diagnosis. However successful atrial capture cannot be determined from the atrial electrogram.

DISLODGMENT OF THE ATRIAL LEAD INTO THE RIGHT VENTRICLE

Forewarned is forearmed !!!

PART 1

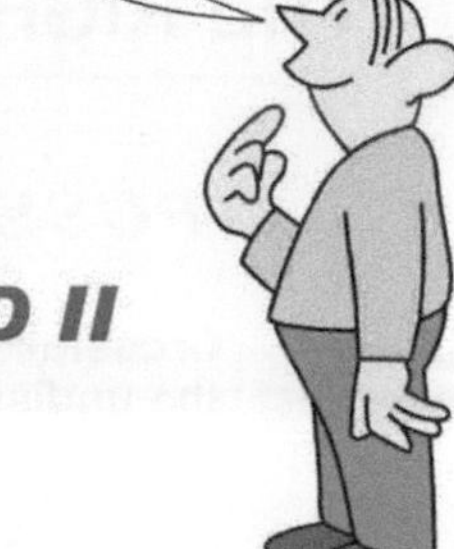

POSSIBLE PATTERNS ON ECG - LEAD II

1. **REFERENCE. Normal AV sequential pacing with programmed AVI and AEI**

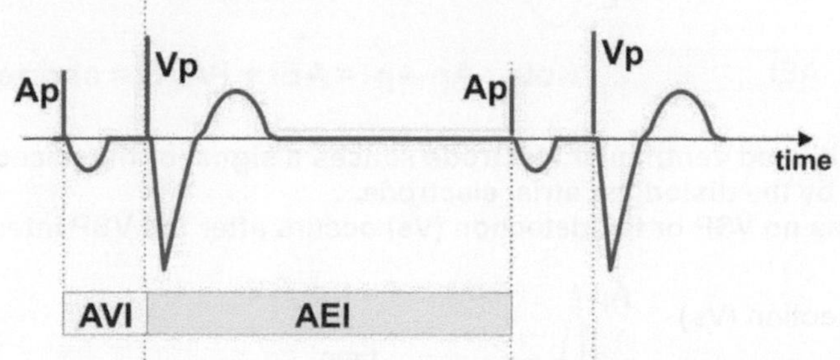

DISLODGED ATRIAL ELECTRODE

CORRECTLY POSITIONED VENTRICULAR ELECTRODE

2. **When neither the atrial stimulus nor the paced QRS complex (generated by the atrial channel) is seen by the undisplaced ventricular electrode. Ap paces the RV**

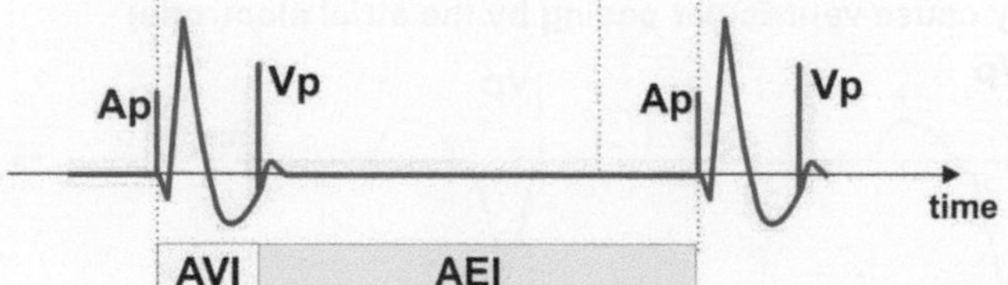

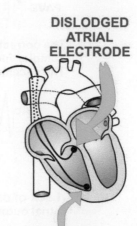

3. **Crosstalk : if the atrial stimulus or the paced QRS complex generated by the displaced atrial electrode, is sensed by the undisplaced ventricular electrode, ventricular safety pacing is activated whereupon the Ap-Vp interval shortens**

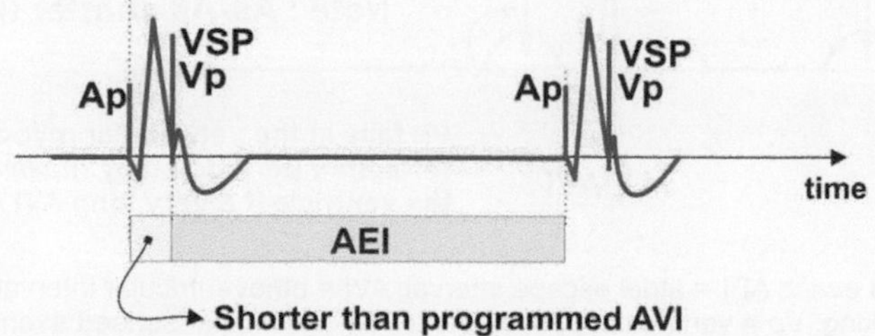

Shorter than programmed AVI

A. F. Sinnaeve

Abbreviations : Ap = atrial paced event; Vp = ventricular paced event; AVI = programmed AV delay; AEI = atrial escape interval; VSP = ventricular safety pacing

DISLODGMENT OF THE ATRIAL LEAD INTO THE RIGHT VENTRICLE

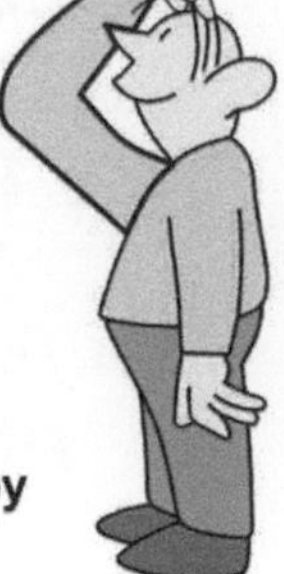

PART 2

POSSIBLE PATTERNS ON ECG - LEAD II

4 **Crosstalk : if the stimulus from the displaced atrial electrode is sensed by the undisplaced ventricular electrode and the pacemaker has no VSP**

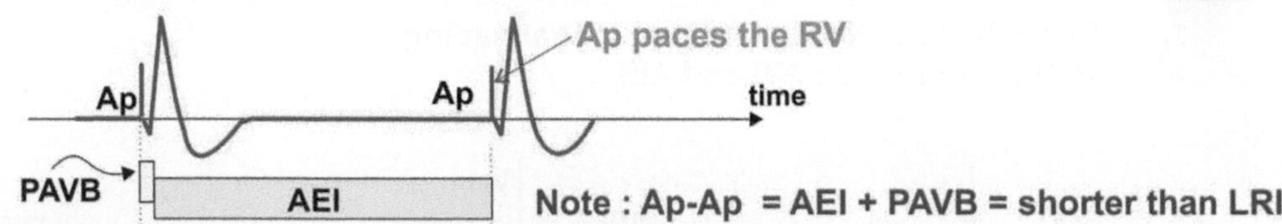

5 **The correctly positioned ventricular electrode senses a signal of the paced QRS complex induced by the dislodged atrial electrode.**
The pacemaker has no VSP or the detection (Vs) occurs after the VSP interval.

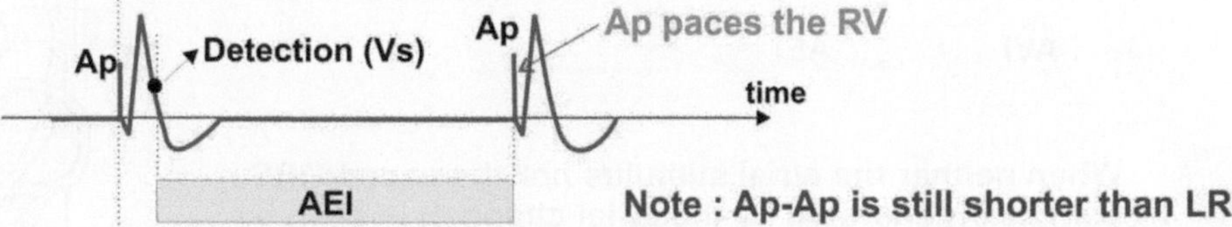

6 **Lack of capture of the displaced atrial lead (however programming the maximal atrial output may cause ventricular pacing by the atrial electrode)**

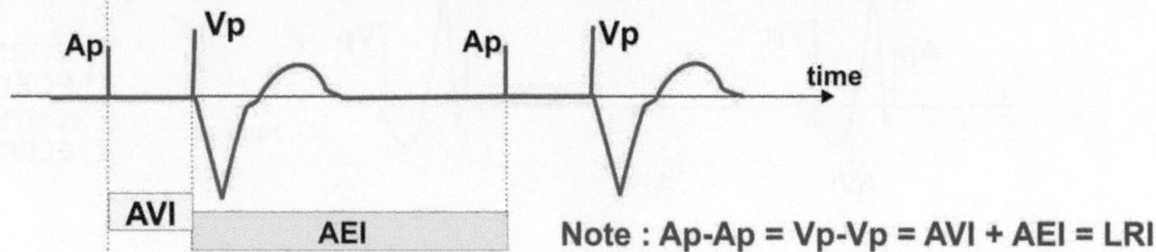

7 **The atrial electrode senses the spontaneous QRS complex and delivers a ventricular stimulus after an AV delay**

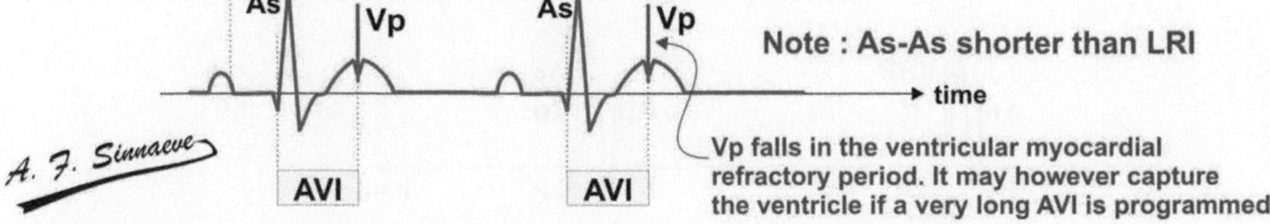

Abbreviations : Ap = atrial paced event; AEI = atrial escape interval; AVI = atrioventricular interval or AV delay; PAVB = postatrial ventricular blanking; Vp = ventricular paced event; Vs = ventricular sensed event; VSP = ventricular safety pacing ; LRI = lower rate interval ;

DISLODGMENT OF THE ATRIAL LEAD INTO THE RIGHT VENTRICLE

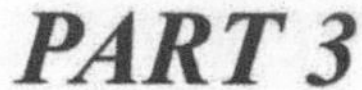

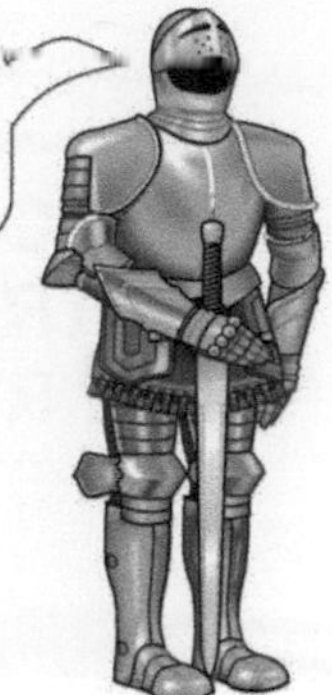

PART 3

Representative ECG

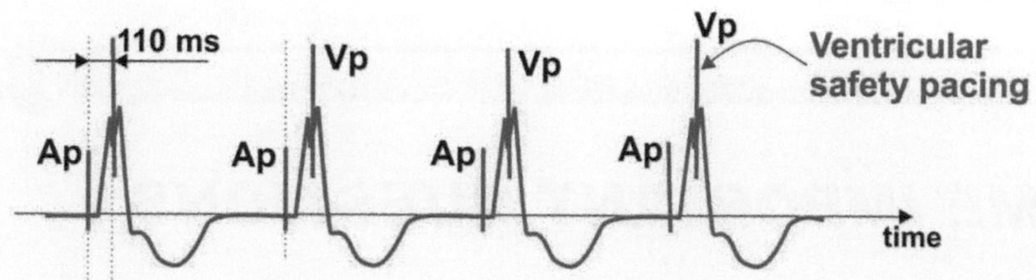

① *Confirm by programming to AAI mode*

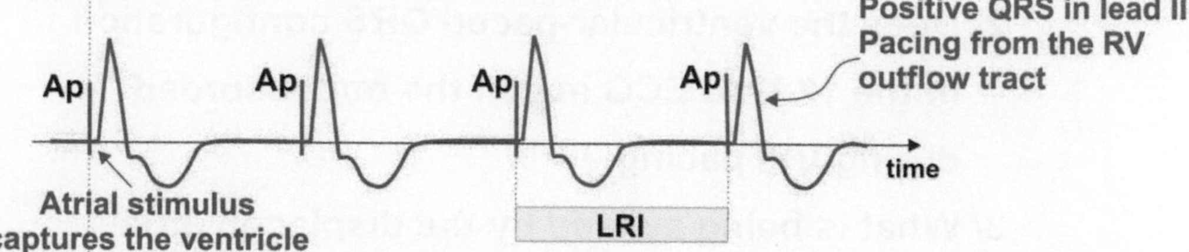

② *and by programming to the VVI mode*

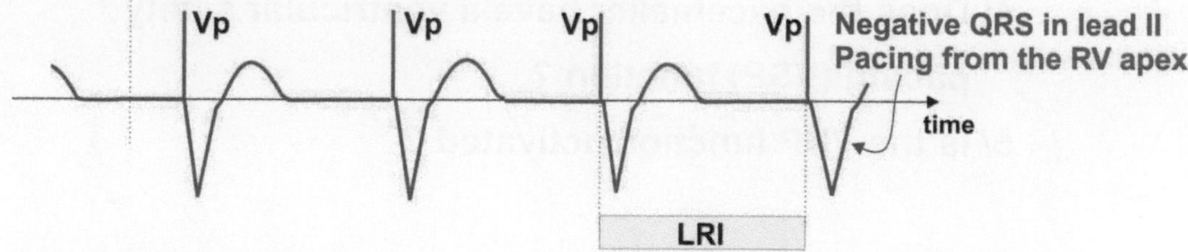

TAKE A CHEST X RAY FOR A DEFINITIVE CONFIRMATION

Abbreviations : Ap = atrial paced event; Vp = ventricular paced event
LRI = lower rate interval

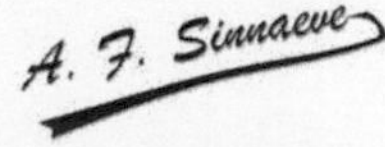

DISLODGMENT OF THE ATRIAL LEAD INTO THE RIGHT VENTRICLE

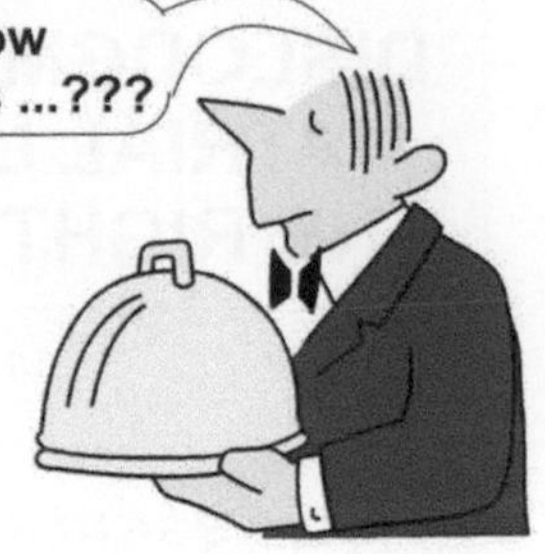
You want to know
what it contains ...???

PART 4

SOME IMPORTANT QUESTIONS :

1/ Does Ap capture the ventricle ?

2/ Does the ventricular-paced QRS configuration in the 12-lead ECG match the one recorded during VVI pacing ?

3/ What is being sensed by the displaced atrial electrode ?

4/ Does the pacemaker have a ventricular safety pacing (VSP) function ?

5/ Is the VSP function activated ?

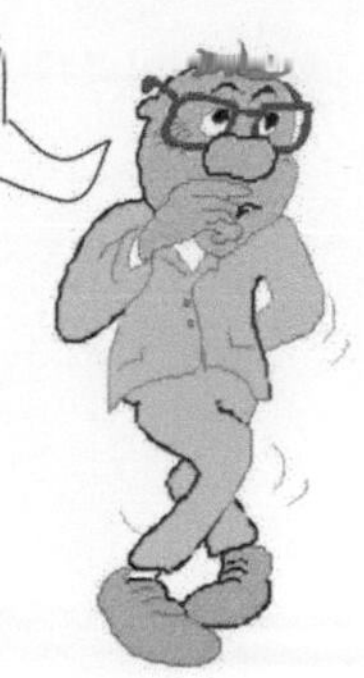
They say I'm a real dummy, just because
I've interchanged a couple of wires

REVERSED CONNECTION OF ATRIAL AND VENTRICULAR LEADS

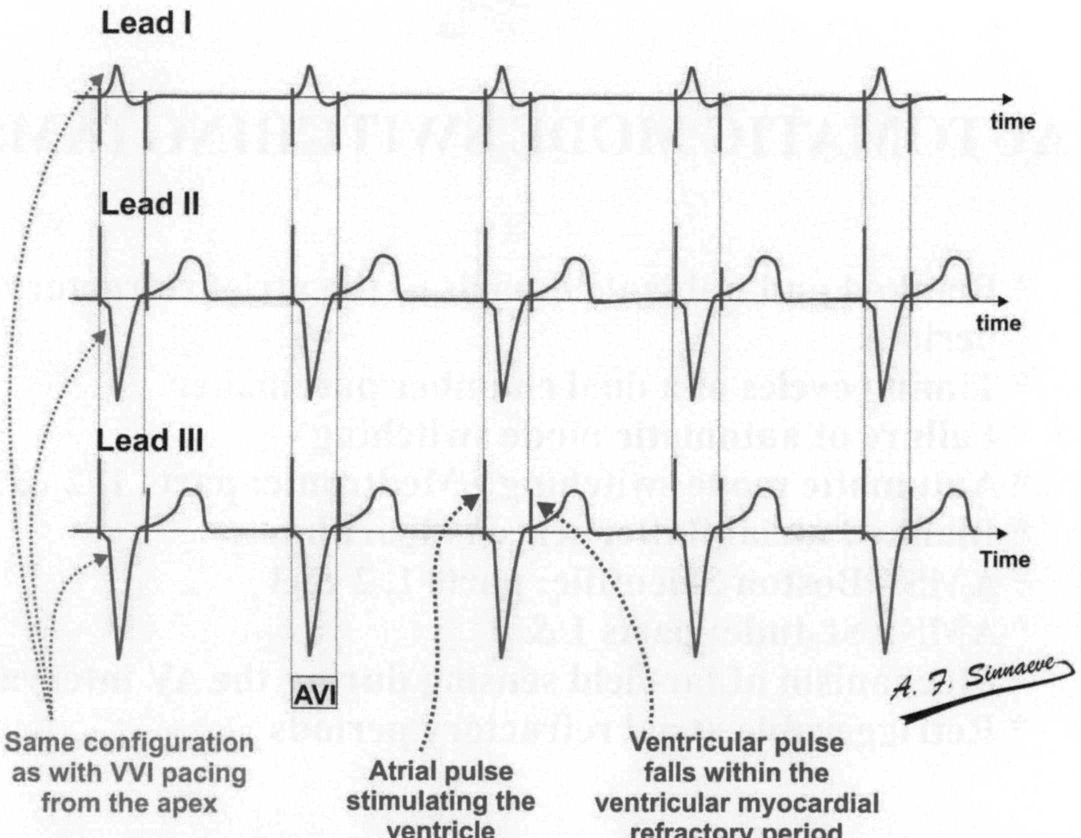

NOTE : * programming to the AAI mode will cause VVI pacing
**   * programming to the VVI mode will cause AAI pacing**

Abbreviations : AVI = programmed AV delay

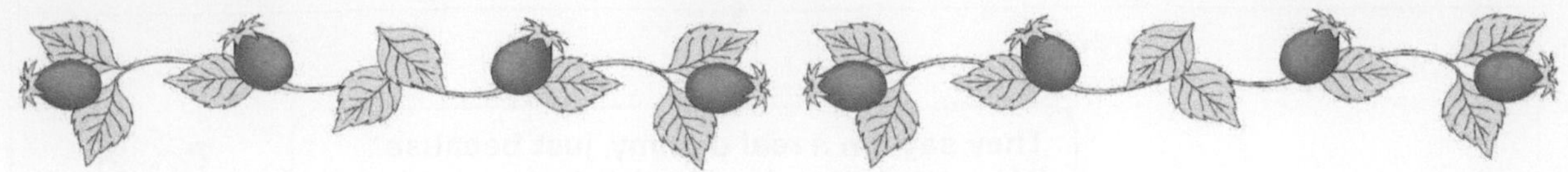

AUTOMATIC MODE SWITCHING (AMS)

* Blanked and unblanked parts of the atrial refractory periods
* Timing cycles of a dual chamber pacemaker
* Failure of automatic mode switching
* Automatic mode switching - Medtronic: parts 1, 2 & 3
* Blanked atrial flutter search algorithm
* AMS - Boston Scientific: parts 1, 2 & 3
* AMS - St Jude: parts 1 & 2
* Mechanism of far-field sensing during the AV interval
* Retriggerable atrial refractory periods

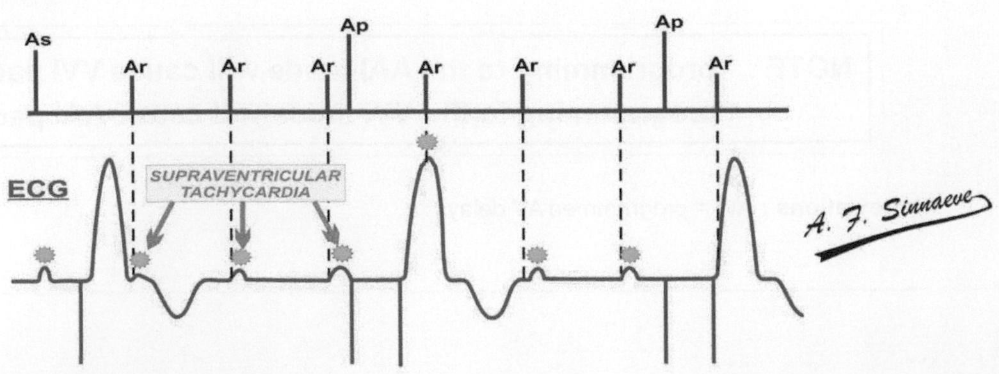

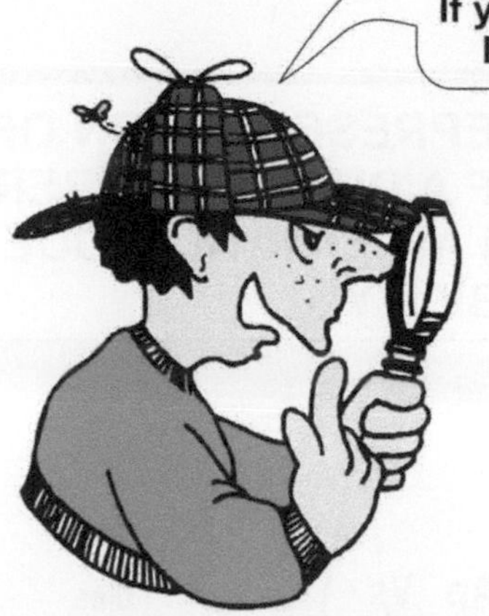
Remember, my dear doctor Watson !
If you want to detect a tachycardia, you have to look in all possible places!

AUTOMATIC MODE SWITCHING
BLANKED and UNBLANKED PARTS of the ATRIAL REFRACTORY PERIODS

ATRIAL REFRACTORY INTERVALS

A signal falling in the refractory period can initiate neither an atrioventricular interval (AVI) nor a lower rate interval (LRI)

TARP = AVI + PVARP

PVARP

AVI

AVI = atrioventricular interval

PVARP = postventricular atrial refractory interval

TARP = total atrial refractory period

ATRIAL BLANKING INTERVALS

During these intervals the atrial channel is insensitive or blind to all signals.
By a special circuit, the electrogram can still be detected and displayed, but cannot influence the function of the pacemaker itself.

AB

PVAB

AB = atrial blanking period

PVAB = postventricular atrial blanking

UNBLANKED ATRIAL REFRACTORY PERIODS

During these intervals signals can be sensed by the atrial channel and used to alter certain pacing timing cycles including the automatic mode switching (AMS), although they are unable to start an AVI or LRI.
Refractory sensed signals are depicted differently by the marker channel (Ar or AR).

AVI-U

PVARP-U

A. F. Sinnaeve

AVI-U = unblanked atrioventricular interval

PVARP-U = unblanked postventricular atrial refractory interval

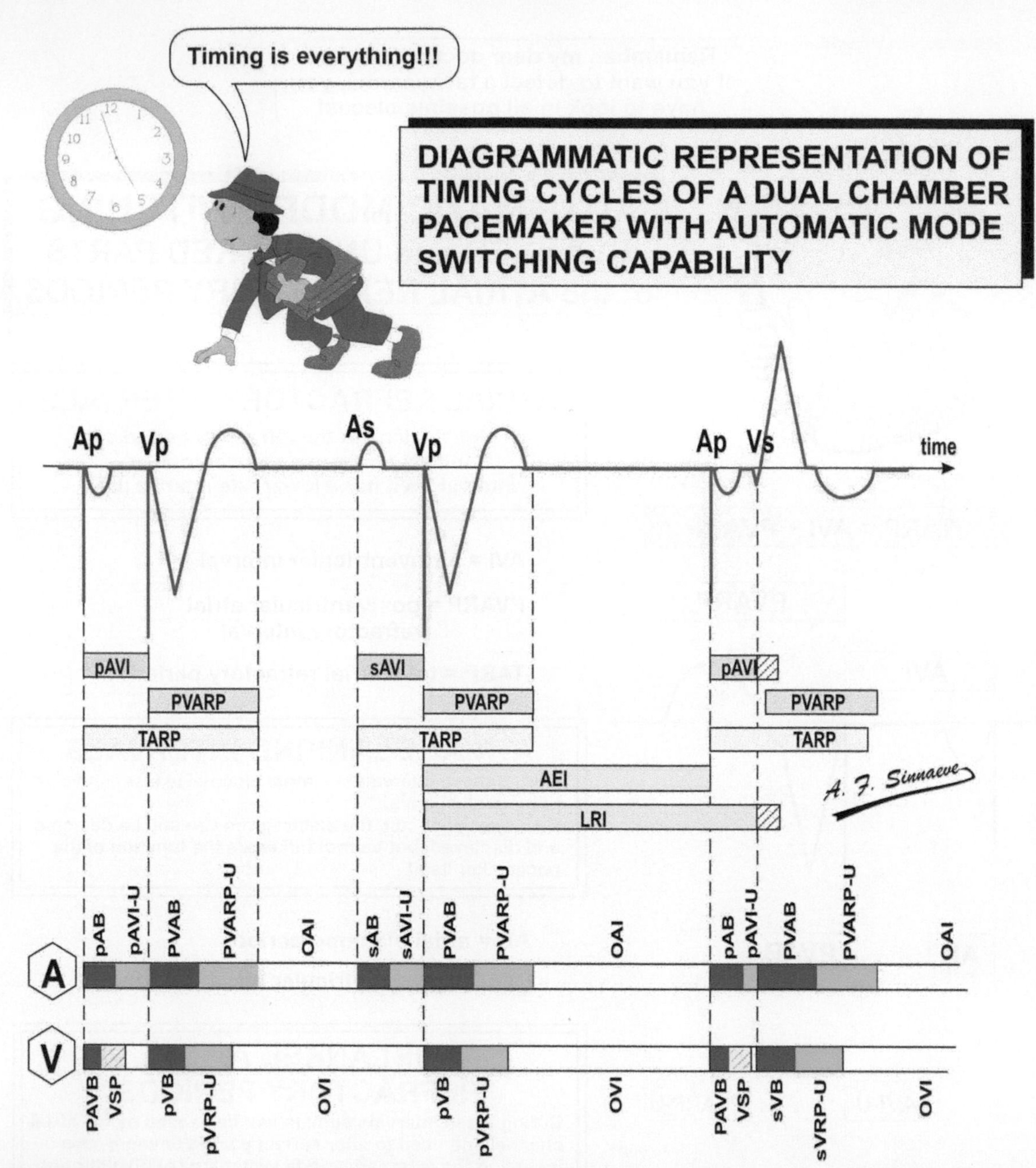

Abbreviations : Ap = atrial paced event; As = atrial sensed event; pAVI = paced atrioventricular interval; sAVI = sensed atrioventricular interval; AB = blanked first part of AVI; AVI-U = unblanked last part of AVI; PVAB = postventricular atrial blanking; PVARP = postventricular atrial refractory period; PVARP-U = unblanked second part of PVARP; TARP = total atrial refractory interval; AEI = atrial escape interval; OAI = open atrial interval;
Vp = ventricular paced event; Vs = ventricular sensed event; PAVB = postatrial ventricular blanking interval; VSP = ventricular safety pacing window ; VB = ventricular blanking period (p: after pacing - s: after sensing); VRP-U = unblanked ventricular refractory period; LRI = lower rate interval (ventricular timing); OVI = open ventricular interval;

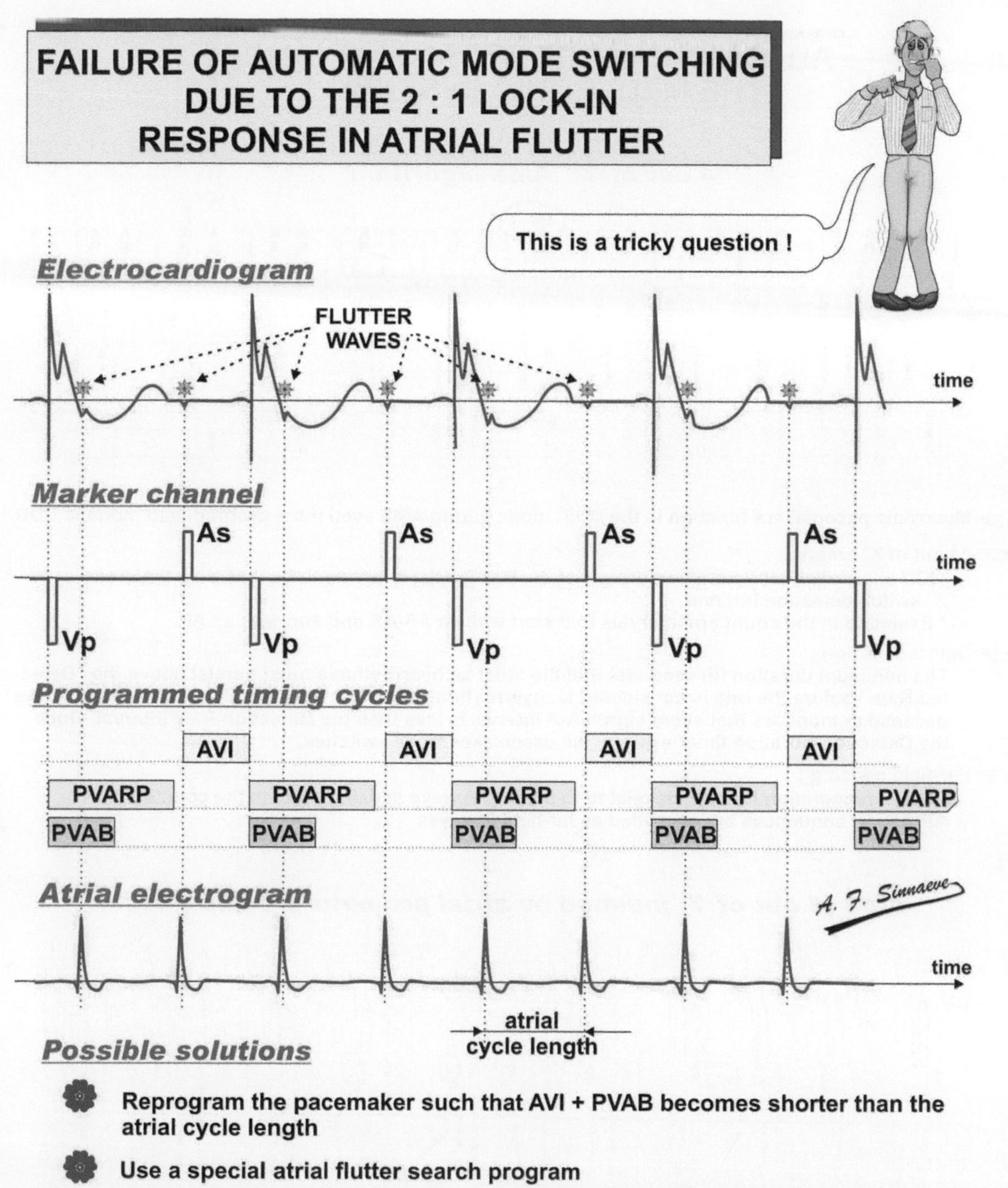

Possible solutions

- **Reprogram the pacemaker such that AVI + PVAB becomes shorter than the atrial cycle length**
- **Use a special atrial flutter search program**

Abbreviations : As = atrial sensed event; Vp = ventricular paced event; AVI = programmed AV delay; PVARP = postventricular atrial refractory period; PVAB = postventricular atrial blanking

AUTOMATIC MODE SWITCHING (AMS) THE MEDTRONIC SYSTEM - 1

"4 out of 7" AMS algorithm

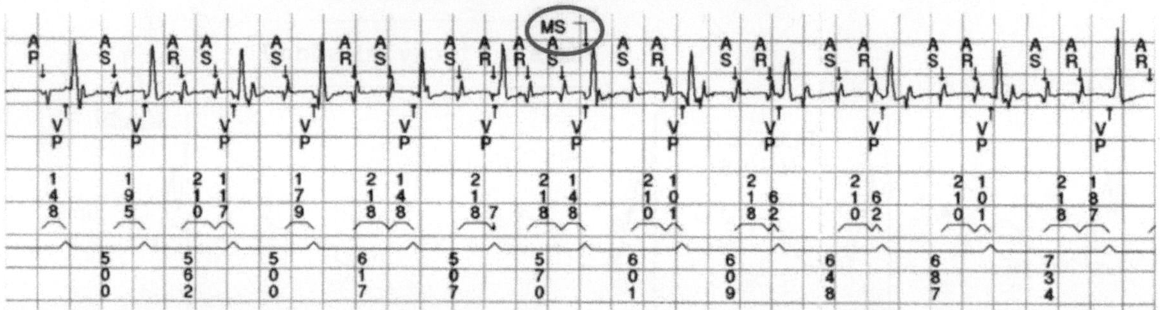

☞ Medtronic pacemakers function in the DDIR mode during AMS even if the programmed mode is DDD

☞ "4 out of 7" criteria :

- * ICD like statistical criteria requiring 4 of the last 7 atrial intervals to be less than the mode switch detection interval.
- * Excluded in the count are intervals that start with an AS/AR and end with an AP.

☞ Detect Duration :

The minimum duration (in seconds) that the atrial tachyarrhythmia must persist above the "Detected Rate" before the rate is considered tachyarrhythmic. To meet the Detection Duration delay, the pacemaker monitors that every eighth A-A interval is less than the Detection Rate interval. Once the Detection Duration timer expires, the pacemaker mode switches.

☞ Far-field sensing :

Pattern recognition for signals related to far-field R wave sensing adjusts the counters. AP-AR-AP sequences are classified as far-field R waves

AMS (4 out of 7) induced by atrial premature complexes

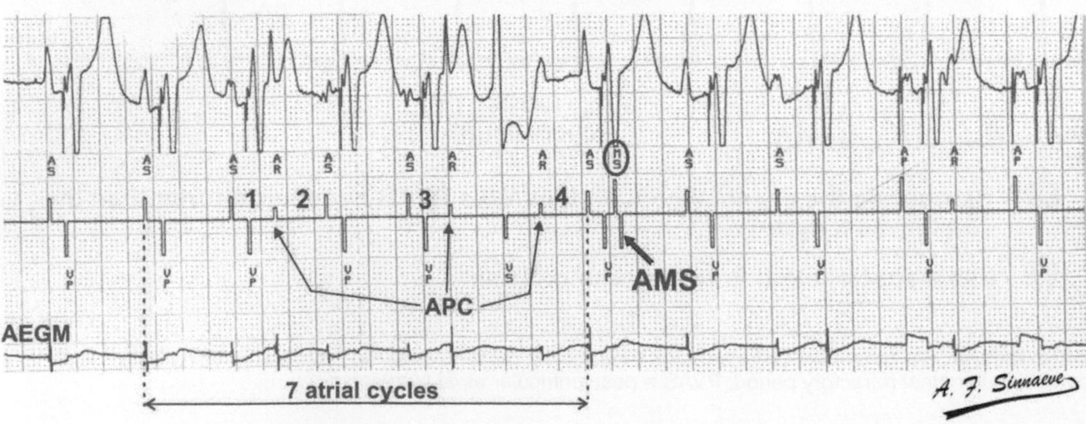

Abbreviatios : AEGM = atrial electrogram ; AMS = automatic mode switching ; AS = sensed atrial event ; AR = sensed atrial event during refractory period ; AP = atrial paced event ; APC = atrial premature complex ; VP = ventricular paced event ;

AUTOMATIC MODE SWITCHING (AMS) THE MEDTRONIC SYSTEM - 2

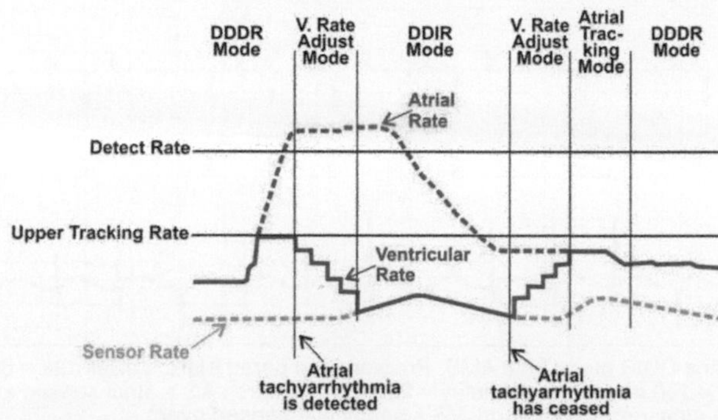

If "Post Mode Switch Overdrive Pacing" (PMOP) is not programmed, after the atrial tachyarrhythmia ends, the pacing rate is smoothly varied until the rate corresponds to the intrinsic atrial rate. Then the pacemaker switches to the programmed atrial tracking mode.
To avoid an abrupt drop in the ventricular rate at the onset of AMS, the pacemaker smoothly reduces the pacing rate from the atrial synchronous rate to the sensor-indicated rate over several pacing cycles.
AMS termination : when at least seven A-A intervals longer than the upper tracking rate interval or when five consecutive atrial paces occur, the pacemaker assumes atrial tachyarrhythmia has ceased and begins to switch back to the programmed atrial tracking mode.

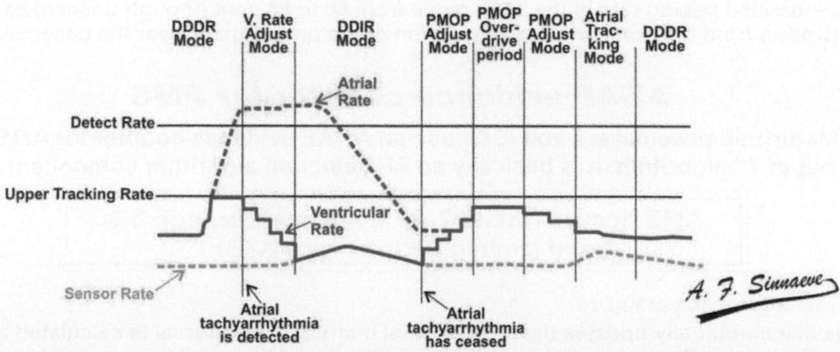

"Post Mode Switch Overdrive Pacing" (PMOP) allows mode switch to provide extended DDIR pacing at a higher rate after the atrial arrhythmia subsides. In PMOP, after the programmed Overdrive Period (at a programmed Overdrive Rate) has elapsed, the pacemaker returns to tracking in the atrium in DDDR or DDD mode as originally programmed.
If PMOP is programmed, after the atrial tachyarrhythmia ends, the pacing rate is smoothly modulated until the programmed Overdrive Rate is reached. The pacemaker maintains the Overdrive Rate in DDIR mode for a programmed duration (Overdrive Period). When the Overdrive period expires, the rate is gradually modulated until the Lower Rate or Sensor Rate is reached, and then the pacemaker switches back to the programmed atrial tracking mode.

AUTOMATIC MODE SWITCHING (AMS) THE MEDTRONIC SYSTEM - 3

Behavior of the PVARP during automatic mode switching

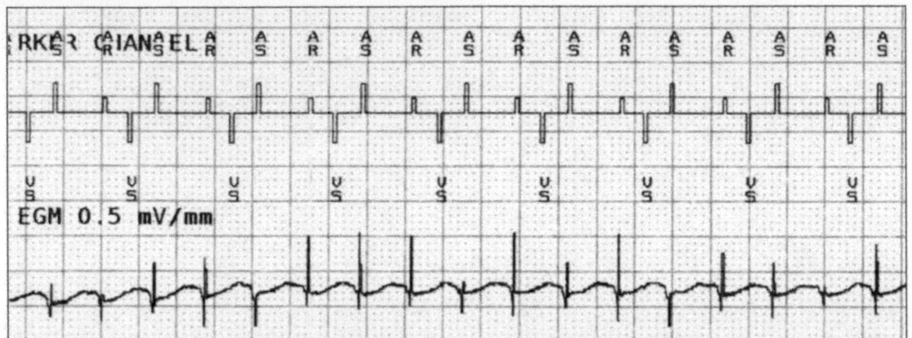

Medtronic pacemaker in the DDIR mode from AMS. Programmed parameters: Lower rate = 80 ppm, PVARP = 250 ms, PVAB = 130 ms, paced AV delay = 220 ms. Markers : AS = atrial sensed event, AR = atrial event sensed in the atrial refractory period, VS = ventricular sensed event.

The pacemaker sees the true atrial flutter rate and mode switching occurred. When the mode switches to DDIR, Medtronic devices use sensor-varied PVARP even if the the original mode was DDD. The sensor-varied PVARP attempts to maintain a 300 ms atrial inhibition window (AIW), i.e. it tries to end the PVARP 300 ms before the scheduled emission of the atrial stimulus. The equation is : PVARP = (escape or sensor-indicated interval) - (paced AV interval) - 300 ms. If the calculation results in a value less than the PVAB, the pacemaker limits the PVARP to the PVAB value. In other words, at this point there would be no actual unblanked PVARP, only a PVAB and the AIW would become shorter than 300 ms. In the case shown in the figure, rate-adaptive AV delay was programmed at 220 ms with a start rate of 100 ppm. Consequently, the parameters permit calculation of the PVAB limit. With the PVAB at 130 ms, sensor-PVARP will reach the PVAB limit at a sensor rate of 92 ppm (interval = 650 ms). The equation is PVARP = 650-220-300 = 130 ms. With a VS-AS interval of about 160 ms as in the tracing, AS is sensed early (beyond the prevailing PVARP which is now shorter in the DDIR mode than the programmed value of 250 ms (but AR is detected in the un-blanked portion of the atrial refractory period during AV (AS-VS) interval initiated by AS). A PVAB ≤ 160 ms would require a sensor-indicated rate of 88 ppm to explain the events in the tracing. The slight increase of the sensor-indicated pacing rate in the DDIR mode from 80 to 88 ppm (though unseen) can be explained by sensor activation from the pressure or manipulation of the programmer over the pacemaker.

AT/AF evidence counter for AMS

Some Medtronic pacemakers and ICDs use an AT/AF evidence counter for AMS rather than the "4 out of 7" algorithm. It is basically an AF detection algorithm component of PR Logic.

AMS occurs when AT/AF Evidence Counter ⩾ 3 and Median PP Interval < ATDI

A. F. Sinnaeve

Median atrial interval :

The device continually updates the median atrial interval. This interval is calculated by finding the median of the 12 most recent atrial intervals. The last 12 intervals are sorted in numerical order, and the median interval is the larger of the middle two values in the set. The median atrial interval must be less than the programmed AT/AF detection interval for AT/AF detection to occur.

AT/AF onset :

AT/AF onset occurs when the median atrial interval is less than the AT/AF detection interval and the AT/AF evidence counter has counted (using PR Logic) at least three ventricular events in which the A:V pattern shows evidence of an atrial tachyarrhythmia. The device begins storing episode data after AT/AF onset occurs.

AMS termination :

The device identifies sinus rhythm using the sinus rhythm criterion of PR Logic. The termination sequence is more complex when there is an unclassified rhythm with a median atrial interval greater than the AT/AF detection interval.

Abbreviations : PVAB = postventricular atrial blanking ; PVARP = postventricular atrial refractory period ;

BLANKED FLUTTER SEARCH ALGORITHM

When 8 consecutive atrial intervals measure less than 2 times the (AVI + PVAB) interval and less than 2 times the tachycardia detection interval, the device extends the PVARP for 1 beat to search of atrial flutter signals.

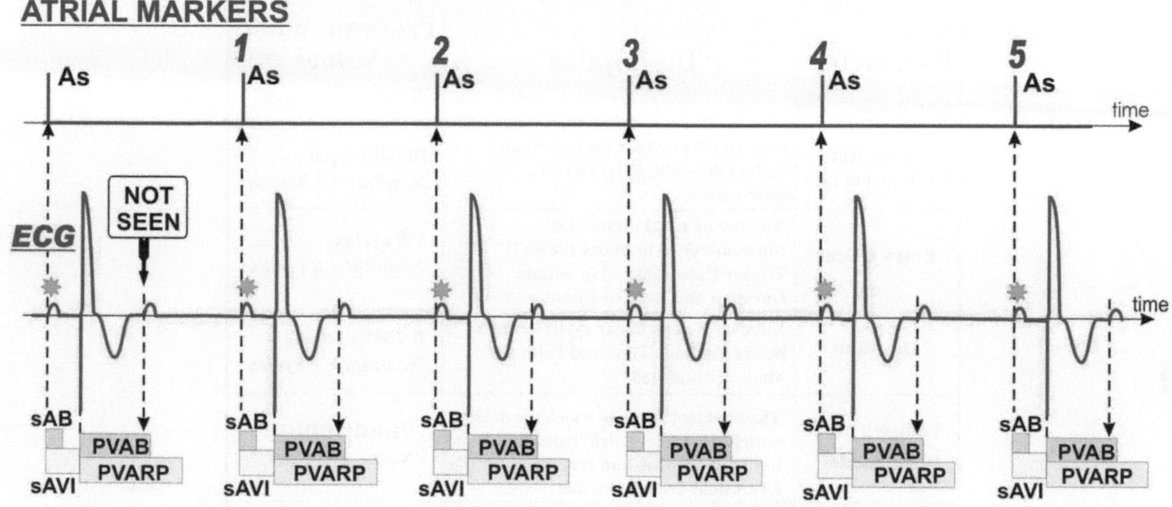

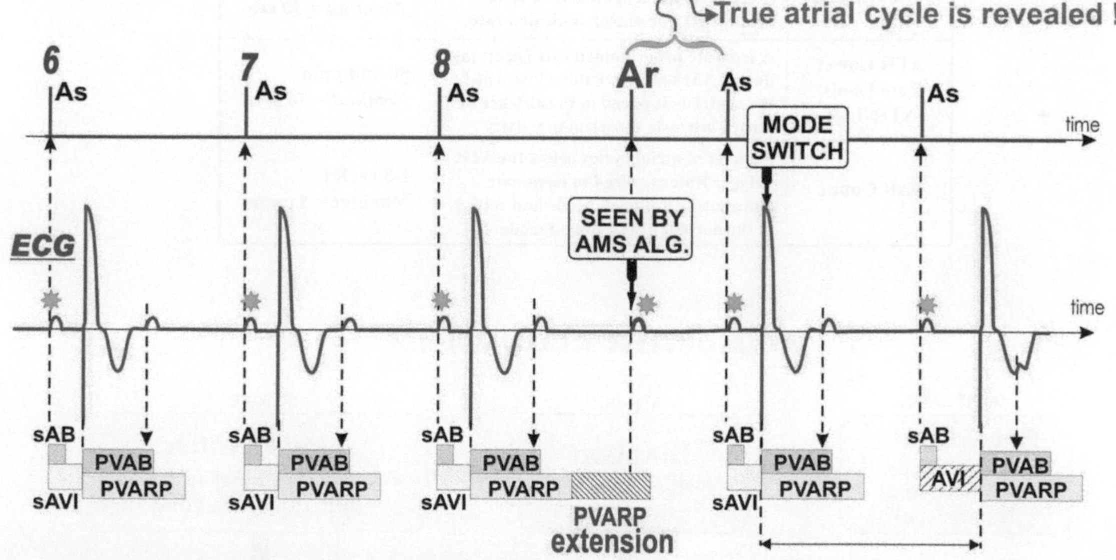

Abbreviations : As = atrial sensed event; Ar =atrial refractory sensed event; sAVI = sensed atrioventricular interval; sAB = blanked first part of sAVI; PVARP = postventricular atrial refractory period; PVAB = postventricular atrial blanking

A. F. Sinnaeve

Blanked Flutter Search Algorithm is from Medtronic Inc.

AUTOMATIC MODE SWITCHING BOSTON SCIENTIFIC

AMS or ATR Programmable Parameters

Parameter	Description	Programmable Values (Insignia model)
Trigger Rate AT detection rate	Rate cutoff at which the pacemaker defines detected atrial rate as a tachycardia	100-200 ppm *Nominal = 170 ppm*
Entry Count	Number of atrial cycles (not consecutive) at or above the ATR Trigger Rate required to initiate Duration and the Exit Counter	1-8 cycles *Nominal = 8 cycles*
Duration	Number of ventricular cycles counted before Fallback Time and Fallback Mode are initiated	0-2048 cycles *Nominal = 8 cycles*
Fallback Mode (AMS mode)	The inhibited mode to which the device switches ("mode switch") once Duration has been fulfilled, and remains in until Exit Count criteria are met	VDI(R), DDI(R) *Nominal = VDI*
Fallback Time	The time that the ventricular paced rate decelerates to the ATR Lower Rate Limit (LRL) or sensor-indicated rate	0-120 sec *Nominal = 30 sec*
ATR Lower Rate Limit (ATR-LRL)	A separate programmed rate occurring during AMS (ATR). Fallback at which the ventricle is paced in the absence of sensed intrinsic ventricular activity	30-150 ppm *Nominal = 70 ppm*
Exit Count	Number of atrial cycles below the ATR Trigger Rate required to terminate Duration or Fallback Mode and return to the normal programmed mode	1-8 cycles *Nominal = 8 cycles*

AMS or ATR ALGORITHM

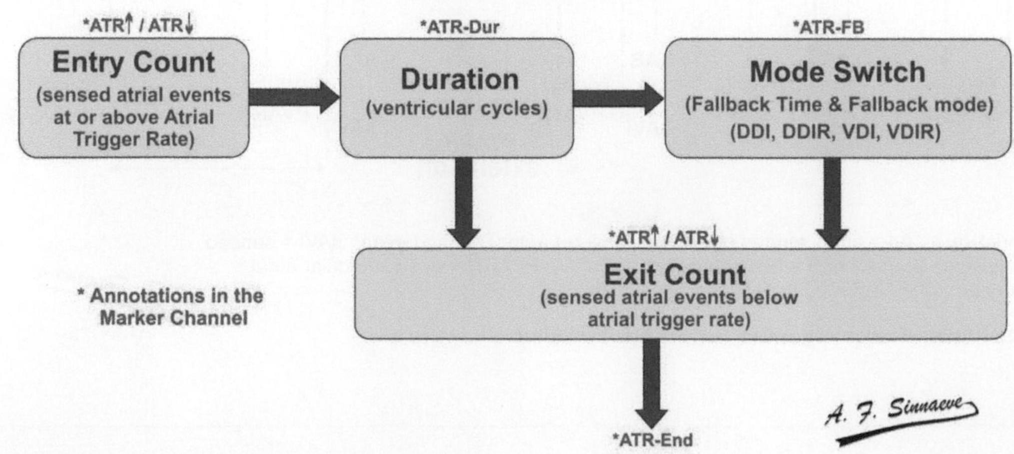

Abbreviations : AMS = automatic mode switching ; AT = atrial tachycardia ; ATR = atrial tachycardia response ;

AUTOMATIC MODE SWITCHING BOSTON SCIENTIFIC - part 2

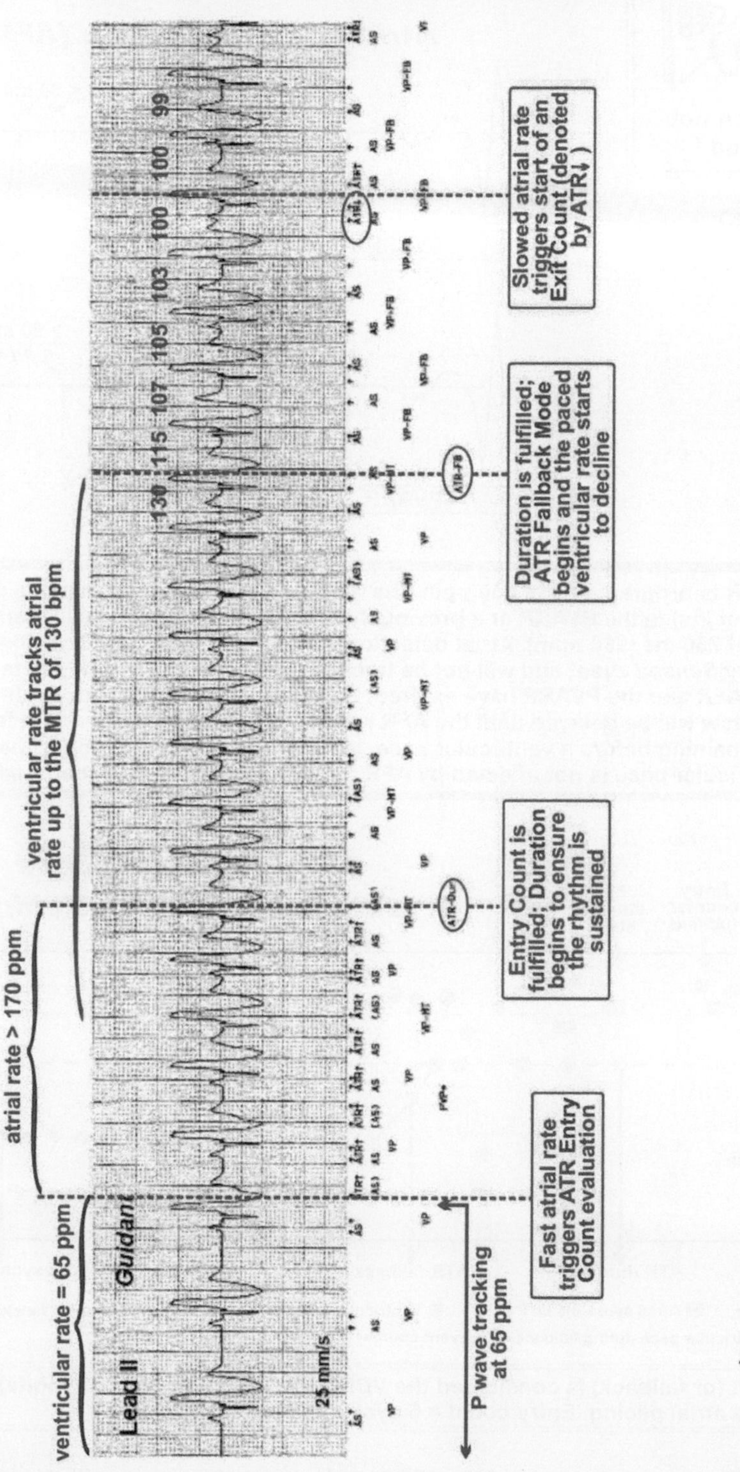

ventricular rate = 65 ppm
atrial rate > 170 ppm
ventricular rate tracks atrial rate up to the MTR of 130 bpm
Lead II
Guidant
25 mm/s
130
115
107
105
103
100
100
99
P wave tracking at 65 ppm
Fast atrial rate triggers ATR Entry Count evaluation
Entry Count is fulfilled; Duration begins to ensure the rhythm is sustained
Duration is fulfilled; ATR Fallback Mode begins and the paced ventricular rate starts to decline
Slowed atrial rate triggers start of an Exit Count (denoted by ATR↓)
A. F. Sinnaeve

Abbreviations : AMS = automatic mode switching ; ATR = atrial tachycardia response ;

Switching seems to be a simple task...
... but it is often not well understood !
A. F. Sinnaeve

AUTOMATIC MODE SWITCHING BOSTON SCIENTIFIC - part 3

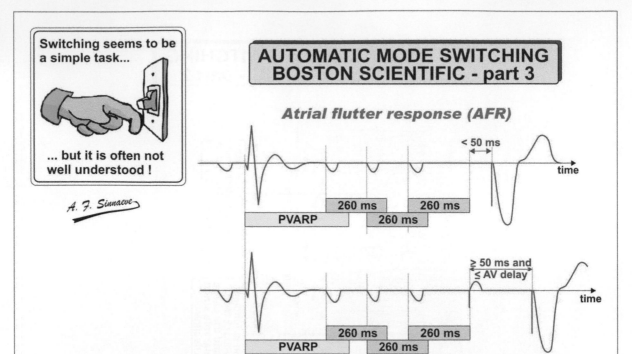

Atrial flutter response (AFR)

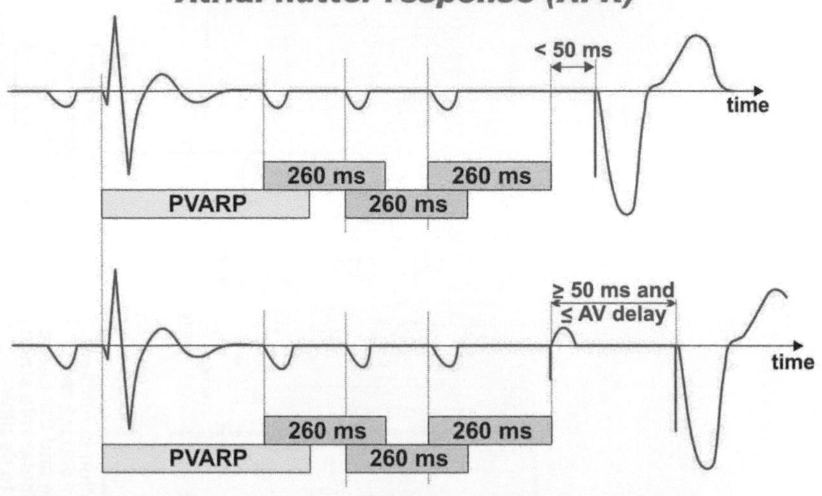

When AFR is programmed to 230 ppm (the maximum value), for example, a detected atrial event inside the PVARP or a previously triggered AFR interval will start an AFR window of 260 ms (230 ppm). Atrial detection inside the AFR will be classified as *Refractory Sensed* event and will not be tracked. The sensing window starts only after both the AFR and the PVARP have expired. Paced atrial events scheduled inside an AFR window will be delayed until the AFR window has expired. If there are fewer than 50 ms remaining before a ventricular pace, the atrial pace is inhibited for the cycle. The ventricular pace is not affected by AFR and will take place as scheduled.

Atrial tachy response (automatic mode switching)

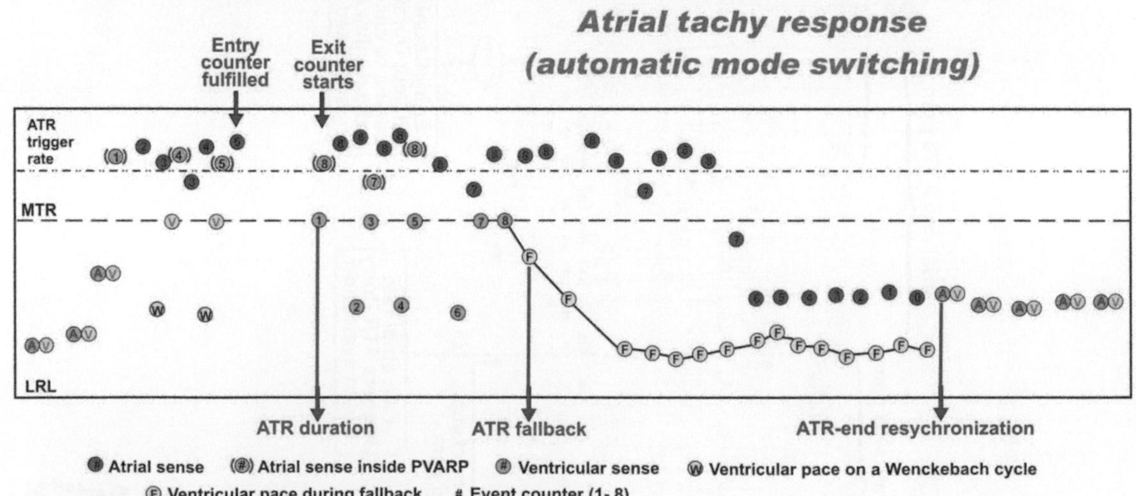

The switch (or fallback) is considered the VDI mode (similar to the DDI mode) because there is no atrial pacing. Entry count = 6 cycles ; duration = 8 cycles.

Abbreviations : AMS = automatic mode switching ; ATR = atrial tachycardia response ; LRL = lower rate limit ; MTR = maximum tracking rate ; PVARP = postventricular refractory period ;

AUTOMATIC MODE SWITCHING - St JUDE ALGORITHM 1

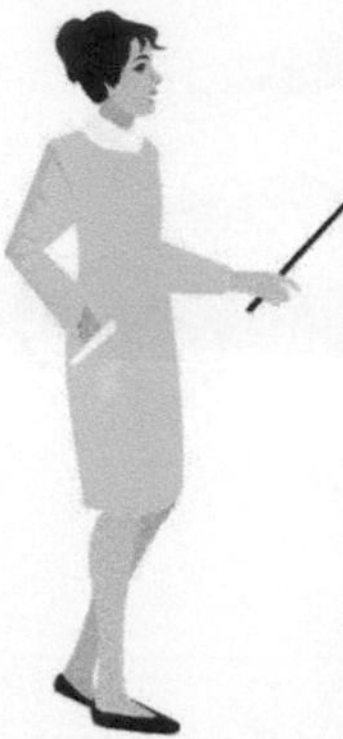

The algorithm in St Jude's devices uses a "running average" rate (also known as the mean atrial rate, filtered or matched atrial rate). This process moves towards AMS by continuously monitoring the P-P interval and generating a filtered heart rate interval (FARI) that changes according to the duration of the prevailing sensed atrial cycle (ARI). AMS will occur when the FARI shortens to a predetermined duration equal to the atrial detection rate interval (ATDI). Because the process is gradual, the rapidity of reaching AMS will depend not only on the ATDI, but also on the pre-existing sinus rate. The FARI reaches the ATDI faster when atrial tachycardia occurs in the setting of a higher resting sinus rate than from a sinus bradycardia. When the baseline is relatively short, the FARI starts from a shorter baseline duration on its gradual way to reach the ATDI. All atrial intervals (AP-AP, AS-AP, AP-AS, AS-AS) are counted towards the FARI. The averaging algorithm shortens FARI by 39 ms for every atrial interval shorter than FARI. It lengthens FARI by 25 ms for every atrial interval longer than FARI.

A similar algorithm was used in the Medtronic Thera DR, Kappa 400 and Gem DR devices

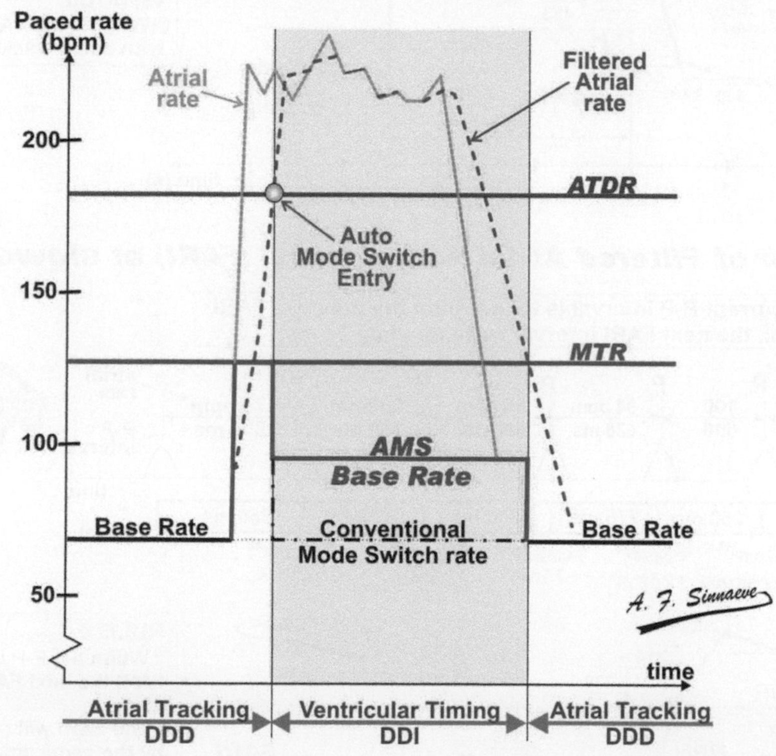

The AMS base rate is programmable and is the pacing rate during AMS. If this parameter is not programmed, the AMS rate will equal the programmed lower rate.

Abbreviations : AMS = automatic mode switching; AP = atrial paced event; AS = atrial sensed event; ARI = atrial rate interval; ATDI = atrial tachycardia detection interval; ATDR = atrial tachycardia detection rate; FARI = filtered atrial rate; MTR = maximum tracking rate;

AUTOMATIC MODE SWITCHING - St JUDE ALGORITHM 2

Behavior of Filtered Atrial Rate Interval (FARI) at fast rates

If the current P-P interval is shorter than the previous FARI interval, the next FARI interval will decrease by 38 ms.

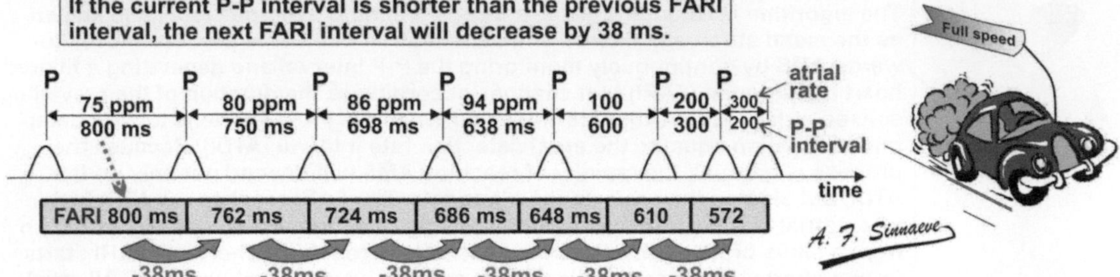

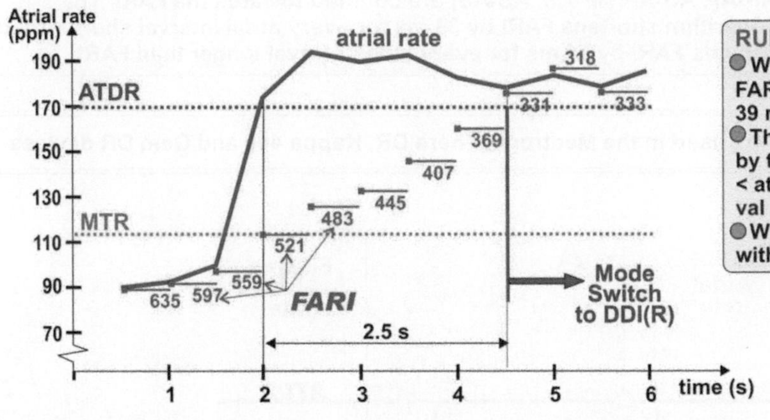

RULE 1 :

- When the P-P interval < previous FARI the next FARI will shorten by 39 ms (38 ms in older devices).
- The FARI will continue to shorten by the same amount until the FARI < atrial tachycardia detection interval (ATDI).
- When FARI < ATDI, AMS occurs with a non-tracking mode (DDI/R)

Behavior of Filtered Atrial Rate Interval (FARI) at slower rates

If the current P-P interval is longer than the previous FARI interval, the next FARI interval will extend by 25 ms.

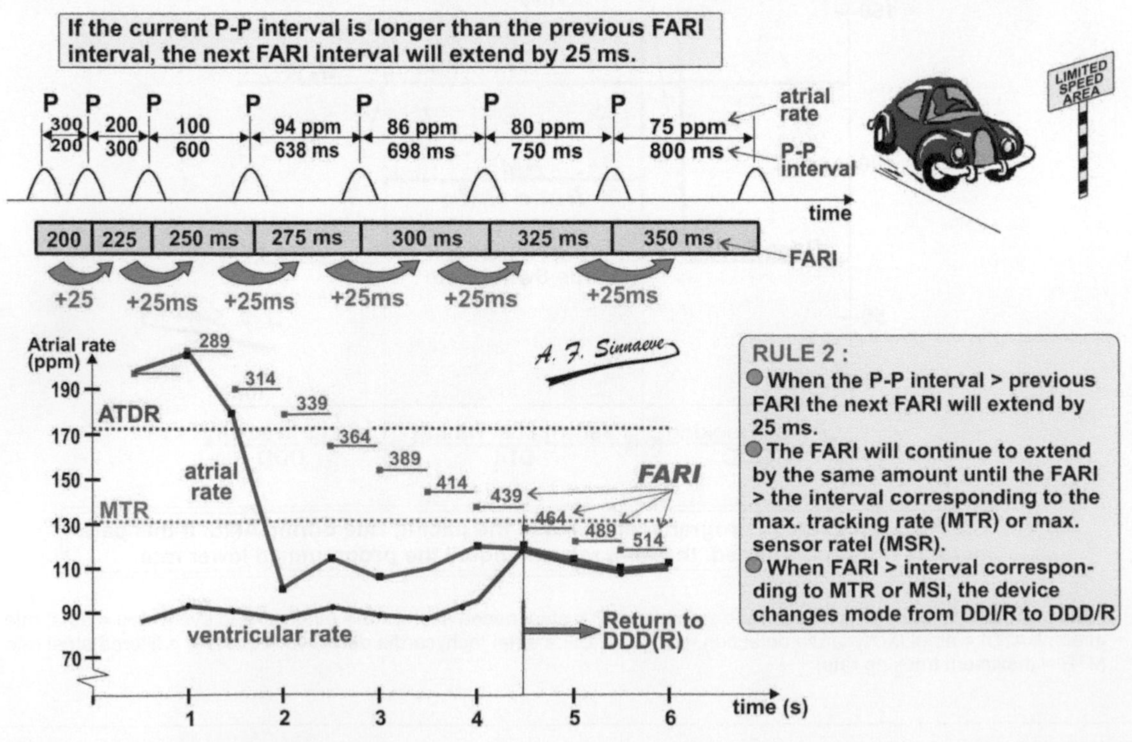

RULE 2 :

- When the P-P interval > previous FARI the next FARI will extend by 25 ms.
- The FARI will continue to extend by the same amount until the FARI > the interval corresponding to the max. tracking rate (MTR) or max. sensor ratel (MSR).
- When FARI > interval corresponding to MTR or MSI, the device changes mode from DDI/R to DDD/R

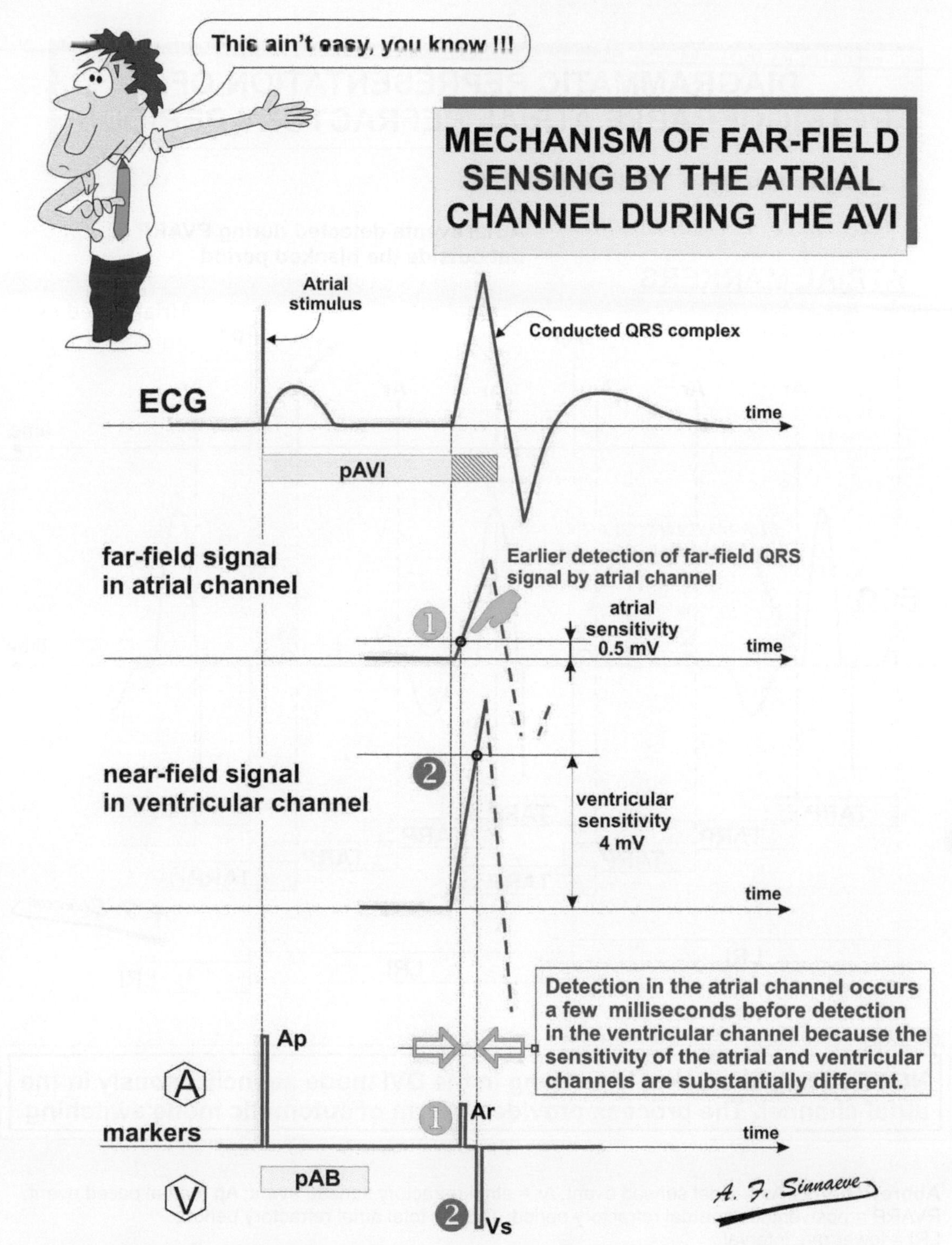

Abbreviations : Ap = atrial paced event; Ar = atrial refractory sensed event; Vs = ventricular sensed event; pAVI = paced atrioventricular interval; pAB = blanked first part of pAVI; AVI = programmed AV delay

DIAGRAMMATIC REPRESENTATION OF RETRIGGERABLE ATRIAL REFRACTORY PERIODS

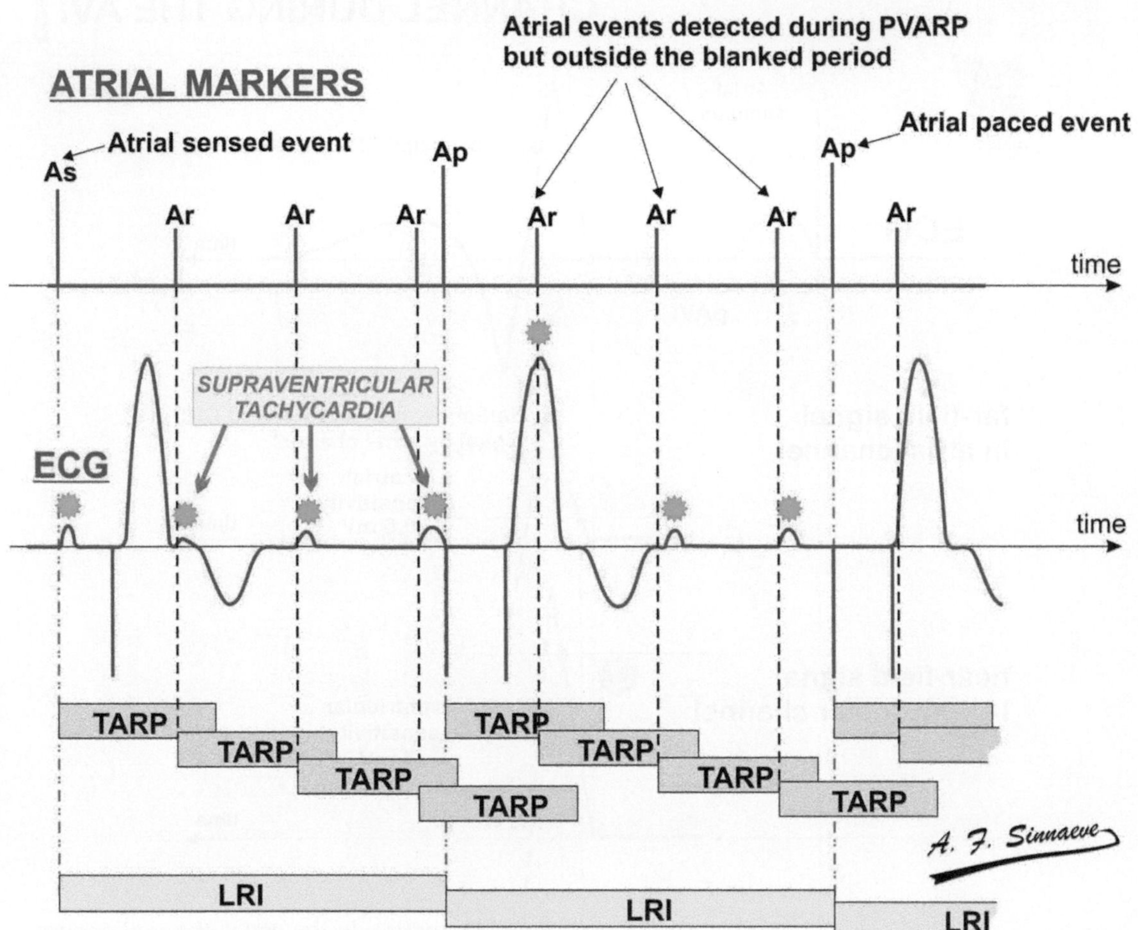

NOTE : The pacemaker is working in the DVI mode asynchronously in the atrial channel. The process provides a form of automatic mode switching.

Abbreviations : As = atrial sensed event; Ar = atrial refractory sensed event; Ap = atrial paced event; PVARP = postventricular atrial refractory period; TARP = total atrial refractory period; LRI = lower rate interval

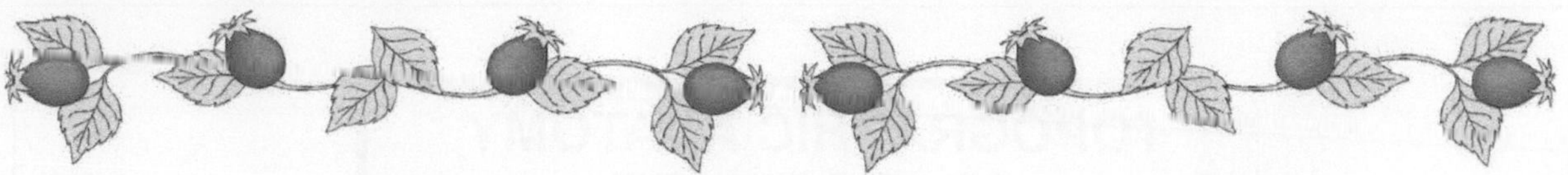

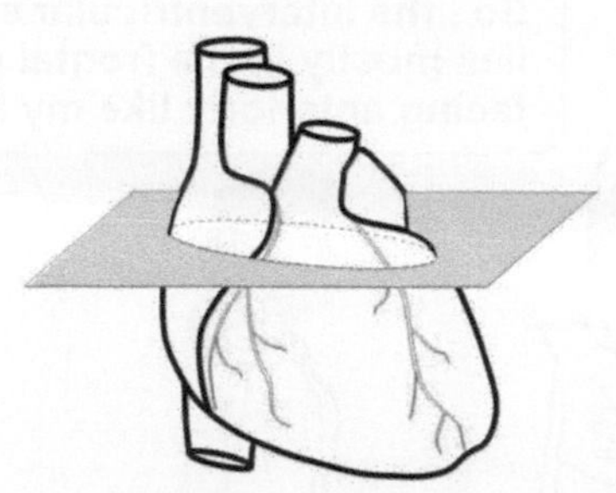

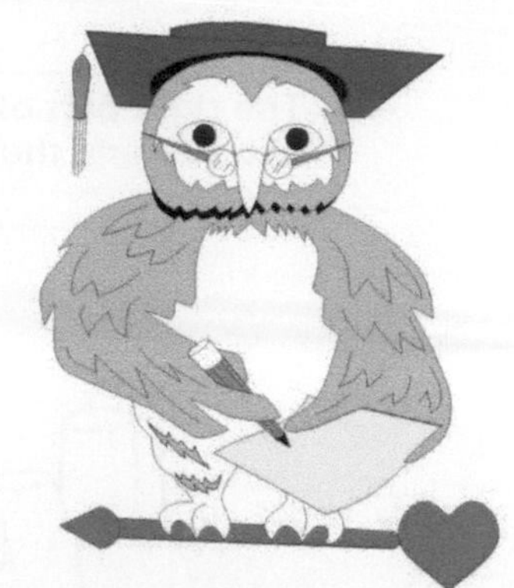

PACEMAKER RADIOGRAPHY

* Topographic anatomy of the heart
* Lead position for VVI pacing
* Lead position for dual chamber pacing - part 1
* Lead position for dual chamber pacing - part 2

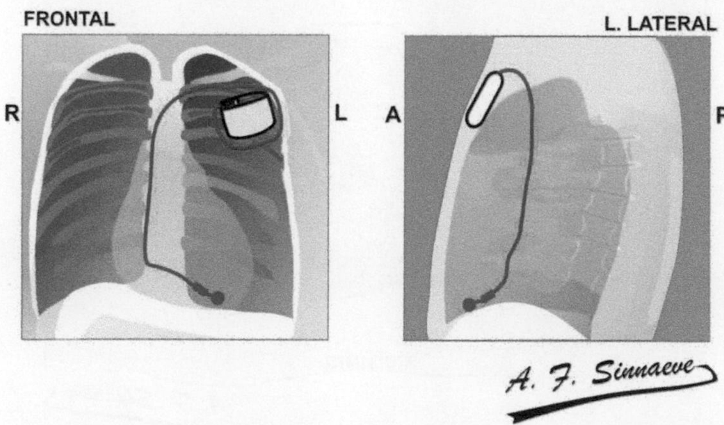

A. F. Sinnaeve

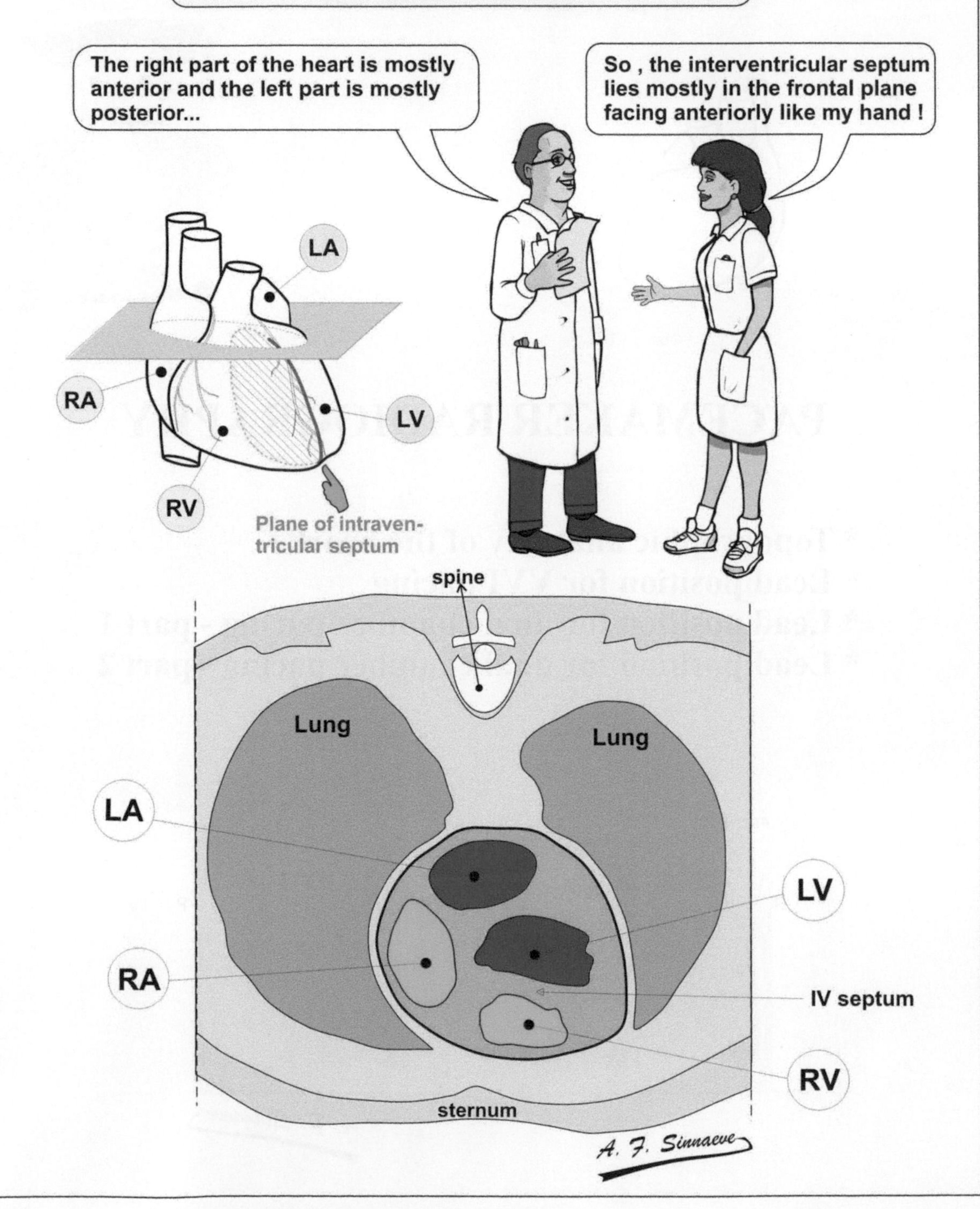
TOPOGRAPHIC ANATOMY OF THE HEART
The right part of the heart is mostly anterior and the left part is mostly posterior...
So , the interventricular septum lies mostly in the frontal plane facing anteriorly like my hand !
LA
RA
LV
RV
Plane of intraven-tricular septum
spine
Lung
Lung
LA
LV
RA
IV septum
RV
sternum
A. F. Sinnaeve

SCHEMATIC REPRESENTATION OF LEAD POSITION FOR VVI PACING

Ventricular lead in right ventricular apex

FRONTAL

L. LATERAL

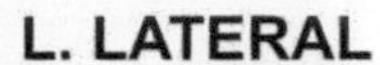

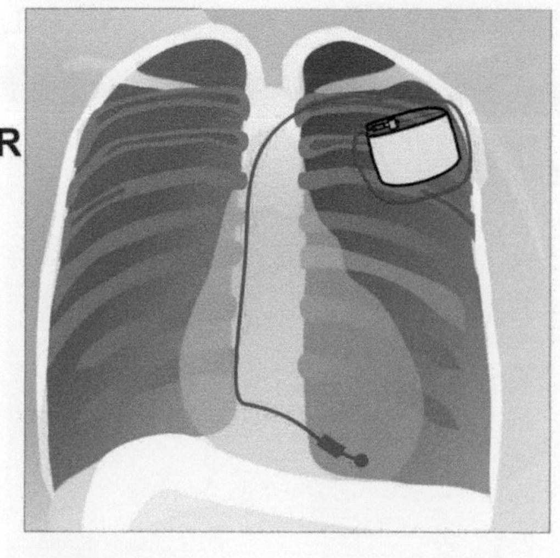

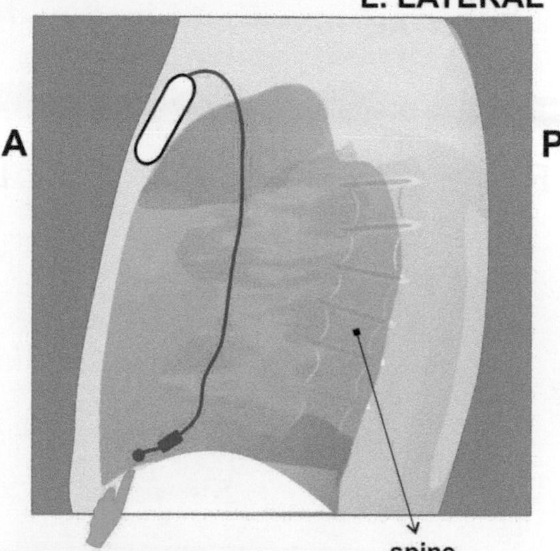

The RV lead is anterior because the right ventricle is anterior

FRONTAL

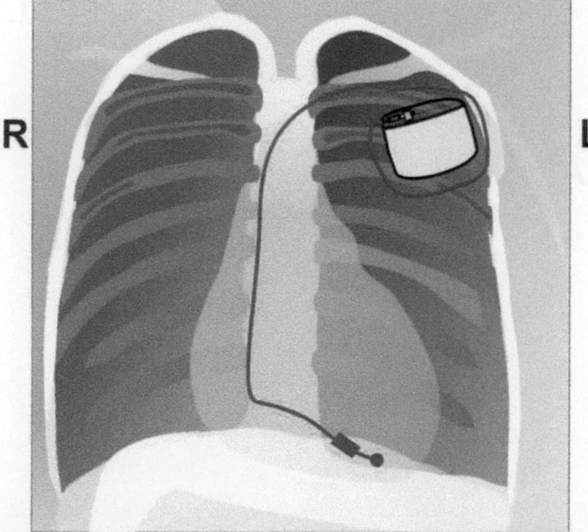

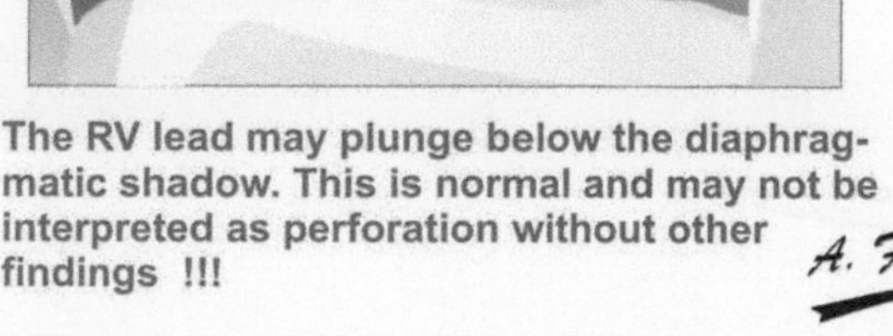

The RV lead may plunge below the diaphragmatic shadow. This is normal and may not be interpreted as perforation without other findings !!!

FRONTAL

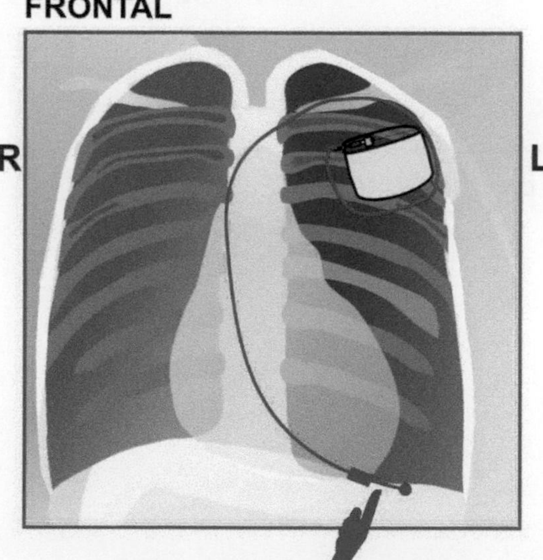

PERFORATION !

The lead is clearly beyond the cardiac shadow !

A. F. Sinnaeve

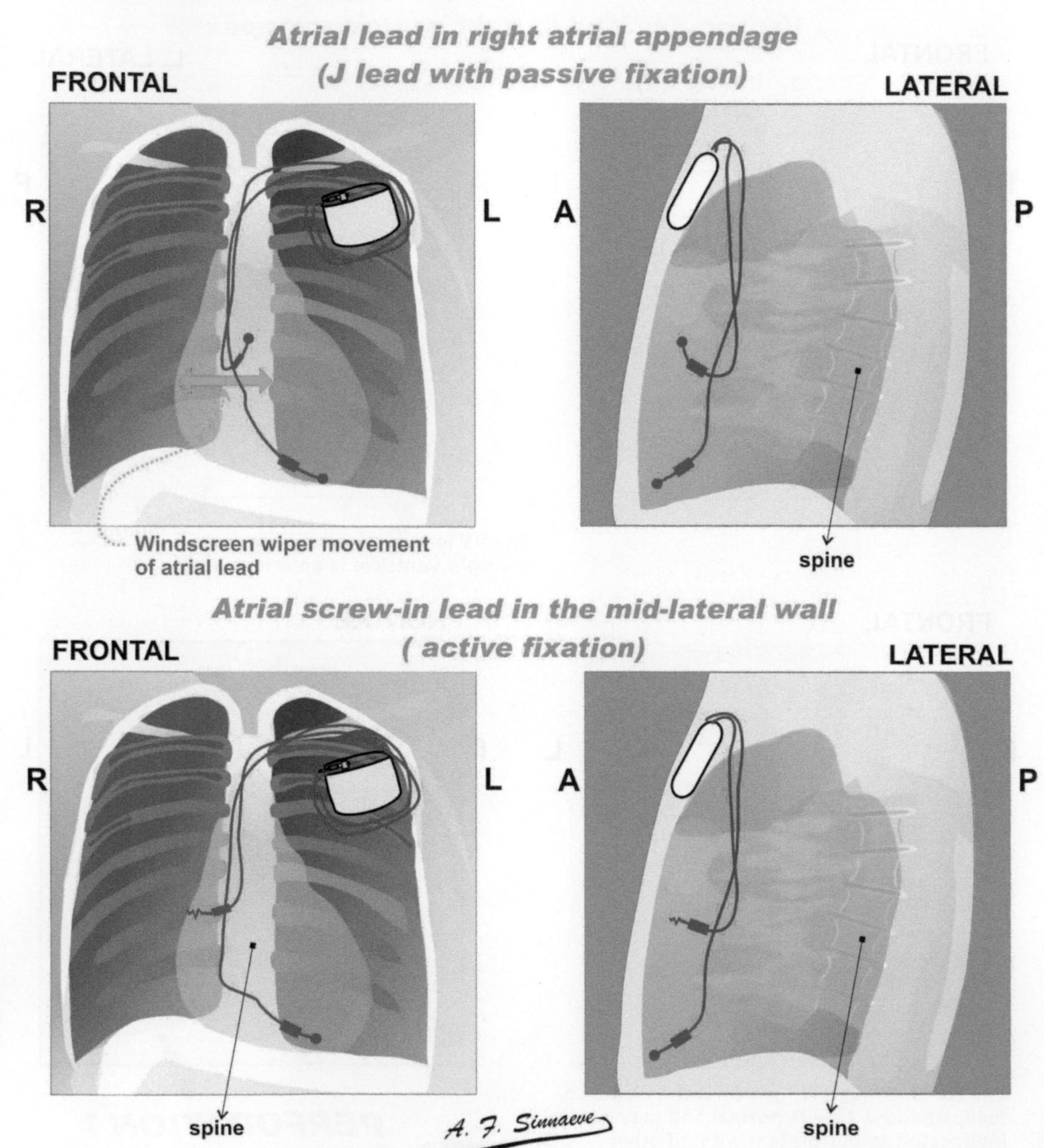
SCHEMATIC REPRESENTATION OF LEAD POSITIONS FOR DUAL CHAMBER PACING
Atrial lead in right atrial appendage
(J lead with passive fixation)
FRONTAL
LATERAL
R
L
A
P
Windscreen wiper movement
of atrial lead
spine
Atrial screw-in lead in the mid-lateral wall
(active fixation)
FRONTAL
LATERAL
R
L
A
P
spine
spine
A. F. Sinnaeve

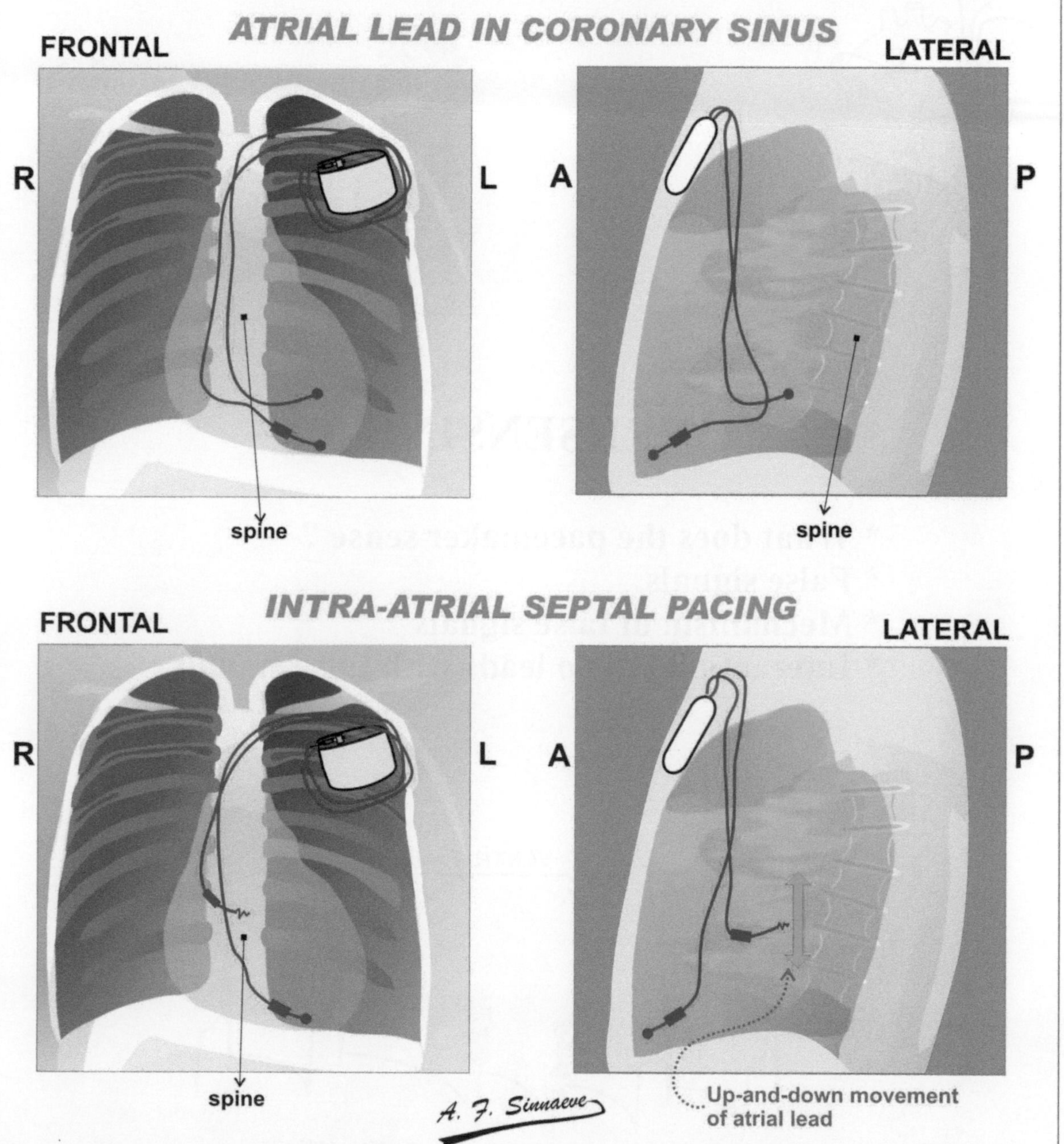
SCHEMATIC REPRESENTATION OF LEAD POSITIONS FOR DUAL CHAMBER PACING
ATRIAL LEAD IN CORONARY SINUS
FRONTAL
LATERAL
R
L
A
P
spine
spine
INTRA-ATRIAL SEPTAL PACING
FRONTAL
LATERAL
R
L
A
P
spine
A. F. Sinnaeve
Up-and-down movement of atrial lead

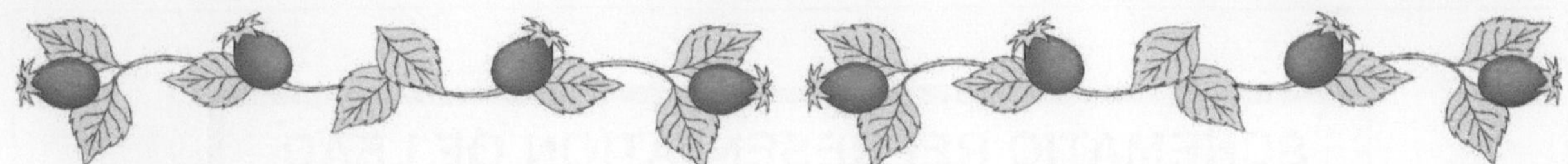

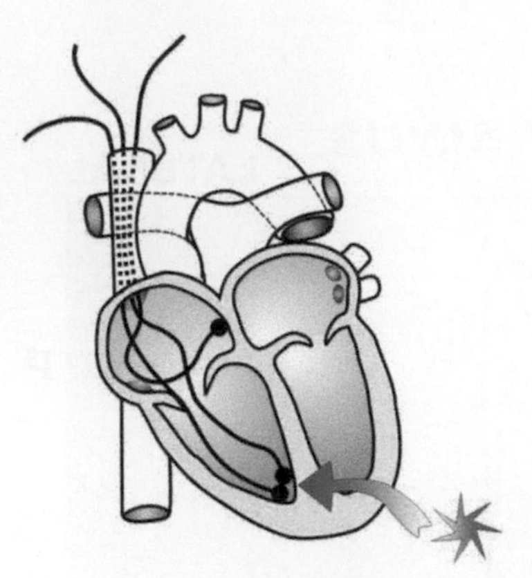

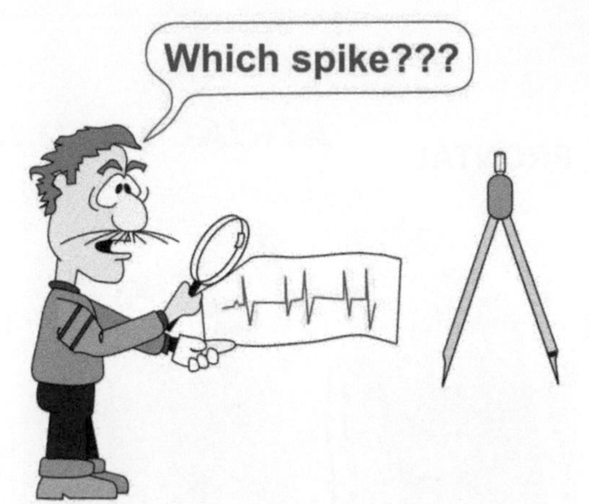

OVERSENSING

* What does the pacemaker sense ?
* False signals
* Mechanism of false signals
* Interaction of two leads with false signals

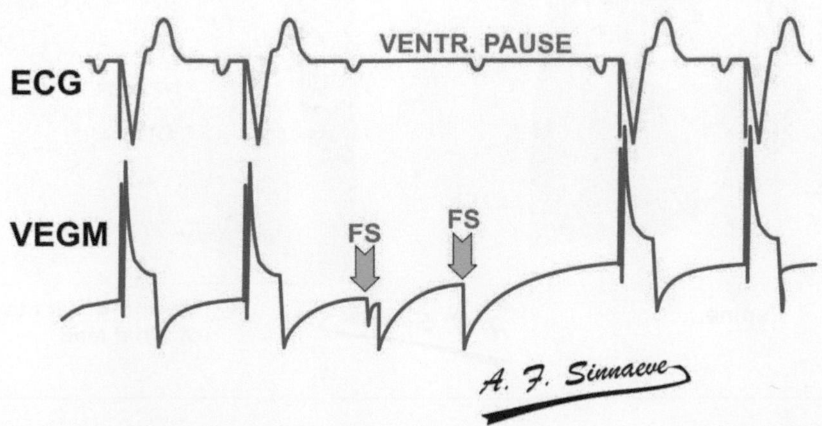

WHAT DOES THE VENTRICULAR CHANNEL OF THE PACEMAKER SENSE ?
T wave, afterpotential, false signal, ... ?

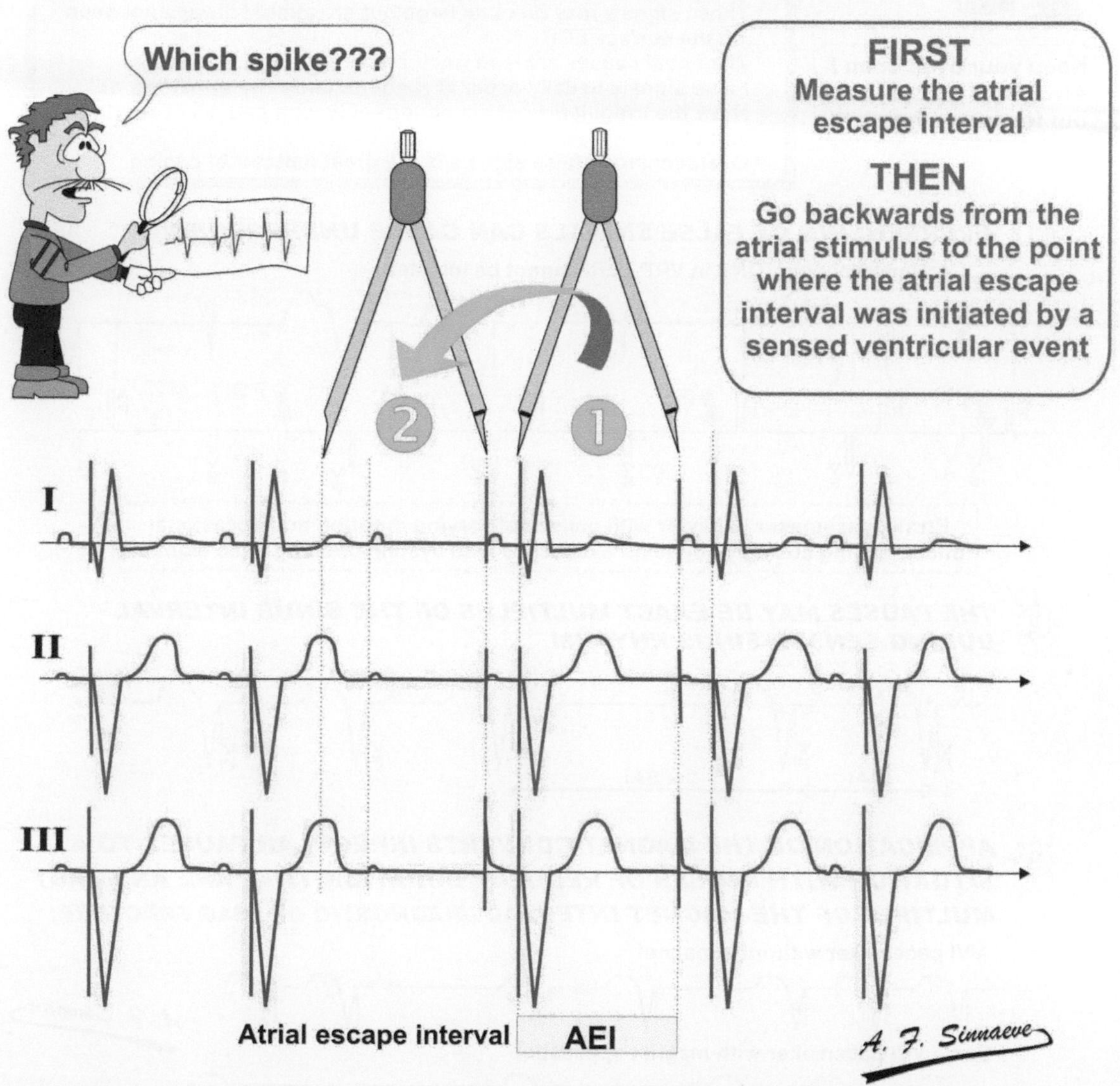
Which spike???
FIRST
Measure the atrial escape interval
THEN
Go backwards from the atrial stimulus to the point where the atrial escape interval was initiated by a sensed ventricular event
2
1
I
II
III
Atrial escape interval
AEI
A. F. Sinnaeve

* In ventricular-based sensing, the atrial escape interval (AEI) always remains constant.
* Measure backwards from an atrial stimulus to the preceding point of sensing because a ventricular event (paced or sensed) always initiates an AEI

This method cannot be used in pacemakers with atrial-based lower rate timing

FALSE SIGNALS
FROM INTERMITTENT DERANGEMENT OF LEAD FUNCTION

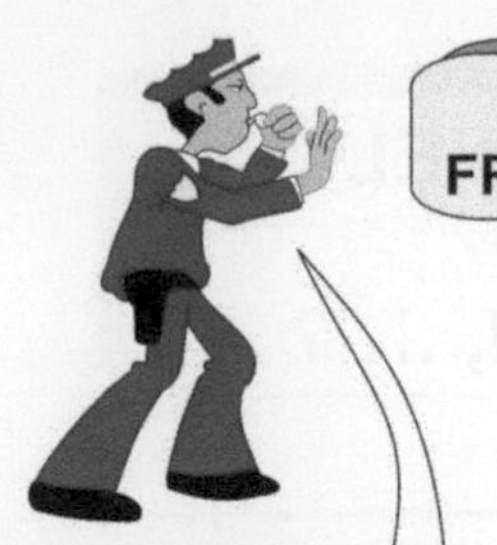

Keep your eyes open ! Always be on the look-out for false signals !!!

Abrupt and large changes in resistance within a pacing system can cause corresponding voltage changes between the electrodes. These signals are called “false signals” or transients.

* These signals may be quite large but are almost always not seen on the surface ECG
* The usual causes are lead fractures and insulation defects
* False signals usually occur at random. Long rhythm strips will show the irregularirty of the abnormality with pauses of varying duration
* Oversensing of false signals is the great imitator of pacing

1 OVERSENSING OF FALSE SIGNALS CAN CAUSE UNDERSENSING

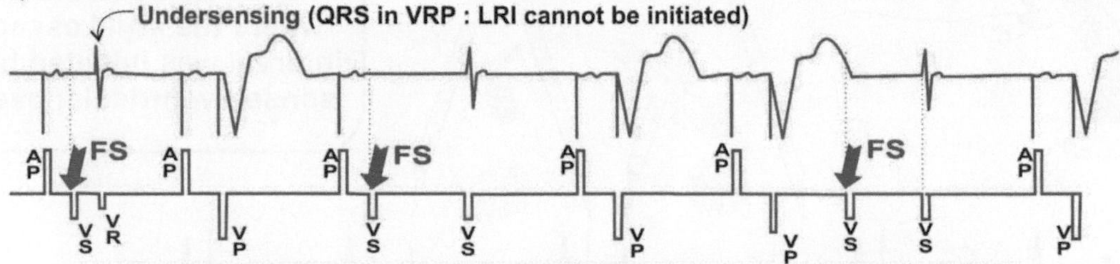

Erratic pacemaker behavior with pauses of varying duration and occasional undersensing strongly suggests a defective lead system creating false signals

2 THE PAUSES MAY BE EXACT MULTIPLES OF THE SINUS INTERVAL DURING SENSED SINUS RHYTHM

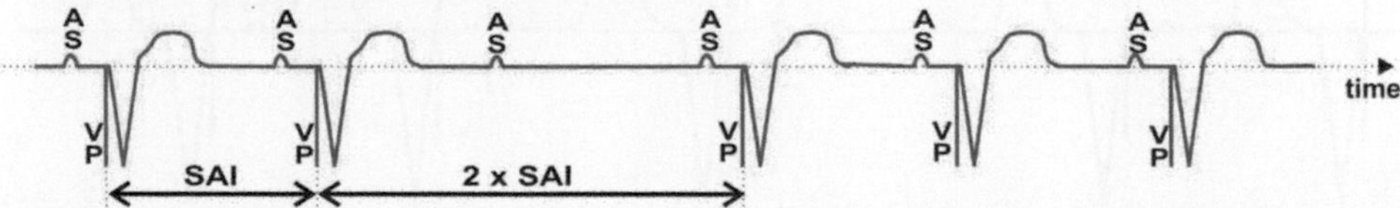

3 APPLICATION OF THE MAGNET CONVERTS IRREGULAR PAUSES TO A SITUATION WITH PAUSES OF REGULAR DURATION THAT ARE AN EXACT MULTIPLE OF THE MAGNET INTERVAL (DIAGNOSTIC OF LEAD FRACTURE)

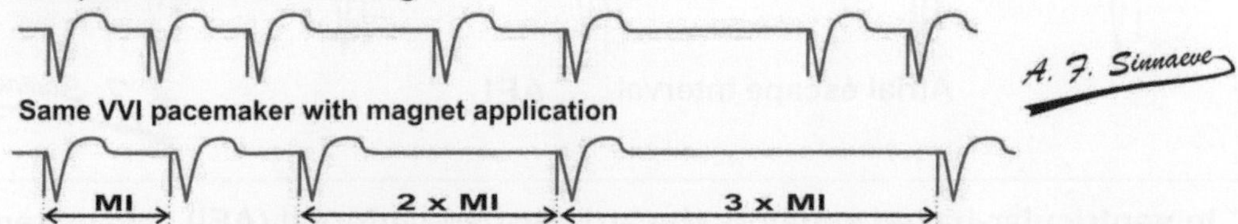

A. F. Sinnaeve

A lead problem can resemble T wave oversensing if mechanical systole creates false signals (making and breaking the circuit) only at a specific part of the cardiac cycle. Such an abnormality can be identical to T wave sensing even after application of the magnet. The diagnosis can be made by the configuration of the false signal in the telemetered EGM

Abbreviatons : AP = atrial pace; AS = atrial sense; FS = false signal; MI = magnet interval; SAI = spontaneous atrial interval; VP = ventricular pace; VS = ventricular sense; VR = ventricular sense in refractory period; LRI = lower rate interval

MECHANISM OF FALSE SIGNALS FROM INTERMITTENT CIRCUIT DISRUPTION

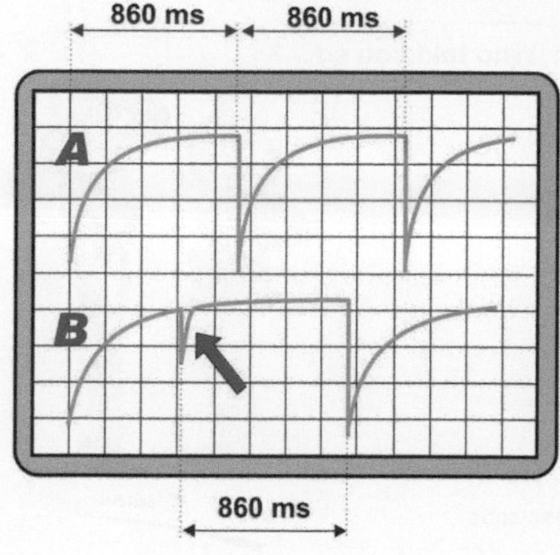

Voltage waveforms on an oscilloscope of a VVI pacemaker connected to a pacing lead in normal saline solution. The recording shows the mechanism of production of "false signals" from intermittent derangement of the pacemaker circuit. A shows an automatic interval of 860ms. In B, a false signal is deliberately created by manually breaking the connection between pacemaker and electrode for an instant. The disturbance causes a rapidly rising voltage of almost 200mV, well outside the refractory period of the pacemaker, which therefore senses it and recycles with an escape interval of 860ms. The reciprocal signal, caused by the return of voltage to the "baseline", because it occurs about 100ms after the initial signal, falls inside the refractory period of the pacemaker. Consequently it is not sensed.

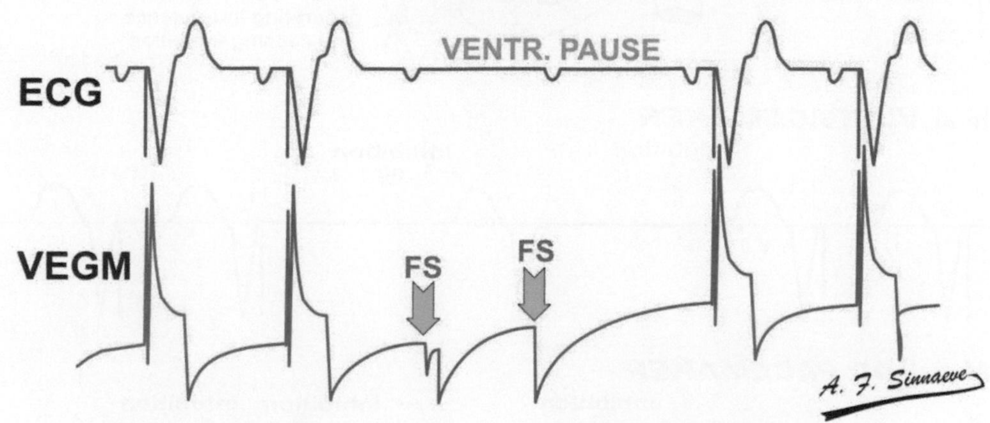

LEAD PROBLEMS CREATE FALSE SIGNALS

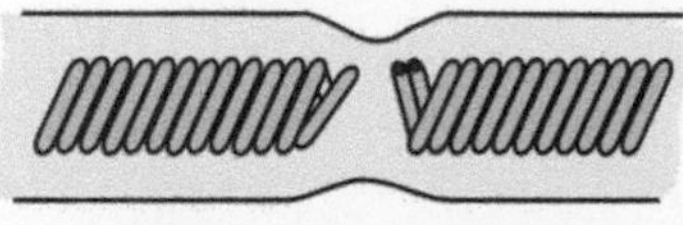
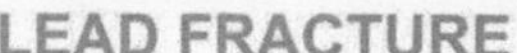

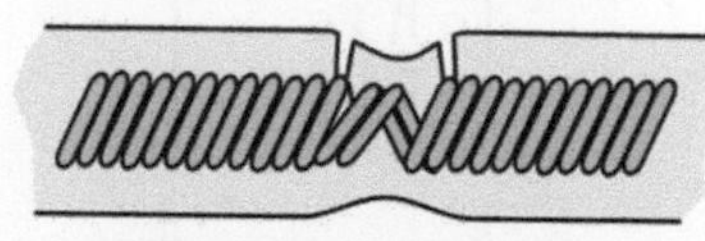

Abbreviations : ECG = surface electrocardiogram ; VEGM = ventricular electrogram ; FS = false signal

INTERACTION OF ACTIVE AND INACTIVE ELECTRODES LYING SIDE-BY-SIDE

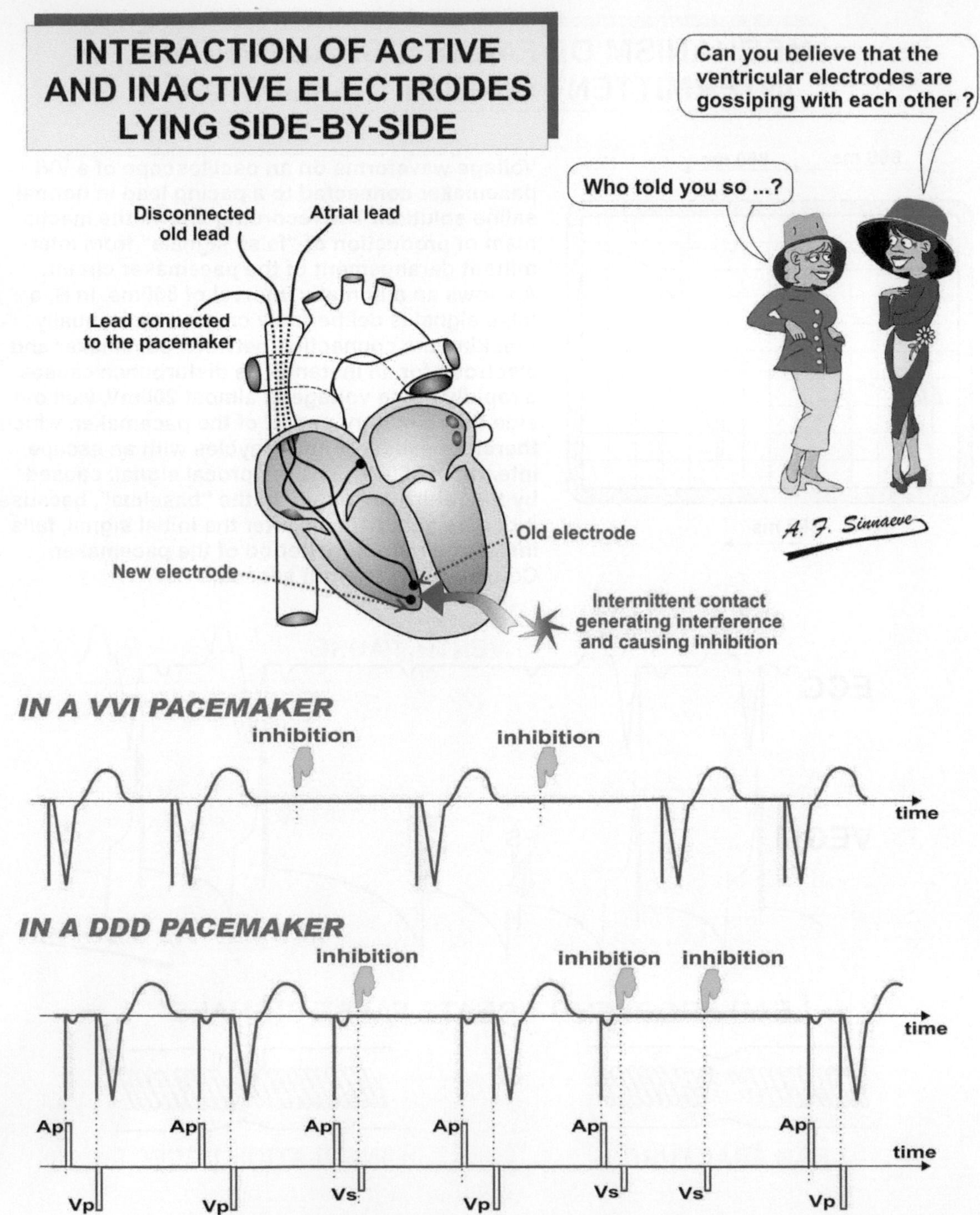

*** Application of the magnet over the pacemaker eliminates the pauses related to oversensing and restores regular pacing at magnet rate.**

*** The false signals created by intermittent contact of the electrodes are invisible on the surface ECG. However, they can be seen in the intracardiac electrogram transmitted by telemetry.**

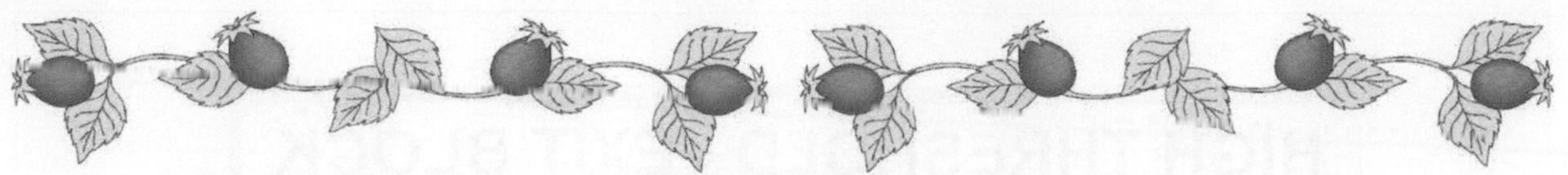

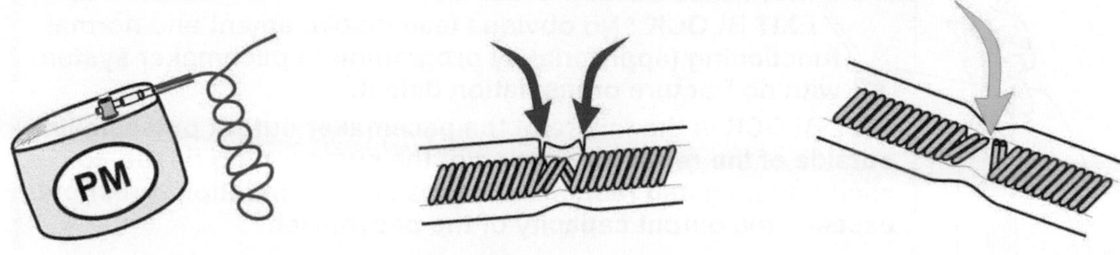

TROUBLESHOOTING

* High threshold - Exit block
* Loss of ventricular capture by visible pacemaker stimuli
* Missing stimuli during VVI pacing
* Lead insulation defect
* Lead fracture
* Analysis of lead problems
* Lead fracture - Conversion from bipolar to unipolar
* Subclavian crush syndrome
* Twiddler's syndrome
* Diaphragmatic stimulation
* Muscle stimulation
* Runaway pacemaker

A. F. Sinnaeve

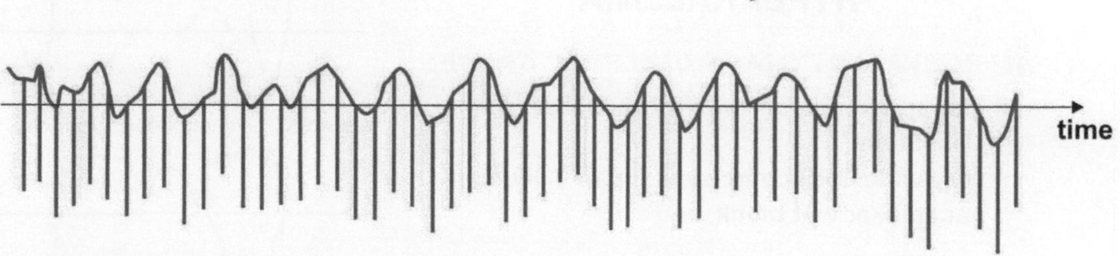

HIGH THRESHOLD - EXIT BLOCK

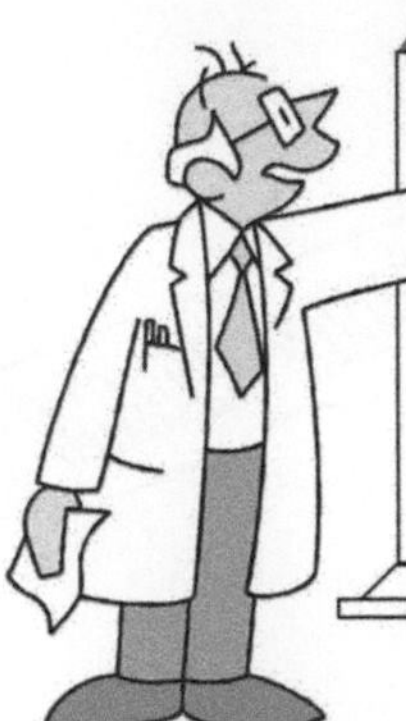

EXIT BLOCK : No obvious lead displacement and normal functioning (appropriately programmed) pacemaker system with no fracture or insulation defect.

EXIT BLOCK is the failure of the pacemaker output pulse, falling outside of the refractory period of the surrounding tissue, to elicit a propagated response because the stimulation threshold exceeds the output capacity of the pacemaker.

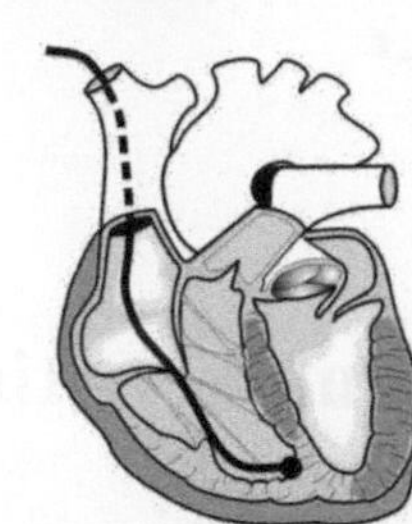

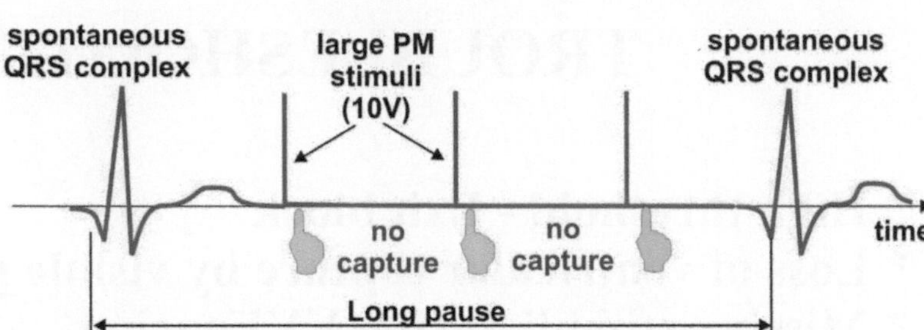

CAUSES :
* excessive tissue reaction around the lead tip
* various antiarhythmic drugs (e.g. flecainide)
* electrolyte abnormality (e.g. hyperkalemia, acidosis and hypothyroidism)
* myocardial infarction & tissue damage from defibrillation, electrocautery and radiotherapy

HYPERKALEMIA

AN ELEVATED POTASSIUM LEVEL CAUSES :
* disappearance of P waves due to atrial asystole
* very wide QRS complexes (up to 3OOms)
* pacemaker exit block

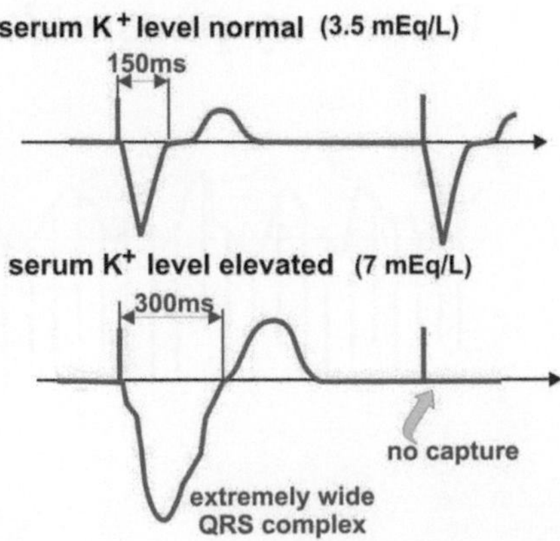

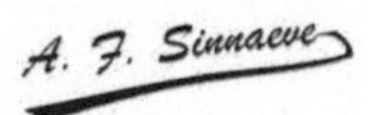

LOSS OF VENTRICULAR CAPTURE BY VISIBLE PACEMAKER STIMULI

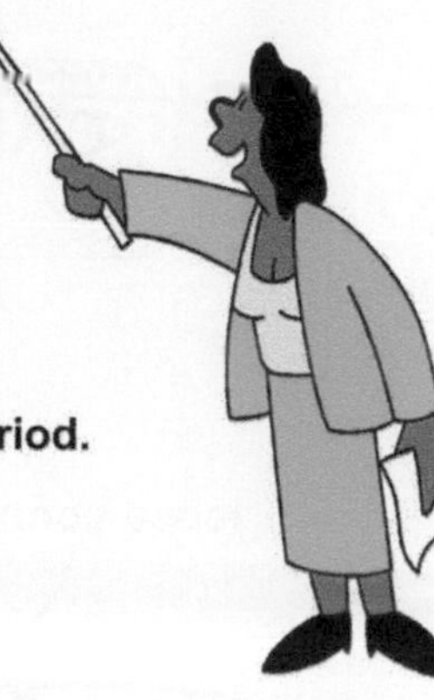

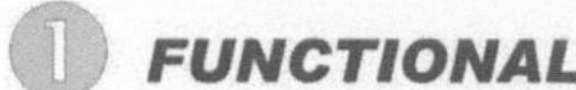

1 FUNCTIONAL

- ✓ Normal situation : stimuli in myocardial refractory period.

2 ELECTRODE-TISSUE INTERFACE

☞ LEAD DISPLACEMENT

- ✓ Early displacement or unstable position of pacing leads (commonest cause).
- ✓ Malposition into the coronary venous system.
- ✓ Twiddler's syndrome causing late displacement.
- ✓ Perforation of right ventricle by ventricular lead.

☞ NO APPARENT LEAD DISPLACEMENT

- ✓ Microdislodgment (a diagnosis of exclusion) causes a marked rise in capture threshold but displacement is not apparent on a chest x-ray.
- ✓ Elevated pacing threshold without obvious lead displacement (exit block) : Acute or chronic reaction at the electrode-tissue interface.
- ✓ Subcutaneous emphysema.
- ✓ Myocardial infarction or ischemia, hypoxia.
- ✓ Hypothyroidism.
- ✓ Elevation of pacing threshold after defibrillation or cardioversion. This is usually transient for a few minutes or less.
- ✓ Electrolyte abnormalities usually hyperkalemia, severe acidosis.
- ✓ Drug effect : Flecainide and propafenone can elevate the pacing threshold with therapeutic doses.

3 ELECTRODE

- ✓ Fracture, short circuit or insulation break.

4 PULSE GENERATOR

- ✓ Normal pacemaker with incorrect programming of parameters.
- ✓ Pacemaker failure from exhaustion or component failure.
- ✓ Iatrogenic causes : Component failure after defibrillation, electrocautery and therapeutic radiation.

A. F. Sinnaeve

CAUSES OF MISSING STIMULI DURING VVI PACING

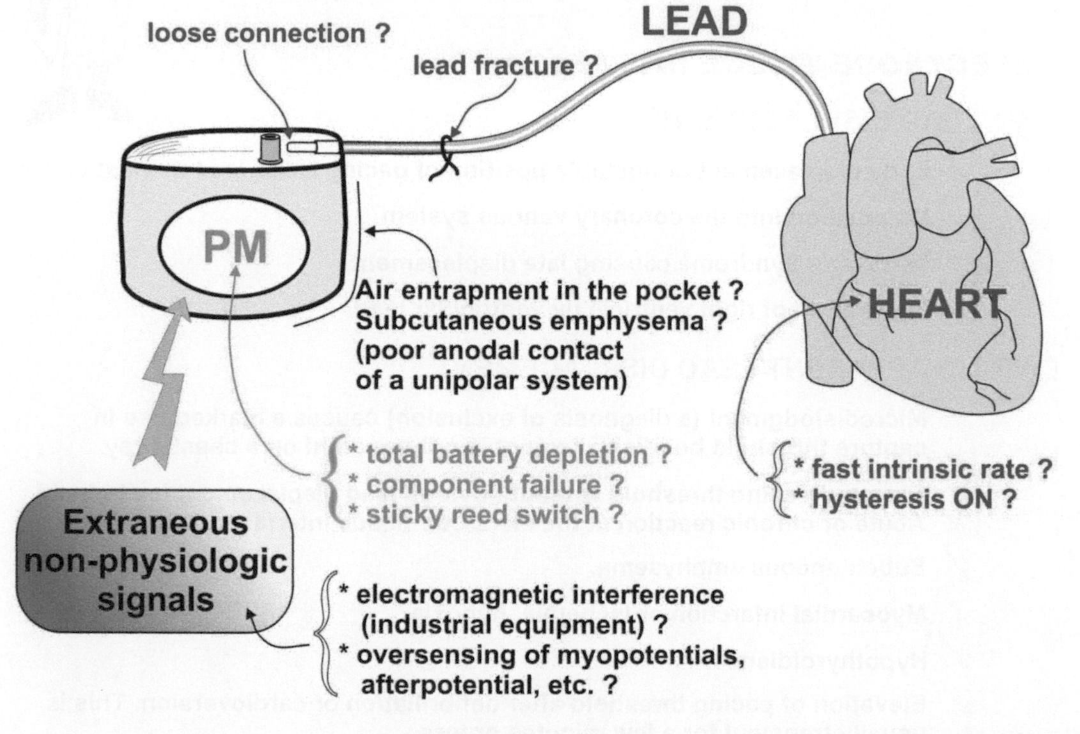

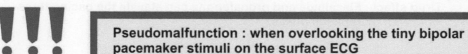

Pseudomalfunction : when overlooking the tiny bipolar pacemaker stimuli on the surface ECG

LEAD INSULATION DEFECTS

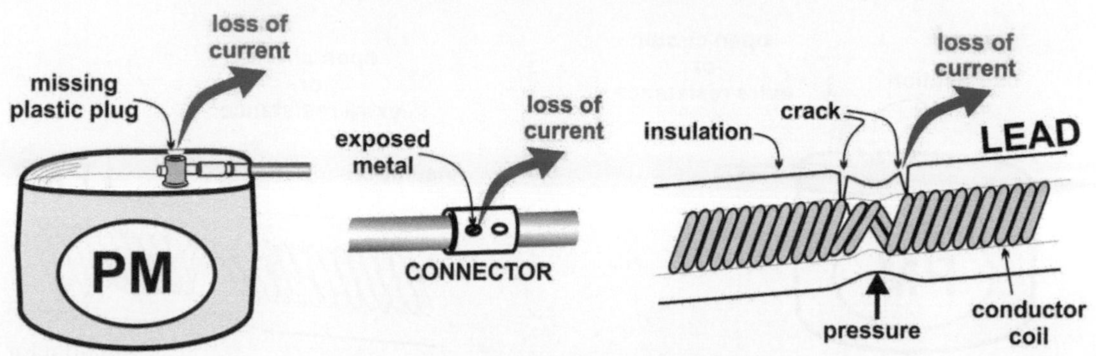

POSSIBLE CONSEQUENCES

* pacing may or may not be preserved
* stimuli are always present
* the pacing impedance is decreased
* excessive current loss leads to premature battery depletion

PACING IS PRESERVED

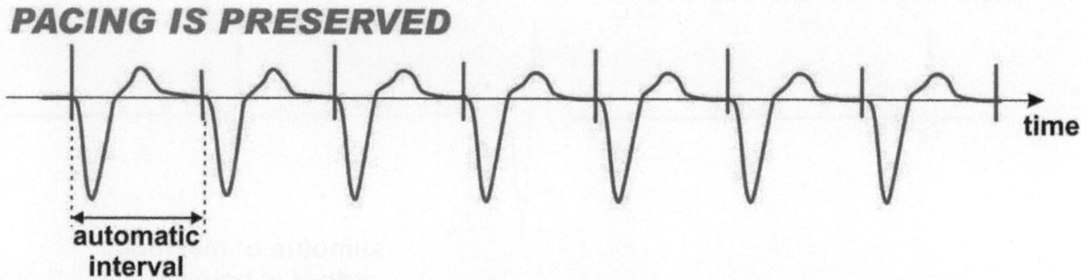

STIMULI, BUT FAIL TO CAPTURE

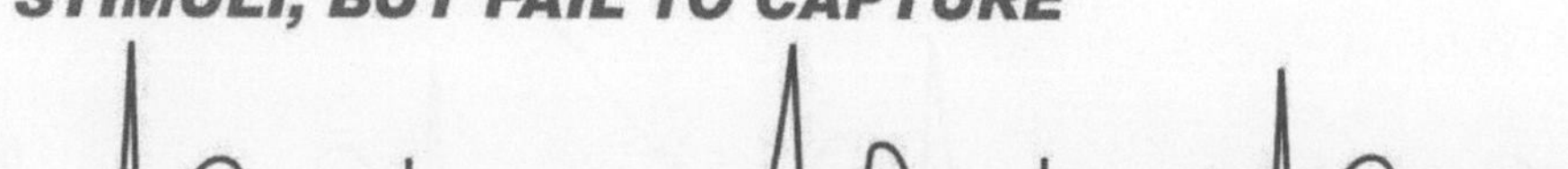

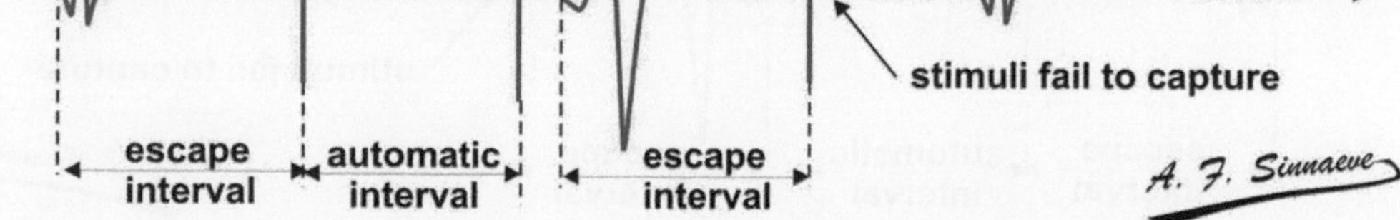

LEAD FRACTURE

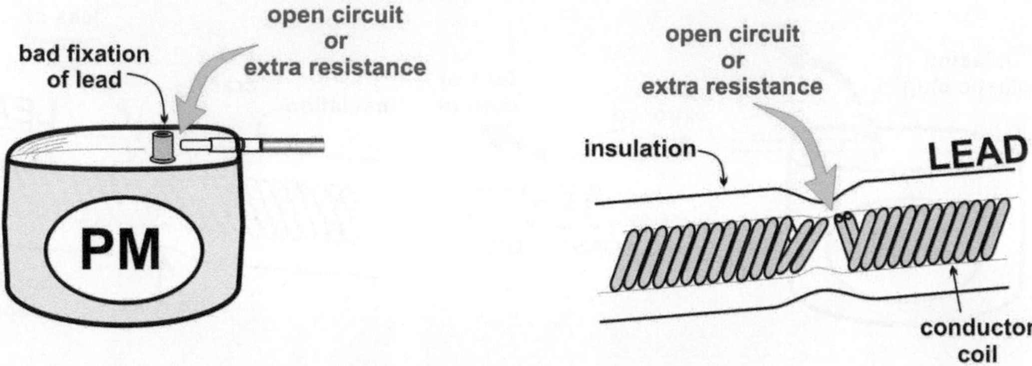

POSSIBLE CONSEQUENCES

* Stimuli may and may not be absent
* The voltage threshold is high
* The pacing impedance is increased

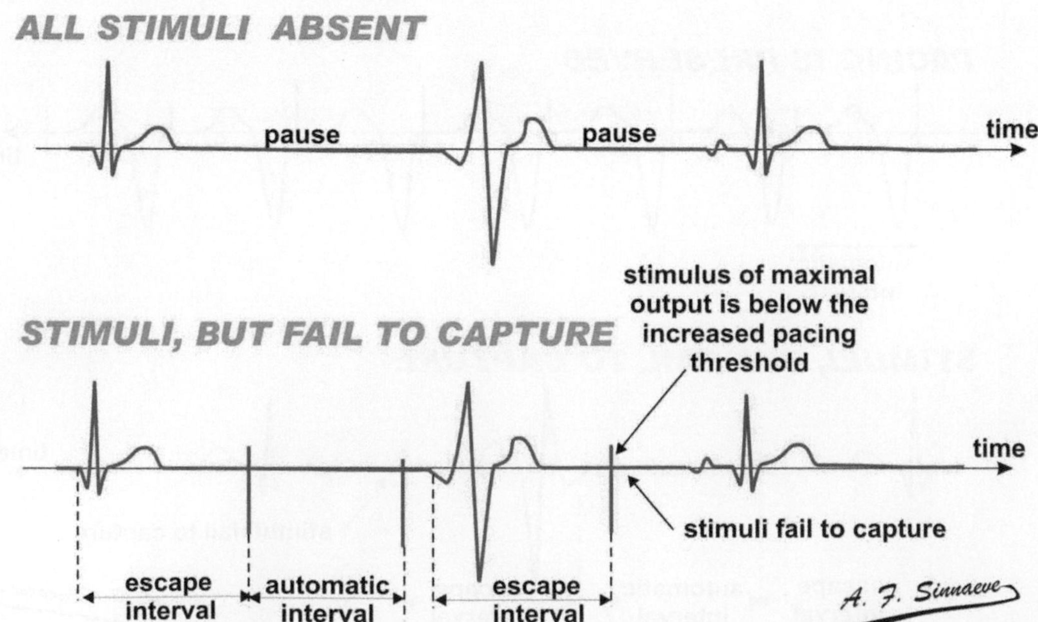

ANALYSIS OF LEAD PROBLEMS

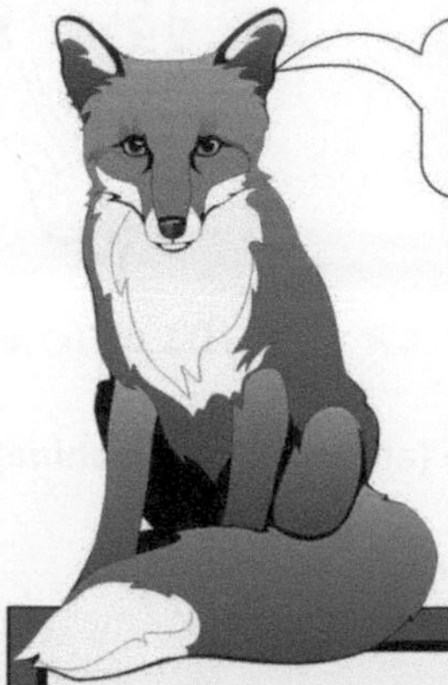

Be cunning as a fox ! You can get a lot of information about the leads, just by looking at the pacing impedance and the voltage threshold. The secret is to look at both !

	IMPEDANCE	*VOLTAGE THRESHOLD*
NORMAL LEAD PLACEMENT	NORMAL	NORMAL
LEAD DISPLACEMENT OR EXIT BLOCK	NORMAL	HIGH
LEAD FRACTURE	HIGH	HIGH
LEAD INSULATION DEFECT	LOW	MAY BE MODERATELY INCREASED

A. F. Sinnaeve

LEAD FRACTURE WITH CONVERSION FROM BIPOLAR TO UNIPOLAR MODE

You know, some broken bipolar leads can still be used ... At least temporarily !!!

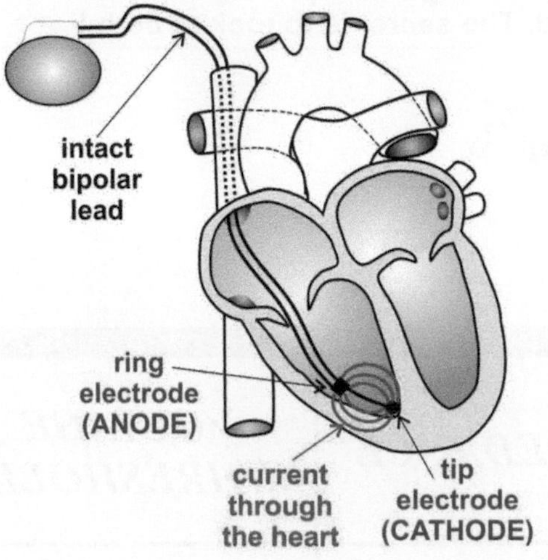

NORMAL BIPOLAR STIMULATION

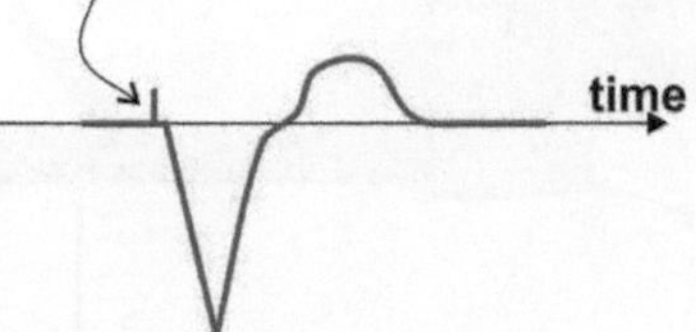

* normal pacing impedance (Z = about 500 ohm)

If one of the conductors in the bipolar lead is fractured, the pacing impedance becomes high !!!

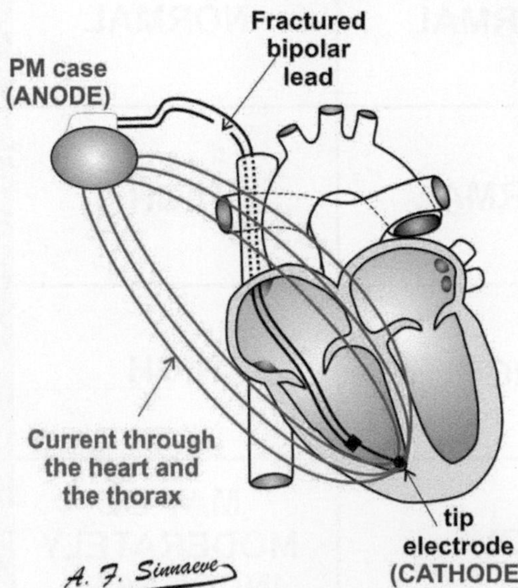

UNIPOLAR STIMULATION (via the distal tip electrode of a bipolar lead)

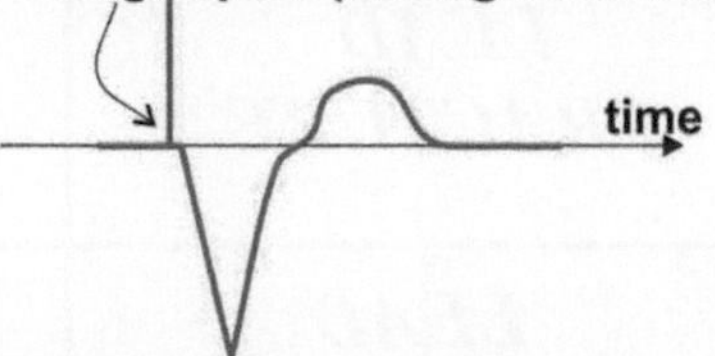

* normal pacing impedance (Z = about 500 ohm)

Some contemporary pacemakers can measure lead impedance periodically and store the data which can be eventually retrieved by telemetry.
Some pacemakers are designed to detect the high impedance of an electrode fracture whereupon the device automatically converts its function from the bipolar to the unipolar mode of pacing and sensing (using the intact electrode as the cathode).
During follow-up, application of a magnet will temporarily restore bipolar function with resultant loss of capture.

SUBCLAVIAN CRUSH SYNDROME

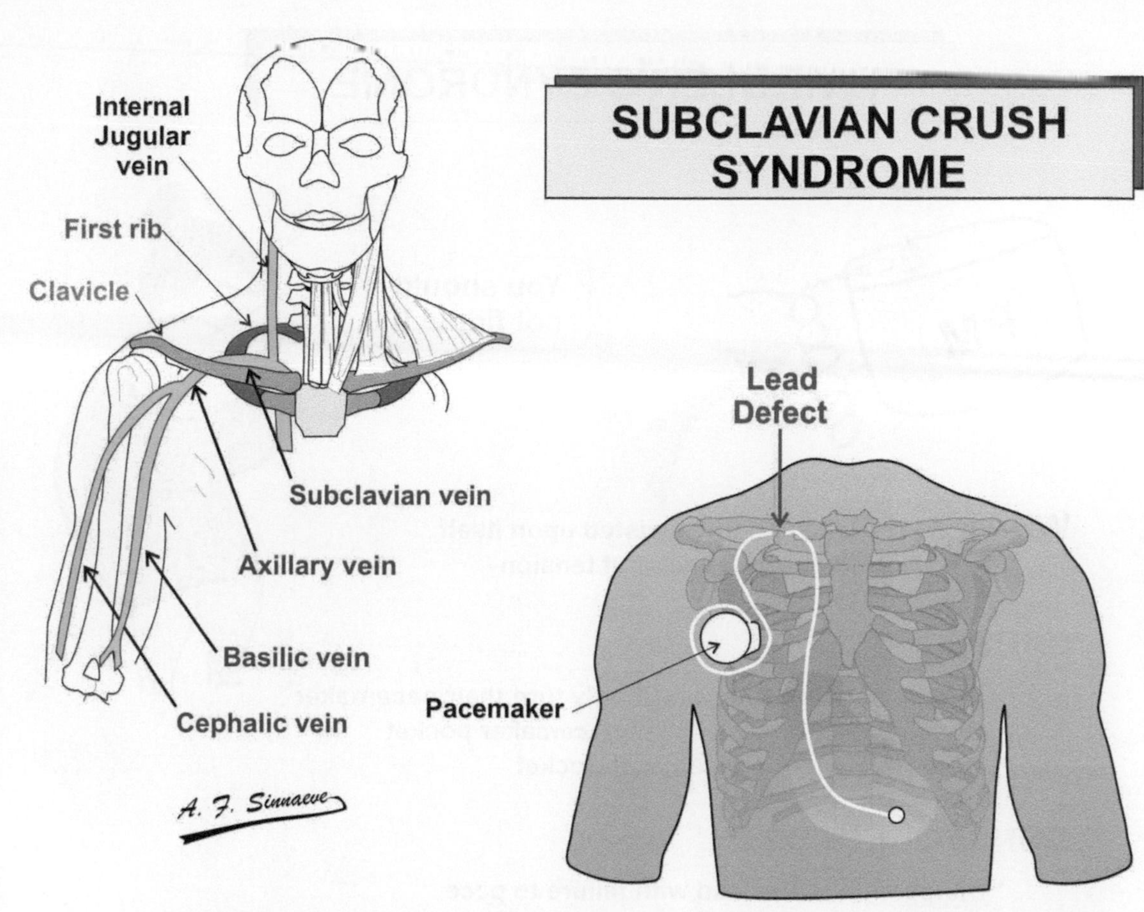

DEFINITION :

The subclavian crush syndrome is described with pacemaker leads implanted via subclavian puncture. This may occur when conductor fractures and insulation breaches develop by compression of a lead between the first rib and the clavicle.

PREVENTION :

The subclavian crush syndrome occurs when the puncture is too medial and may be avoided by a more lateral subclavian puncture or by using the axillary vein or even the cephalic vein.

TWIDDLER'S SYNDROME

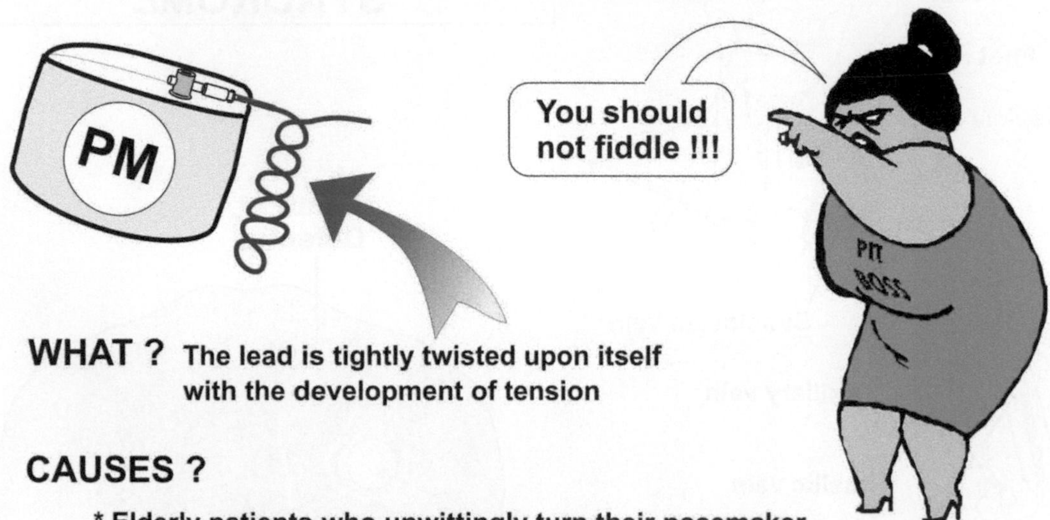

WHAT ? The lead is tightly twisted upon itself with the development of tension

CAUSES ?

* Elderly patients who unwittingly turn their pacemaker
* Obese patients with a loose pacemaker pocket
* Excessively large pacemaker pocket

CONSEQUENCES ?

* Dislocation of the lead with failure to pace
* Lead fracture
* Insulation defect

DIAGNOSIS ?

* The diagnosis is obvious on a standard chest X-ray

PREVENTION :

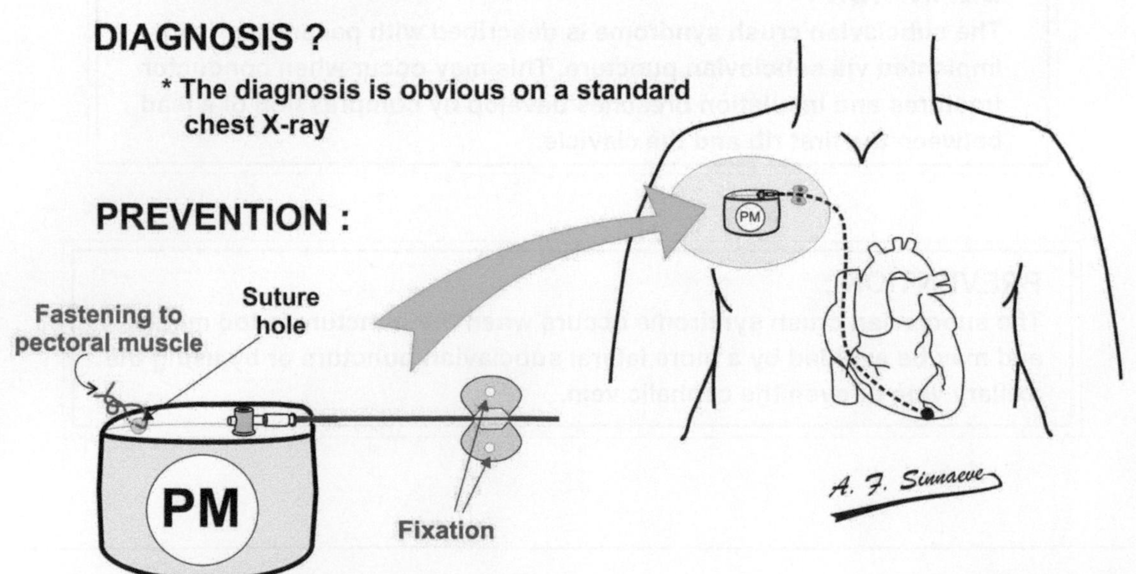

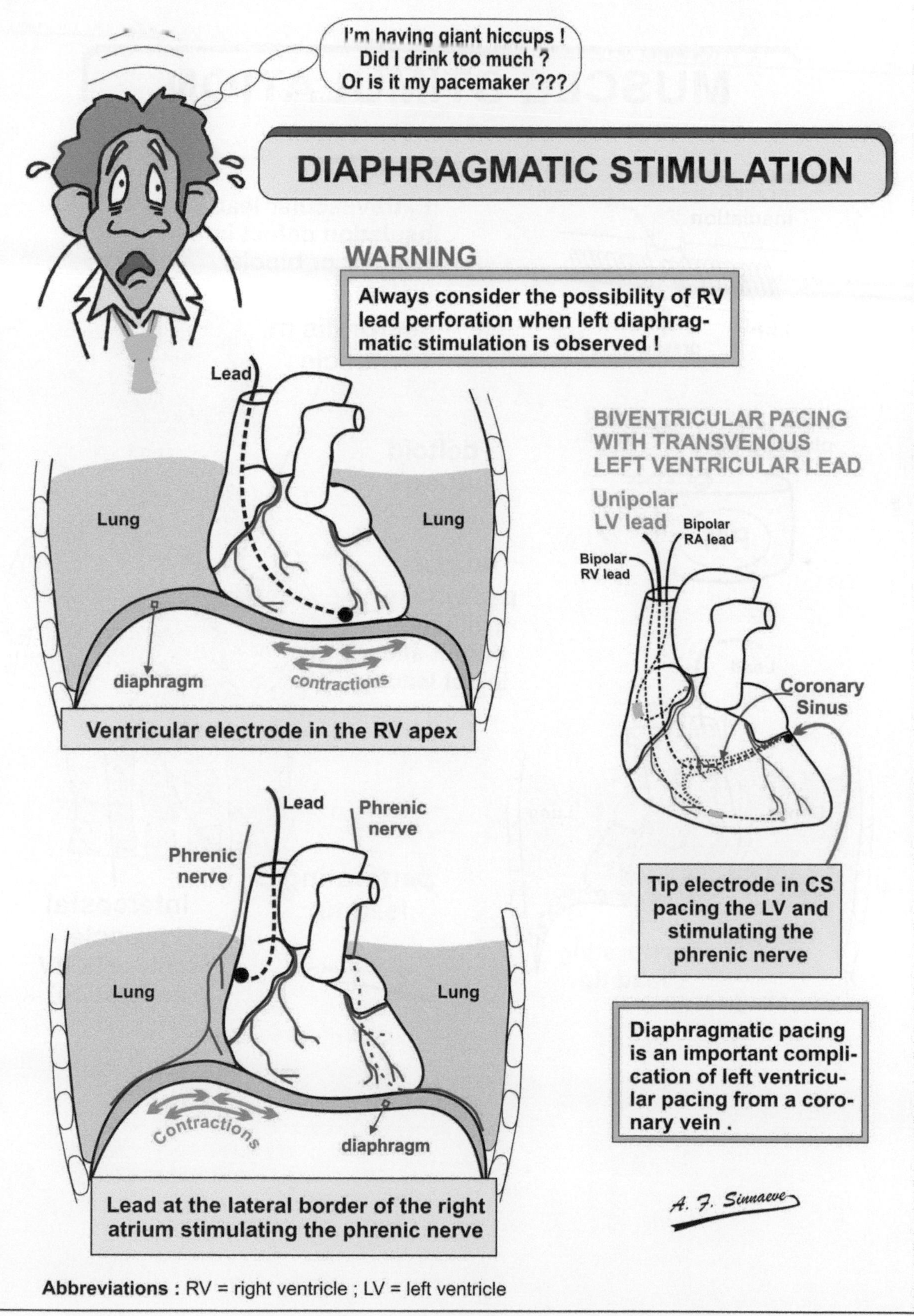
I'm having giant hiccups !
Did I drink too much ?
Or is it my pacemaker ???
DIAPHRAGMATIC STIMULATION
WARNING
Always consider the possibility of RV lead perforation when left diaphragmatic stimulation is observed !
Lead
Lung
Lung
diaphragm
contractions
Ventricular electrode in the RV apex
Lead
Phrenic nerve
Phrenic nerve
Lung
Lung
contractions
diaphragm
Lead at the lateral border of the right atrium stimulating the phrenic nerve
BIVENTRICULAR PACING WITH TRANSVENOUS LEFT VENTRICULAR LEAD
Unipolar LV lead
Bipolar RA lead
Bipolar RV lead
Coronary Sinus
Tip electrode in CS pacing the LV and stimulating the phrenic nerve
Diaphragmatic pacing is an important complication of left ventricular pacing from a coronary vein .
A. F. Sinnaeve
Abbreviations : RV = right ventricle ; LV = left ventricle

MUSCLE STIMULATION

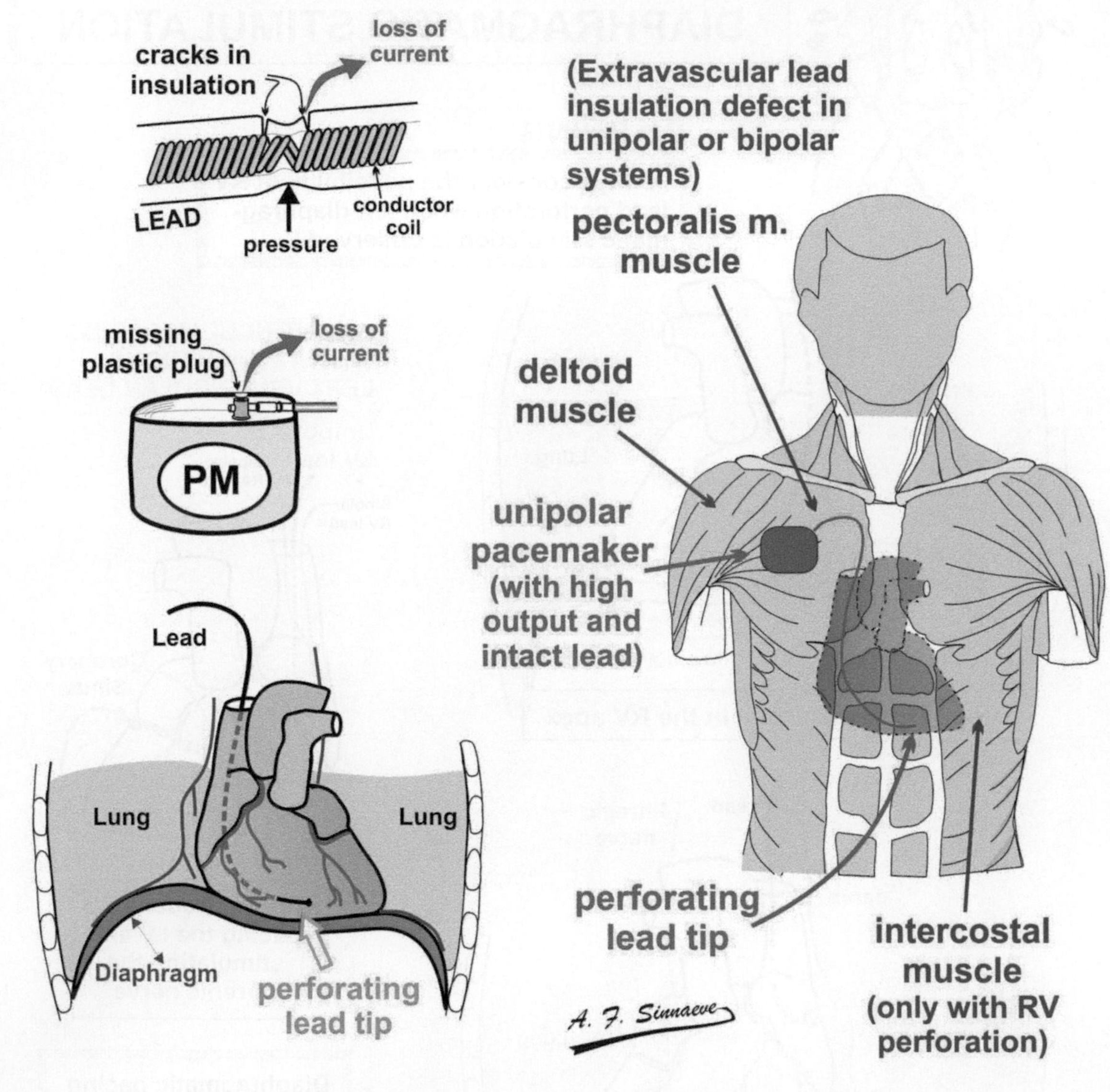

cracks in insulation
loss of current
LEAD
pressure
conductor coil
(Extravascular lead insulation defect in unipolar or bipolar systems)
pectoralis m. muscle
missing plastic plug
loss of current
PM
deltoid muscle
unipolar pacemaker (with high output and intact lead)
Lead
Lung
Lung
Diaphragm
perforating lead tip
perforating lead tip
intercostal muscle (only with RV perforation)
A. F. Sinnaeve

PACEMAKER RUNAWAY

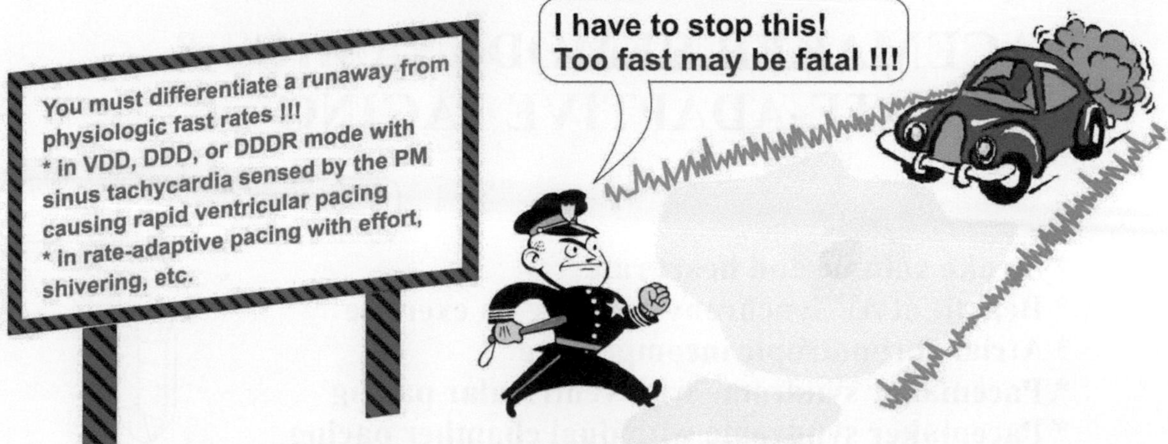

RUNAWAY OF AN OLD PACEMAKER AT 475 ppm

The VVI pacemaker emits stimuli at a rate of 475 ppm, too fast to cause 1:1 capture because of the ventricular myocardial refractory period. Such a situation may induce ventricular fibrillation. Emergency treatment consists of cutting the pacing lead.

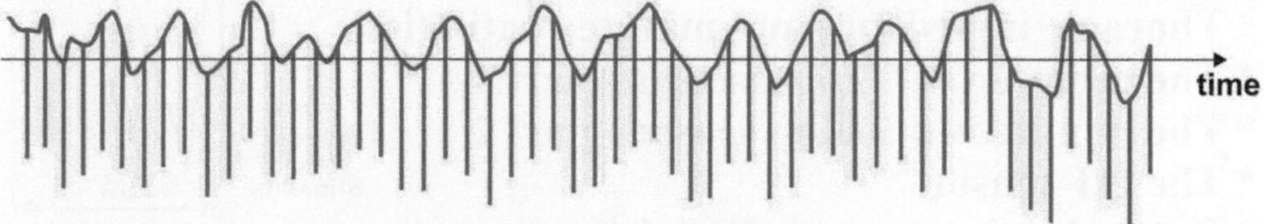

RUNAWAY OF A RECENT VVI PACEMAKER

The pacemaker was programmed at 70 ppm and paced at 145 ppm.
(The patient presented with palpitations and dyspnea until the unit was removed)

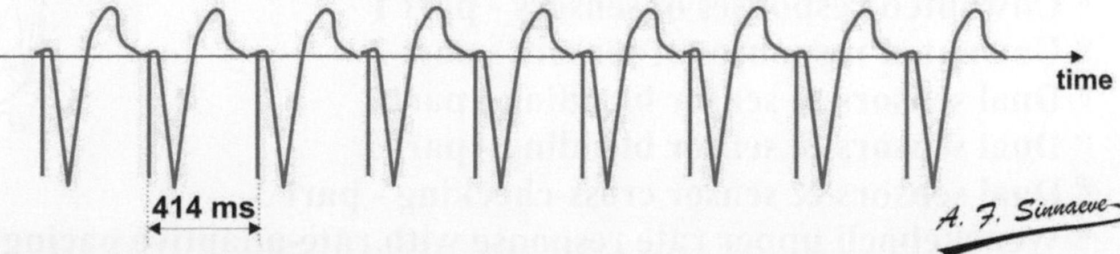

Runaway is a serious component malfunction of pacemakers. It is now rare because of improved technology. All contemporary pacemakers are equipped with a "runaway protection circuit", usually limiting the maximum pacing rate to 150 - 180 bpm.

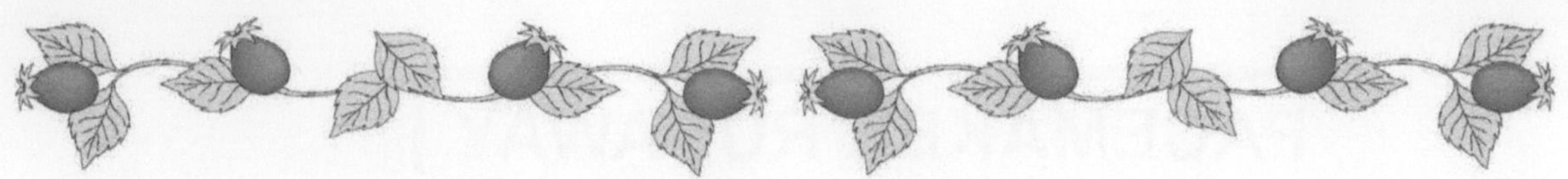

PACEMAKER HEMODYNAMICS & RATE-ADAPTIVE PACING

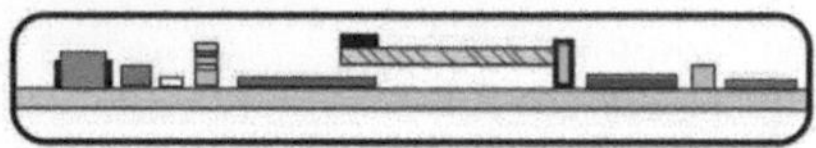

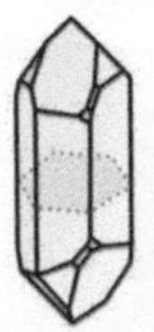

* Stroke volume and heart rate
* Benefit of AV synchrony and rate on exercise
* Atrial chronotropic incompetence
* Pacemaker syndrome with ventricular pacing
* Pacemaker syndrome with dual chamber pacing
* Maintenance of normal depolarization
* Indicators for rate-adaptive pacing
* Open loop rate-adaptive pacing
* Sensors of body motion
* Pressure on activity sensors
* Thoracic impedance and minute ventilation
* The minute ventilation sensor - part 1
* The minute ventilation sensor - part 2
* The QT sensor
* Rate-adaptive pacing - Definitions
* Algorithms for rate-adaptive pacing - part 1
* Algorithms for rate-adaptive pacing - part 2
* Sensor-driven and atrial-driven upper rates
* Unwanted responses of sensors - part 1
* Unwanted responses of sensors - part 2
* Dual sensors & sensor blending - part 1
* Dual sensors & sensor blending - part 2
* Dual sensors & sensor cross-checking - part 3
* Wenckebach upper rate response with rate-adaptive pacing
* Fixed-ratio block with rate-adaptive pacing
* The rate-adaptive postventricular atrial refractory period (PVARP)
* Non-competitive atrial pacing (NCAP)

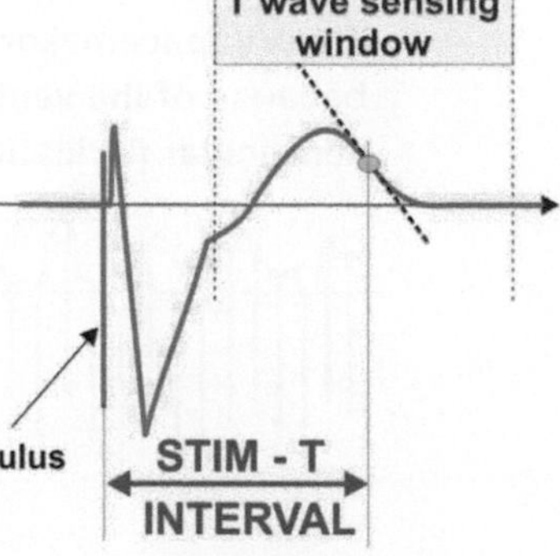

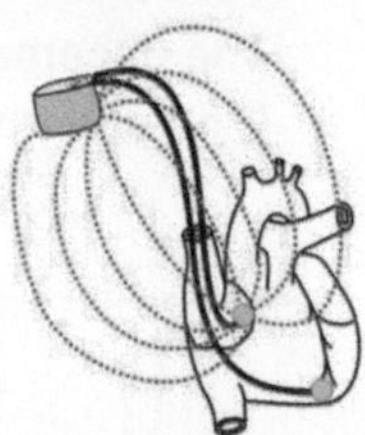

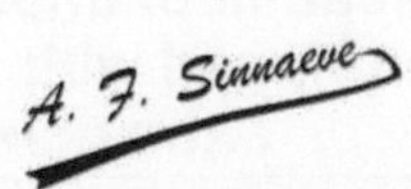

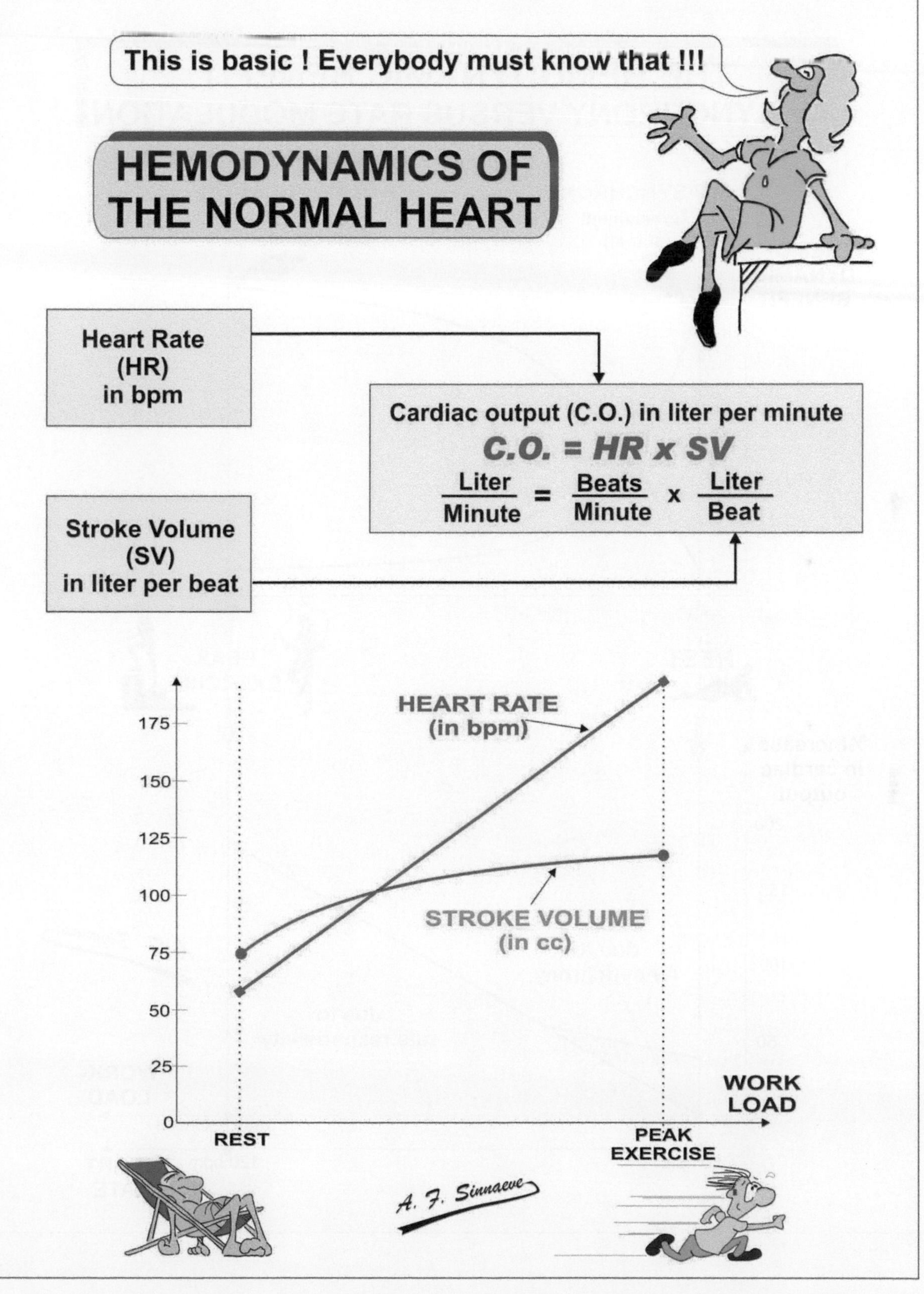
This is basic ! Everybody must know that !!!
HEMODYNAMICS OF THE NORMAL HEART
Heart Rate (HR) in bpm
Cardiac output (C.O.) in liter per minute
C.O. = HR x SV
Liter / Minute = Beats / Minute x Liter / Beat
Stroke Volume (SV) in liter per beat
175
150
125
100
75
50
25
0
HEART RATE (in bpm)
STROKE VOLUME (in cc)
WORK LOAD
REST
PEAK EXERCISE
A. F. Sinnaeve

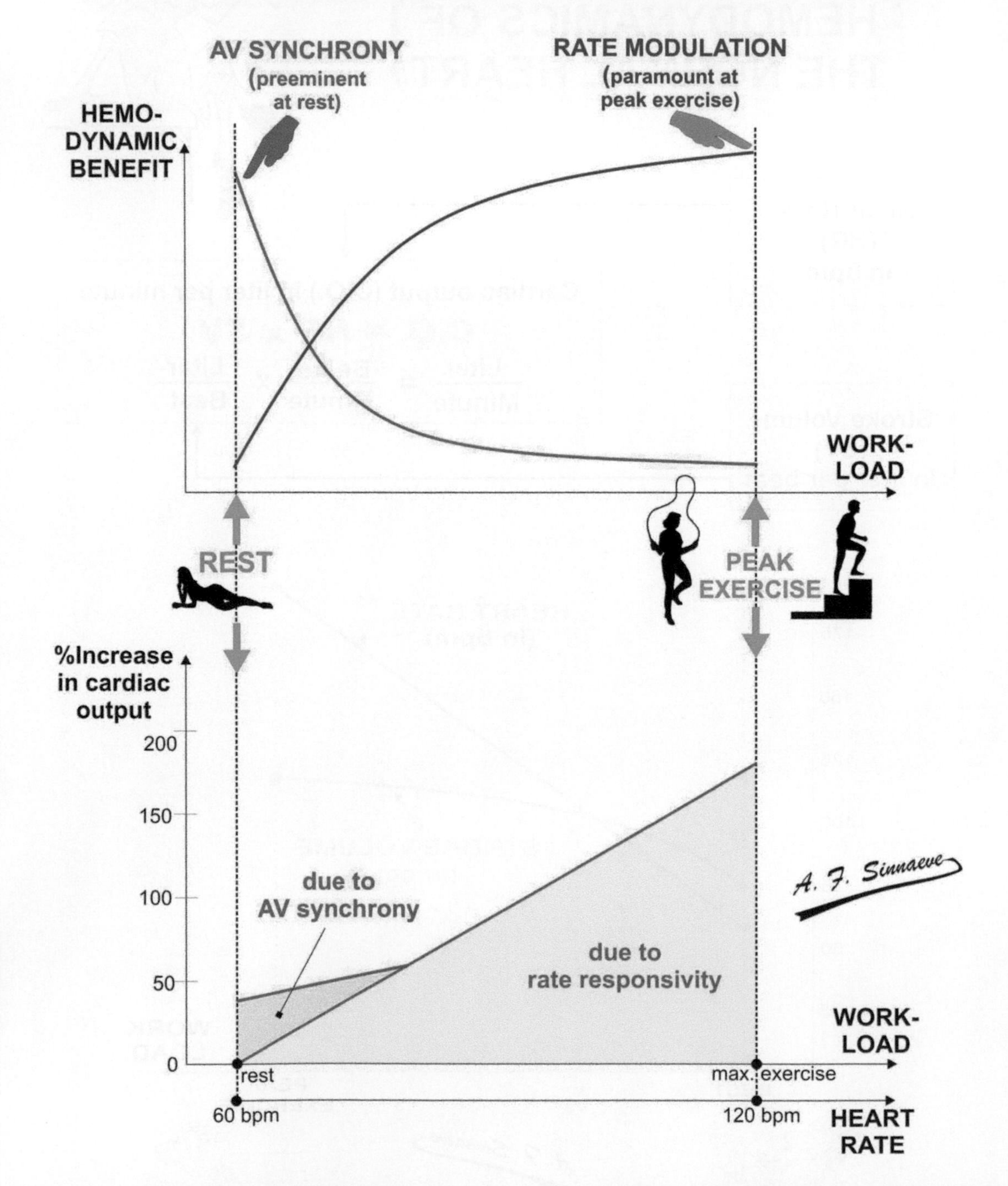
THE HEMODYNAMIC BENEFIT
AV SYNCHRONY VERSUS RATE MODULATION
AV SYNCHRONY
(preeminent at rest)
RATE MODULATION
(paramount at peak exercise)
HEMO-DYNAMIC BENEFIT
WORK-LOAD
REST
PEAK EXERCISE
%Increase in cardiac output
200
150
100
50
0
due to AV synchrony
due to rate responsivity
A. F. Sinnaeve
WORK-LOAD
rest
max. exercise
60 bpm
120 bpm
HEART RATE

RATE - ADAPTIVE PACING AND CHRONOTROPIC INCOMPETENCE

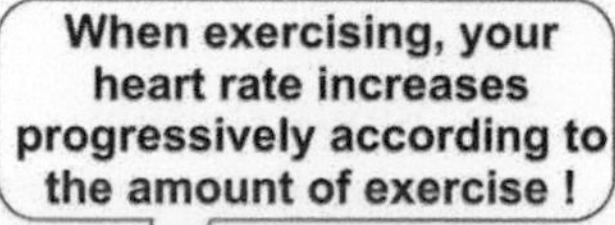

When exercising, your heart rate increases progressively according to the amount of exercise !

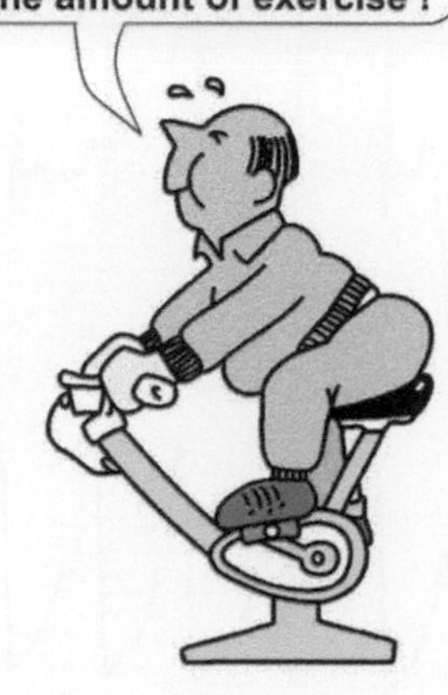

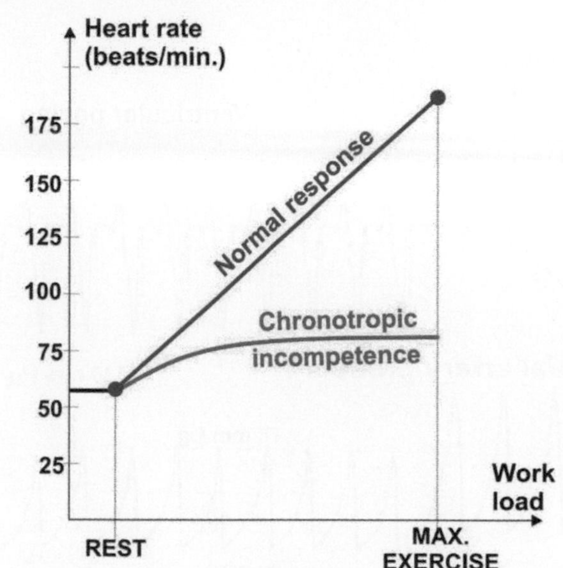

With a VVI pacemaker the ventricular pacing rate remains constant

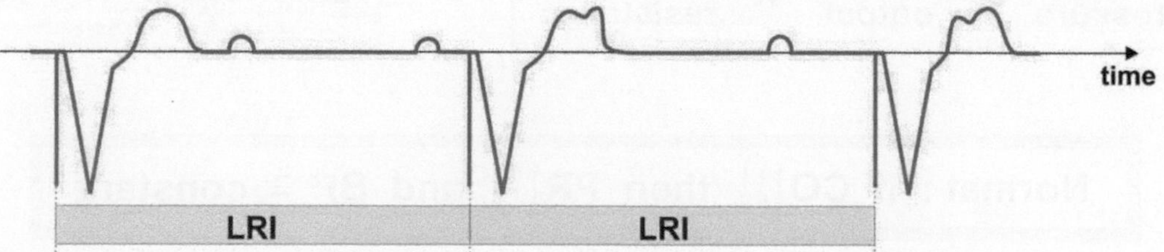

With a VVIR pacemaker the ventricular pacing rate increases when the workload increases

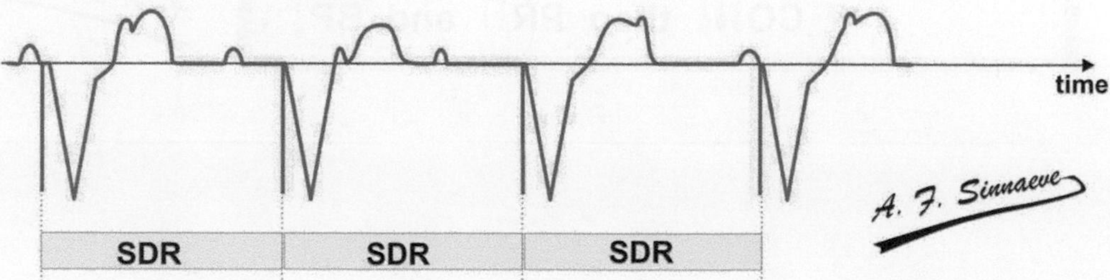

Abbreviations : LRI = lower rate interval ; SDR = sensor-driven interval

VVI PACING AND THE PACEMAKER SYNDROME

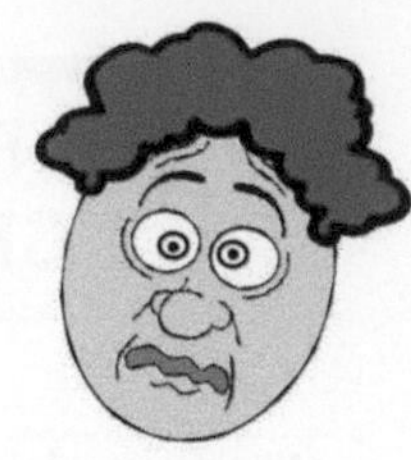

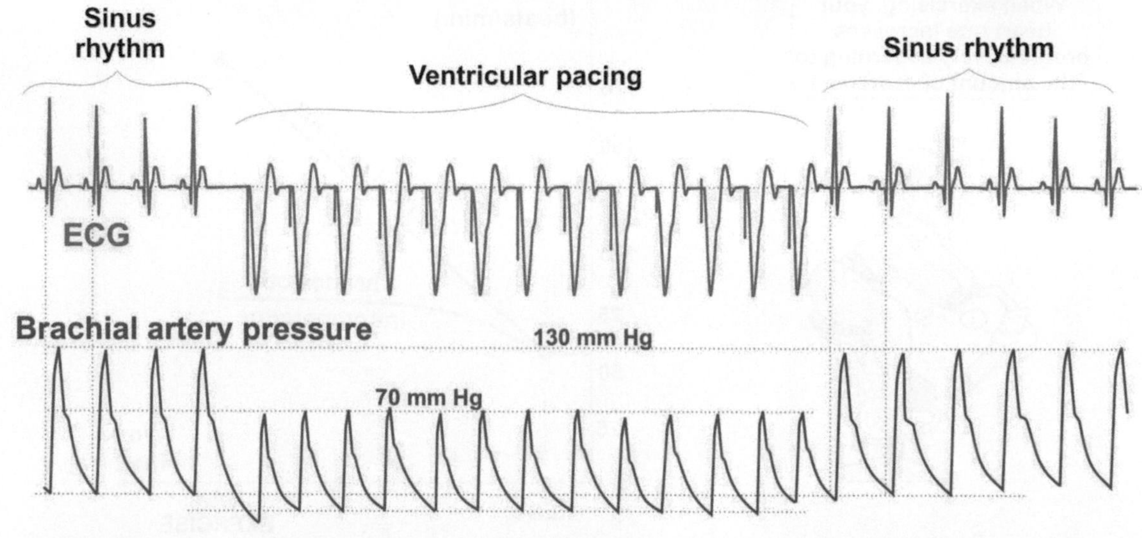

Blood pressure	=	Cardiac output	X	Peripheral resistance	or	BP = CO x PR

Normal : if CO↓↓↓ then PR↑↑↑ and BP ≅ constant

With pacemaker syndrome :
If CO↓↓↓ then PR↑↑ and BP↓

A. F. Sinnaeve

My doctor says I have a very sophisticated dual chamber pacemaker...
But I'm not feeling well...

PACEMAKER SYNDROME WITH DUAL CHAMBER PACEMAKERS

The pacemaker syndrome refers to symptoms and signs present in the pacemaker patient which are caused by inadequate timing of atrial and ventricular contractions.

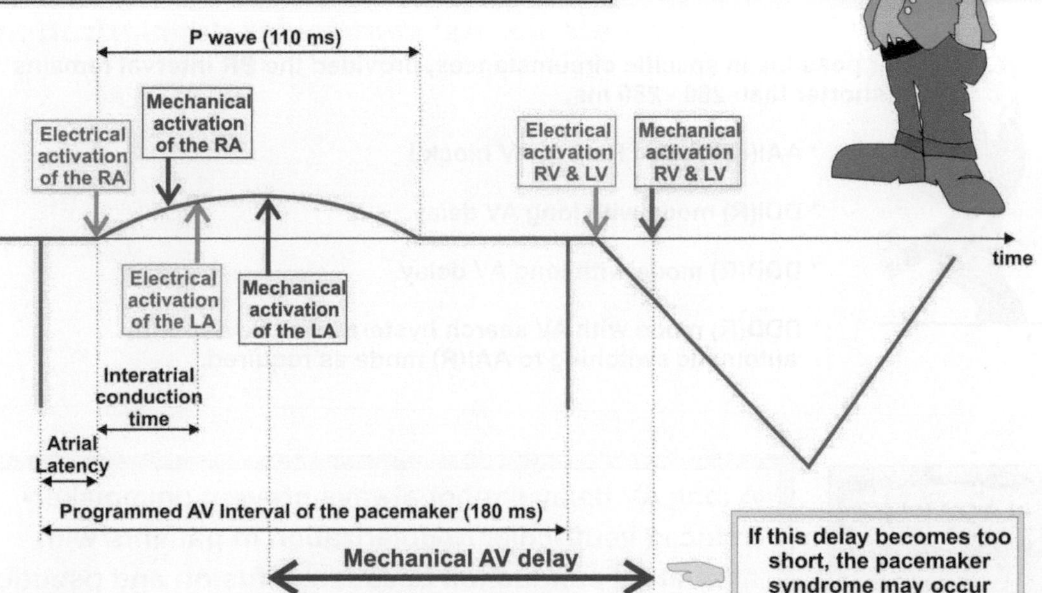

PM syndrome in atrial tracking pacemakers

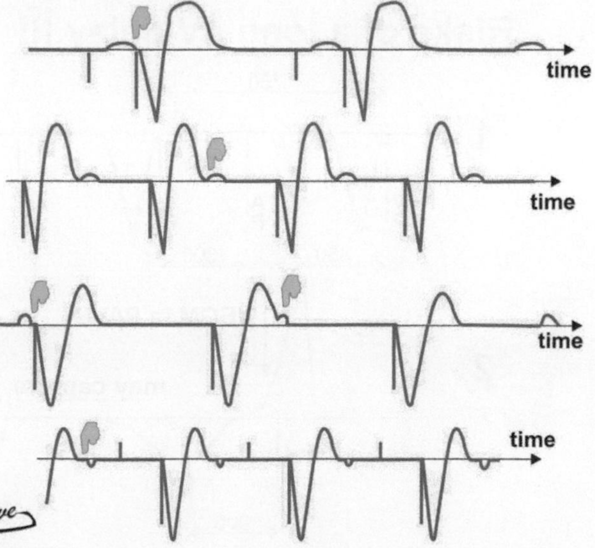

A. F. Sinnaeve

MAINTENANCE OF NORMAL VENTRICULAR DEPOLARIZATION

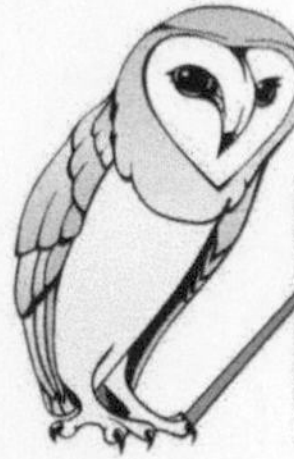

Ventricular depolarization via the normal pathway is hemodynamically superior to pacemaker induced depolarization on a short-term as well as on a long-term basis

Attempt to promote normal ventricular depolarization
if possible in specific circumstances, provided the PR interval remains shorter than 260 - 280 ms.

- **AAI(R) mode . Risk of AV block !**
- **DDI(R) mode with long AV delay.**
- **DDD(R) mode with long AV delay.**
- **DDD(R) mode with AV search hysteresis or device with automatic switching to AAI(R) mode as required.**

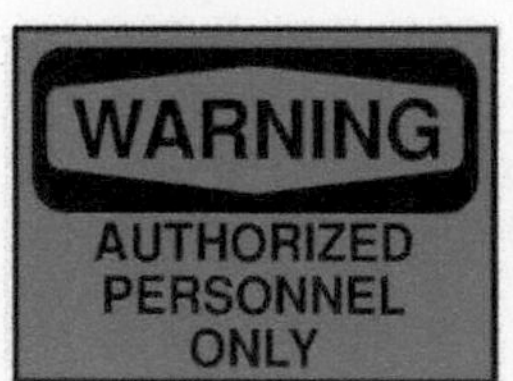

A long AV delay cannot always prevent pacemaker-induced ventricular depolarization in patients with normal AV conduction because of fusion and pseudo-fusion beats and other circumstances.

Risks of a long AV delay !!!

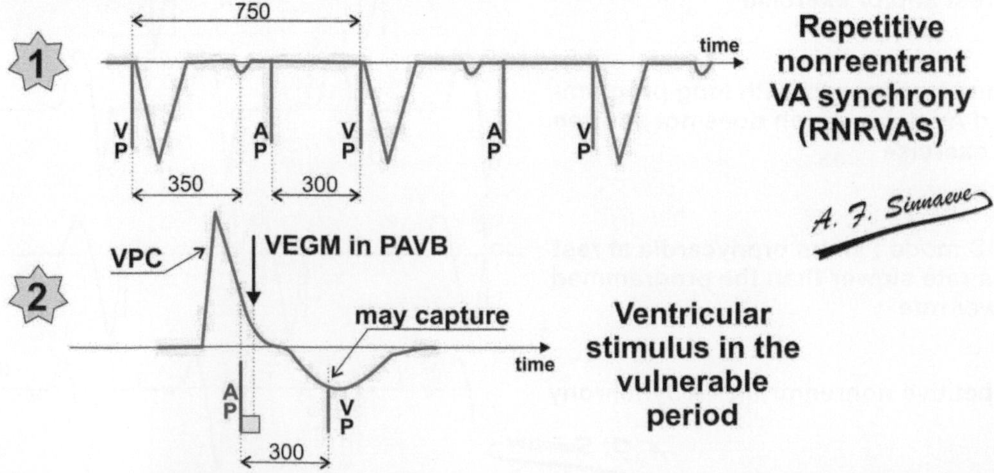

Abbreviations : AP = atrial pace; VP = ventricular pace; VPC = ventricular premature complex; VEGM = ventricular electrogram ; PAVB = postatrial ventricular blanking

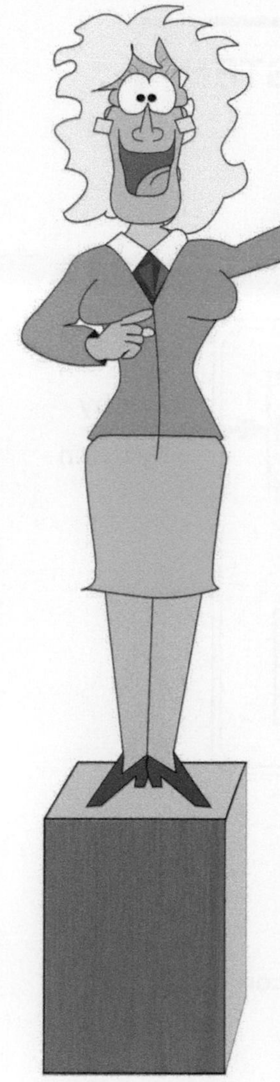
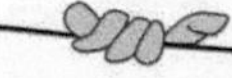

INDICATORS FOR RATE-ADAPTIVE PACING

1. NON - PHYSIOLOGIC

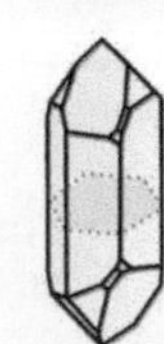

* Vibration (Activity)
* Acceleration

2. PHYSIOLOGIC

A/ Non-cardiac parameters
Indirect metabolic

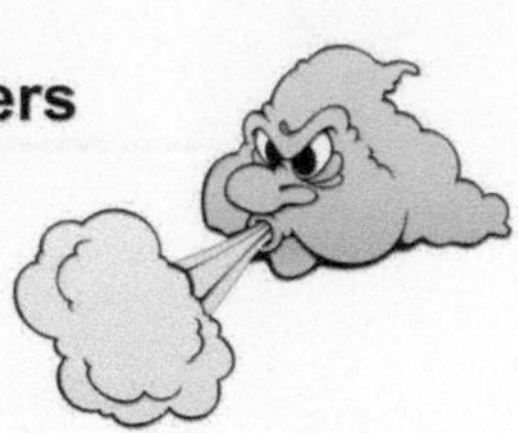

* Minute ventilation

B/ Cardiac parameters

* QT interval

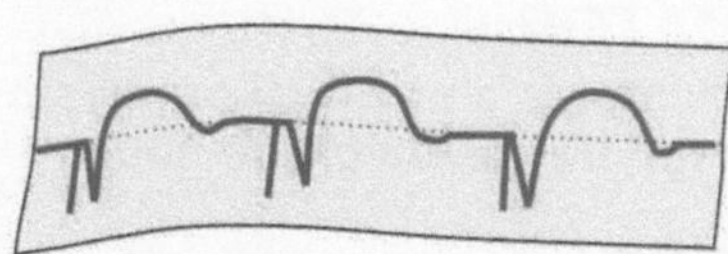

A. F. Sinnaeve

OPEN LOOP RATE - ADAPTIVE PM SYSTEM

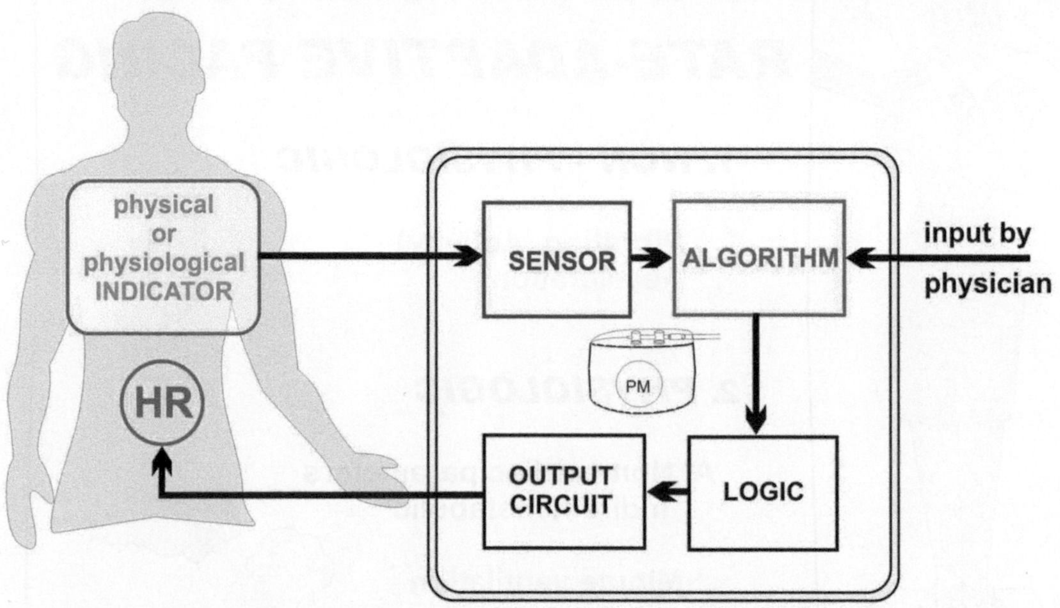

HEART RATE (HR) :

The heart rate should be adapted to the need of the body

INDICATOR :

An indicator is a physical or physiological parameter, changing according to the metabolic needs of the body

SENSOR :

A sensor is a device that converts non-electrical data (i.e. an indicator) into electrical signals. The response of the indicator to the body function determines the magnitude and frequency of the electrical signals

ALGORITHM :

The algorithm is the software function of the pacemaker that converts the electrical signals from the sensor into an appropriate pacing response by the device

A. F. Sinnaeve

SENSORS OF BODY MOTION

① THE PIEZOELECTRIC EFFECT

Some crystals (e.g. quartz) generate an electric voltage when they are subjected to mechanical stress.

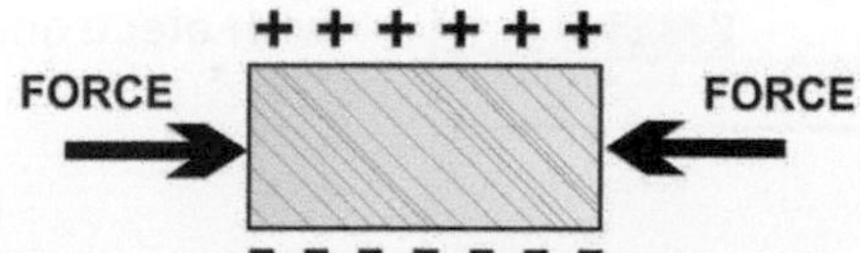

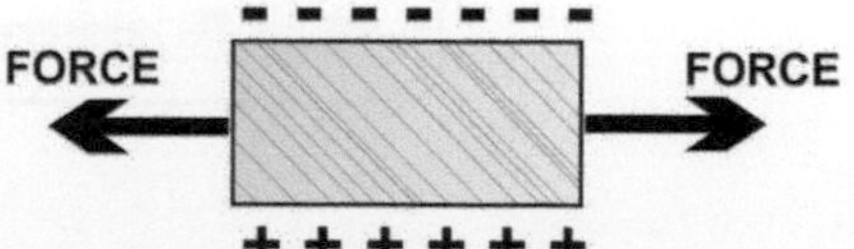

② THE ACTIVITY SENSOR

Responds to body vibrations.
Reacts to external stimuli that should not increase the pacing rate e.g. pressure on the device.

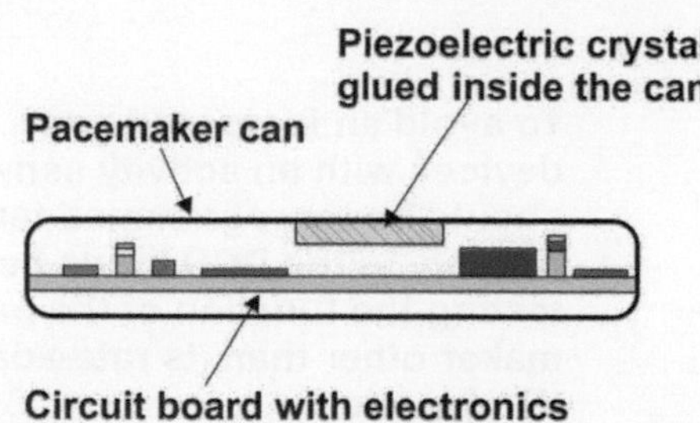

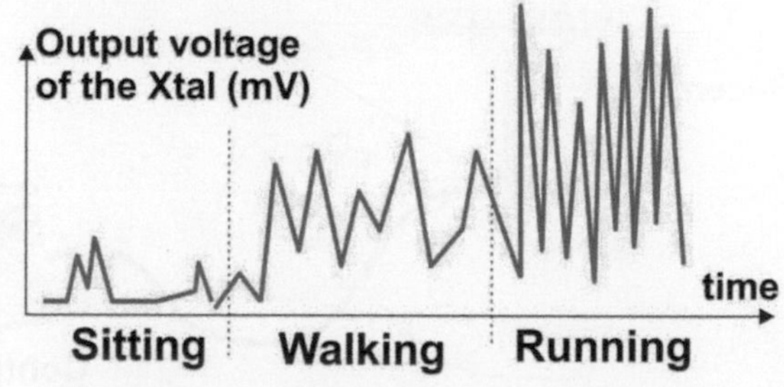

③ THE ACCELEROMETER

A very small mass in the pacemaker reacts upon acceleration and deforms the crystal which generates a voltage. This system has greater specificity than the activity sensor above, i.e. less false positive responses.

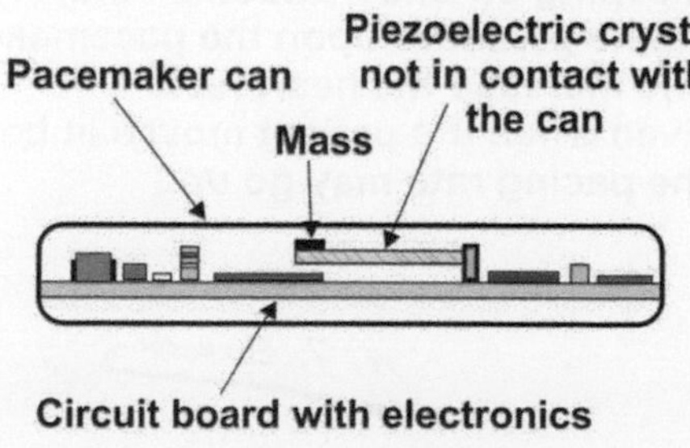

Both the activity sensor and the accelerometer react very fast upon the onset of any movement. The capability of early exercise detection makes the activity sensor a good component of dual sensor systems : e.g. activity + minute ventilation or activity + QT sensing

A. F. Sinnaeve

Abbreviations : mV = millivolt ; Xtal = crystal

PRESSURE ON DEVICES EQUIPPED WITH AN ACTIVITY SENSOR

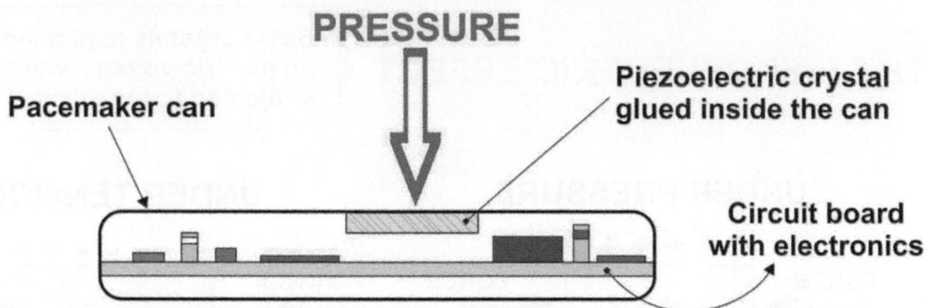

Since the crystal is in contact with the pacemaker can, pressure on the device may increase the heart rate without any exercise of the patient !!!

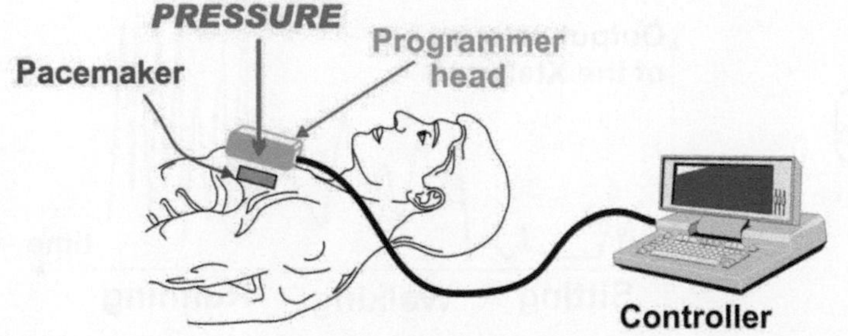

To avoid an increased rate, devices with an activity sensor should be reprogrammed temporarily to the DDD mode before testing the function of the pacemaker other than its rate-adaptive function.

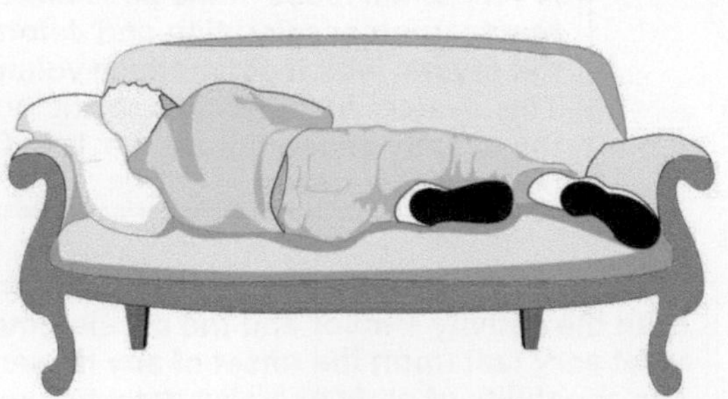

Sleeping on one's abdomen may create pressure upon the pacemaker and increase the heart rate. Even when the patient moves in bed, the pacing rate may go up.

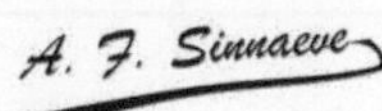

ARRANGEMENT OF MINUTE VENTILATION SENSORS

SINGLE CHAMBER SYSTEM (VVIR)
with bipolar pacing & sensing

DUAL CHAMBER SYSTEM (DDDR)
with two unipolar leads

Thoracic impedance $Z = \frac{V}{I}$
Proportional to the minute ventilation

1 Bipolar pacing lead

Current I for measurement of Z

Ring

Tip

2 Unipolar pacing leads

Current I for measurement of Z

Atrial electrode

Ventricular electrode

Current injection(I) between PM can and ring electrode
Voltage measurement (V) between PM can and tip electrode

Current injection(I) between PM can and atrial electrode
Voltage measurement (V) between PM can and ventricular electrode

* the current pulses I for impedance measurement are subthreshold, they have a low amplitude and are very short (pulse duration 5 to 15 µs)
* the measurement is frequently repeated (480 to 1200 times per minute)

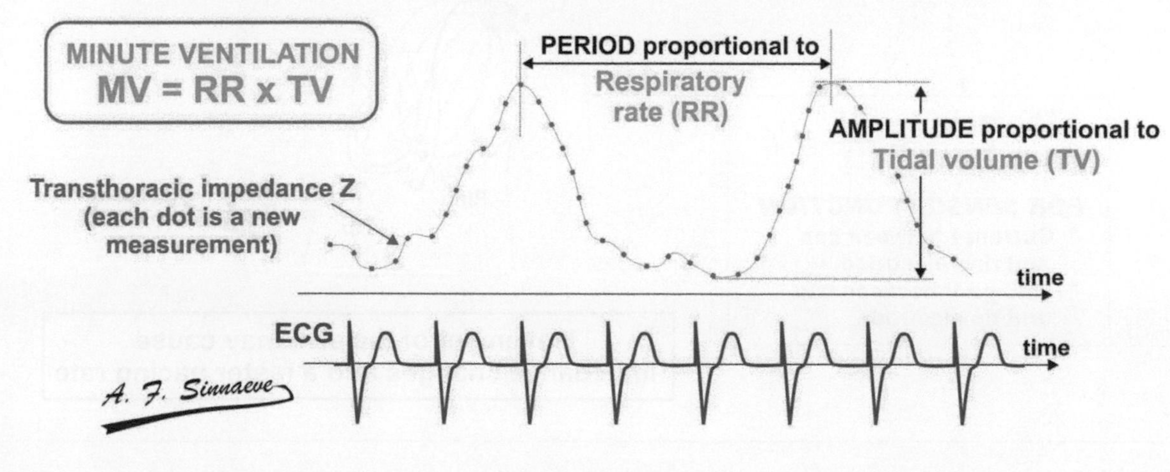

MINUTE VENTILATION SENSOR

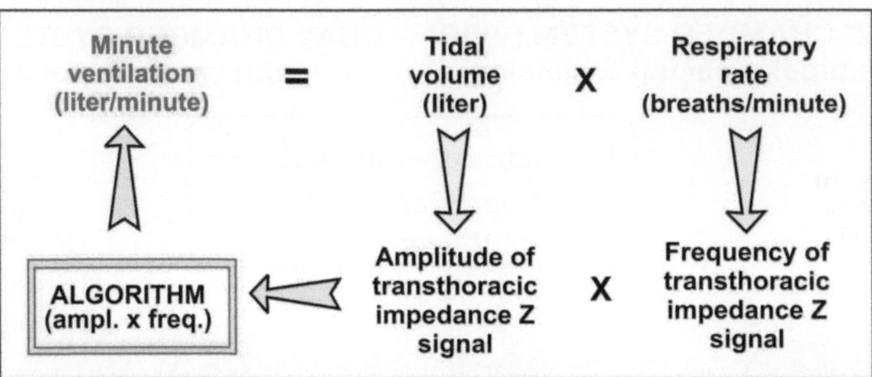

A special circuit inside the pacemaker sends very short subthreshold current pulses I of known amplitude through the thorax. The device measures the voltage V between 2 thoracic sites as shown in the diagram below. This voltage is proporional to the transthoracic impedance Z

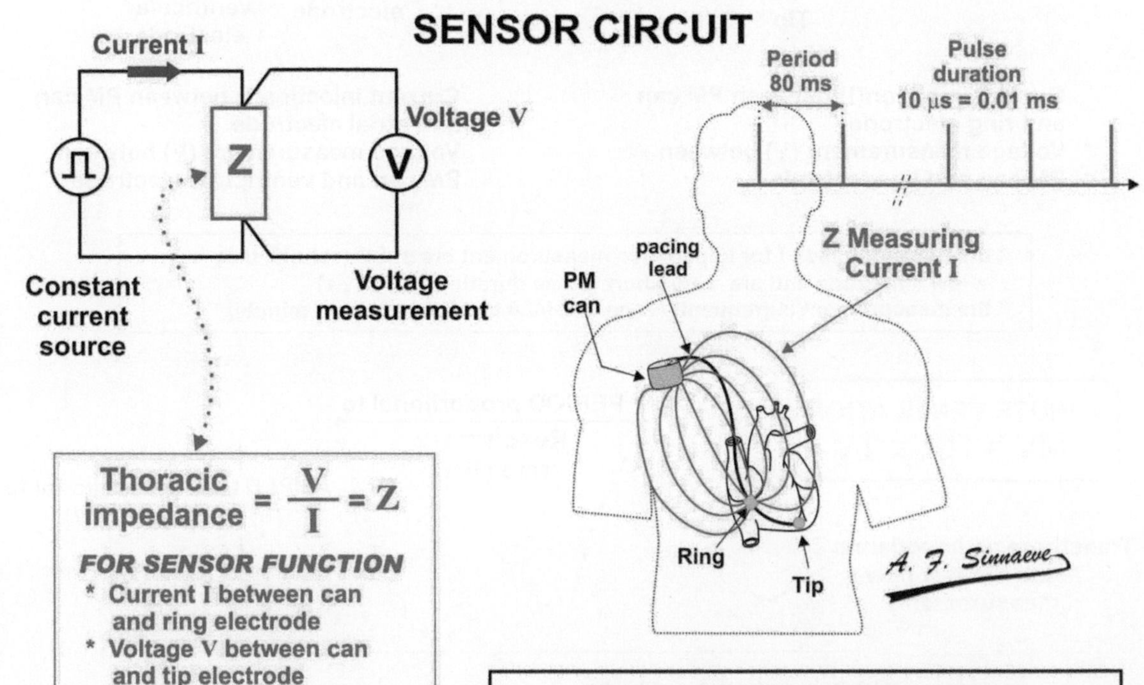

Movement of the arm may cause impedance changes and a faster pacing rate

MINUTE VENTILATION SENSOR - PART 2

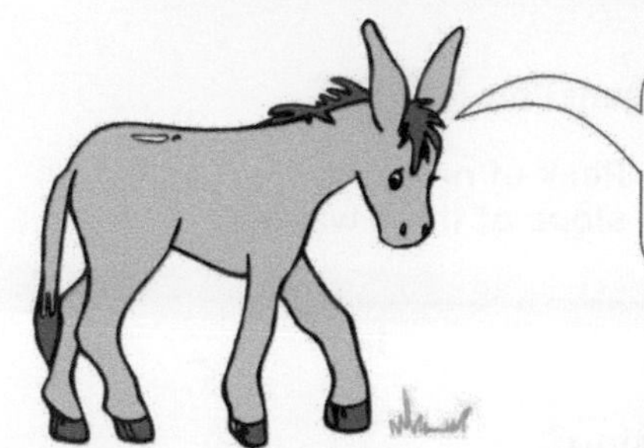
According to the engineers it's a piece of cake... and I don't even understand what they are talking about !!! But I am only a little donkey...

NOTE THE DIFFERENCE !!!
THERE ARE 2 SEPARATE ELECTRIC CIRCUITS INVOLVED

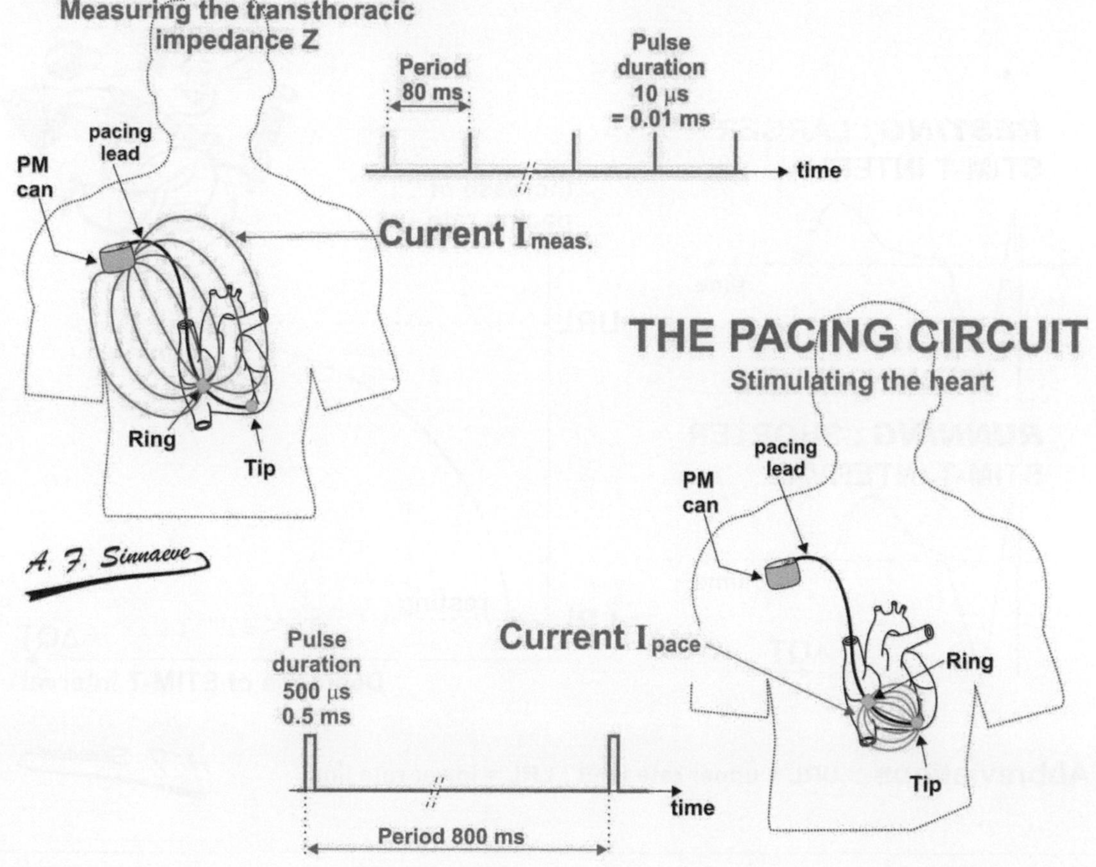

SENSING the QT or STIMULUS - T INTERVAL

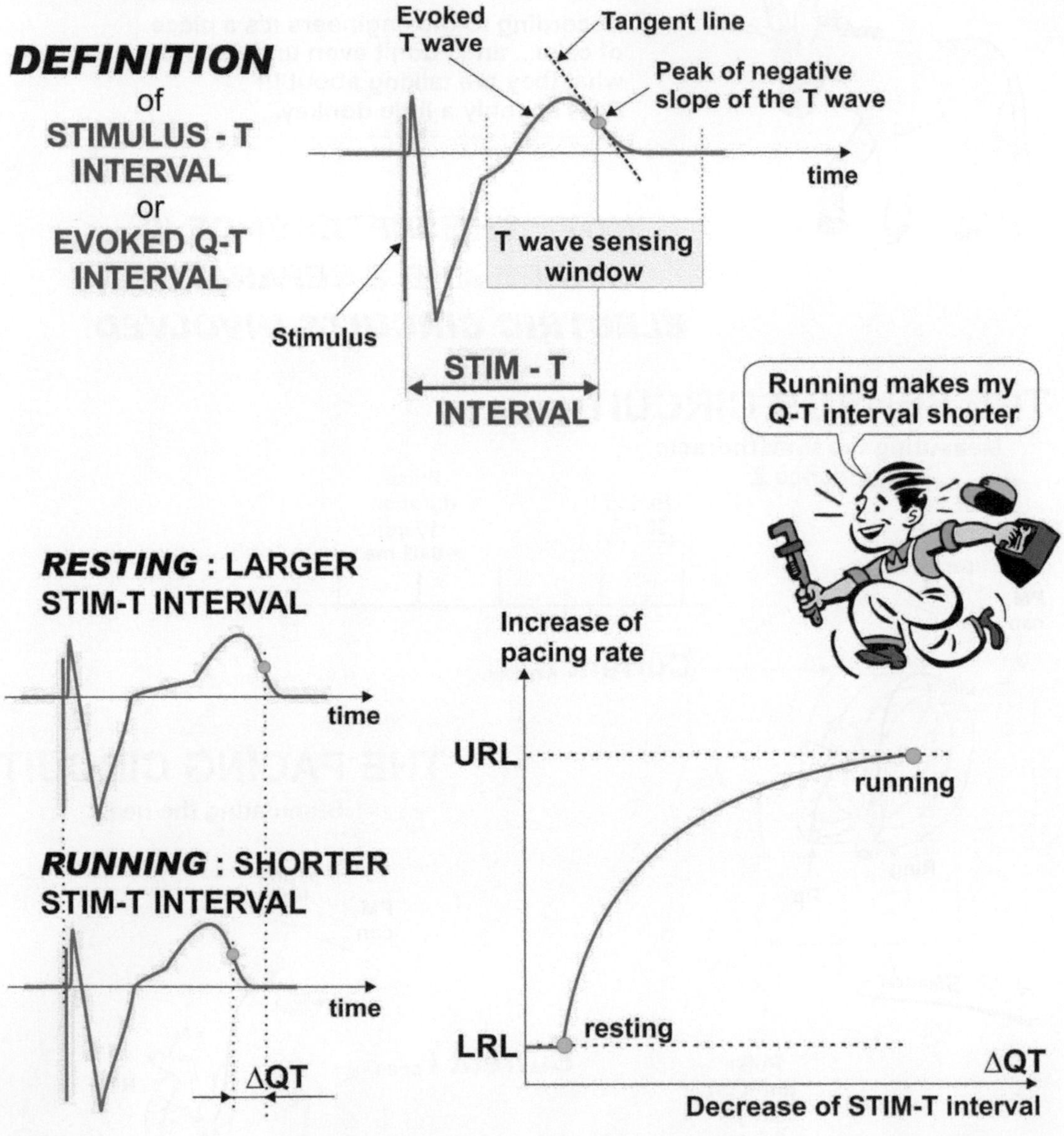

DEFINITION of STIMULUS - T INTERVAL or EVOKED Q-T INTERVAL

RESTING : LARGER STIM-T INTERVAL

RUNNING : SHORTER STIM-T INTERVAL

Abbreviations : URL = upper rate limit ; LRL = lower rate limit

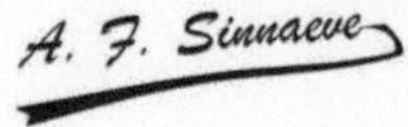

RATE-ADAPTIVE PACING DEFINITIONS

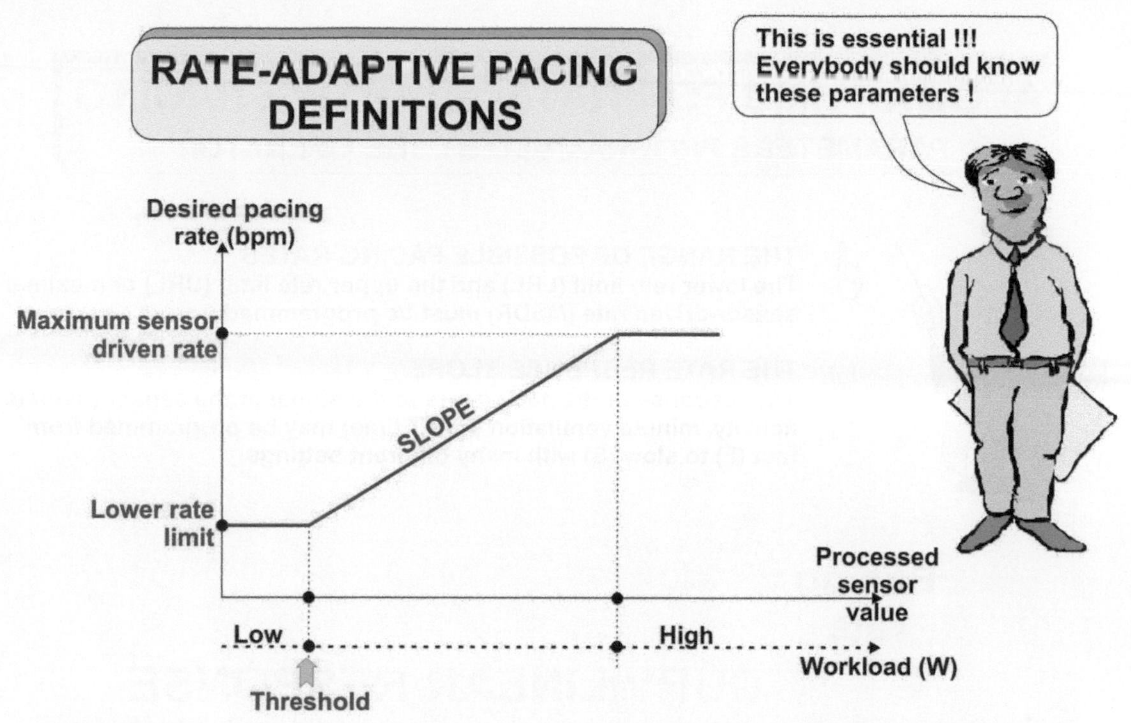

LOWER RATE LIMIT : the minimum desired resting heart rate of the patient (average 65 bpm)

THRESHOLD : minimum workload (or minimum activity) at which the sensor driven pacing rate increases above the lower rate limit or resting rate

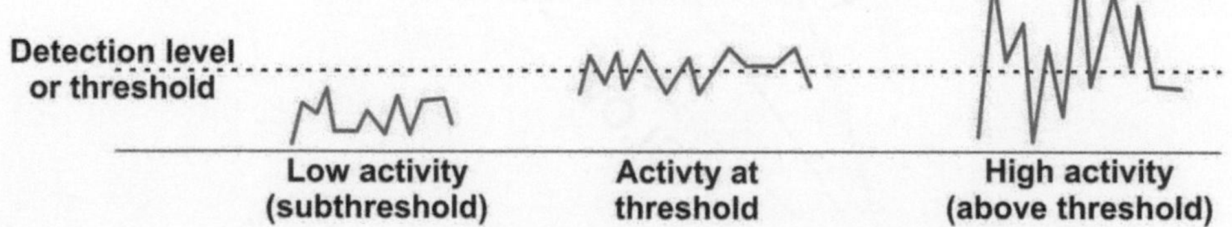

MAXIMUM SENSOR DRIVEN RATE : maximum pacing rate induced by the sensor

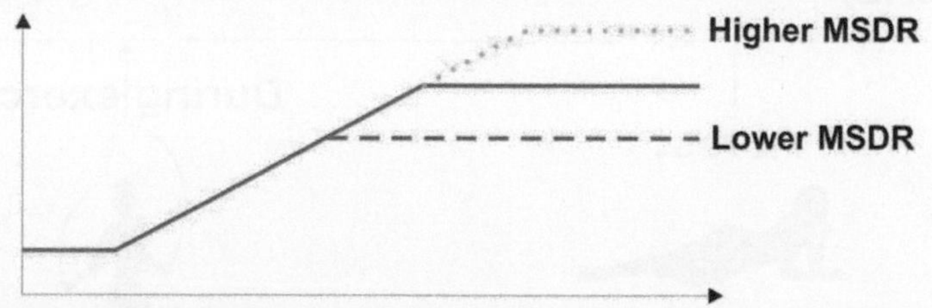

SLOPE : how fast the sensor driven pacing rate increases in response to the increasing workload (or increasing sensor output signal)

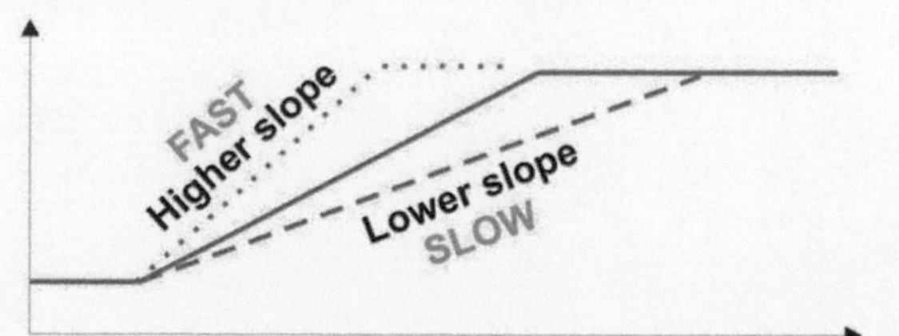

A. F. Sinnaeve

ALGORITHMS FOR RATE-ADAPTIVE PACING

PARAMETERS PROGRAMMED BY THE OPERATOR

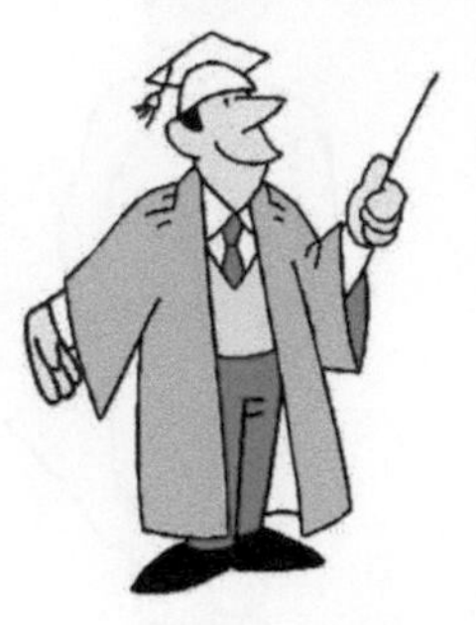

THE RANGE OF POSSIBLE PACING RATES
The lower rate limit (LRL) and the upper rate limit (URL) or maximal sensor-driven rate (MSDR) must be programmed

THE RATE RESPONSE SLOPE
The response of the pacing rate to the signal of the sensor (detected activity, minute ventilation or Q-T time) may be programmed from fast (F) to slow (S) with many different settings

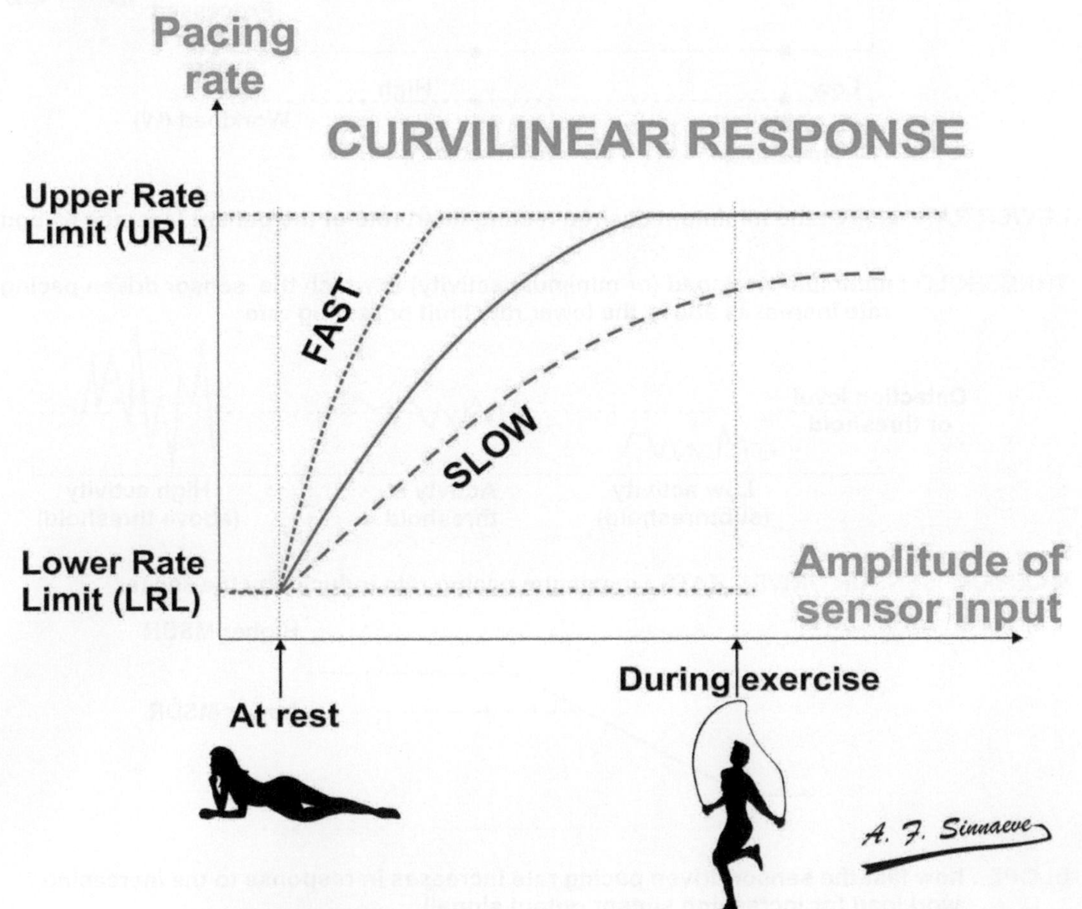

ALGORITHMS FOR RATE-ADAPTIVE PACING

PARAMETERS PROGRAMMED BY THE OPERATOR - PART 2

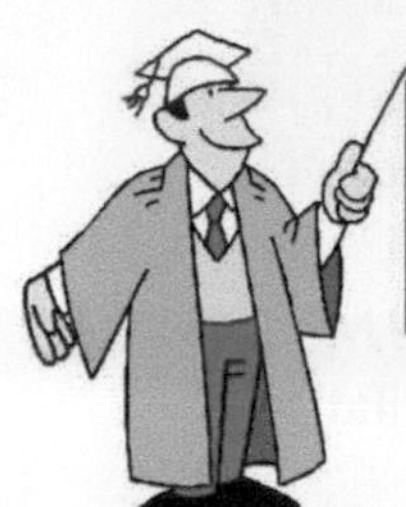

Many rate adaptive pacemakers use different sets of curves for the post-exercise recovery. The slope of these deceleration curves may be programmed by the operator.

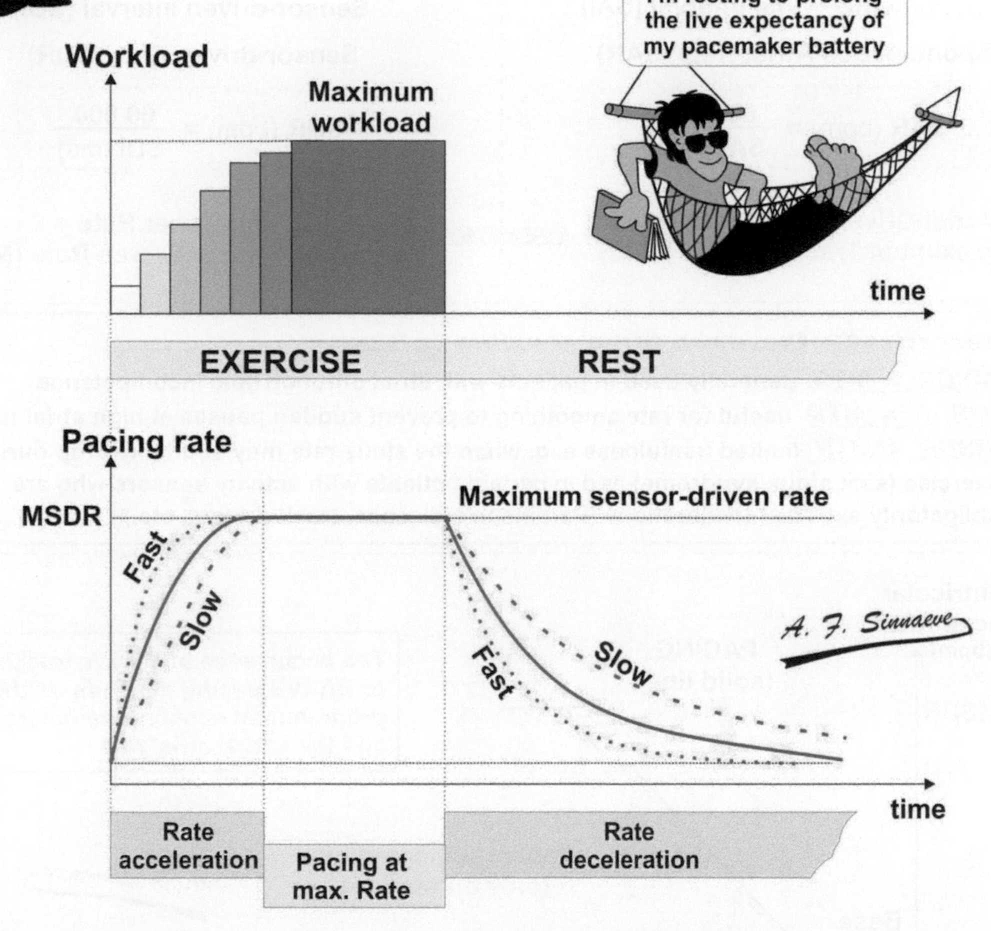

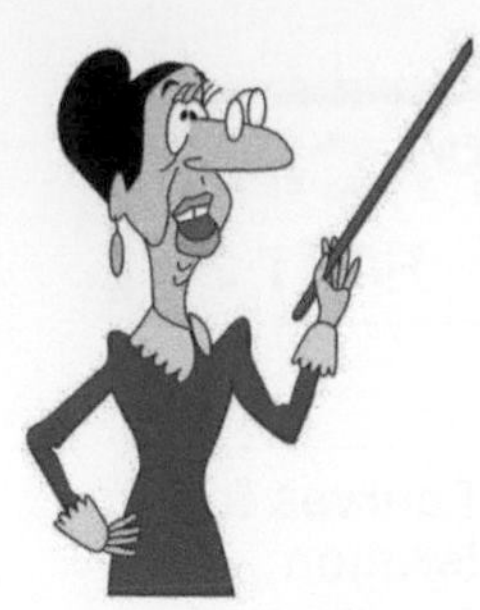

PAY ATTENTION !!! NOTE THE DIFFERENCE BETWEEN ATRIAL-DRIVEN RATE AND SENSOR-DRIVEN RATE

DUE TO INTRINSIC ATRIAL ACTIVITY (e.g. Sinus Node)	***DUE TO THE SIGNAL OF THE SENSOR*** (e.g. Minute Ventilation)
Spontaneous Atrial Interval (SAI)	**Sensor-driven Interval (SDI)**
Spontaneous Atrial Rate (SAR)	**Sensor-driven Rate (SDR)**
$\mathbf{SAR}\ (\text{bpm}) = \frac{60\,000}{\mathbf{SAI}\ (\text{ms})}$	$\mathbf{SDR}\ (\text{bpm}) = \frac{60\,000}{\mathbf{SDI}\ (\text{ms})}$
Atrial-Driven Upper Rate = Maximum Tracking Rate (MTR)	**Sensor-Driven Upper Rate = Maximum Sensor-Driven Rate (MSDR)**

Theoretically, there are three possible settings :

* *MSDR > MTR* generally used in patients with atrial chronotropic incompetence
* *MSDR = MTR* useful for rate smoothing to prevent sudden pauses at high atrial rates
* *MSDR < MTR* limited usefulness e. g. when the sinus rate may suddenly drop during exercise (sick sinus syndrome) and in certain patients with activity sensors who are obligatorily exposed to vibrations (Parkinson's disease, truck drivers, etc.)

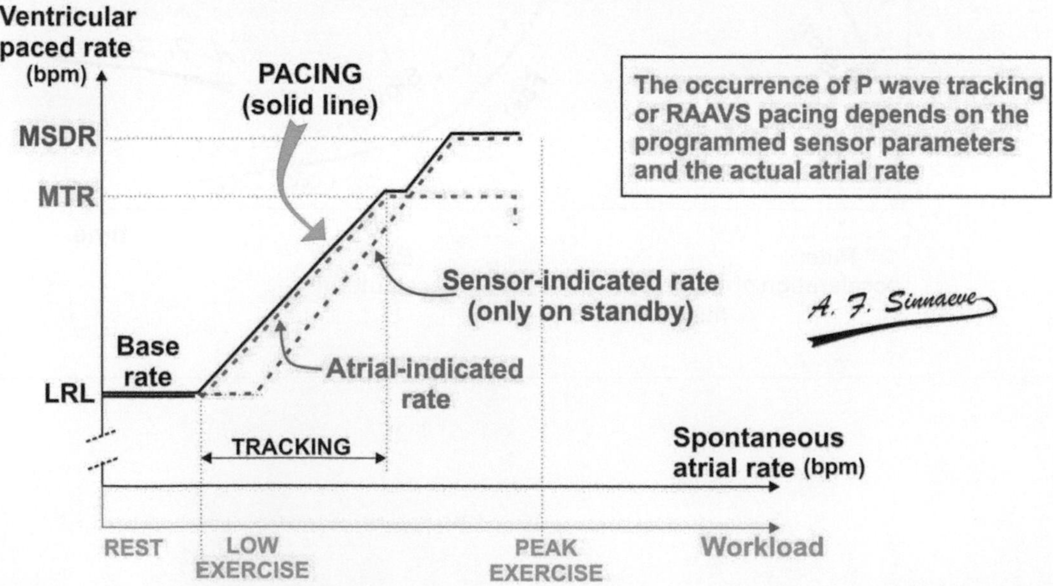

Abbreviations : LRL = lower rate limit; MSDR = maximum sensor-driven rate; MTR = maximum tracking rate; RAAVS = rate-adaptive AV sequential pacing; SAI = spontaneous atrial interval; SAR = spontaneous atrial rate; SDI = sensor-driven interval; SDR = sensor-driven rate.

UNWANTED RESPONSES OF SENSORS - PART 1

1 SENSORS OF BODY MOTION

The pacing rate of devices with an activity sensor or an accelerometer depends on the type of activity and does not correlate well with the level of exertion or the amount of work, i.e. body vibration is not proportional to the level of energy expenditure

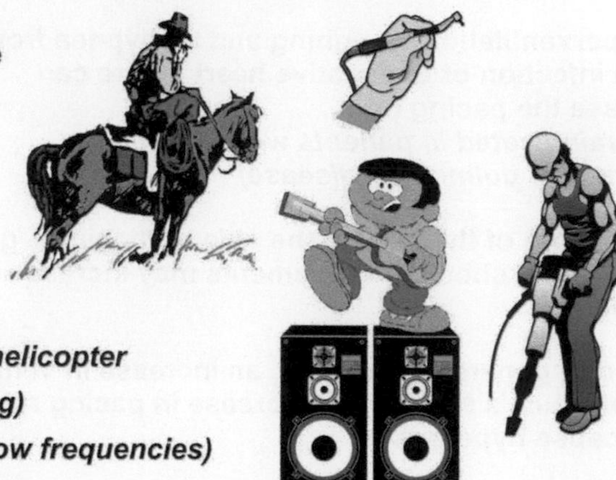

1/ Environmental interference may cause an unwanted increase in pacing rate (less pronounced for devices equipped with an accelerometer) :

* ***riding on horseback***
* ***driving in a car on rough terrain***
* ***riding on a motorcycle on a bad road***
* ***flying in a small-engine aircraft or in a helicopter***
* ***the use of drills (including dental drilling)***
* ***very loud rock music (especially ultra-low frequencies)***

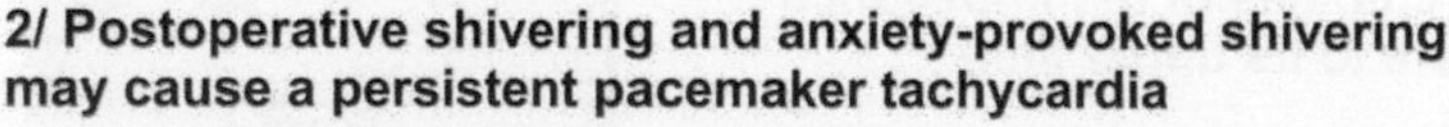

2/ Postoperative shivering and anxiety-provoked shivering may cause a persistent pacemaker tachycardia

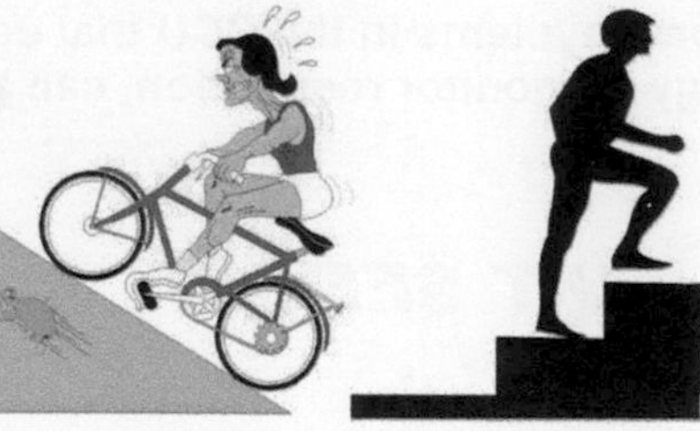

3/ Epileptic seizures and myotonic jerking with chorea can increase the pacing rate

4/ When bicycling the condition of the road influences the rate response excessively, while walking downstairs may cause a larger rate increase than walking upstairs

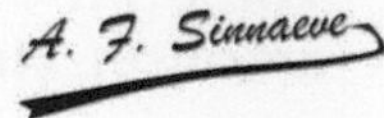

UNWANTED RESPONSES OF SENSORS - PART 2

SENSORS OF MINUTE VENTILATION

Systems with a minute ventilation sensor are highly physiologic and therefore highly specific. Occasionally the reaction to the onset of exercise may be delayed and the rate may be too fast after the end of exercise

1/ Hyperventilation, coughing and tachypnea from chest infection or congestive heart failure can increase the pacing rate *(contraindicated in patients with chronic obstructive pulmonary disease)*

2/ Swinging of the arm on the side of the pulse generator and rotating shoulder movements may increase the pacing rate

3/ During general anesthesia, an increase in ventilation can produce a substantial increase in pacing rate that may cause hypotension

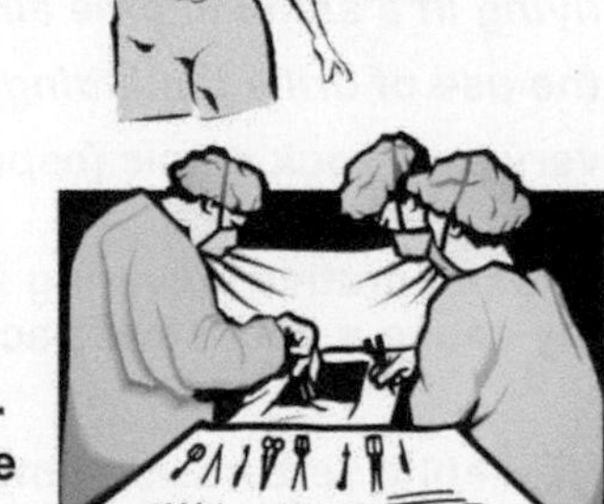

4/ Electrocautery may provoke changes of the impedance and thus increase the pacing rate to its upper limit

5/ Some systems in the CCU that use similar impedance technology to monitor respiration, can also disturb the pacing rate

Q-T SENSOR

The Stim-T interval not only responds to exercise, but also to emotion. However, the QT interval reacts rather slowly.

1/ T wave detection may be hampered by frequent ventricular ectopy, by ventricular fusion beats and by substantial lead polarization

2/ The Q-T interval may be affected by electrolyte disturbances, some medications and coronary artery disease with myocardial ischemia or infarction

A. F. Sinnaeve

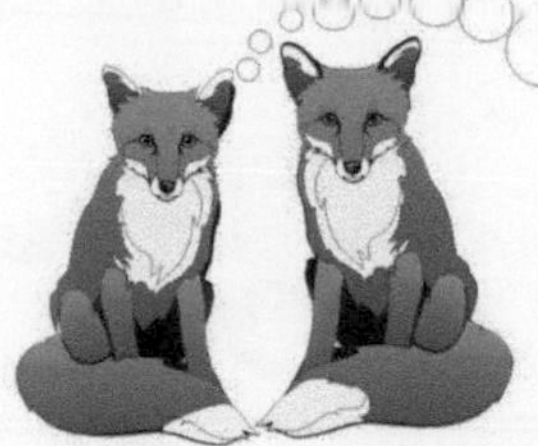

We are an excellent smart couple !
We are combining our merits!!!

DUAL SENSORS & SENSOR BLENDING PART 1

A combination of two sensors is used to improve the correlation to workload for various forms of exercise and to minimize paradoxical responses

NON-PHYSIOLOGIC OR MECHANICAL INDICATORS	PHYSIOLOGIC OR METABOLIC INDICATORS
SENSORS : Activity sensors, Accelerometers	*SENSORS* : Minute Ventilation, QT- interval
PRO : fast responding	*CONTRA* : slow responding
CONTRA : low specificity i.e. Increased incidence of false positive responses unrelated to actual exercise	*PRO* : high specificity i.e. Lesser incidence of false positive responses unrelated to actual exercise

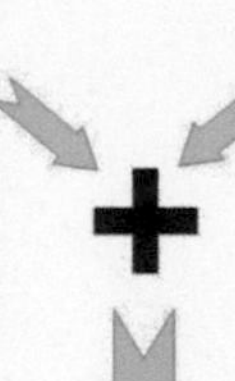

The combination of a physiologic and a non-physiologic sensor results in a rate response that mimics normal sinus node response closely and that to a great extent ignores false positive sensor information

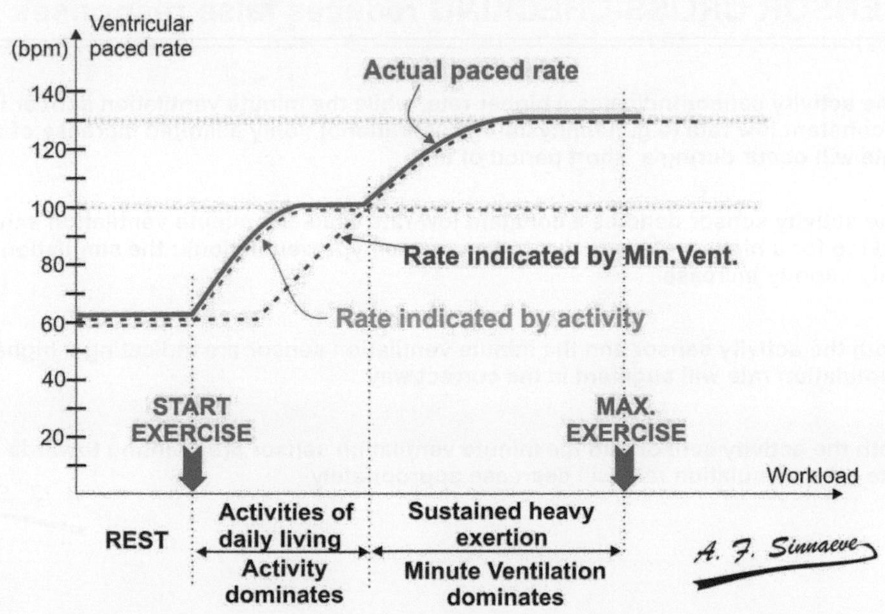

A. F. Sinnaeve

DUAL SENSOR PACING PART 2

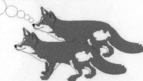

We are cunning foxes and so is a pacing system with two sensors

SENSOR BLENDING determines the relative influence of each sensor upon the pacing rate.

Depending upon the sophistication of the algorithm, the blending may be programmed in fixed steps (0/100 - 30/70 - 50/50 - 70/30 - 100/0) or the relative contribution of each sensor may vary automatically across the rate response range

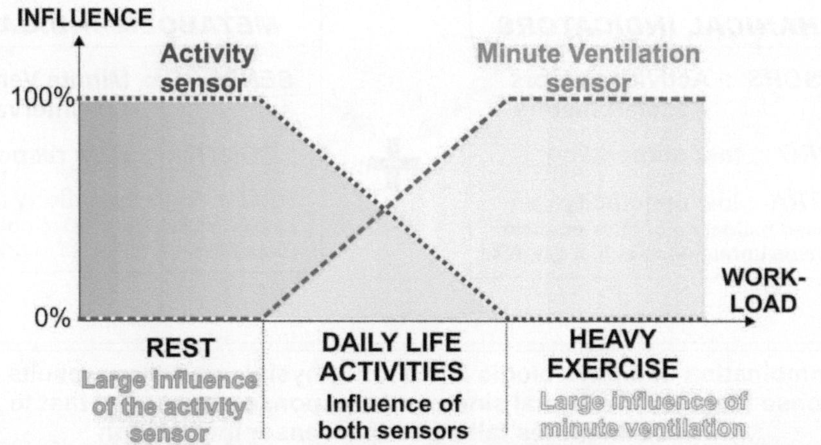

SENSOR CROSS-CHECKING reduces false responses

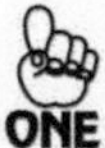
ONE

The activity sensor indicates a higher rate, while the minute ventilation sensor indicates a constant low rate (e.g. nonphysiologic vibrations) : only a limited increase of stimulation rate will occur during a short period of time

TWO

The activity sensor denotes a constant low rate while the minute ventilation sensor is asking for a higher rate (e.g. due to fever or to hyperventilation) : the simulation rate will only slightly increase

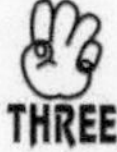
THREE

Both the activity sensor and the minute ventilation sensor are indicating a higher rate : the stimulation rate will augment in the correct way

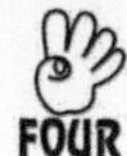
FOUR

Both the activity sensor and the minute ventilation sensor are pointing towards a lower rate : the stimulation rate will decrease appropriately

A. F. Sinnaeve

DUAL SENSOR PACING
PART 3 : SENSOR CROSS-CHECKING

We are cunning foxes and so is a pacing system with two sensors

I had a pacemaker with an activity sensor. Every time I drove on this bumpy road, my heart rate went up a lot ... !!!

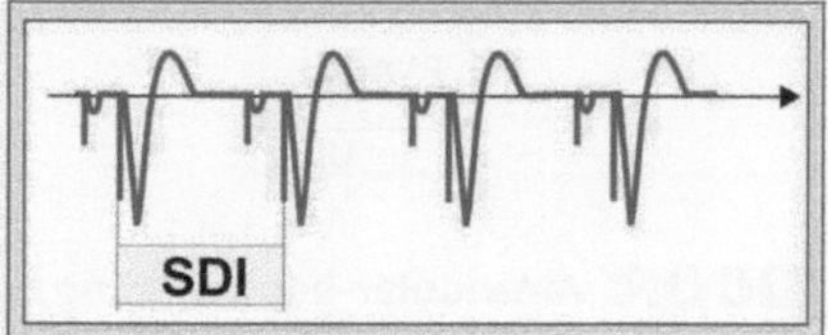

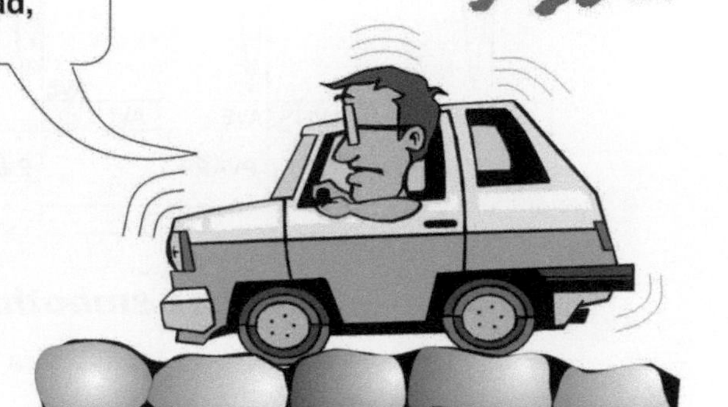

Now I have a pacemaker with two sensors, activity and QT. Even driving faster on the same bumpy road, my heart rate goes up only slightly!!!

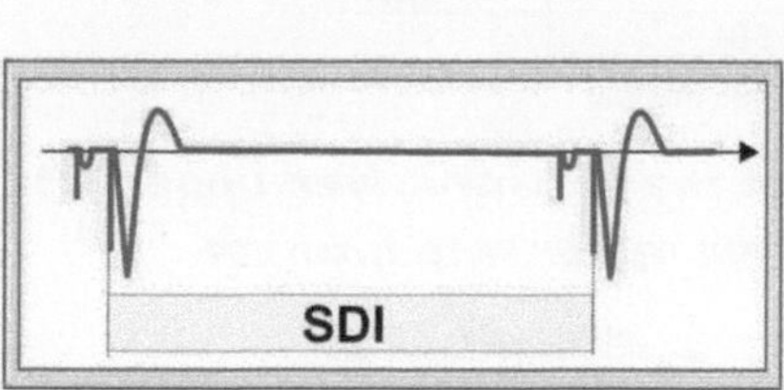

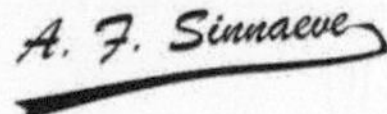

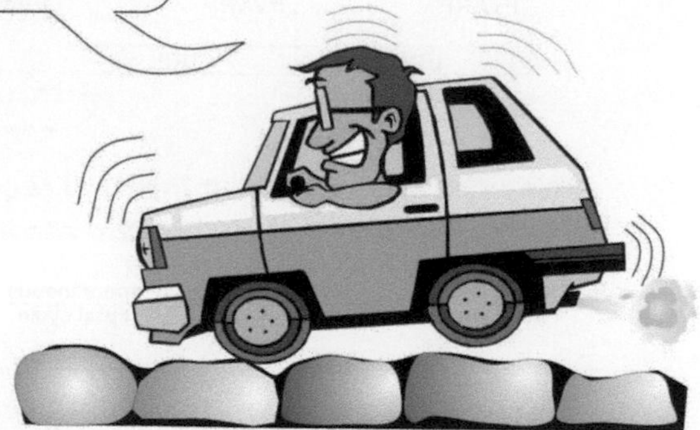

Abbreviations : SDI = sensor driven interval

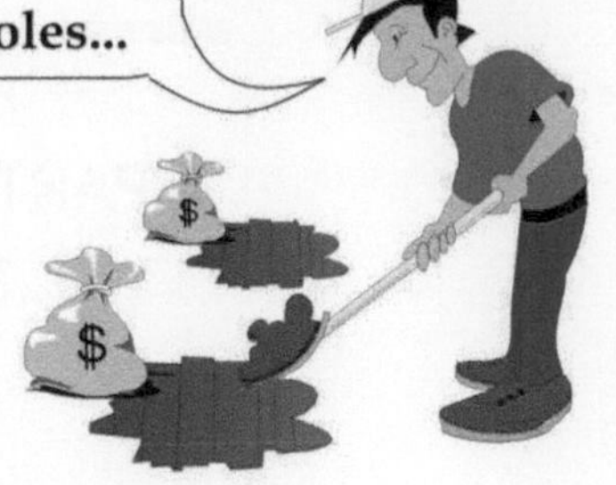

WENCKEBACH UPPER RATE BEHAVIOR DURING RATE - ADAPTIVE PACING

1. *DDD pacing* (ventricular-based timing)

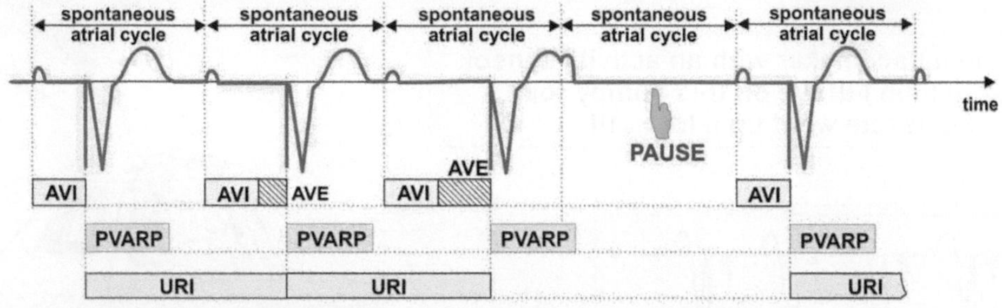

2. *Sensor-driven rate smoothing (DDDR* ventricular-based timing*)*

When the sensor-driven interval is longer than the atrial-driven upper rate interval

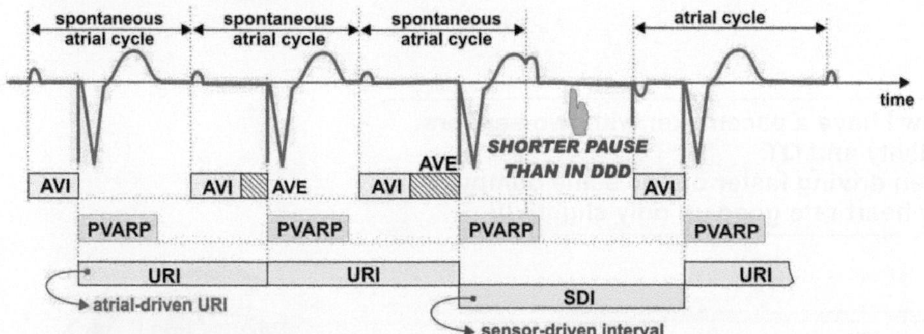

When the sensor-driven interval (equal to the sensor-driven upper rate interval SDURI) is equal to the atrial-driven upper rate interval

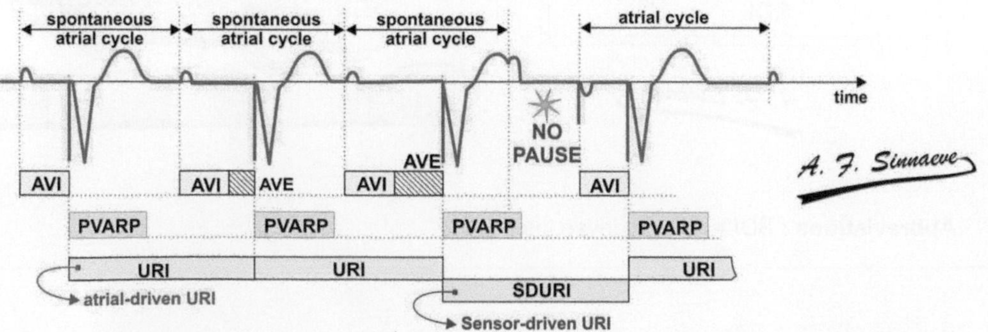

Abbreviations : AVI = programmed AV delay ; AVE = AV extension ; PVARP = postventricular atrial refractory period ; URI = atrial-driven upper rate interval ; SDI = sensor driven interval ; SDURI = sensor-driven upper rate interval

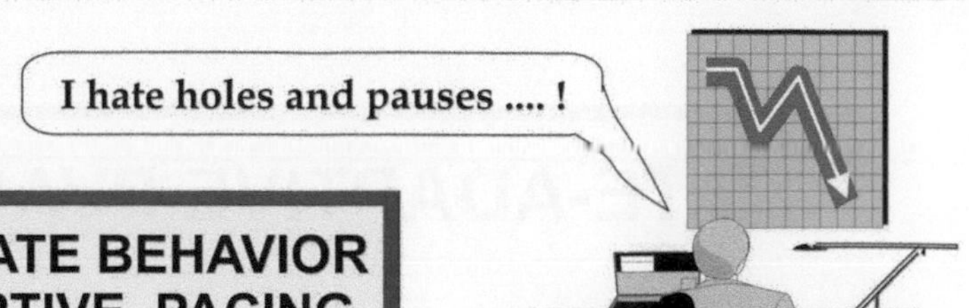

2 :1 BLOCK UPPER RATE BEHAVIOR DURING RATE - ADAPTIVE PACING

1. *DDD pacing* (ventricular-based timing)

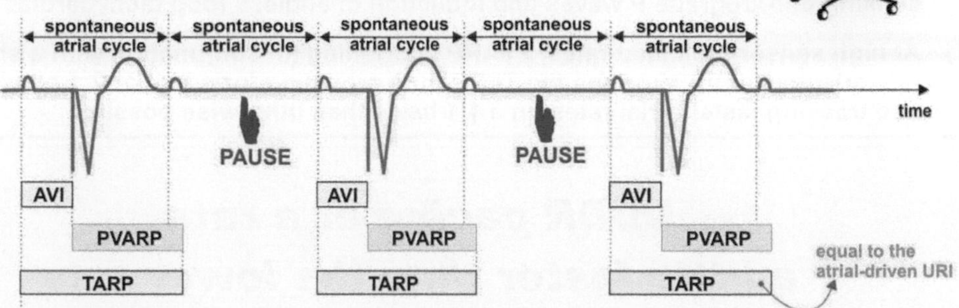

2. *Sensor-driven rate-smoothing (DDDR* ventricular-based timing*)*

When the sensor-driven interval is longer than the atrial-driven upper rate interval

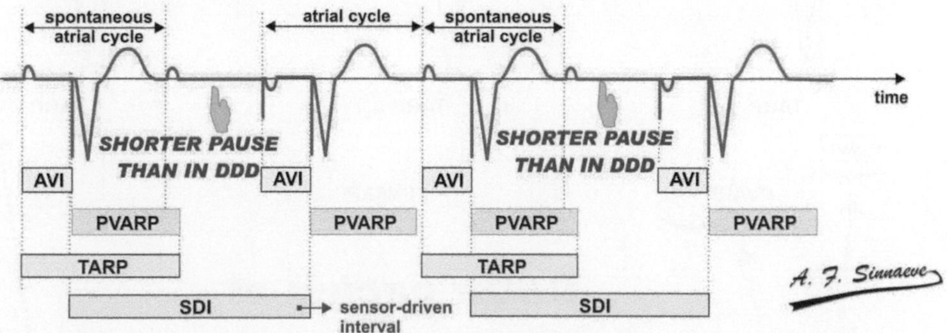

When the sensor-driven interval (equal to the sensor-driven upper rate interval SDURI) is equal to the atrial-driven upper rate interval

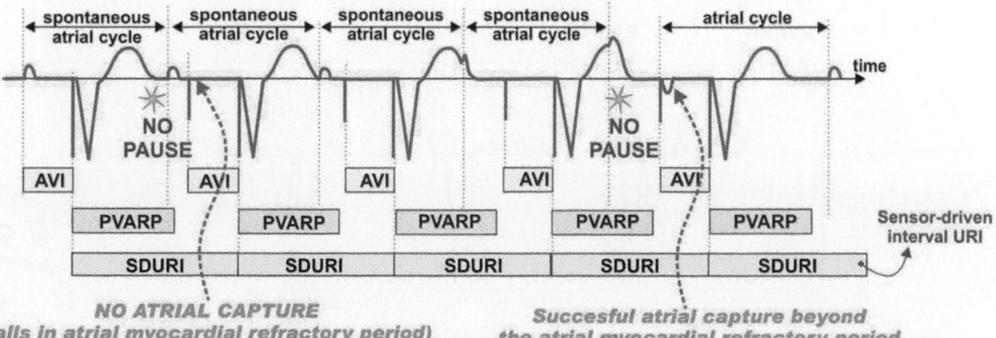

Abbreviations : AVI = programmed AV delay ; AVE = AV extension ; PVARP = postventricular atrial refractory period ; URI = atrial-driven upper rate interval ; SDI = sensor driven interval ; SDURI = sensor-driven upper rate interval ; TARP = total atrial refractory interval

RATE-ADAPTIVE PVARP

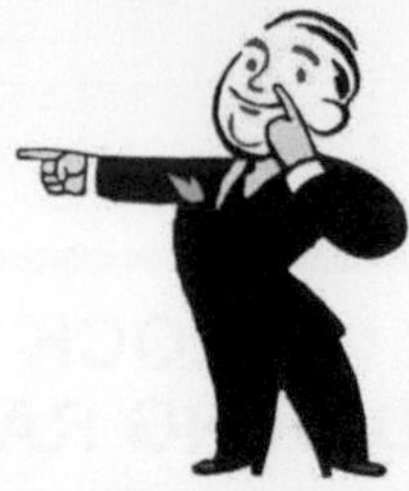

- At low rates, the PVARP is longer. A long PVARP enhances protection against sensing of retrograde P waves and induction of endless loop tachycardia.
- At high sensor-indicated rates, PVARP shortening (in conjunction with a shorter rate adaptive sAVI) shortens the TARP thus providing for a higher 2:1 block rate and tracking faster atrial rates on a 1:1 basis than otherwise possible

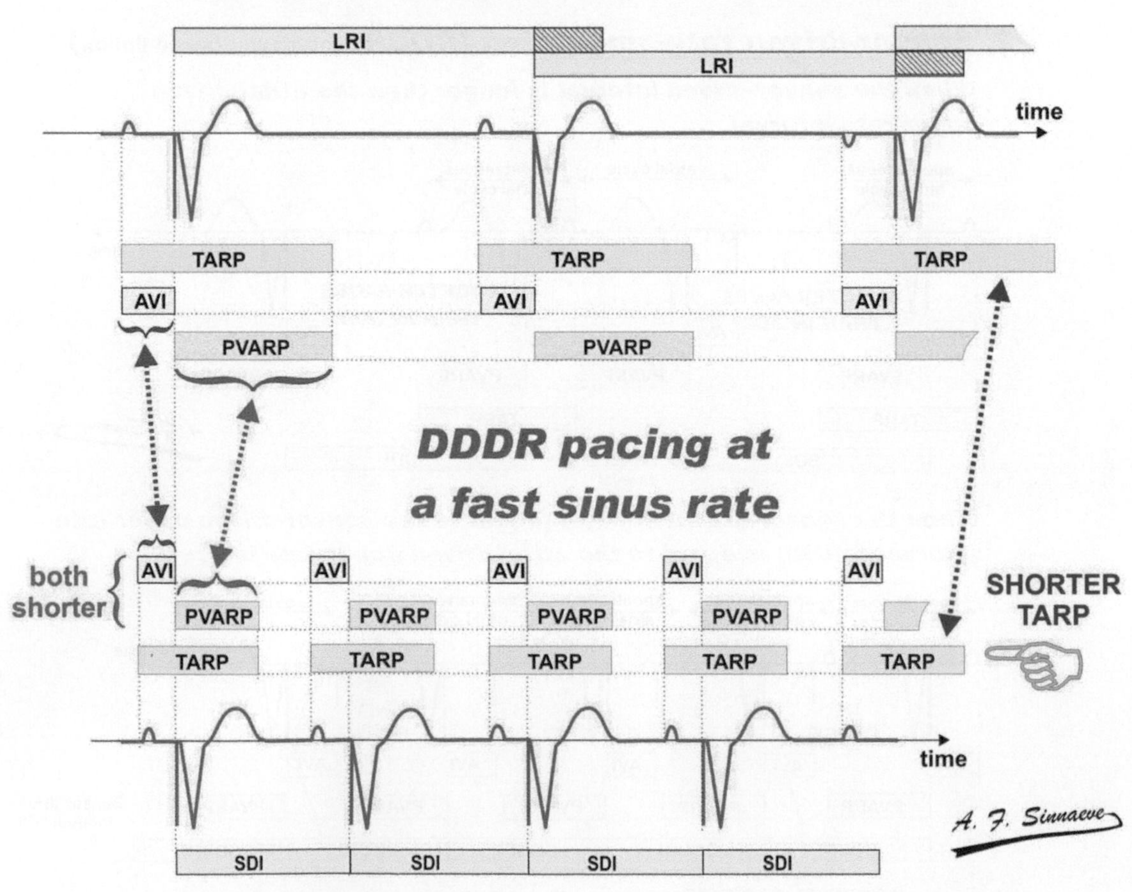

Abbreviations : AVI = programmed AV delay; PVARP = postventricular atrial refractory period; SDI = sensor-driven interval; LRI = lower rate interval; TARP = total atrial refractory period

NON-COMPETITIVE ATRIAL PACING (NCAP)

The NCAP interval is a period of time when the pacemaker is prevented from delivering an atrial stimulus. This function was designed to prevent the induction of atrial tachyarrhythmias by an atrial pacing stimulus falling into the atrial relative refractory period and the vulnerable period of the atrium.

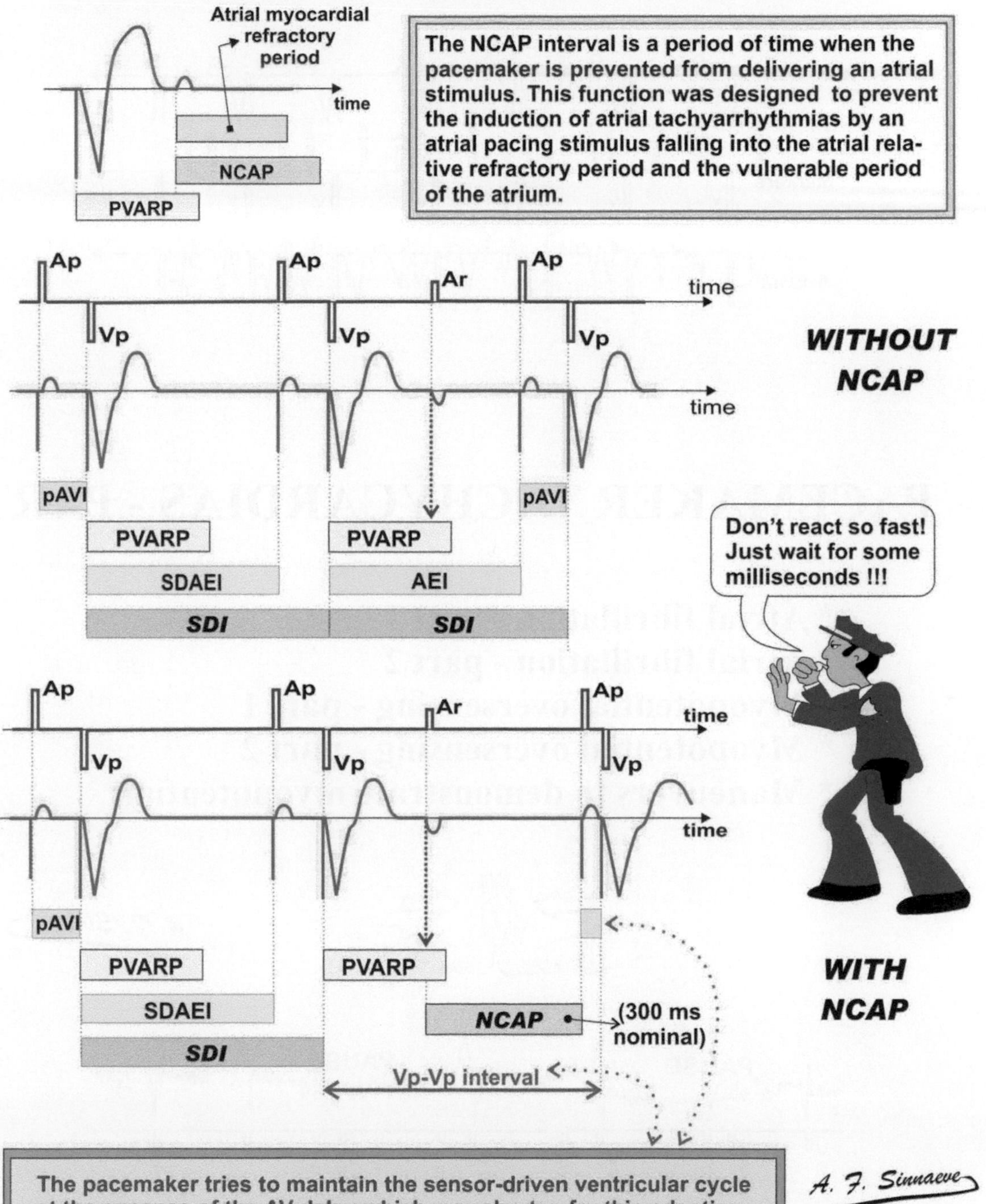

The pacemaker tries to maintain the sensor-driven ventricular cycle at the expense of the AV delay which may shorten for this adaption

A. F. Sinnaeve

Abbreviations : Ap = atrial paced event; Ar = atrial refractory sensed event; Vp = ventricular paced event; pAVI = paced atrioventricular interval; PVARP = postventricular atrial refractory period; SDAEI = sensor driven atrial escape interval; SDI = sensor driven interval; NCAP = non-competitive atrial pacing period.

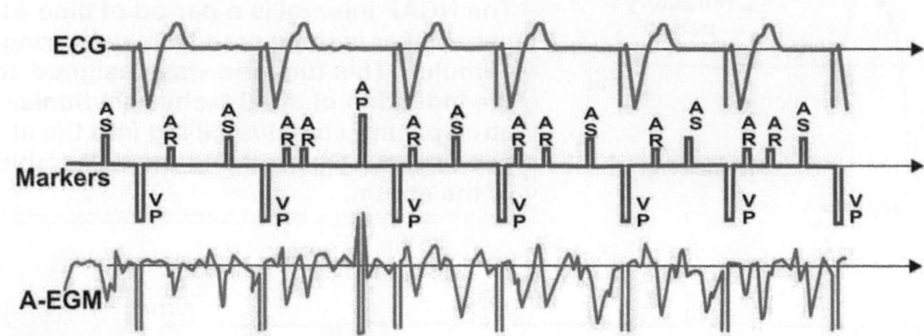

PACEMAKER TACHYCARDIAS - PART 1

- **Atrial fibrillation - part 1**
- **Atrial fibrillation - part 2**
- **Myopotential oversensing - part 1**
- **Myopotential oversensing - part 2**
- **Maneuvers to demonstrate myopotentials**

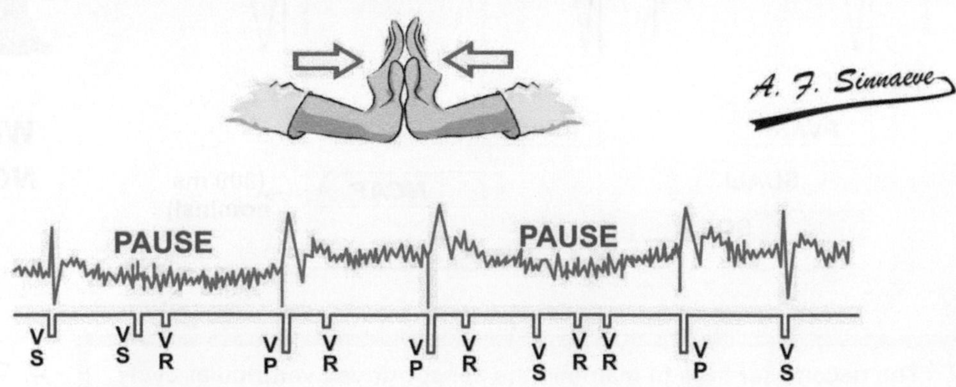

DDD PACEMAKERS AND ATRIAL FIBRILLATION - Part 1

1 A FIB may provoke a fast ventricular response (regular or irregular)

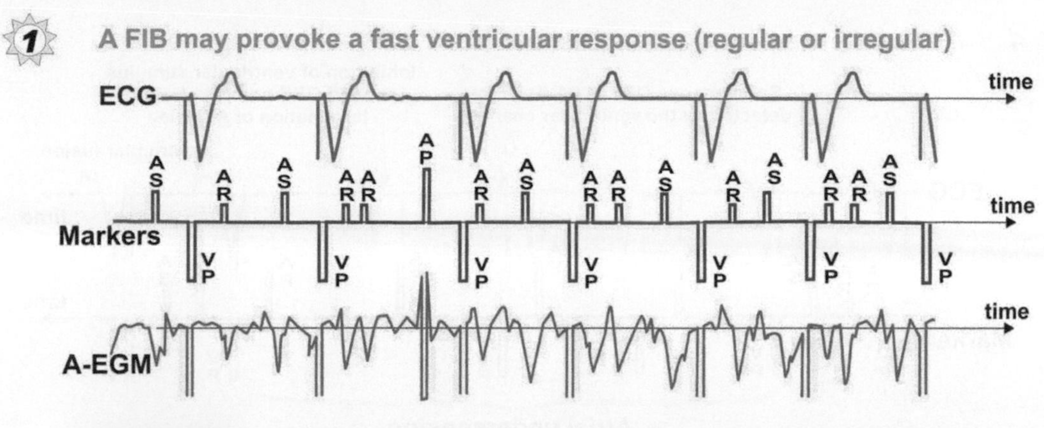

CAUTION
ELIMINATE DOUBT...LOCK IT OUT

A fast and irregular pacemaker tachycardia is almost always due to atrial fibrillation !!!

2 Intermittent sensing of f waves ; mixed response

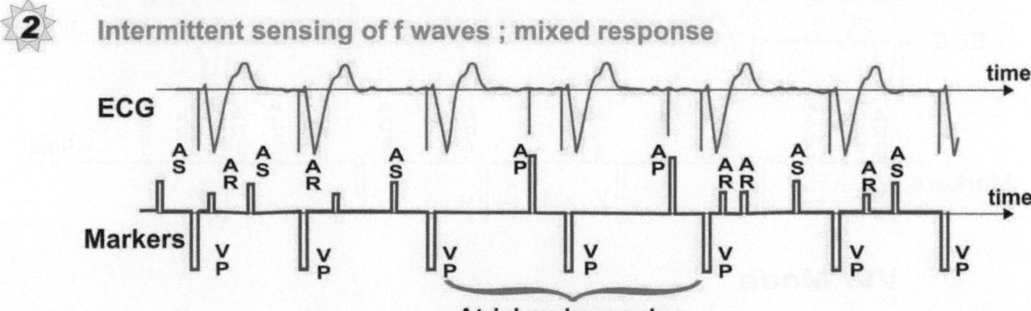

3 Ventricular safety pacing when f waves are unsensed **(VSP occurs with a spontaneous QRS complex or an EMI signal that comes after AP but before the expected VP)**

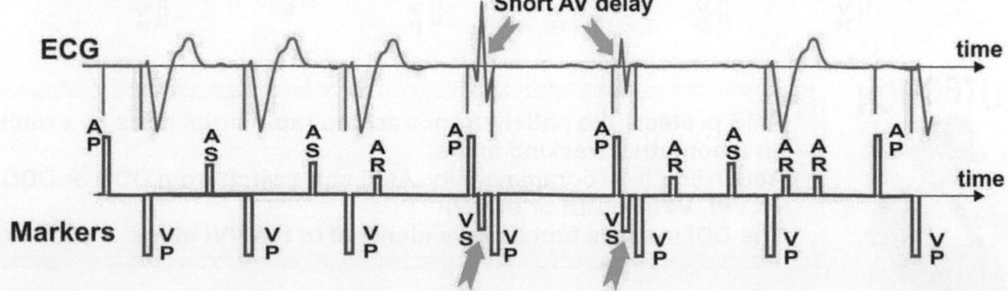

Abbreviations : AS = sensed atrial event; AR = atrial sense in refractory period; AP = atrial pace; VP = ventricular pace; VS = ventricular sense; SDI = sensor-driven interval; A FIB = atrial fibrillation; AMS = automatic mode switching; PAVB = post-atrial ventricular blanking; VSP = ventricular safety pacing; EMI = electromagnetic interference

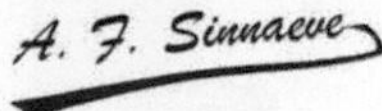

DDD PACEMAKERS AND ATRIAL FIBRILLATION - Part 2

A FIB may create confusion (VSP switched OFF)

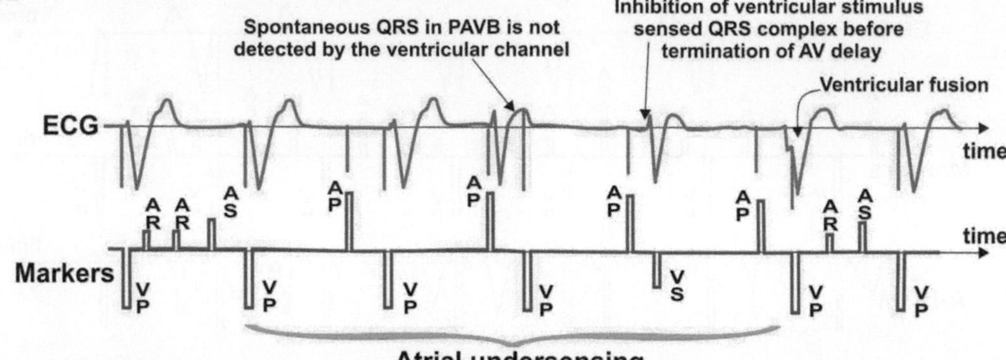

A FIB and Automatic Mode Switching (AMS)

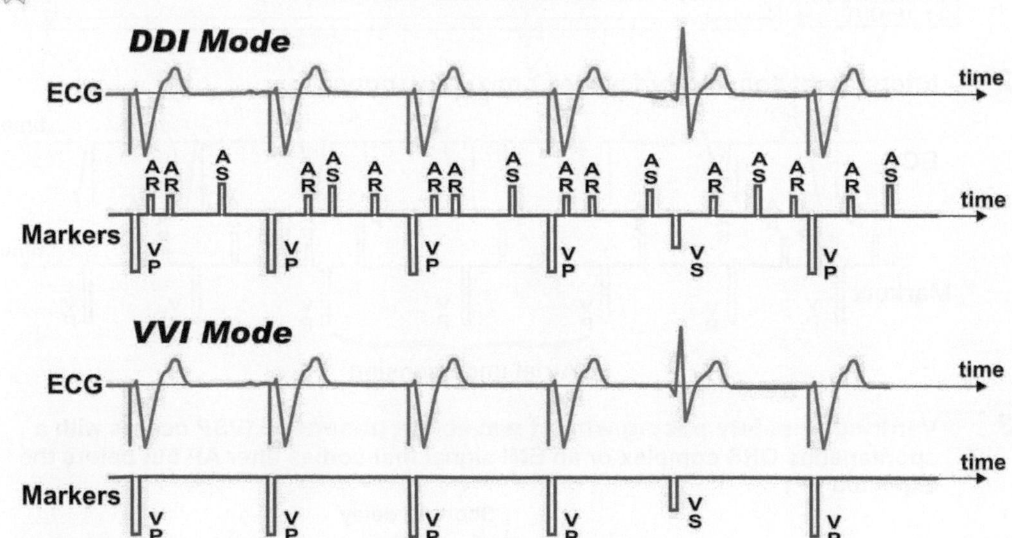

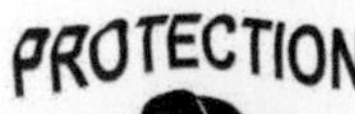

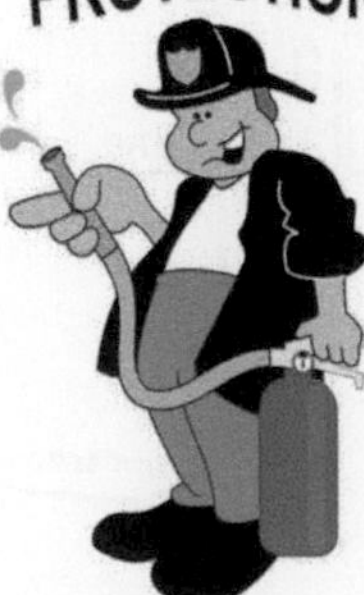

* AMS protects the patient from tracking rapid atrial rates by switching to a non-atrial tracking mode.
* According to programmability, AMS can switch from DDD or DDD(R) to VVI, VVI(R), DDI or DDI(R)
* The DDI mode is functionally identical to the VVI mode

Abbreviations : AS = sensed atrial event; AR = atrial sense in refractory period; AP = atrial pace; VP = ventricular pace; VS = ventricular sense; SDI = sensor-driven interval; A FIB = atrial fibrillation; AMS = automatic mode switching; PAVB = post-atrial ventricular blanking; VSP = ventricular safety pacing

A. F. Sinnaeve

MYOPOTENTIAL SENSING DURING UNIPOLAR DDD PACING - Part 1

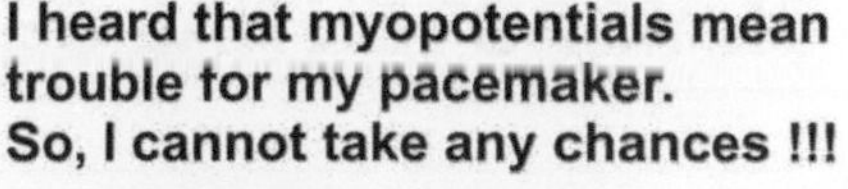

I heard that myopotentials mean trouble for my pacemaker.
So, I cannot take any chances !!!

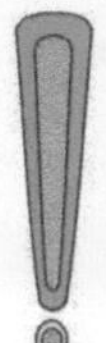

Baseline interference of the surface ECG is characteristic of myopotential oversensing

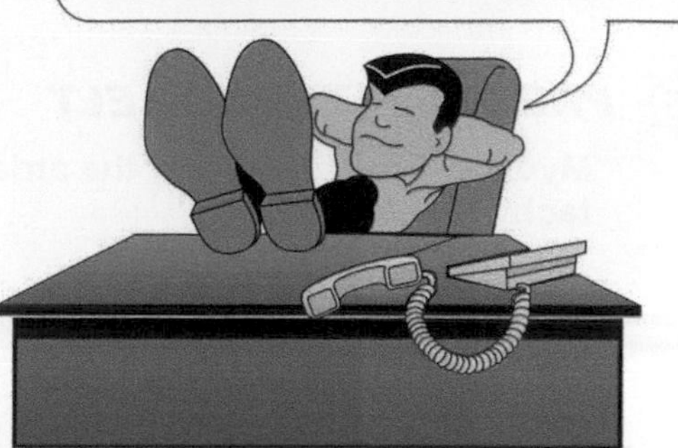

INHIBITION OF THE VENTRICULAR CHANNEL

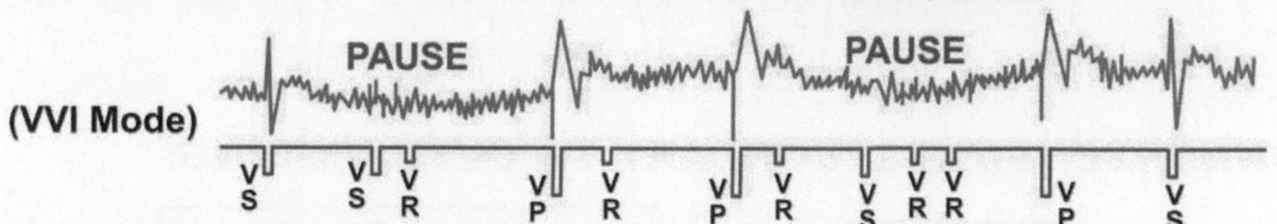

TRIGGERING OF RAPID VENTRICULAR RATES

Sensing by the atrial channel with resultant triggering of ventricular pacing and increase in the paced ventricular rate : tachycardia which can cause symptoms of uncomfortable palpitations, angina, dyspnea, etc.

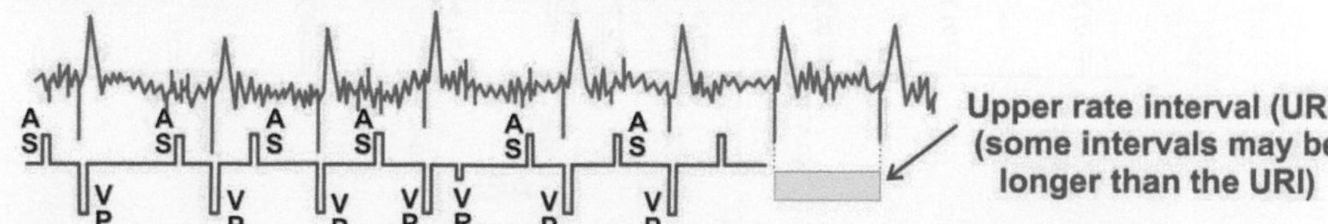

MIXED RESPONSE WITH INHIBITION & TRIGGERING

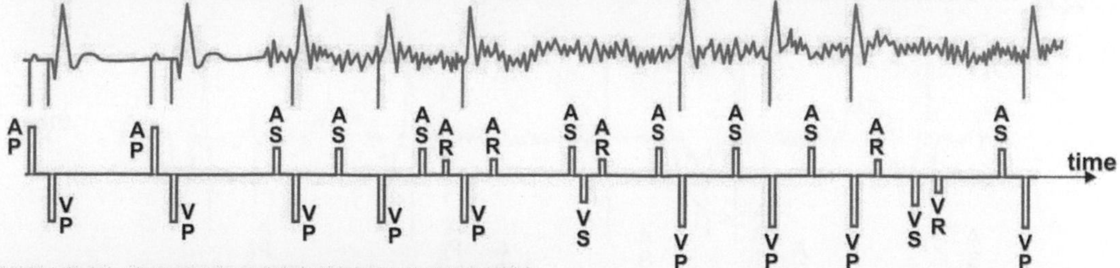

NOISE INTERFERENCE MODE

Reversion to the asynchronous noise interference mode is possible for 1 or more cycles (often at the same rate as the programmed lower rate)

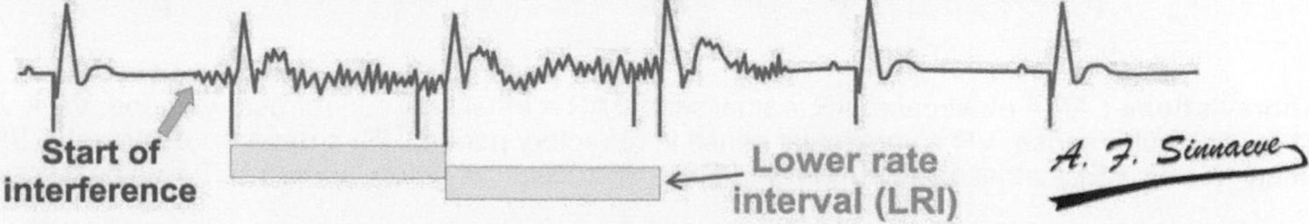

A. F. Sinnaeve

Abbreviations : AP = atrial pace; AS = atrial sense; AR = atrial sense in refractory period; VP = ventricular pace; VS = ventricular sense; VR = ventricular sense in refractory period; URI = upper rate interval

MYOPOTENTIAL SENSING DURING DDD PACING Part 2

5 PRECIPITATION OF ELT

Myopotential sensing by the atrial channel can precipitate an endless-loop tachycardia

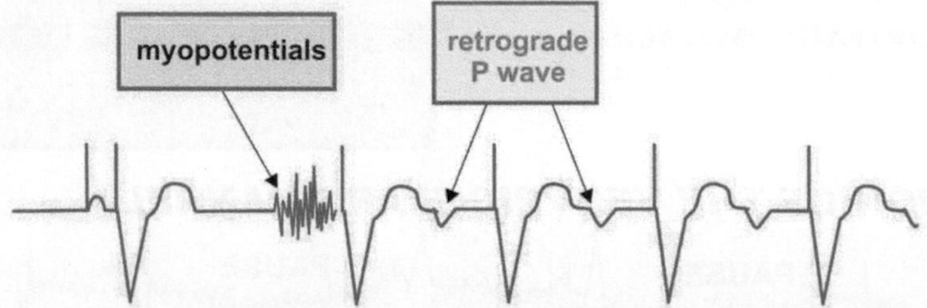

6 UNDERSENSING SECONDARY TO OVERSENSING

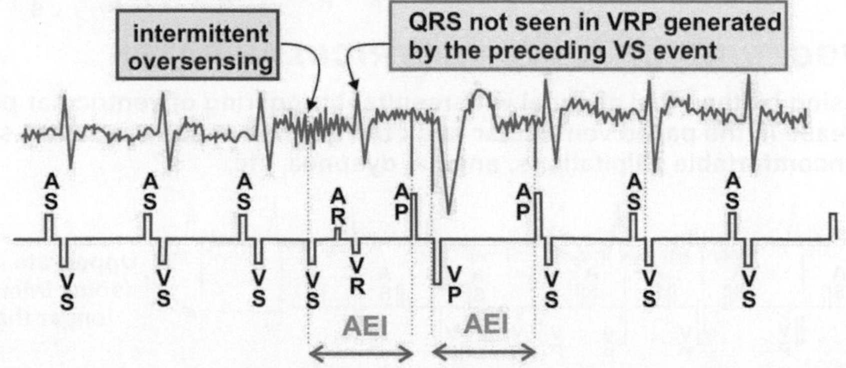

7 MIXED RESPONSE WITH VENTRICULAR SAFETY PACING

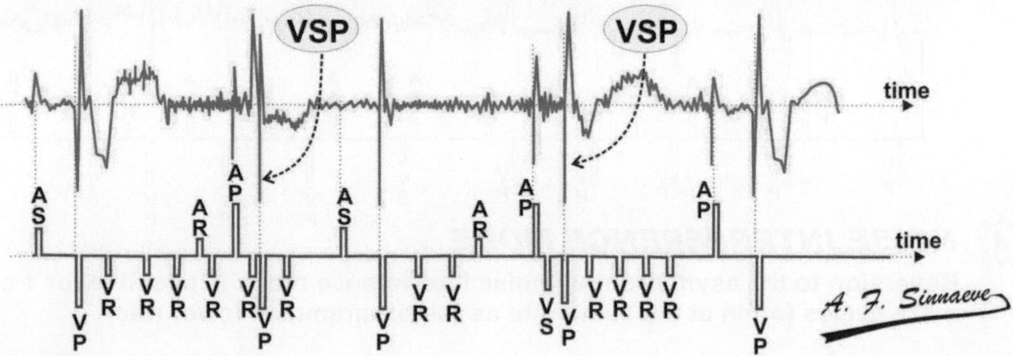

Abbreviations : AP = atrial pace; AS = atrial sense; AR = atrial sense in refractory period; VP = ventricular pace; VS = ventricular sense; VR = ventricular sense in refractory period; URI = upper rate interval; VSP = ventricular safety pacing; AEI = atrial escape interval; VRP = ventricular refractory period; ELT = endless-loop tachycardia.

COMMONLY USED MANEUVERS TO DEMONSTRATE MYOPOTENTIALS

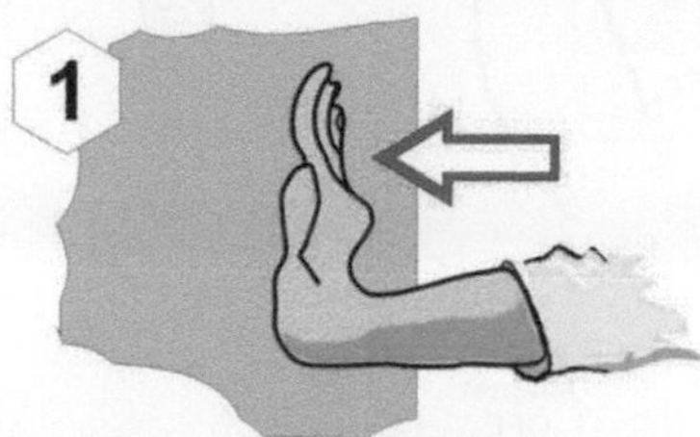

Pressing against a wall

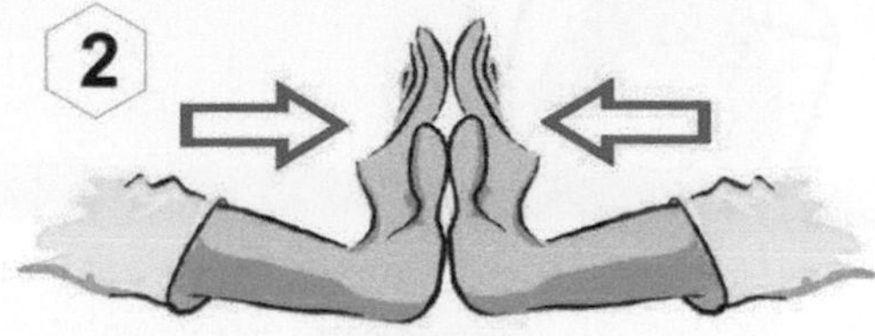

Pressing hands against each other

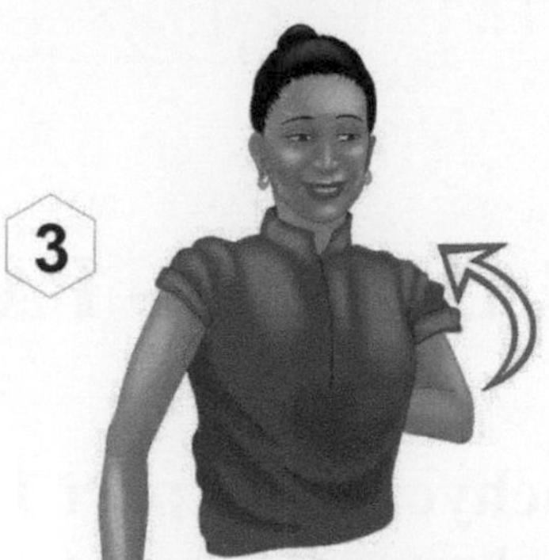

Hyperadduction reach test
or
Adduction of arm against resistance

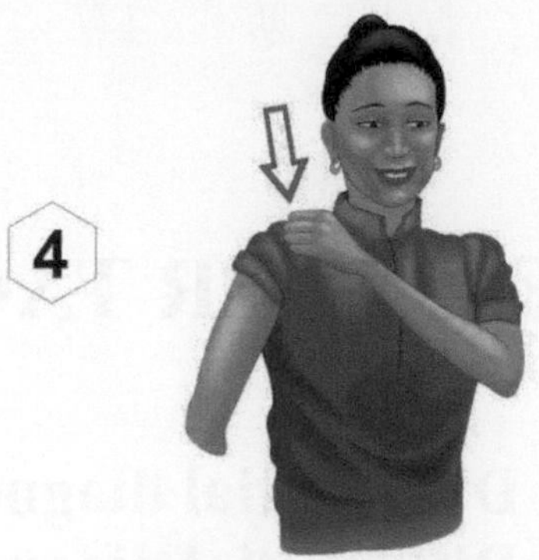

Cup the hand over the shoulder and exert firm and sustained downward pressure

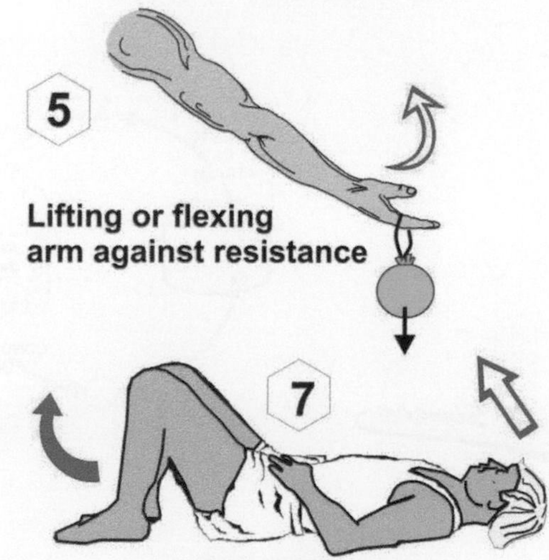

Lifting or flexing arm against resistance

Trunk lifting or
Lifting & holding legs

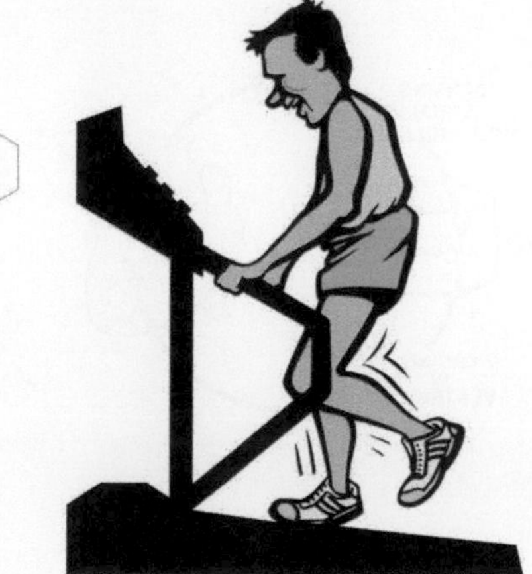

Treadmill stress test

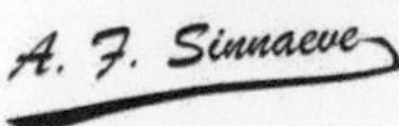

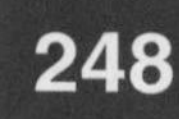

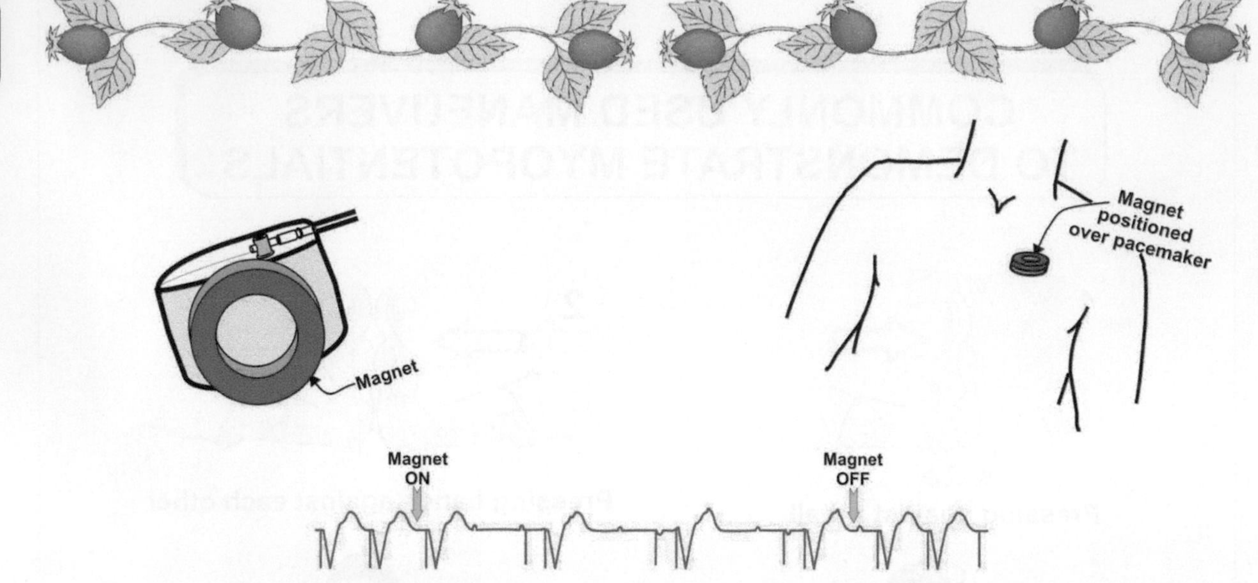

PACEMAKER TACHYCARDIAS - PART 2

* **Differential diagnosis of tachycardia - part 1**
* **Differential diagnosis of tachycardia - part 2**
* **Orthodromic tachycardia**

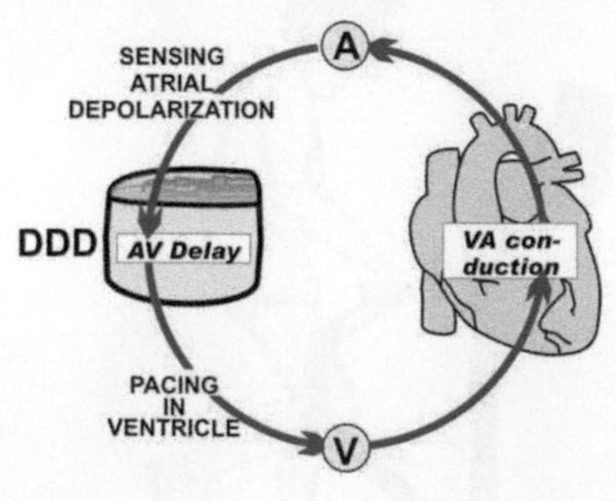

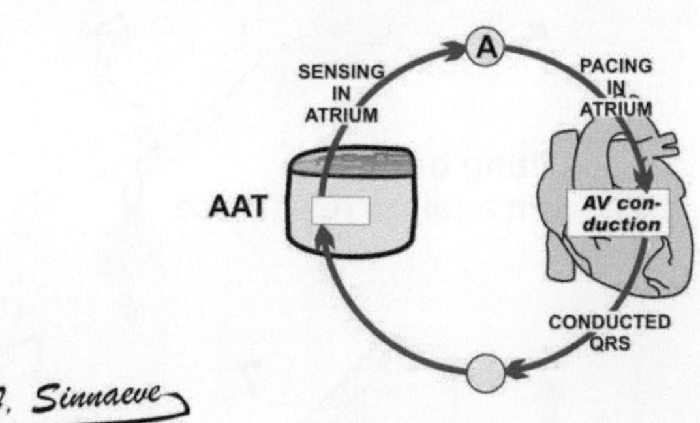

A. F. Sinnaeve

DIFFERENTIAL DIAGNOSIS OF TACHYCARDIA DURING DDD(R) PACING part 1

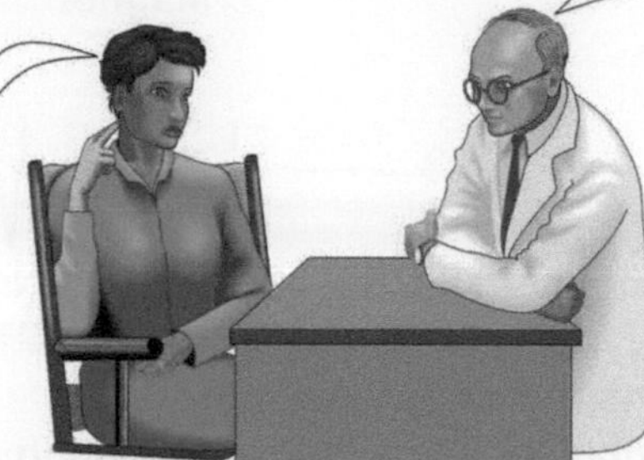

Doctor, I have palpitations all the time ! I cannot stand it any longer !

Well, there are many causes of palpitations, we have to differentiate :

* Rapid paced ventricular rates without a specific arrhythmia :atrial-driven or sensor-driven
* Tracking of atrial arrhythmias with rapid ventricular pacing
* Endless-loop tachycardia (or pacemaker mediated tachycardia)
* Special sensor related tachycardia
* Myopotential triggering
* EMI triggering
* VVI or VVIR pacing with retrograde conduction (without endless-loop tachycardia) or AV dissociation in susceptible patients. Maybe pacemaker syndrome ?
* Native arrhythmias

1 SINUS TACHYCARDIA

* Application of the magnet (slower DOO mode) may reveal P waves. The tachycardia returns upon withdrawal of the magnet.

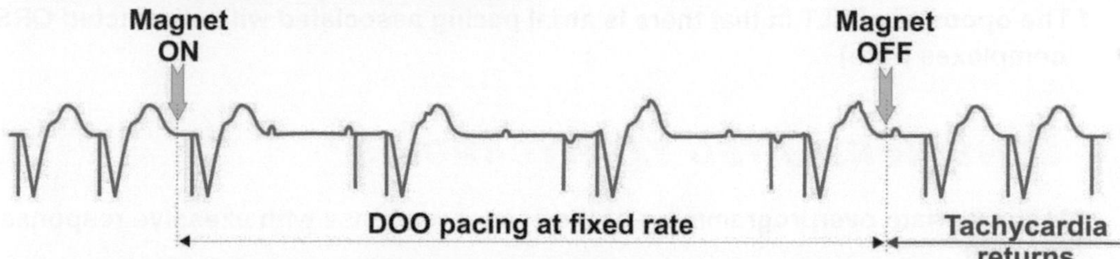

* Atrial electrogram and markers will also reveal a regular atrial rate
* Pacemaker Wenckebach upper rate response suggests a regular rate faster than the programmed upper rate. In this case it could also be an atrial tachycardia ! A Wenckebach upper rate response effectively rules out endless loop tachycardia.

2 ATRIAL FLUTTER & FIBRILLATION

* The paced ventricular rate is fast and may be regular or irregular
* Diagnosis is suggested when the ventricular pacing rate is fast and irregular and may be confirmed by recording the telemetered atrial electrogram

3 MYOPOTENTIAL TRIGGERING

* A pacemaker tachycardia can be triggered by myopotentials sensed by the atrial channel of pacemakers with unipolar sensing
* The tachycardia may be regular or irregular, with pacing cycles often at the upper rate interval. The tachycardia is mostly short-lived and pacing quickly returns to baseline
* Diagnosis : the tachycardia is reproducible by standard maneuvers to bring out myopotentials. A decrease in atrial sensitivity followed by a repeat of the maneuvers often shows elimination of the tachycardia.

A. F. Sinnaeve

Abbreviations : EMI = electromagnetic interference; DOO = asynchronous dual chamber pacemaker

DIFFERENTIAL DIAGNOSIS OF TACHYCARDIA DURING DDD(R) PACING - part 2

4 ENDLESS LOOP TACHYCARDIA

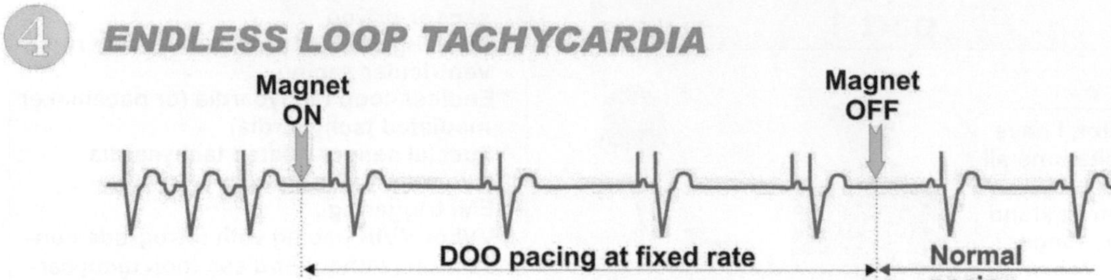

* The telemetered markers show a constant VA (Vs-As) interval
* Disappears upon application of the magnet and with programming a longer PVARP
* There are two types : near-field and far-field (rare)

5 ORTHODROMIC PACEMAKER TACHYCARDIA

* The opposite of ELT in that there is atrial pacing associated with conducted QRS complexes (rare)

6 SENSOR RELATED TACHYCARDIAS

* Inappropriate overprogramming of the sensor response with exessive response to effort
* Minute ventilation sensor in patients with CHF and in patients undergoing electro-cautery during a surgical intervention
* ECG monitors, etc. using the same high frequency low amplitude signals as the minute ventilation sensor of the pacemaker, may cause pacing at upper rate
* Excessive shivering or post-epileptic state of patients with activity sensors
* Firm pressure over an activity-driven pacemaker

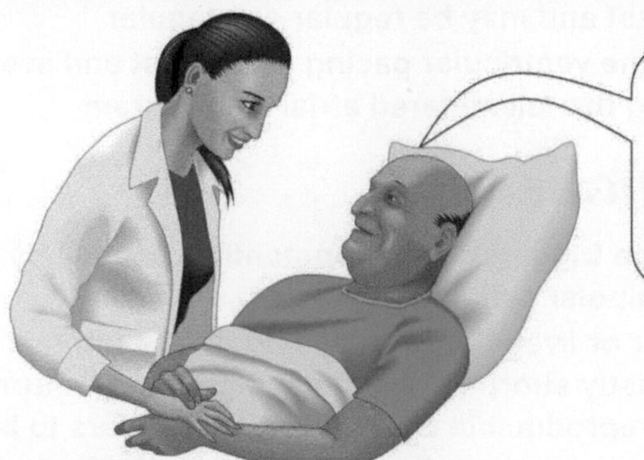

Nurse, I'm feeling palpitations when I turn over in bed and lie on my belly.
Can you ask my doctor if it may be related to the activity sensor of my pacemaker ???
A. F. Sinnaeve

Abbreviations : ELT = endless-loop tachycardia; CHF = congestive heart faillure; DOO = asynchronous dual chamber pacemaker.

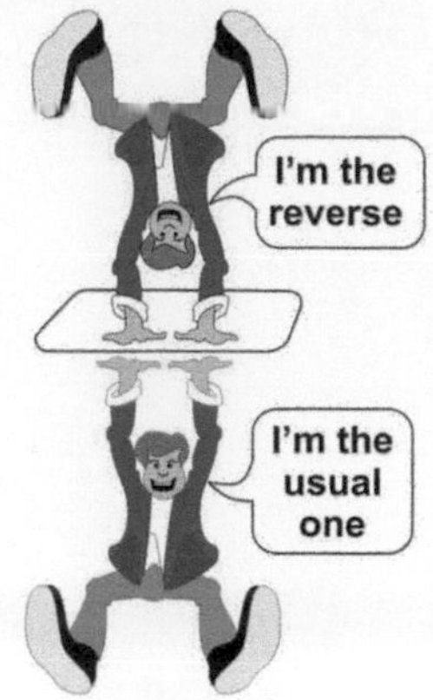

ORTHODROMIC MACRO-REENTRANT PACEMAKER TACHYCARDIA

Orthodromic pacemaker tachycardia has been called "reverse endless loop tachycardia". There is anterograde conduction across the AV junction and the QRS is conducted and not paced. This is the opposite of ELT where there is ventricular pacing. The return pathway is via the pacemaker by producing atrial pacing in contrast to ELT where there is atrial sensing !

Endless loop tachycardia or ELT

Orthodromic macro-reentrant pacemaker tachycardia

Near-field dual chamber

Far-field single chamber

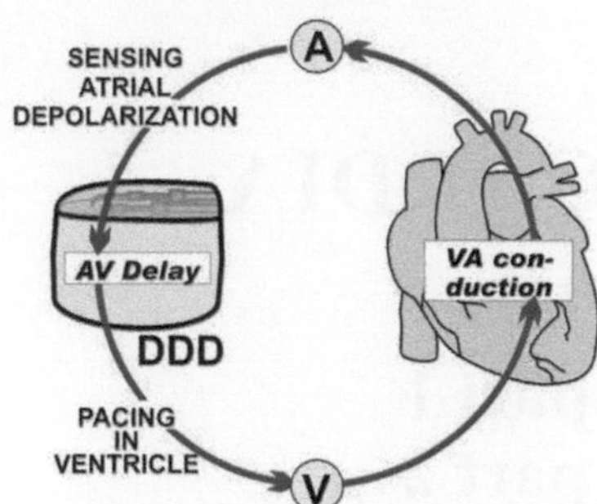

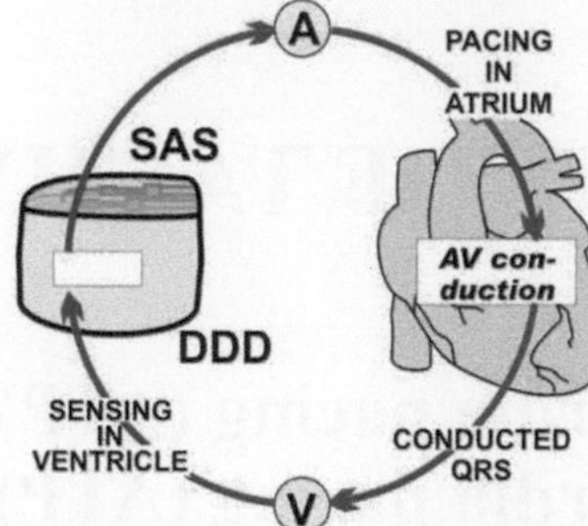

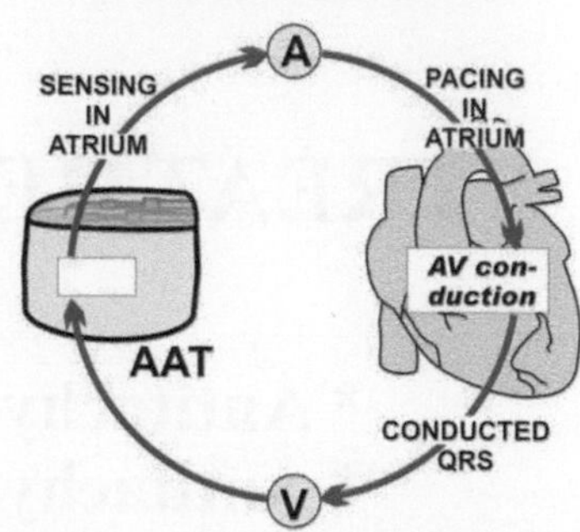

Dual chamber orthodromic PM tachycardia

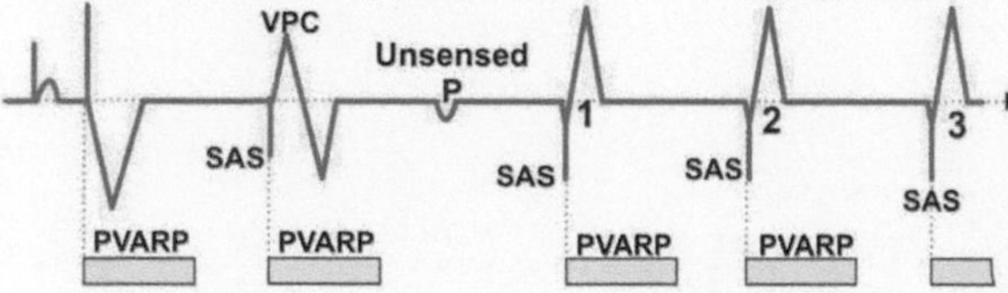

Mechanism of orthodromic pacemaker tachycardia during DDD pacing with synchronous atrial stimulation (SAS) algorithm to prevent ELT. SAS delivers an atrial stimulus on detection of a VPC. In this way, retrograde VA conduction engendered by a VPC cannot cause atrial depolarization because it is pre-empted by SAS that renders the atrium refractory. A VPC is sensed by the ventricular electrode, thereby triggering SAS. This is followed by an unsensed P wave outside the PVARP. The unsensed P wave is conducted and gives rise to the first conducted QRS complex that is sensed beyond the ventricular refractory period of the PM. The pulse generator interprets this conducted QRS complex as a VPC and delivers SAS. This again leads to a conducted QRS complex (2) with a very long PR interval. The second QRS complex causes SAS 2, and SAS 2 causes QRS 3, etc...

AAT single chamber orthodromic PM tachycardia

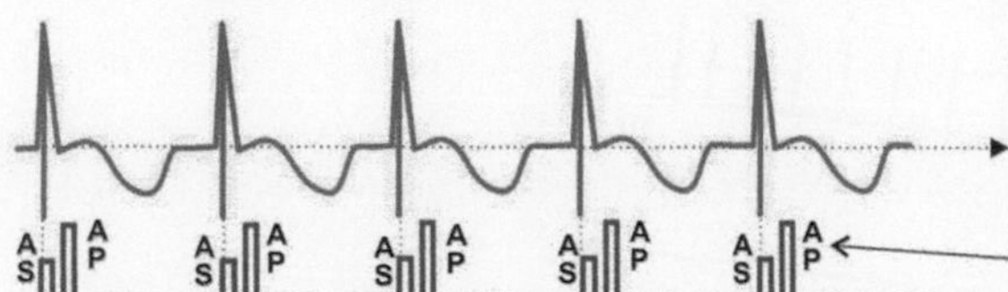

Far-field sensing of the R wave triggers an atrial stimulus which captures the atrium. The P wave is conducted to the ventricle. The conducted QRS is again sensed by the atrial lead as a far-field signal and the process perpetuates itself.

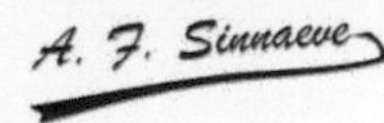

Abbreviations : AAT = an atrial stimulus is promptly delivered upon sensing in the atrium; ELT = endless-loop tachycardia; SAS = synchronous atrial stimulation; PVARP = postventricular atrial refractory period; VPC = ventricular premature coplex; AS = atrial sensed event; AP = atrial pacing; PM = pacemaker

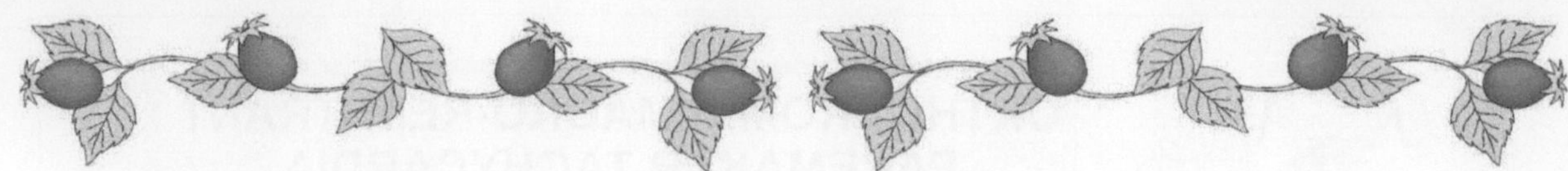

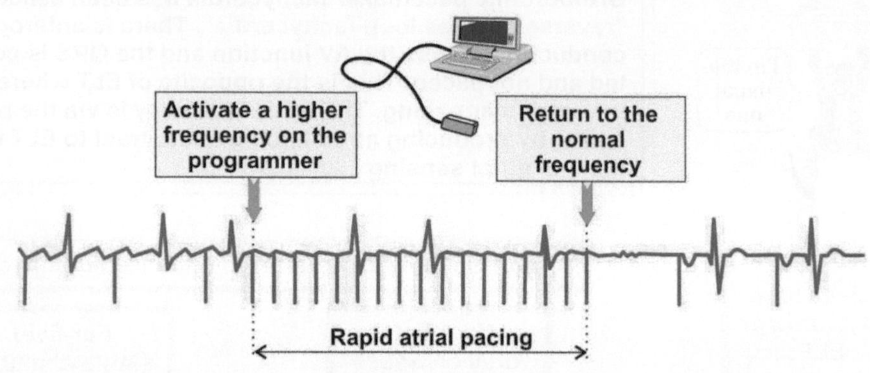

TREATMENT OF TACHYCARDIA

* Antitachycardia pacing (ATP) - part 1
* Antitachycardia pacing (ATP) - part 2
* Prevention of atrial fibrillation

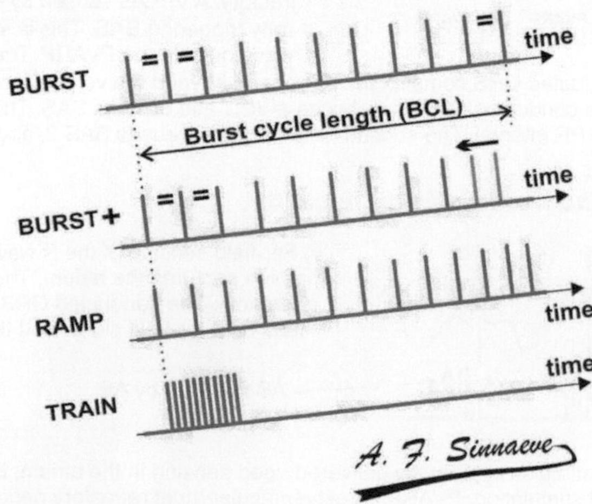

TREATMENT OF TACHYCARDIA WITH PACING PART 1

Manual procedure with the programmer : Overdrive pacing

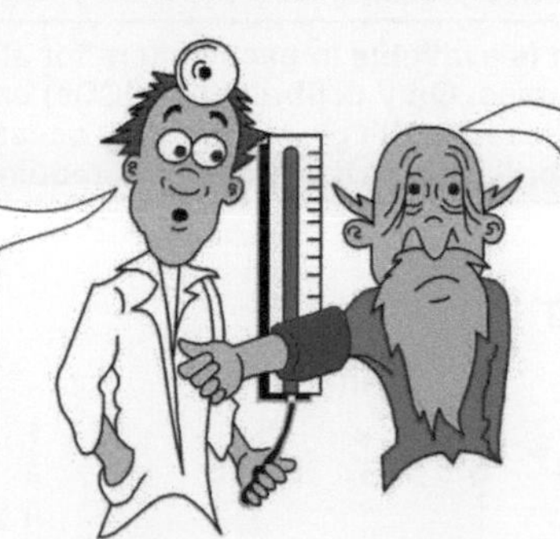
Overdrive pacing at a fast rate is easy to perform.
Put the head of the programmer over the pacemaker and temporarily program a pacing rate faster than the heart rate. Upon termination of the tachycardia, return to the normal pacing rate.
I don't trust those machines !
My physician has to do it himself !!!

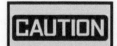

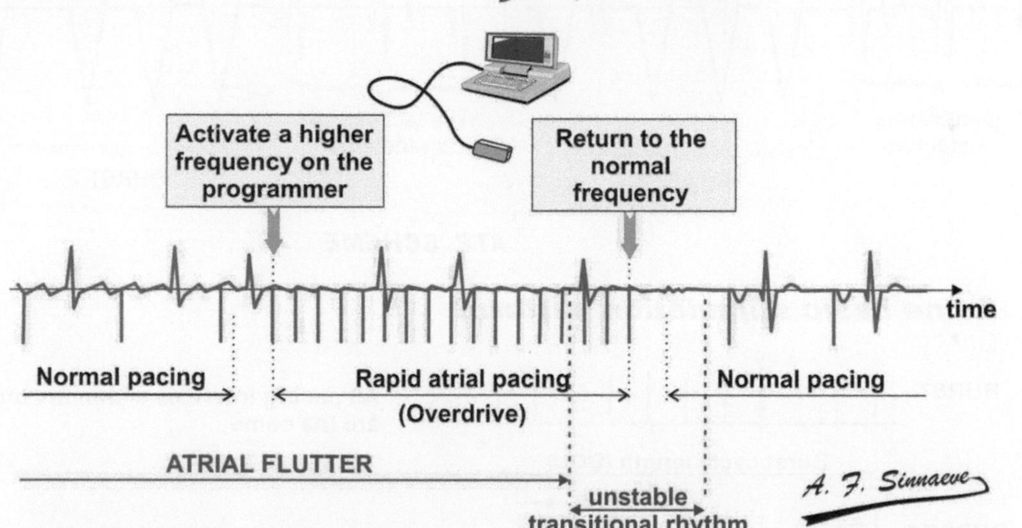

CAUTION

The procedure requires a standby defibrillator in the rare case of a complication

Rapid overdrive pacing is important for the treatment of reentrant supraventricular tachyarhythmias such as atrial flutter and other organized atrial tachycardias. It is ineffectual for atrial fibrillation.

TREATMENT OF TACHYCARDIA WITH PACING PART 2

Automatic : Antitachycardia Pacing (ATP)

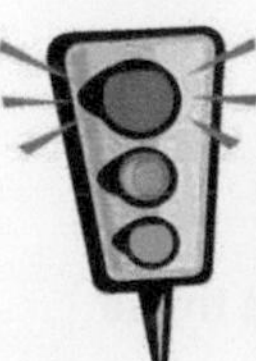

This function is available in pacemakers for atrial pacing in the treatment of supraventricular tachyarrhythmias. Only defibrillators (ICDs) can deliver rapid ventricular pacing for ventricular tachycardia because the procedure may occasionally accelerate the tachycardia or precipitate ventricular fibrillation, arrhythmias that require immediate defibrillation !!!

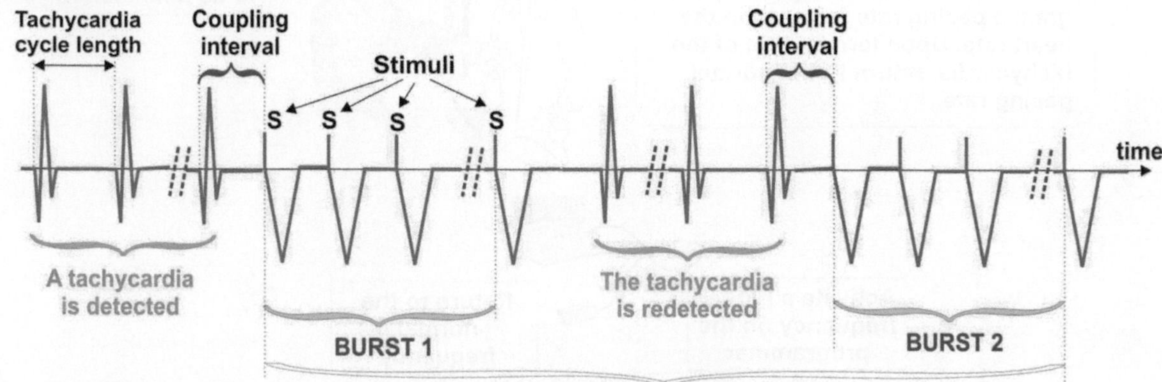

ATP SCHEME

Some basic stimulation patterns

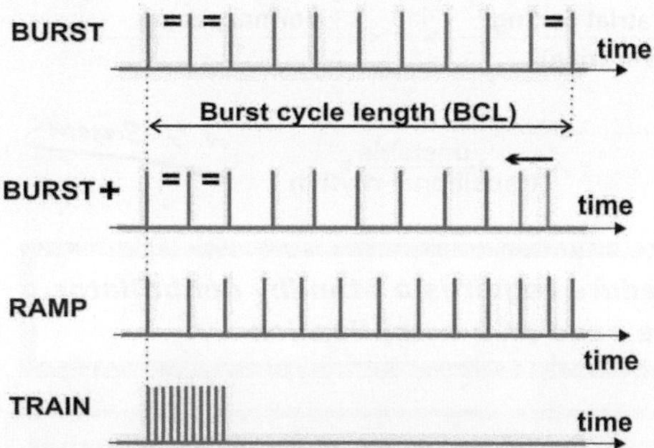

BURST: All pacing intervals within the burst are the same

BURST+: A burst followed by 2 stimuli with a decremental coupling interval

RAMP: The pacing intervals within the burst are continuously decreased (or increased in some pacemakers)

TRAIN: A high frequency burst pacing at 50Hz (3000bpm) during 0.5 - 3 seconds

WHAT CAN BE PROGRAMMED ?

* The number of bursts delivered
* The number of pulses within each burst
* The coupling interval as a % of the tachycardia cycle length
* The burst cycle length
* A minimum pacing interval

Many combinations are possible and different terminology is used by different manufacturers !

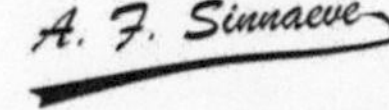

It is well-known that conventional dual chamber pacemakers can prevent atrial fibrillation in patients with underlying bradycardia in the sick sinus syndrome
OK, you are both right, but... These new algorithms from a variety of manufacturers are very complex, especially when more than one is used in a given patient....
Yes, but according to new developments, we can now consider new atrial sites and/or new pacing algorithms for the prevention of atrial fibrillation

THE PREVENTION OF ATRIAL FIBRILLATION

- **Continuous overdrive of sinus rate at a dynamic rate.** This ensures atrial pacing without an excessive increase in the rate.
- **Prevention of post-extrasystolic pauses.** This prevents short-long sequences.
- **Overdrive pacing at an increased rate after atrial premature beats.**
- **Overdrive pacing at an increased rate after the termination of atrial fibrillation.** This attempts to reduce the immediate reinitiation of the arrhythmia which is a common clinical problem.

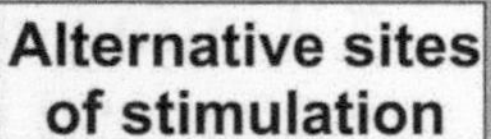

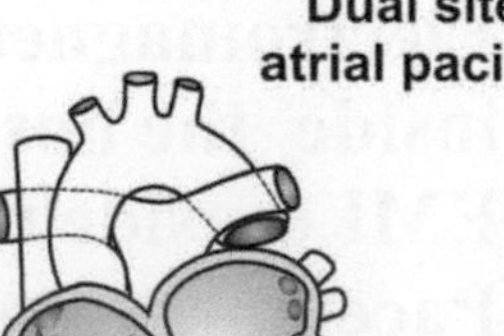

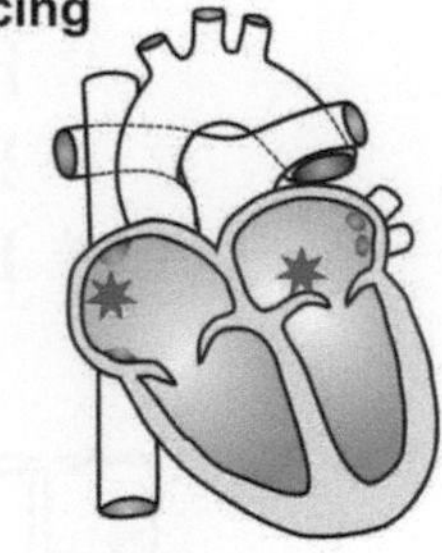

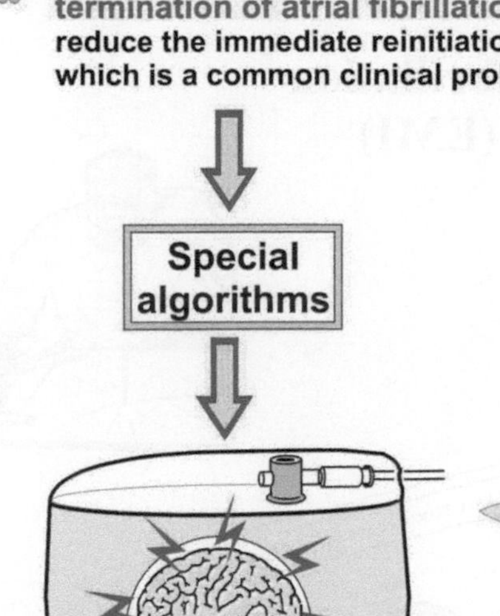

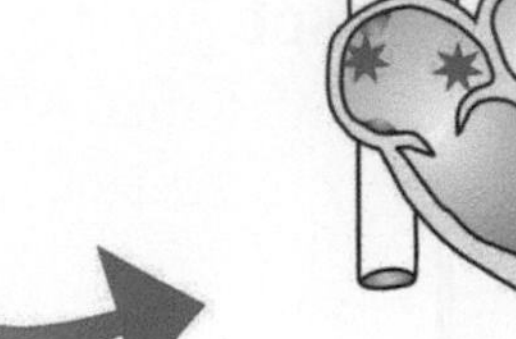

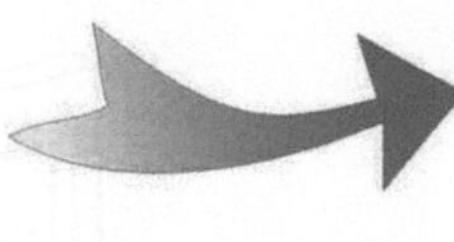

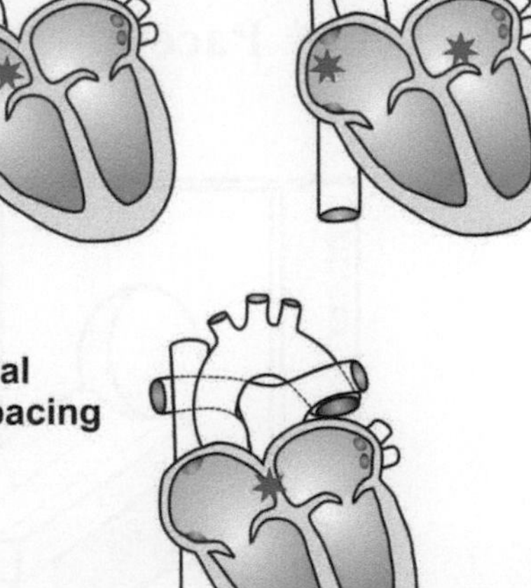

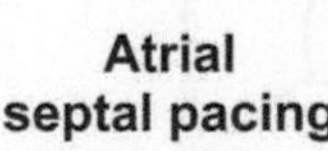

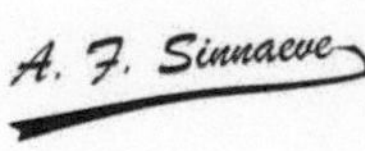

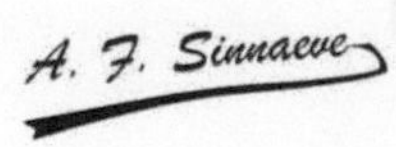

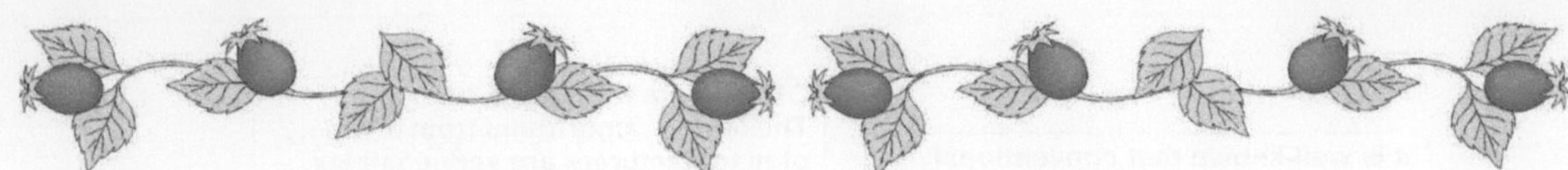

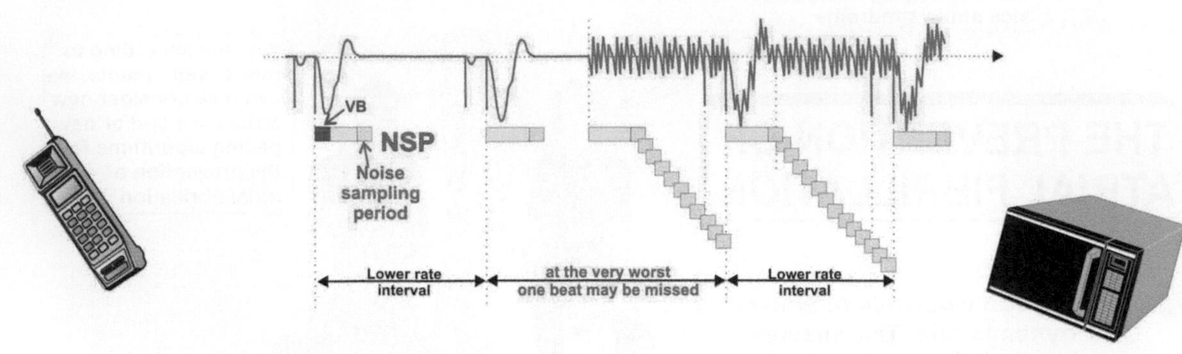

PACEMAKER INTERFERENCE

* Timing cycles - Noise sampling period
* General surgery
* External cardioversion & defibrillation
* Electromagnetic Interference (EMI) inside the hospital
* EMI outside the hospital
* Pacemaker reset

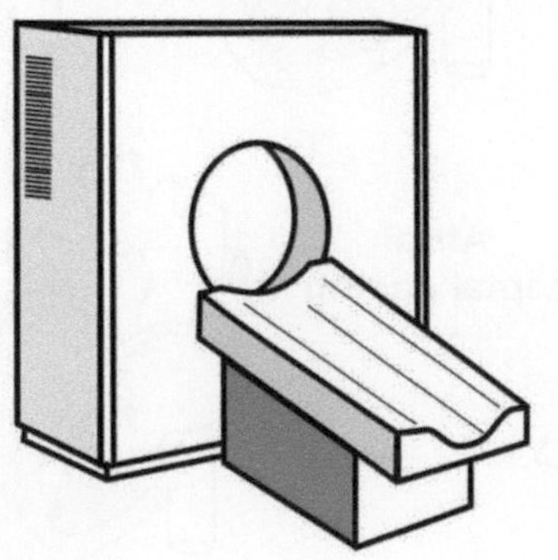

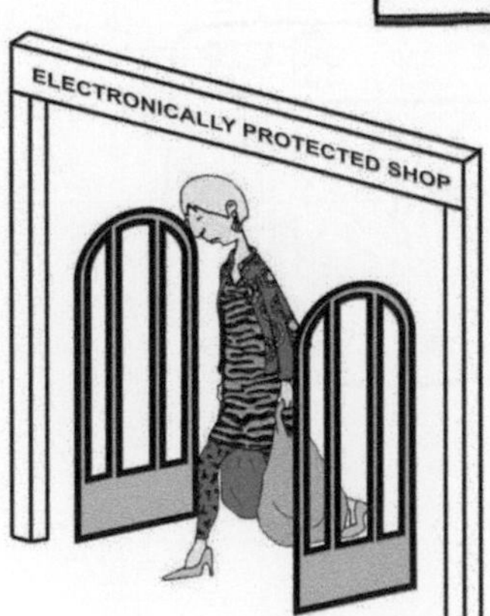

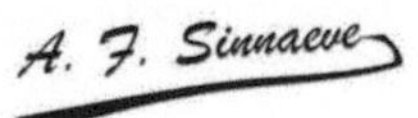

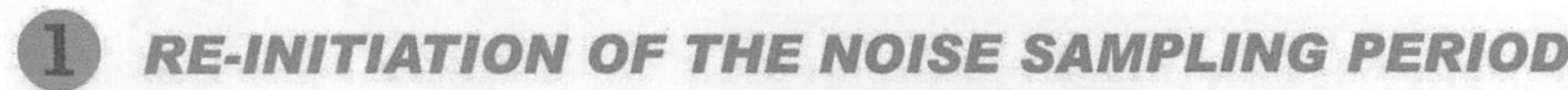

1 RE-INITIATION OF THE NOISE SAMPLING PERIOD

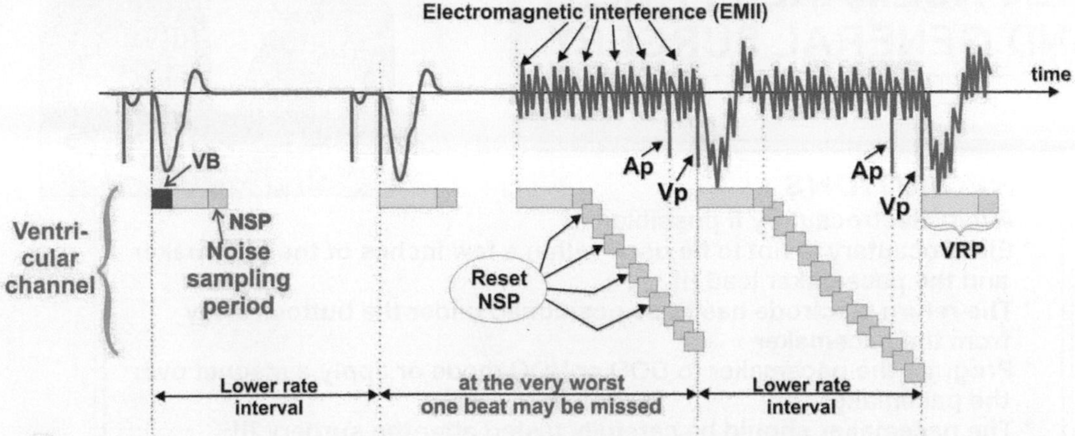

2 RE-INITIATION OF THE TOTAL REFRACTORY PERIOD

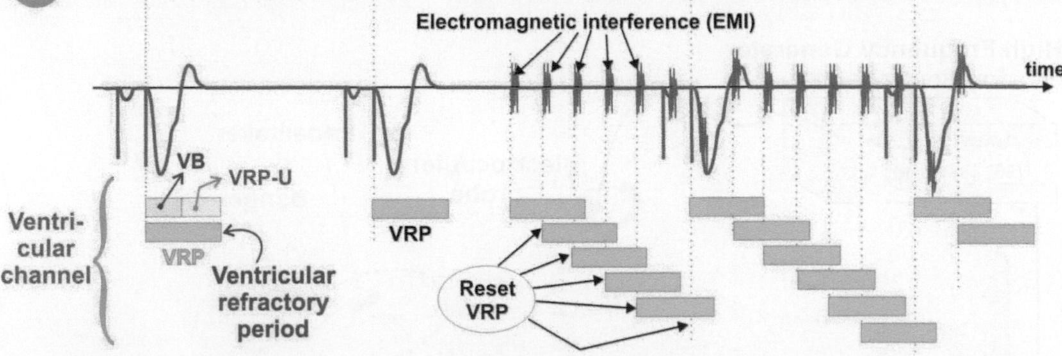

NOTE :
THE HAZARD OF PULSED ELECTROMAGNETIC INTERFERENCE WITH A LOW REPETITION FREQUENCY

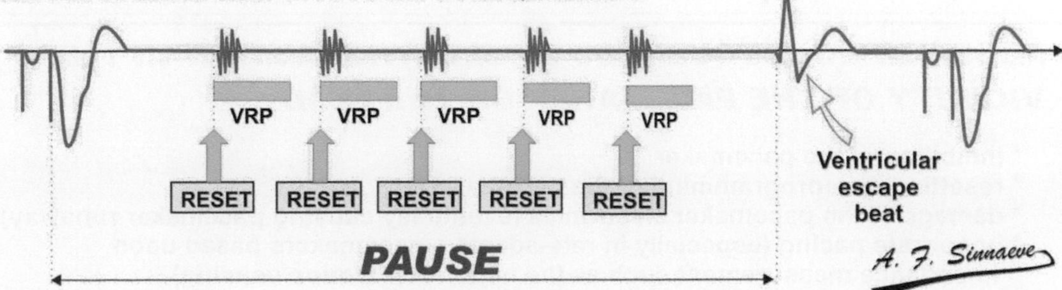

Abbreviations : VB = ventricular blanking period; VRP = ventricular refractory period; VRP-U= unblanked part of VRP; NSP = noise sampling period ; EMI = electromagnetic interference

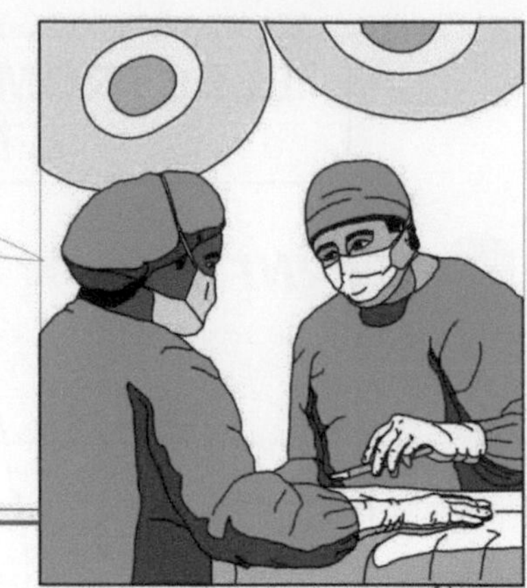

We have to take some extra precautions.
The guy has a pacemaker !
And don't cut in the insulation of the lead!!!

THE PACEMAKER PATIENT AND GENERAL SURGERY

PRECAUTIONS :

* Avoid electrocautery if possible
* Electrocautery is not to be used within a few inches of the pacemaker and the pacemaker lead !!!
* The return electrode has to be positioned under the buttock away from the pacemaker
* Program the pacemaker to DOO or VOO mode or apply a magnet over the pacemaker
* The pacemaker should be carefully tested after the surgery !!!

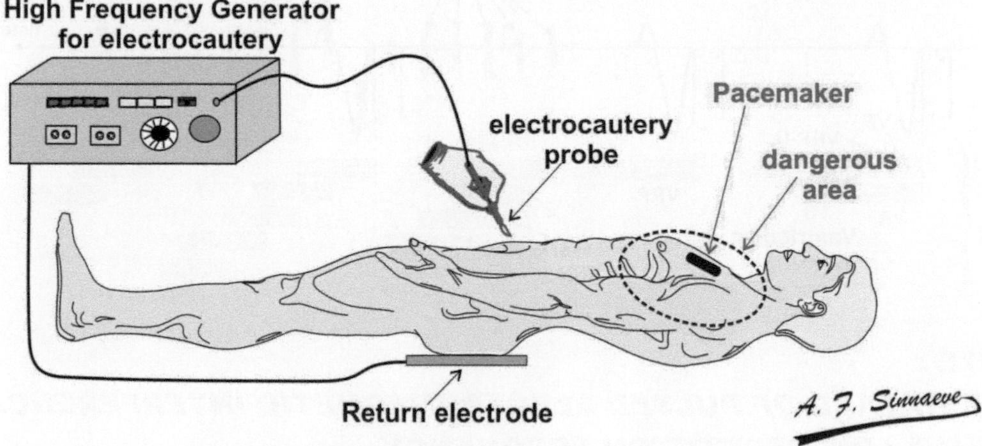

POSSIBLE CONSEQUENCES OF ELECTROCAUTERY IN THE VICINITY OF THE PACEMAKER OR THE LEAD :

* inhibition of the pacemaker
* resetting or reprogramming of the pacemaker
* damage of the pacemaker electronics (eventually causing pacemaker runaway)
* upper rate pacing (especially in rate-adaptive pacemakers based upon impedance measurement such as the minute ventilation sensing)
* current induced in the lead may cause internal burns and scarring, creating a higher pacing threshold or even exit block

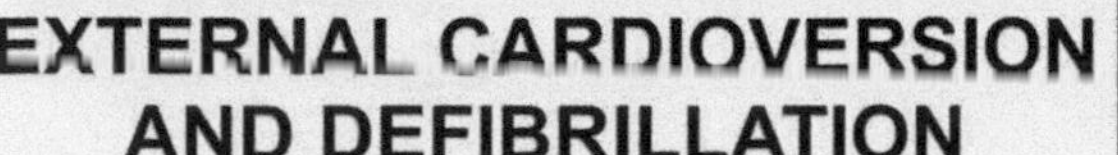

EXTERNAL CARDIOVERSION AND DEFIBRILLATION

Doctor, how should I position the paddles if my patient has a pacemaker ?

External transthoracic defibrillation can damage the pulse generator and the myocardium in contact with the lead. The degree of damage is related to the distance from the paddles to the pacemaker. The paddles should be placed as far as possible from the generator, at least 10 cm away. They should be positioned perpendicular to the axis of the pacemaker lead, in order to minimize the current induced in the lead during defibrillation.

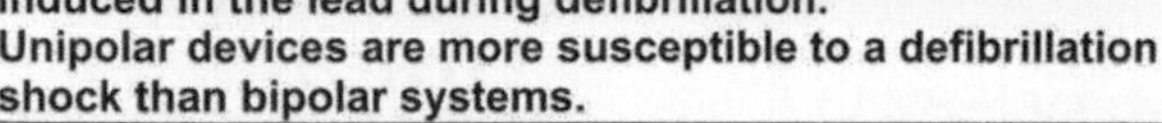

Unipolar devices are more susceptible to a defibrillation shock than bipolar systems.

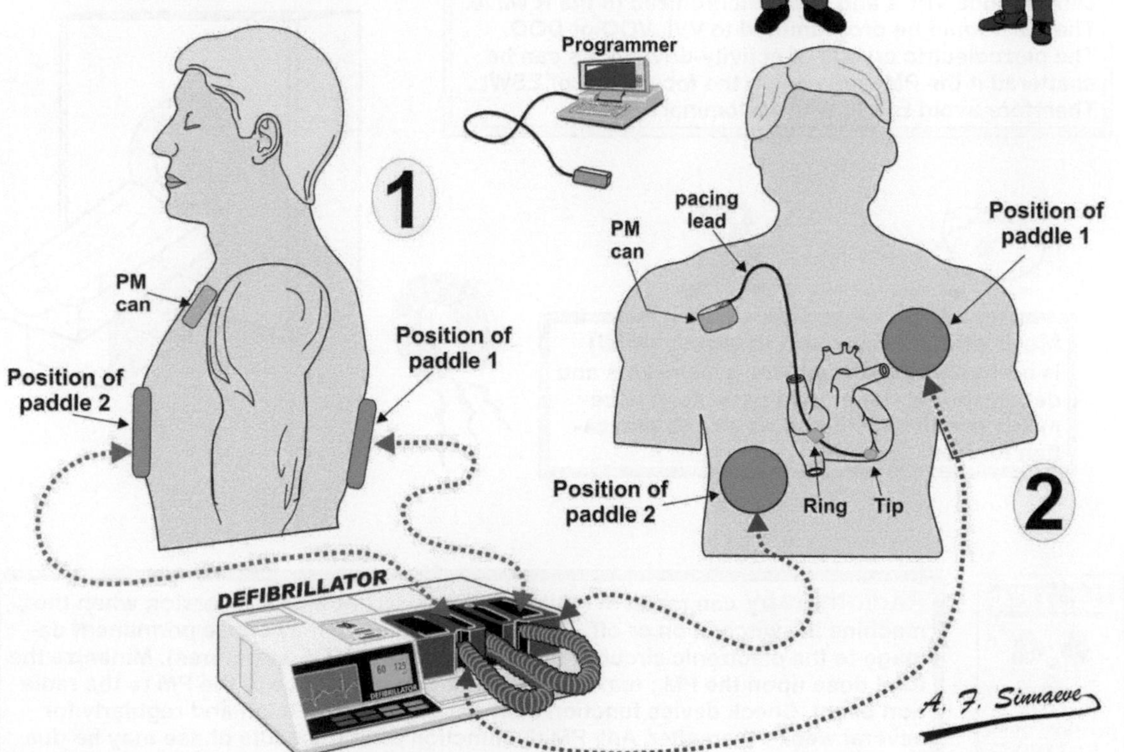

* IMPORTANT : After defibrillation, the device should be interrogated and the programmed parameters compared with those before defibrillation-cardioversion.
* Although all pacemakers have a defibrillation protection circuit, it can be overwhelmed by the extremely high energy of a defibrillation shock. Therefore, it is wise to have a transcutaneous pacemaker nearby.
* A transient rise in threshold can be treated by increasing the output (voltage and pulse duration) of the pacemaker. A prolonged severe increase in ventricular threshold is rare. Transient undersensing is not a serious problem.
* The defibrillation shock can also erase the programmed settings in the memory of the pulse generator. Contemporary devices have a built in protection called “Power On Reset” which automatically reprograms the pacemaker to a safe set of values (normally in VVI mode). The pacemaker is not damaged and can be reprogrammed from the reset mode to its usual parameters.

ELECTROMAGNETIC INTERFERENCE (EMI) INSIDE THE HOSPITAL

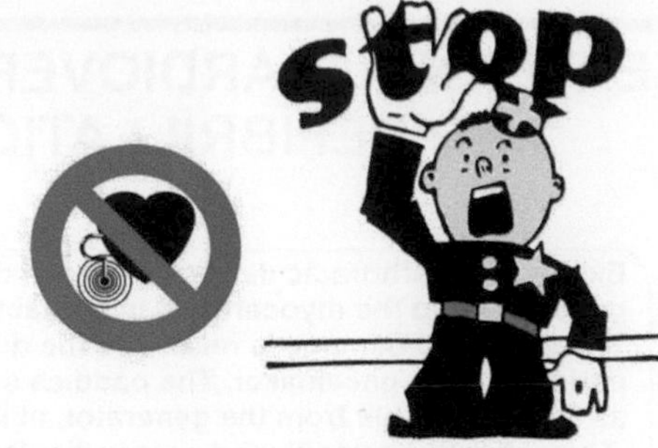

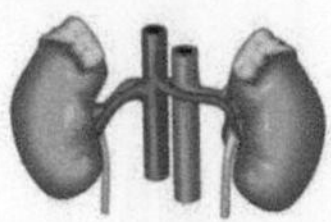

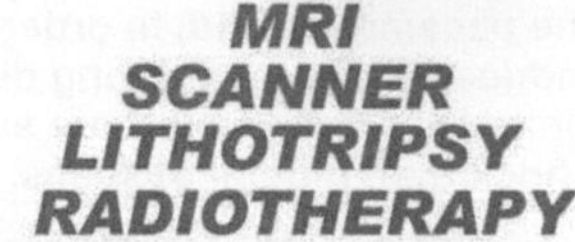

Extracorporeal Shock Wave Lithotripsy (ESWL) can produce VPCs and it is synchronized to the R wave. The PM should be programmed to VVI, VOO or DOO. The piezoelectric crystal of activity-driven PMs can be shattered if the PM is placed in the focal point of ESWL. Therefore avoid ESWL with abdominal PMs.

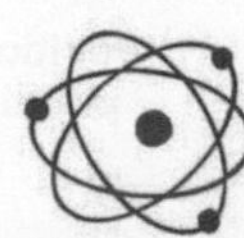

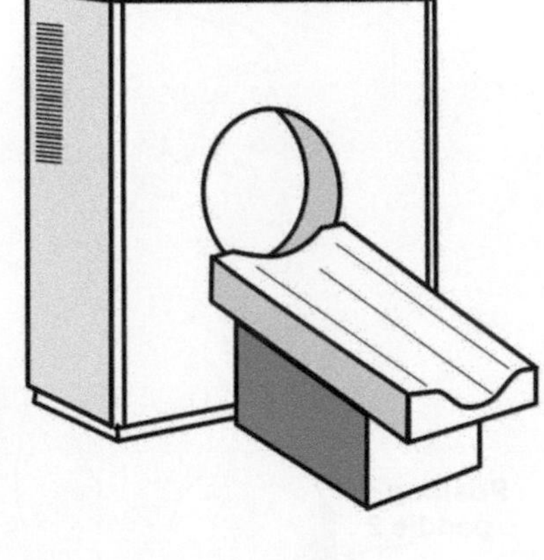

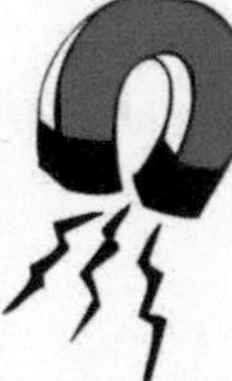

Magnetic Resonance Imaging (MRI) is normally catastrophic for pacemakers and deadly for PM-dependent patients. A pacemaker is still considered as a contraindication for MRI.

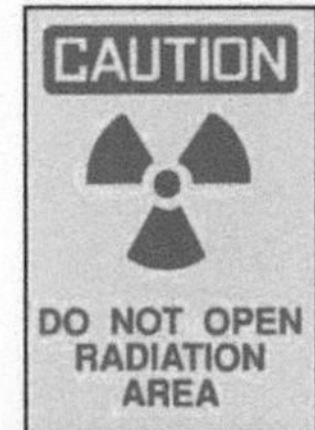

Radiotherapy can result in inhibition, tracking and noise reversion when the machine is switched on or off. The ionizing radiation may cause permanent damage to the electronic circuitry of the generator (CMOS structures). Minimize the total dose upon the PM ; maximize shielding and distance of the PM to the radiation beam. Check device function after each therapy session and regularly for several weeks thereafter. Any PM dysfunction after the acute phase may be due to a potentially serious component failure and requires device replacement.

A. F. Sinnaeve

ELECTROMAGNETIC INTERFERENCE (EMI) OUTSIDE THE HOSPITAL

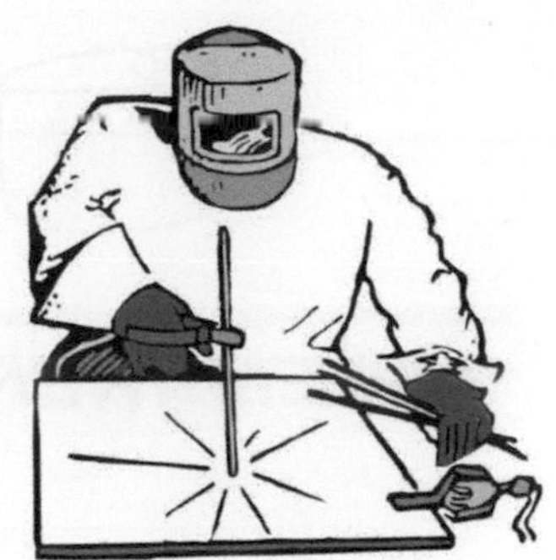

If a PM-dependent patient works in an industrial environment with strong EMI, on-site evaluation may be required. The device manufacturer should be contacted. Holter recordings and pacemaker diagnostics may suffice in non-pacemaker-dependent patients

ELECTRIC ARC WELDING

Most common EMI situations are essentially benign for pacemakers !

Cellular phones :
The highest risk of interference is when the phone is placed directly over the PM. Minimal interference occurs at the ear position and most interference is eliminated if the phone is kept 8 to 10cm (3 to 4 inches) from the device

Metal detector gates :
Asynchronous pacing or inhibition for 1-2 beats without any ill effects

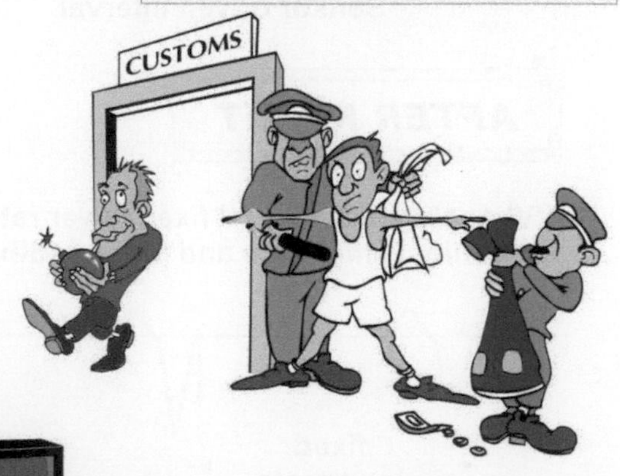

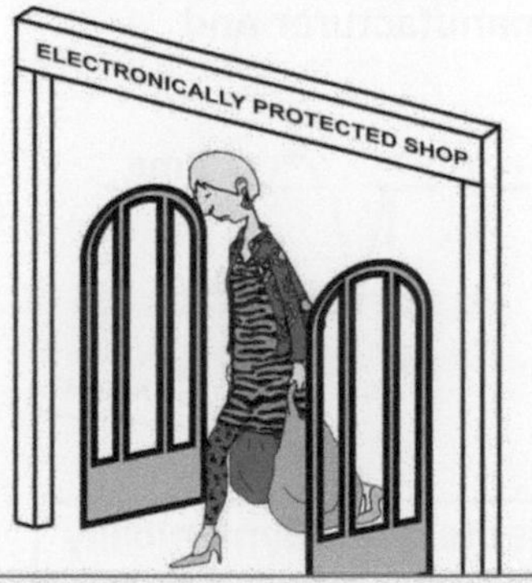

Electronic Article Surveillance
(antitheft) : Asynchronous pacing and inhibition for 1-2 beats without any ill effects in most situations. Possible pacemaker reset on rare occasions.

Appliances and Electronics at home
(microwave oven, TV remote control, etc.) have normally no effect on contemporary pacemakers

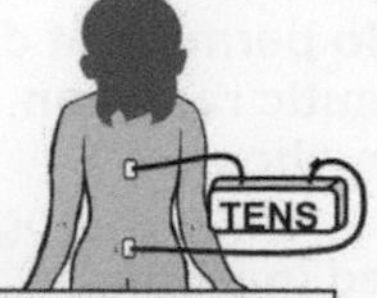

Transcutaneous electrical nerve stimulation may inhibit the pacemaker and require reprogramming of the sensitivity

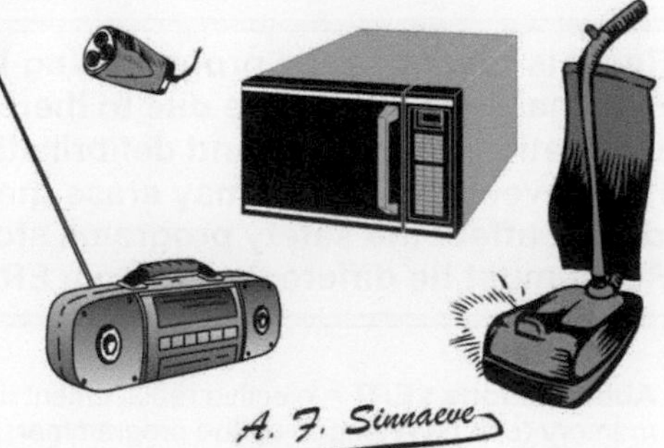

A. F. Sinnaeve

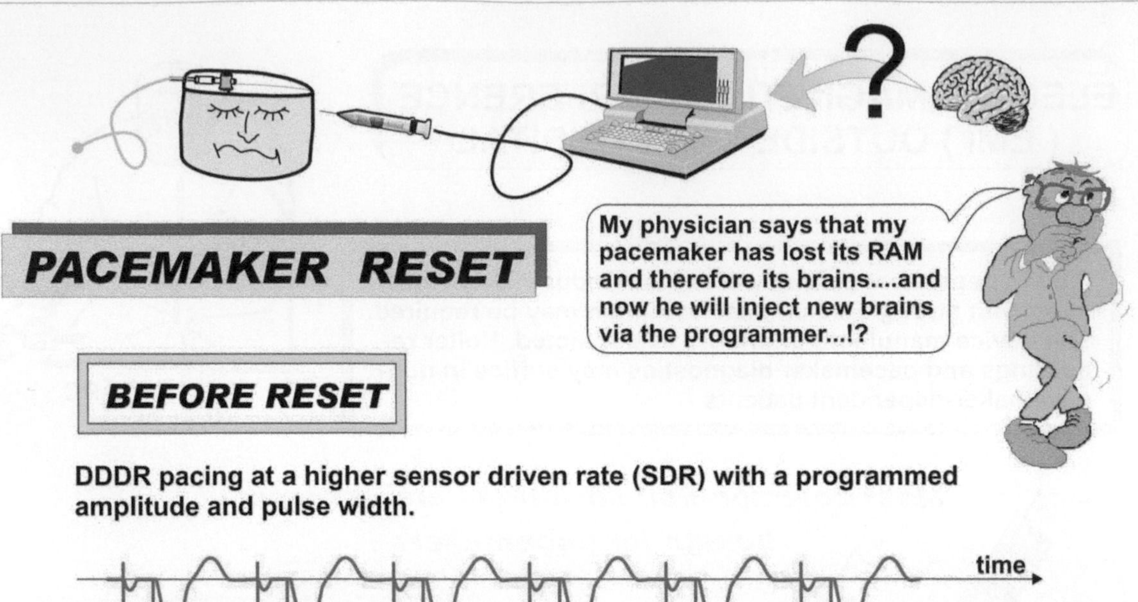

My physician says that my pacemaker has lost its RAM and therefore its brains....and now he will inject new brains via the programmer...!?

PACEMAKER RESET

BEFORE RESET

DDDR pacing at a higher sensor driven rate (SDR) with a programmed amplitude and pulse width.

AFTER RESET

VVI pacing at a special fixed lower rate defined by the manufacturer and at nominal amplitude and pulse width.

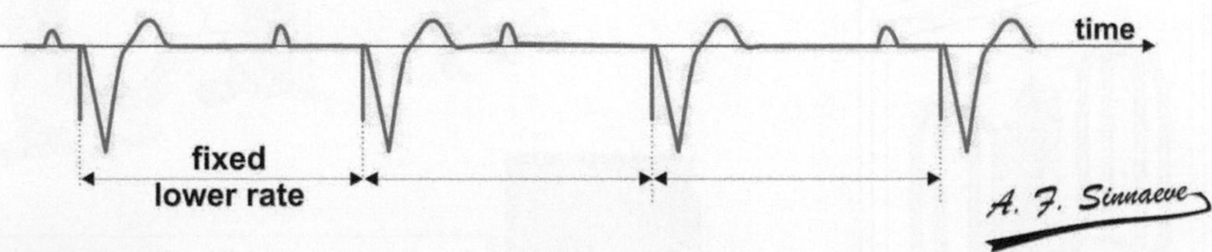

CAUTION Reset may be poorly tolerated in patients hemodynamically dependent on AV synchrony !!!

* Reset is reversible by programming ! No permanent damage is done to the pacemaker.
* Pacemaker reset may be due to therapeutic radiation, electrocautery, heavy electromagnetic interference and defibrillation shock.
* High level interference may erase the pacemaker programs that are stored in RAM, but do not affect the safety programs stored in ROM .
* Reset must be differentiated from ERT (check the battery voltage and impedance !)

Abbreviations : ERT = elective replacement time (just before battery depletion) ; RAM = random access memory (can be changed by the programmer) ; ROM = read only memory (a fixed content that can only be read by the microprocessor inside the pacemaker)

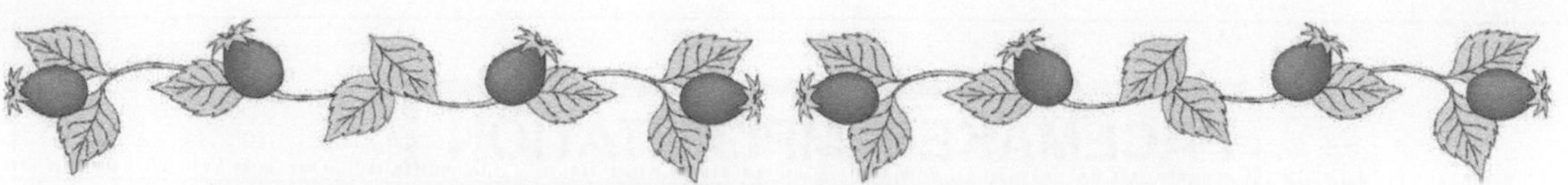

PACEMAKER FOLLOW-UP

* Pacemaker implantation
* Requirements for follow-up
* Central role of ventriculoatrial (VA) conduction
* Central role of postventricular atrial refractory period (PVARP)
* Transtelephonic follow-up
* General approach - parts 1 & 2
* Systematic follow-up - Various steps
* Automatic threshold determination - Initial steps
* Automatic threshold determination - End of active phase
* Follow-up of AAI pacemakers
* Application of the triggered mode
* End-of-life (EOL) and elective replacement indicator (ERI)
* The concept of telemetry - General
* Telemetered ventricular electrogram
* Example of real-time readout
* Telemetry - Interrogation
* Measurement of impedance by telemetry
* Telemetry - Memorized data
* Telemetry - Measured data
* Unidentified pacemaker
* Pacemaker as a Holter recorder
* Memory of a VVI pacemaker
* Pacemaker diagnostics
* The memory train
* Storage of pacing states
* Stored histograms
* P wave amplitude histogram
* Pacemaker diagnostics - sensing thresholds
* Heart rate & sensor indicated histogram
* Beware of stored data
* Arrhythmias & automatic mode switching - parts 1, 2 & 3
* Clinical application of stored atrial EGMs - parts 1 & 2
* The value of stored EGMs - Examples parts 1 & 2
* Automatic capture verification - parts 1 & 2
* Automatic capture verification with non-low polarization leads parts 1 & 2
* Medtronic Atrial Capture Management

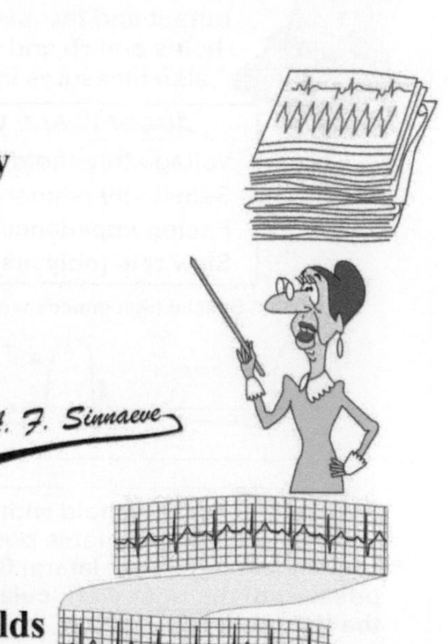

PACEMAKER IMPLANTATION

Have the patient's chart :

* Indication for pacemaker
* Medications
* Allergies
* Laboratory tests (INR, blood group, ...)
* Latest 12-lead ECG and chest X ray

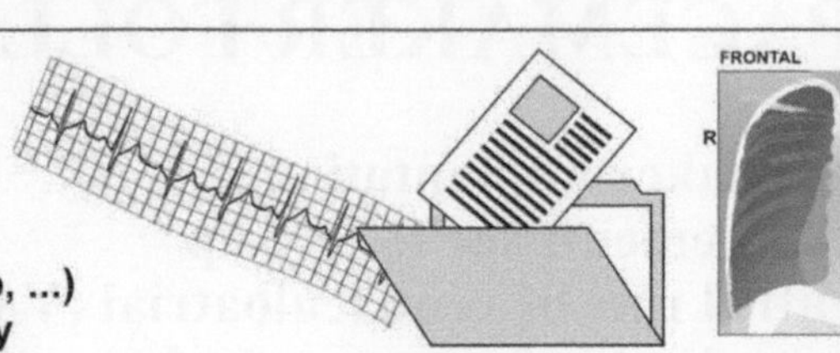

Make sure that the right pacemaker, leads, manual, and programmer are at your disposal

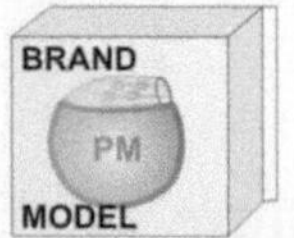

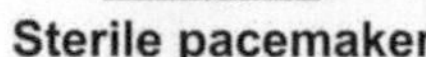
Sterile pacemaker

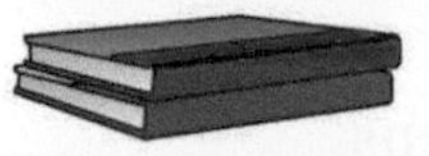
Technical manual provided by the pacemaker manufacturer

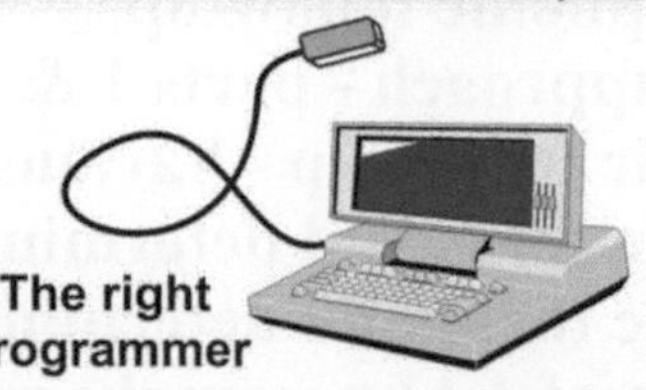
The right programmer

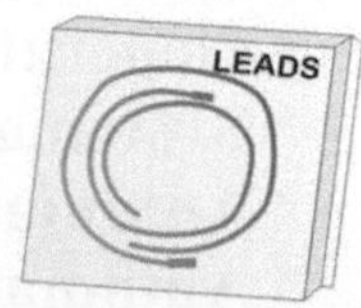

Sterile leads

Measure, verify and adjust

Use a PSA or Pacemaker System Analyzer permitting measurements of the output and the sensitivity of the pacemaker to be implanted and the thresholds and R- and P-wave characteristics of the implanted leads. The PSA also measures impedance

ACCEPTABLE VALUES AT IMPLANTATION	Atrial	Ventricular
Voltage threshold (at 0.5ms pulse width)	<1.5V	<0.5V
Sensitivity (signal amplitude)	>1.5mV	>5mV
Pacing impedance (at 5V and 0.5ms)°	<750Ω	<750Ω
Slew rate (only measured if the amplitude is small)	>0.5V/s	0.5V/s

° Special high impedance leads will register a higher impedance (consult manufacturers notes)

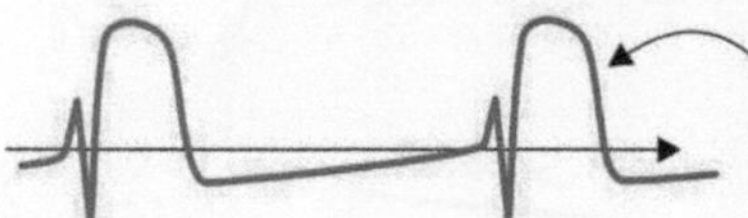

ST-segment shift due to current of injury indicates good endocardial contact of RV. This ensures a low pacing threshold.
(Unipolar electrogram from tip electrode)

* Try pacing near threshold with deep respiration and coughing and look for eventual unstable position of the leads
* Look at lateral or near lateral fluoroscopy to document the anterior position of the right ventricular lead and/or atrial lead if positioned in the right atrial appendage
* If there is sensing when the pacemaker is placed in the subcutaneous tissue, apply the magnet to make sure that both channels are capable of pacing
* Pace both A and V at 10V to rule out diaphragmatic stimulation
* Take a 12-lead ECG to make sure that the ventricular lead does not pace the left ventricle
* Look for retrograde VA conduction at the time of implantation or later before hospital discharge.

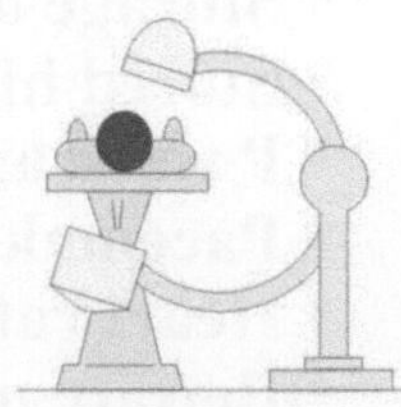

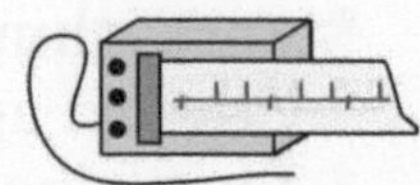

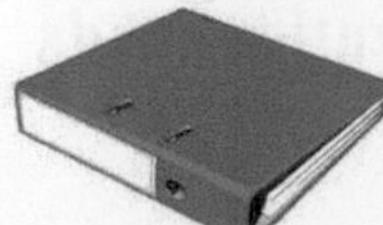

* Take a permanent chest x-ray soon after implantation for lead position and to rule out pneumothorax
* Interrogate the PM and reprogram if necessary; make a print-out for the patient's file
* Document all implantation data in the patient's chart

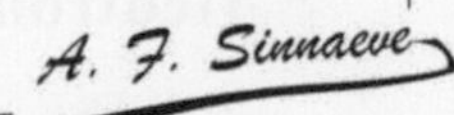

SYSTEMATIC PACEMAKER FOLLOW-UP

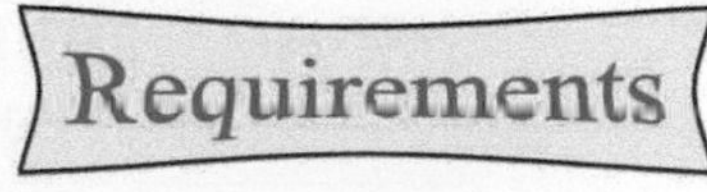

Requirements

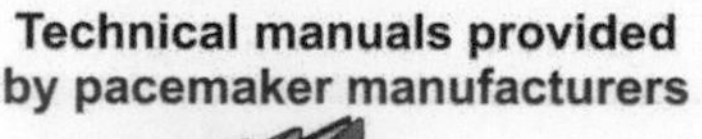

Technical manuals provided by pacemaker manufacturers

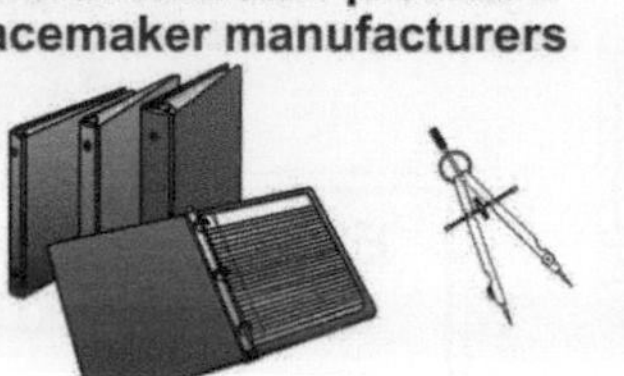

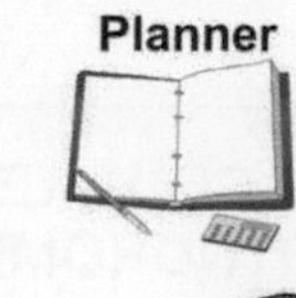

Planner

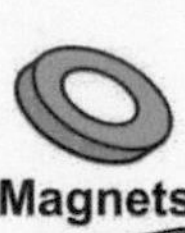

Magnets

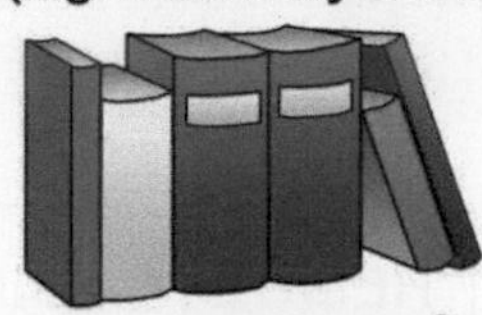

Official guidelines for pacemaker follow-up (e.g. Heart Rhythm Society)

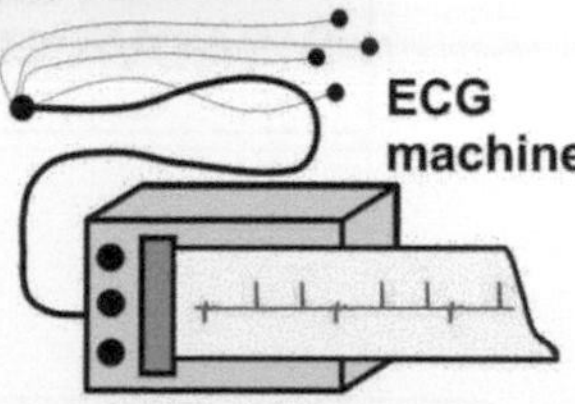

ECG machine

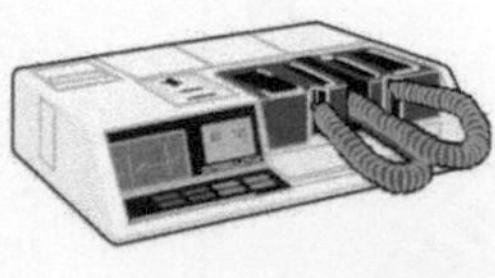

External defibrillator

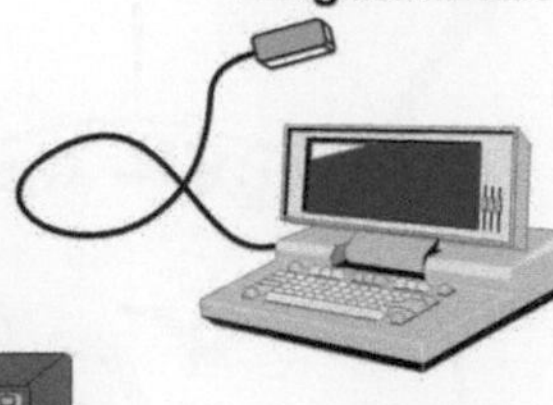

Programmers

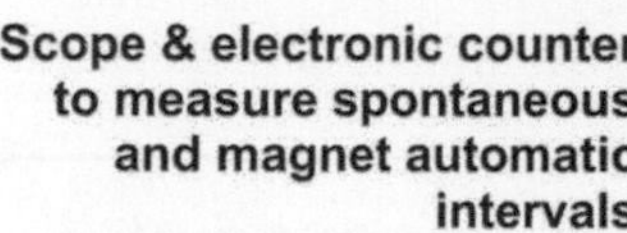

Scope & electronic counter to measure spontaneous and magnet automatic intervals

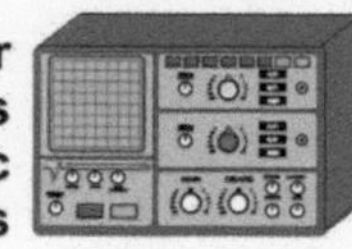

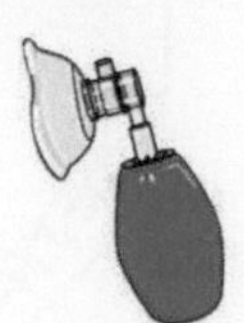

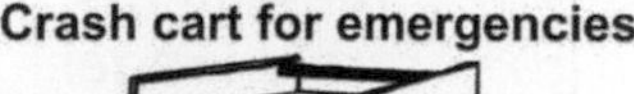

Crash cart for emergencies

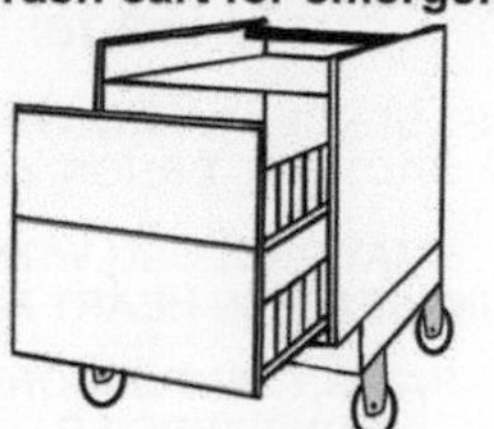

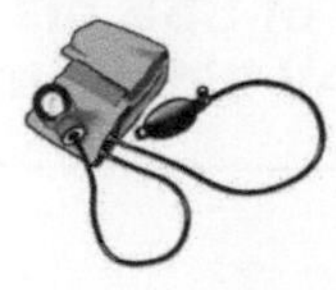

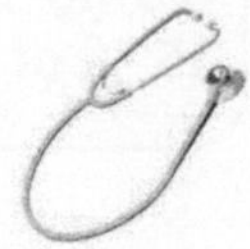

HISTORY & PHYSICAL EXAMINATION are part of pacemaker follow-up

Thou shalt take long rhythm strips and thou shalt be rewarded to the fullness of thy days !

12-LEAD ECG WITH AND WITHOUT MAGNET

1. Verify automatic interval with and without magnet application
2. Estimate degree of pacemaker dependence
3. Verify appropriate depolarization sequence, capture, sensing, fusion and pseudofusion beats

MARKERS & INTRACARDIAC ELECTROGRAMS

Make a simultaneous recording of ECG annotated markers and intracardiac electrograms

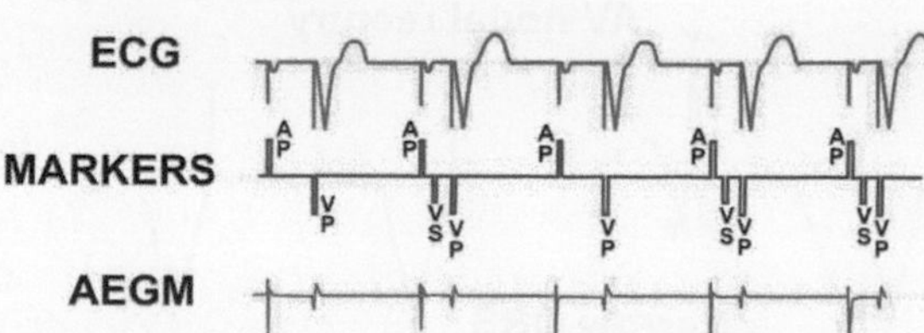

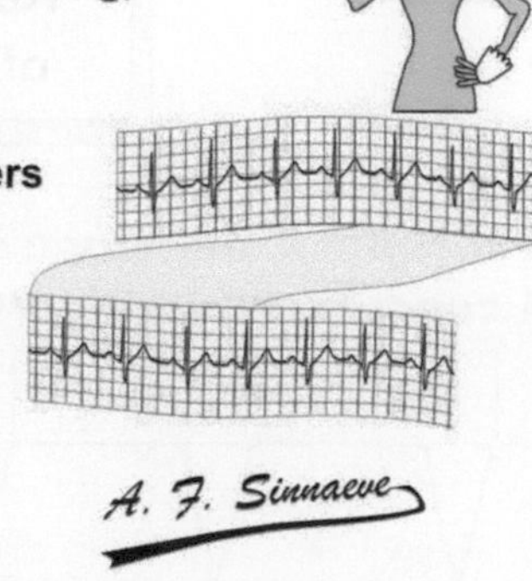

IMPACT OF RETROGRADE CONDUCTION IN CARDIAC PACING

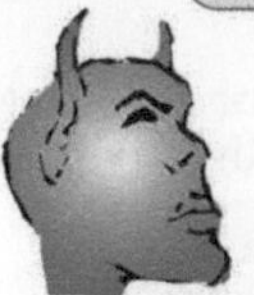

PACEMAKER SYNDROME

HEMODYNAMIC DISADVANTAGE

ENDLESS-LOOP TACHYCARDIA (ELT)

REPETITIVE NONREENTRANT VA SYNCHRONY (RNRVAS)

THE EVIL GENIUS

RETROGRADE P WAVES

VA CONDUCTION
100-400 ms
rarely longer

INFLUENCED BY AUTONOMIC FACTORS, DRUGS, etc.

MAY PROLONG WITH INCREASE IN HEART RATE

RARELY OCCURS ONLY ON EXERCISE

OCCURS IN :
70-80 % of SSS pts
35 % of AV block pts

MANIFESTATIONS OF SUSTAINED VA CONDUCTION

* Regular 1 : 1 VA conduction
* Regular or irregular 2 : 1, 3 : 1 VA conduction
* Regular Wenckebach phenomenon of VA conduction

A. F. Sinnaeve

Wenckebach sequence of retrograde VA conduction during VVI pacing

Abbreviations : AV = atrioventricular (anterograde or orthograde); VA = ventriculoatrial (retrograde); SSS = sick sinus syndrome; pts = patients

THE CENTRAL ROLE OF THE POSTVENTRICULAR ATRIAL REFRACTORY PERIOD (PVARP) IN DUAL CHAMBER PACING

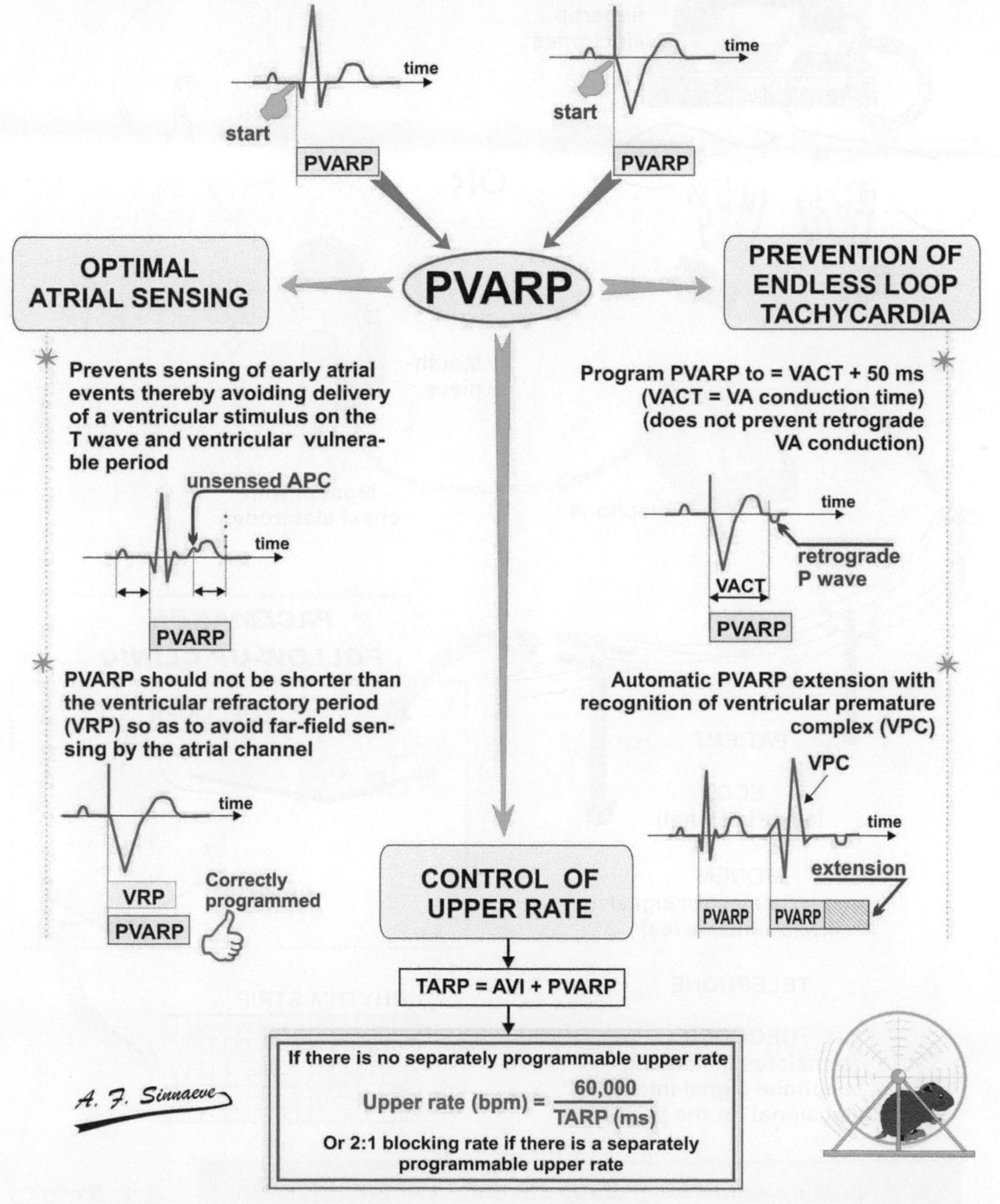

Abbreviations : VA = ventriculoatrial; APC = atrial premature complex; TARP = total atrial refractory period; VRP = ventricular refractory period .

TRANSTELEPHONIC FOLLOW-UP

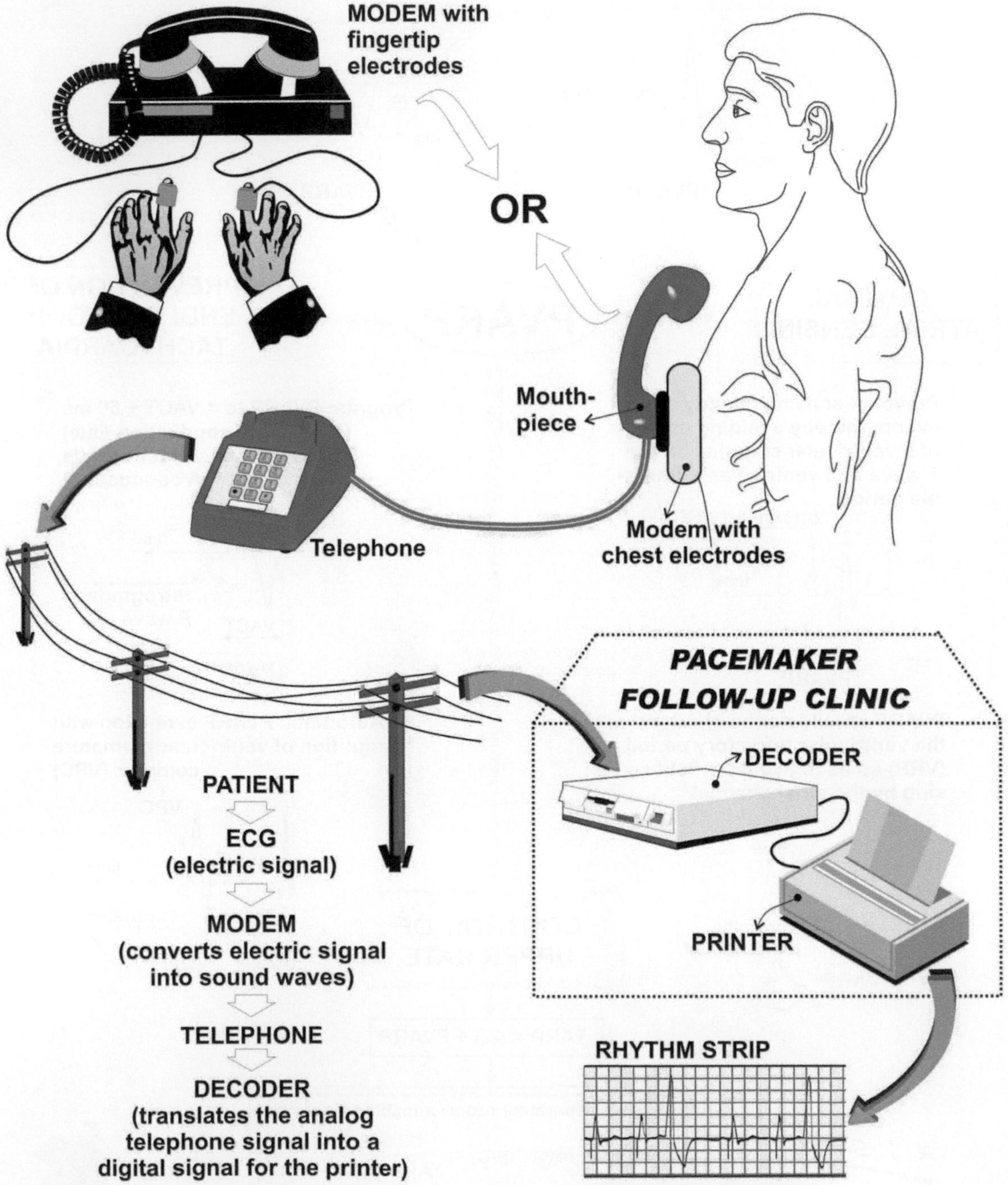

MODEM with
fingertip
electrodes
OR
Mouth-
piece
Telephone
Modem with
chest electrodes
PACEMAKER
FOLLOW-UP CLINIC
DECODER
PRINTER
PATIENT
ECG
(electric signal)
MODEM
(converts electric signal
into sound waves)
TELEPHONE
DECODER
(translates the analog
telephone signal into a
digital signal for the printer)
RHYTHM STRIP

This follow-up mode is virtually obsolete with the advent of pacemaker follow-up via the Internet.

A. F. Sinnaeve

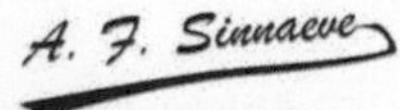

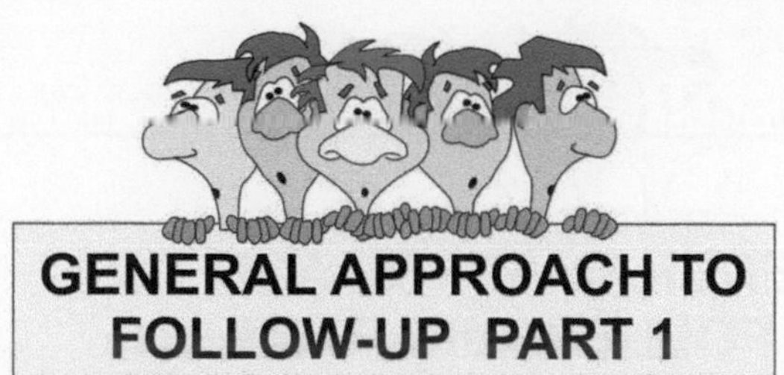

GENERAL APPROACH TO FOLLOW-UP PART 1

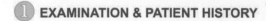

① EXAMINATION & PATIENT HISTORY

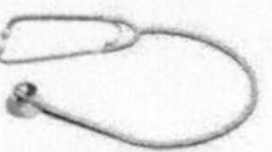

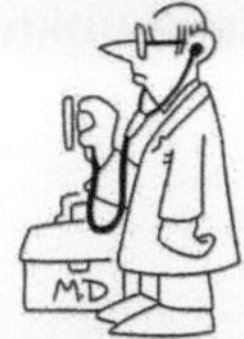

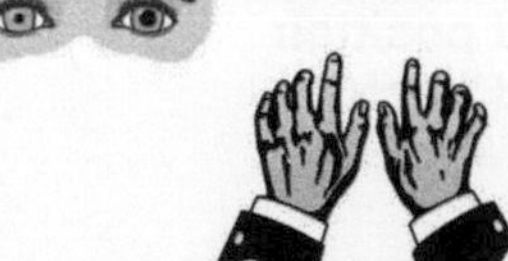

A clinical approach is very important !!!

② BLOOD PRESSURE

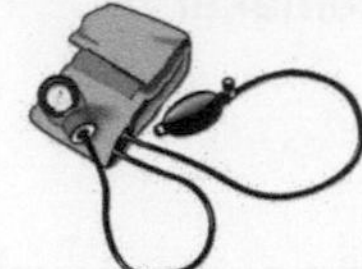

The pacemaker syndrome causes a fall in blood pressure during pacing !!!

③ APPLICATION OF THE MAGNET

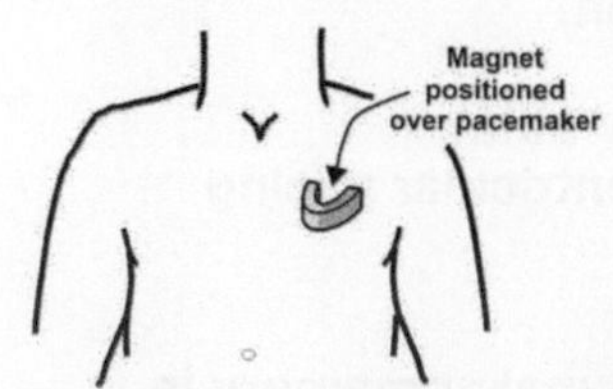

1. **Asynchronous pacing at the magnet rate. The rate and mode (DOO or VOO for dual chamber pacemakers) are device specific.**
2. **AV interval usually shortens**
3. **The magnet rate (which may differ from the programmed rate according to design) reflects the status of the battery and indicates an intensified follow-up period, ERT and EOL**
4. **Some devices allow the magnet response to be programmed on or off**

④ VERIFY THE ECG THOROUGHLY

Never ignore the diagnostic value of the 12-lead ECG !!!
See if myopotentials or lead problems can be demonstrated.

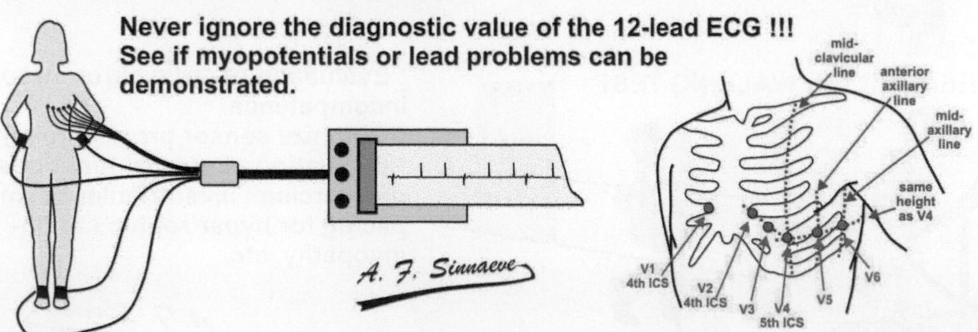

Abbreviations : DOO= Dual chamber AV sequential asynchronous mode; VOO = Ventricular asynchronous pacing mode; ECG = Electrocardiogram; EOL = End-of -Life; ERT = Elective Replacement Time; ICS = intercostal space

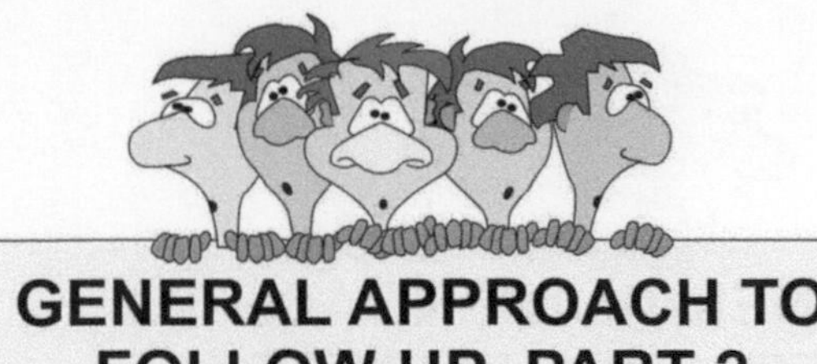

GENERAL APPROACH TO FOLLOW-UP PART 2

5 EXAMINE THE CHEST X- RAY

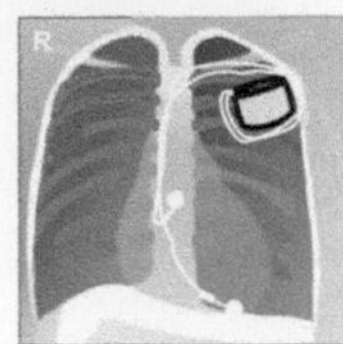

1. Identification of manufacturer and model if unknown
2. Check for lead position
3. Check for lead fracture
4. Check for LV failure

6 USE THE PROGRAMMER

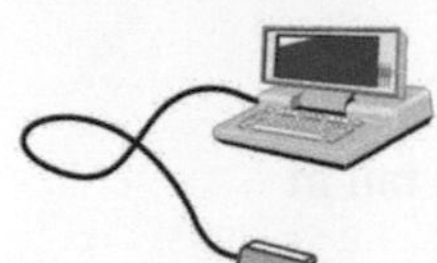

Match the programmer with the pacemaker !!!

7 ECHOCARDIOGRAPHY

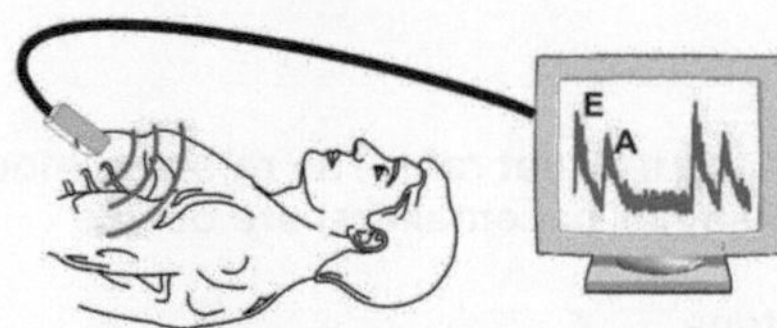

1. Anatomic
   a. Diagnosis of unusual lead position such as LV site best documented by TEE
   b. Ventricular lead perforation (with possible pericardial effusion)
2. Hemodynamic
   a. Optimization of AV delay
   b. Evaluation of biventricular pacing

8 HOLTER MONITORING

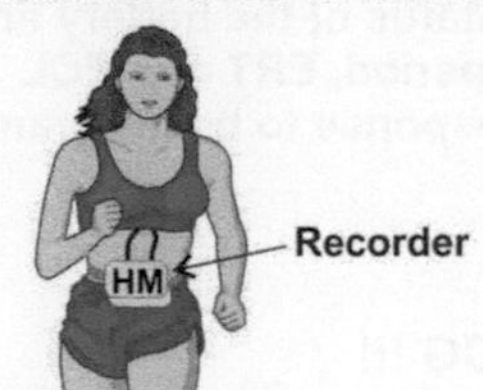

To complement data in pacemaker memory in patients who remain symptomatic

9 TREADMILL or WALKING TEST

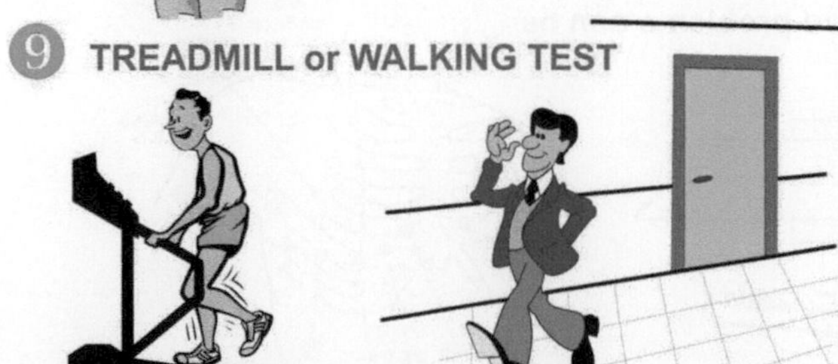

* Evaluation of atrial chronotropic incompetence
* Optimize sensor programming
* Evaluation of special functions on exercise : biventricular pacing, pacing for hypertrophic cardio-myopathy, etc.

A. F. Sinnaeve

Abbreviations : AV = atrioventricular; LV = left ventricular; TEE = transesophageal echocardiography

SYSTEMATIC PACEMAKER FOLLOW-UP

Make sure that the programming head is positioned carefully over the pacemaker

PACEMAKER INTERROGATION

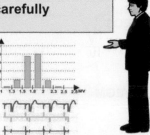

1. Verify the administrative data
2. Check on the programmed data
3. Examine the measured or real-time data { Output ? Battery ? Leads ?
4. Inspect the memorized data

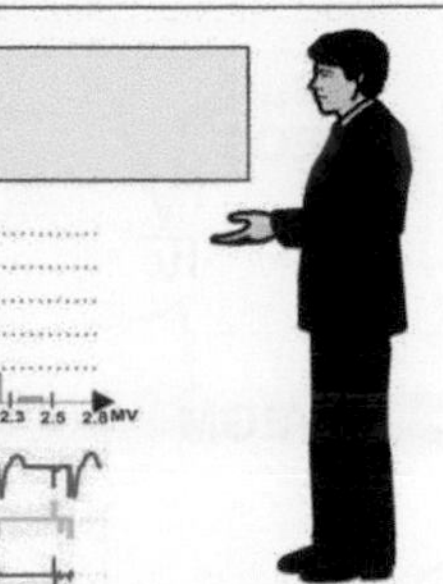

A higher sensitivity means a lower number in mV !

DETERMINATION OF SENSING THRESHOLDS

1. Automated and/or manual determination of sensing thresholds is needed if patient has periods of spontaneous rhythm
2. Reprogram sensitivity as necessary

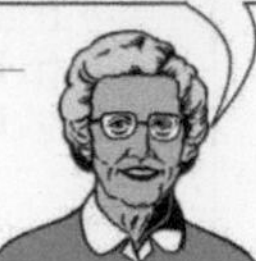
Will my pacemaker still work on demand?

Make sure that the safety margin is adequate !

DETERMINATION OF PACING THRESHOLDS

1. Automated and/or manual determination of pacing thresholds
2. Reprogram voltage and/or pulse duration as necessary

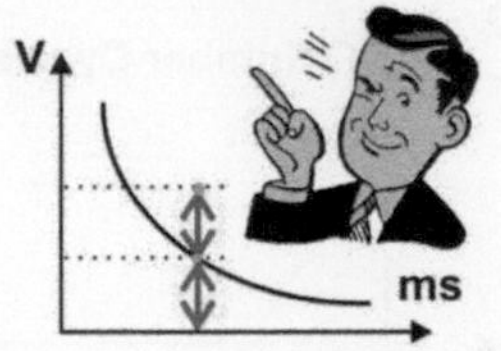
V
ms

CHECK THE SPECIFIC FUNCTIONS

1. Check for crosstalk
2. Evaluate retrograde VA conduction and propensity to endless loop tachycardia
3. Look for eventual myopotential interference interference in unipolar PMs
4. Examine rate-adaptive function, sleep rate, hysteresis, automatic mode switching, histogram settings, etc.

IF NECESSARY ORDER SPECIAL TESTS : Chest X ray, Holter, etc.

PREPARE YOUR REPORT

Meticulous record-keeping is necessary

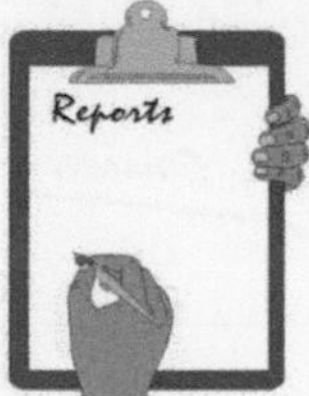
Reports

1. Clear the appropriate memorized data
2. Make the final print-outs
3. Compare final parameters with those at presentation
4. Give the patient a copy of the print-out

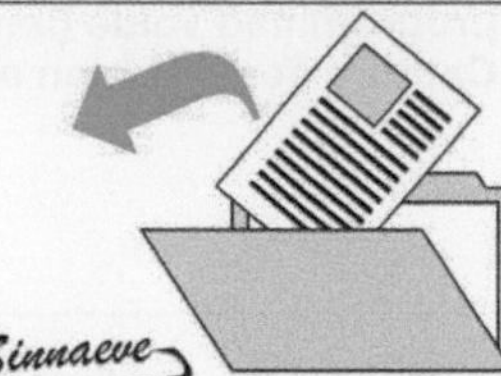

A. F. Sinnaeve

AUTOMATIC DETERMINATION OF THRESHOLD INITIAL STEPS

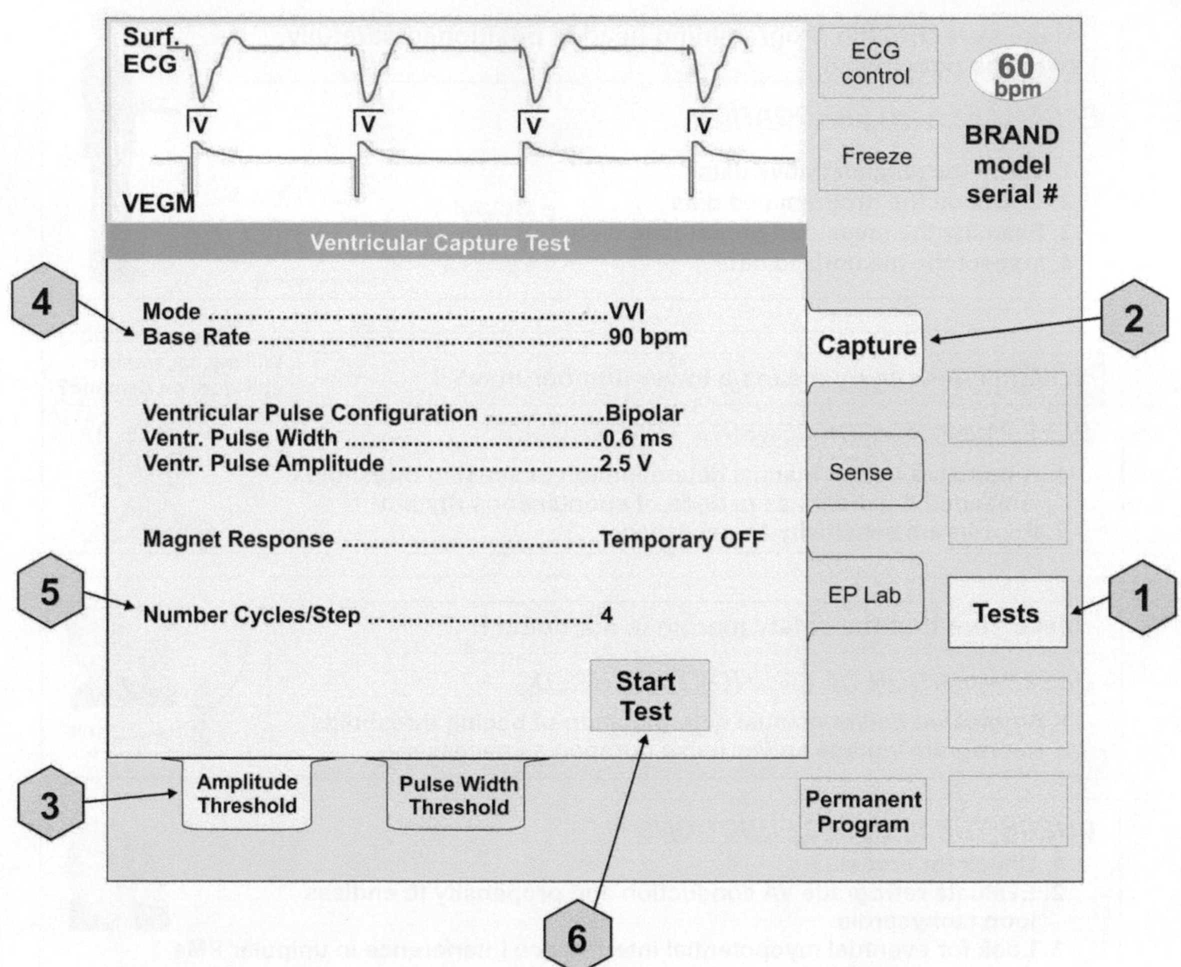

* Initial Step 4 : The actual "Base Rate" (60) indicated in red in the upper right corner is programmed to a higher temporary value (90) above the patient's intrinsic rate to ensure pacing

*Initial Step 6 : When {Start Test} is touched, a "Test in Progress" message will appear with two option buttons {End Test} and {Stop Test}. The {Stop Test} is the emergency button, immediately restoring the settings to the previously programmed values

* When capture is lost, touching {End Test} terminates the test and restores the previously programmed value (amplitude or pulse width). The system then displays the "Confirm Capture Test" screen and stores the test in the memory of the programmer.

A. F. Sinnaeve

AUTOMATIC DETERMINATION OF THRESHOLD
END OF ACTIVE PHASE

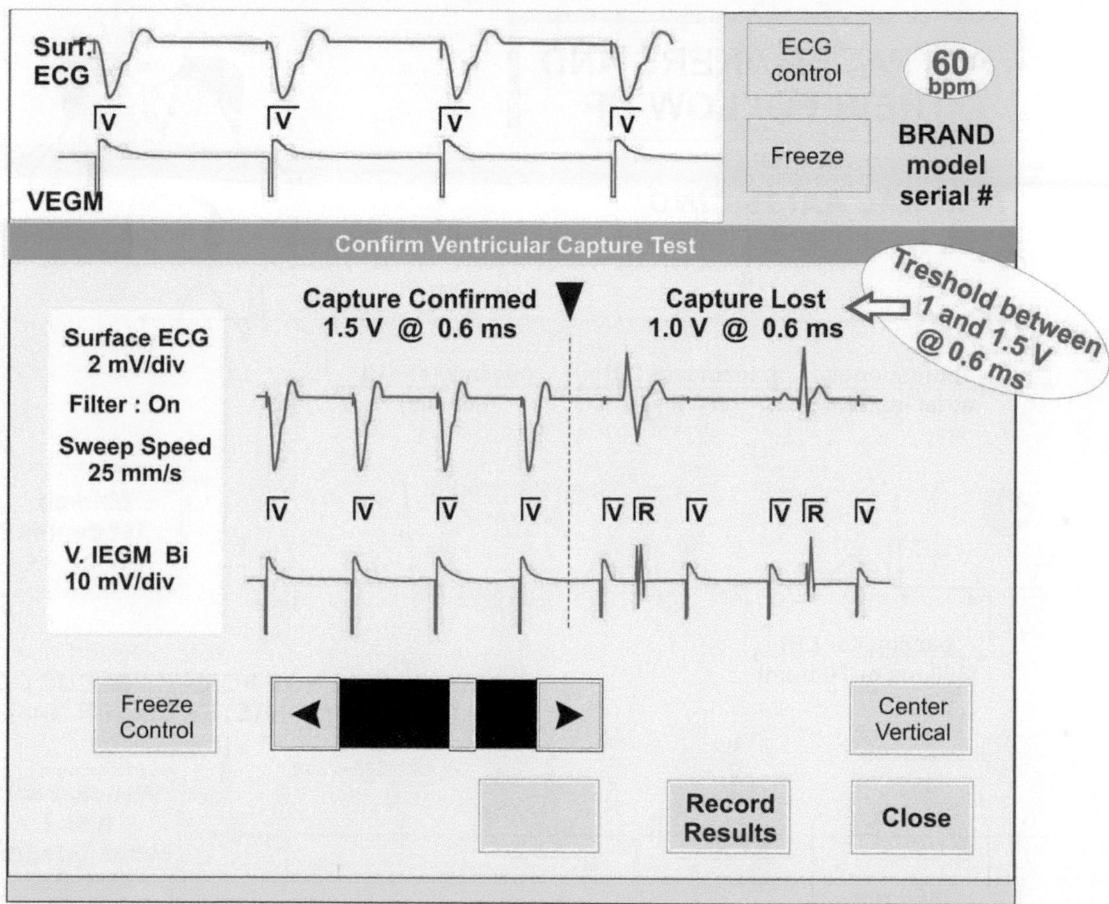

* During the test the temporary actual rate (90) is indicated in red in the upper right corner. At the end of the test, the programmed "Base Rate" (60) is restored.

* The test will start at a value (amplitude or pulse width depending upon choice) one step lower then the prevailing value. After every programmed "Number Cycles/Step", the value of the test parameter will decrease by one step. Each step is indicated by the appearance of a vertical line on the ECG display.

* Pressing {End Test} not only terminates the test, but restores the previously programmed values, i.e. 2.5 V - 0.6 ms - 60 bpm. These settings may be checked in the upper part of the display

* After touching {Close} the pacemaker should be programmed to yield a suitable safety margin for reliable long-term pacing (confirm with {Permanent program})

A. F. Sinnaeve

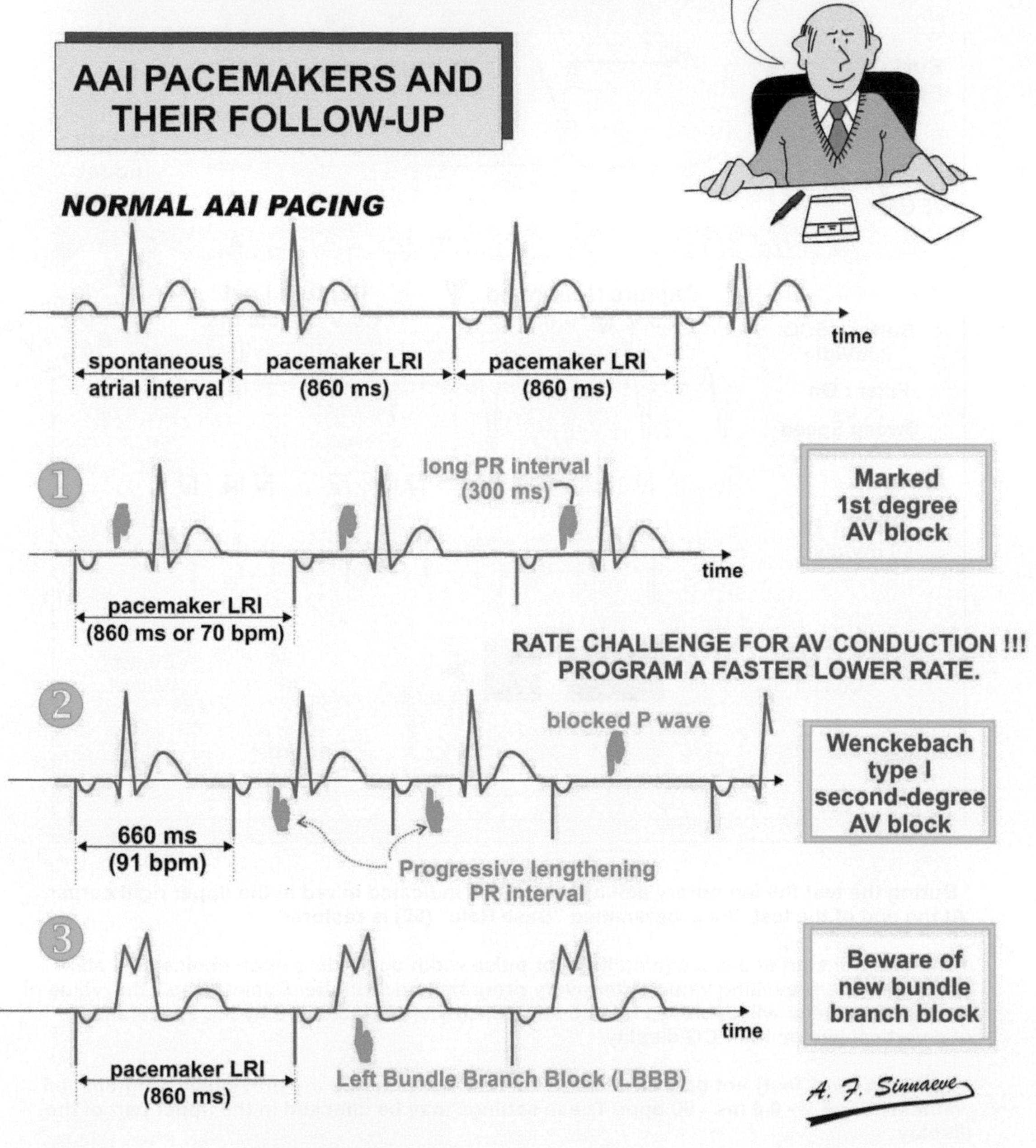

You know, even in carefully selected patients for AAI and AAIR pacemakers, there is always a small but definite risk of second- and third-degree AV block with the passage of time. The status of AV conduction must be carefully evaluated during follow-up to detect the earliest manifestations of potentially serious AV block that may require upgrading to a dual chamber pacemaker.
AAI PACEMAKERS AND THEIR FOLLOW-UP
NORMAL AAI PACING
time
spontaneous atrial interval
pacemaker LRI (860 ms)
pacemaker LRI (860 ms)
1
long PR interval (300 ms)
time
pacemaker LRI (860 ms or 70 bpm)
Marked 1st degree AV block
RATE CHALLENGE FOR AV CONDUCTION !!! PROGRAM A FASTER LOWER RATE.
2
blocked P wave
660 ms (91 bpm)
Progressive lengthening PR interval
Wenckebach type I second-degree AV block
3
time
pacemaker LRI (860 ms)
Left Bundle Branch Block (LBBB)
Beware of new bundle branch block
A. F. Sinnaeve

Abbreviations : LRI = lower rate interval ; LBBB = left bundle branch block ; AAI = atrial demand pacemaker mode ; AAIR = atrial demand rate-adaptive pacemaker mode ;

APPLICATION OF THE TRIGGERED PACING MODE

Remember that a DDD pacemaker functions in the triggered mode in the atrium because atrial sensing triggers a ventricular output after a delay equivalent to the programmed AV interval. In the AAT or VVT modes triggering occurs immediately after sensing without delay so that the pacemaker stimulus falls within the sensed event, P wave or QRS complex.

DDD pacemaker (basic or lower rate 60 bpm) Is the atrial channel correctly sensing ?

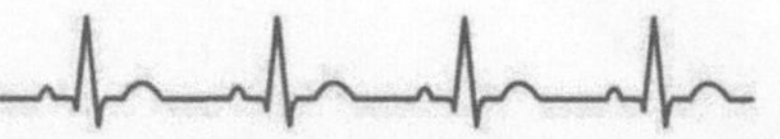

Temporary pacing at the AAT mode (30 bpm) when atrial sensing is properly adjusted

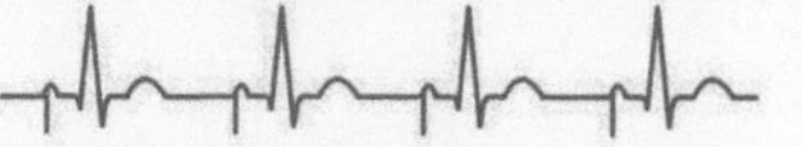

Temporary pacing at the AAT mode (30 bpm) with undersensing of the atrial channel

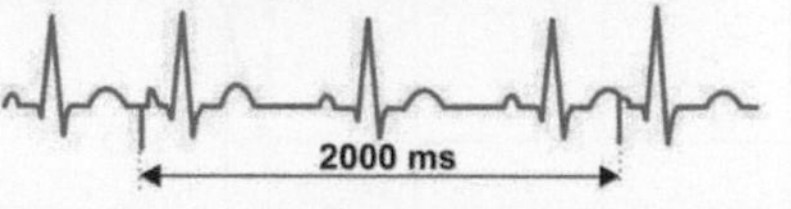

This could be asynchronous pacing, a pseudofusion beat (sensing has not yet occurred) or a triggered response (sensing has already occurred)

Ventricular stimulus

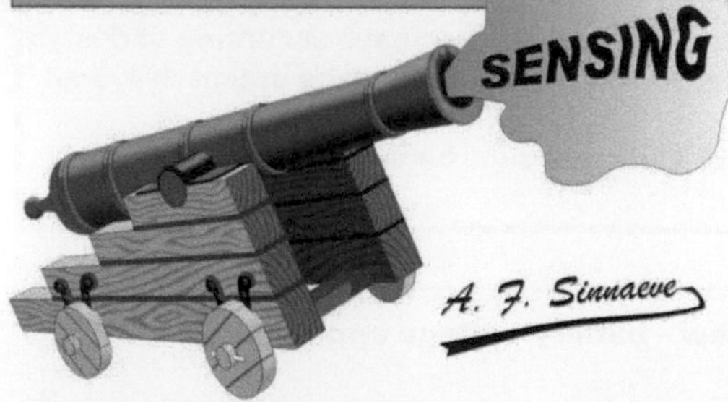

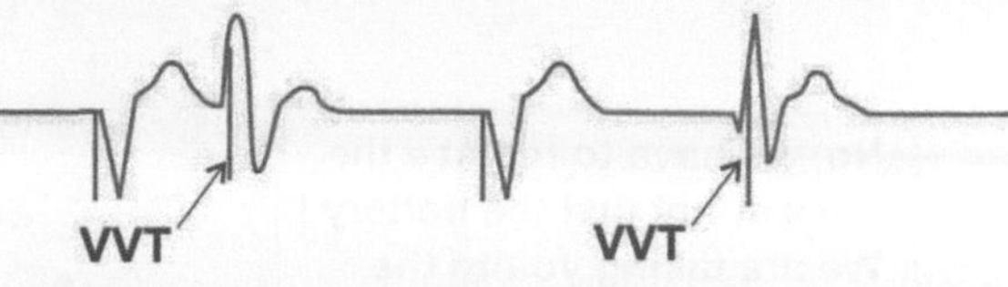

Triggered pacemaker modes are intended mostly for pacemaker diagnostic purposes :

1/ to facilitate identification of sensed events with pacing artifacts e.g. in high noise environment

2/ to correct myopotential oversensing unresponsive to lowering sensitivity (the pacemaker then increases its rate with myopotential sensing)

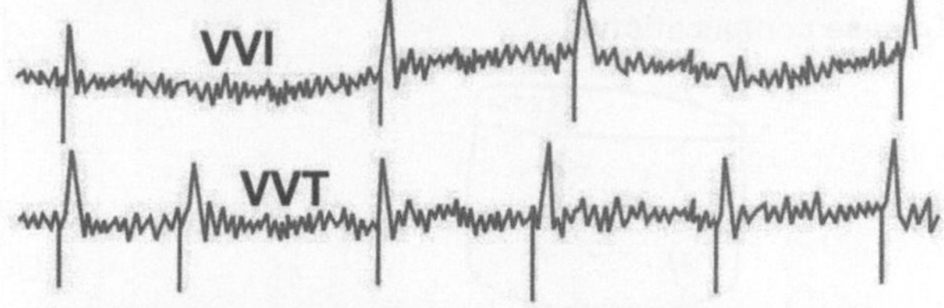

3/ to correct oversensing from noisy leads, until lead replacement can be performed

4/ to show retrograde P waves and to measure the sensed signal in DDT mode

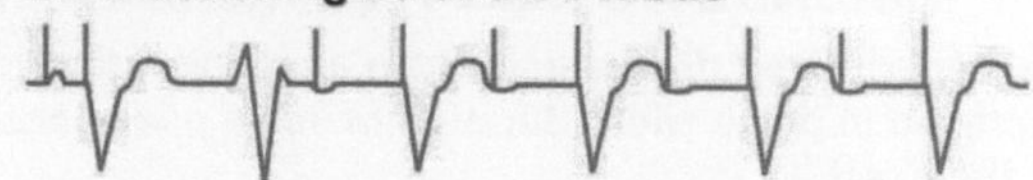

5/ to perform electrophysiologic studies and termination of tachycardias by chest wall stimulation (CWS) in pacemakers without these functions

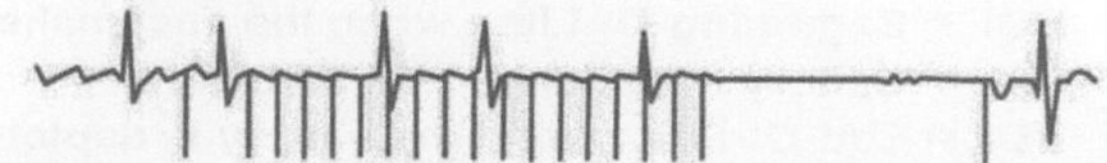

The triggered modes can be used in Holter recordings in patients with suspected oversensing that cannot be demonstrated in the pacemaker clinic with telemetered markers. The triggered impulse represents a marker for the diagnosis and the timing of sensed signals.

Abbreviations : CWS = chest wall stimulation: delivery of pacemaker stiumuli to the chest wall with an external pacemaker (painless procedure unable to capture the heart) to be sensed by an implanted pacemaker; **LRI** = lower rate interval ; **VRP** = ventricular refractory period ; **DDT** mode = a triggered response occurs in the atrium upon atrial sensing and a triggered response also occurs in the ventricle upon ventricular sensing;

BATTERY DEPLETION & END OF LIFE

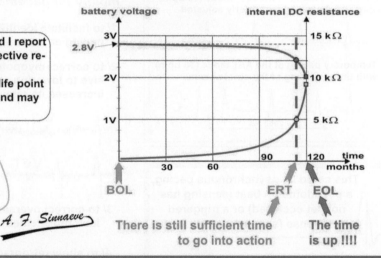

The battery of your pacemaker is almost depleted. The mode of the device is changed and its pacing rate remains low.

Doctor, do you have to change the batteries of my pacemaker ?

No, we have to replace the device, not just the battery ! We are taking you to the operating room.

I can predict the end of my life and I report it to the doctor by a diagnostic elective replacement indicator !
I do not want to reach the end-of-life point when my function will be erratic and may cause complications.

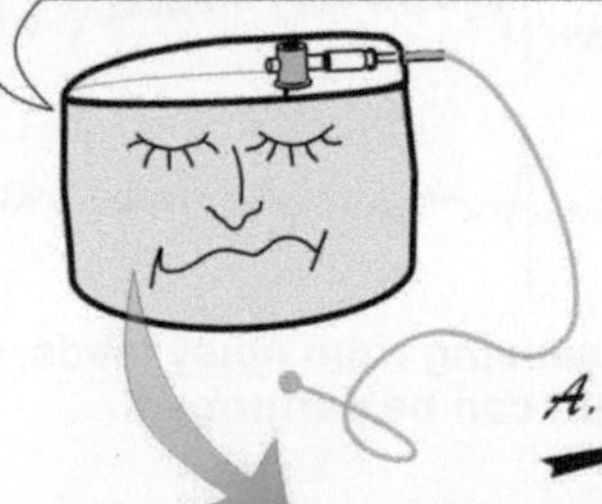

A. F. Sinnaeve

battery voltage
internal DC resistance
3V
2.8V
2V
1V
15 kΩ
10 kΩ
5 kΩ
30
60
90
120
time months
BOL
ERT
EOL
There is still sufficient time to go into action
The time is up !!!!

DIAGNOSTIC ELECTIVE REPLACEMENT INDICATORS

1. Percent or fixed decrease in the magnet rate; the free-running rate may also decrease according to design
2. Increase in pulse width duration in some pacemakers to compensate for a lower voltage output delivered to the heart.
3. Change to simpler pacing mode : DDDR to VVI, VVIR to VVI or VOO to reduce battery current drain and delay the time to end of life.

BOL = Beginning-Of-Life : when the pacemaker is new - battery voltage approx. 2.8V and battery impedance less than 1kΩ

EOL = End-Of-Life : when the battery is depleted and the basic pacer functions not longer supported - battery voltage lower than approx. 2.1 - 2.4V and battery impedance higher than 5 - 10kΩ

ERT = Elective Replacement Time : generator replacement should be considered well in advance of end of life - battery voltage is reduced but still able to support basic or all pacer functions

ERI = Elective Replacement Indicator : battery voltage approx. 2.1 - 2.4V and battery impedance approx. 5 - 10kΩ

SPECIFIC VALUES OF EOL & ERI WILL VARY FROM MANUFACTURER TO MANUFACTURER

THE CONCEPT OF TELEMETRY

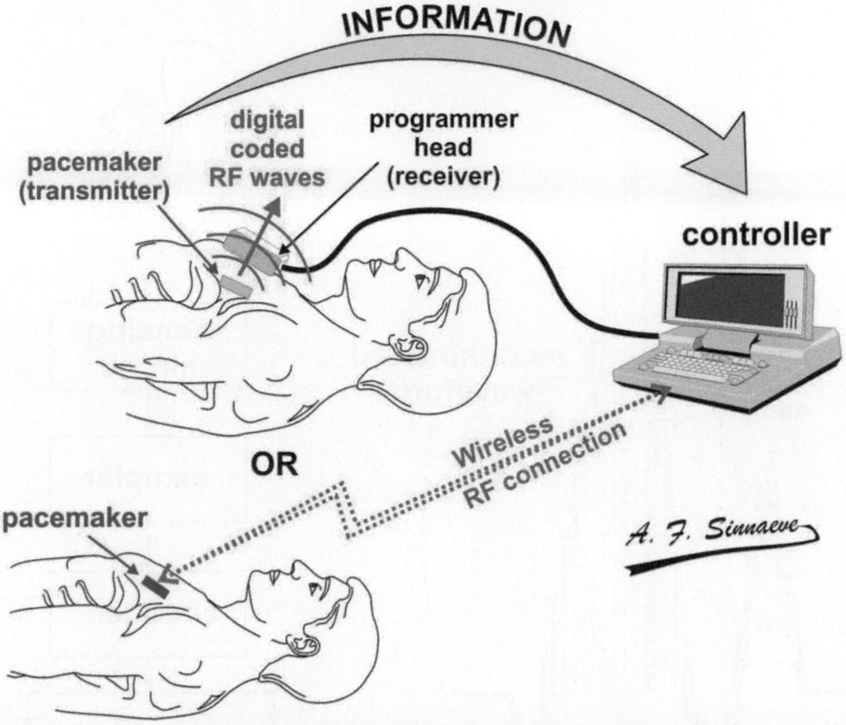

DATA OBTAINABLE BY TELEMETRY

* **ADMINISTRATIVE DATA** (model, serial number, patient's name, date of implantation, indication for implantation)
* **PROGRAMMED DATA** (mode, rate, refractory period, hysteresis on/off, pulse amplitude & width, sensitivity)
* **MEASURED DATA** (rate, pulse amplitude, pulse current, pulse energy, pulse charge, lead impedance, battery impedance, battery voltage, battery current drain)
* **STORED DATA** (Holter function, rhythm histogram, ...)
* **MARKER SIGNALS** for ECG interpretation
* **INTRACARDIAC ELECTROGRAM**

TELEMETERED VENTRICULAR ELECTROGRAM

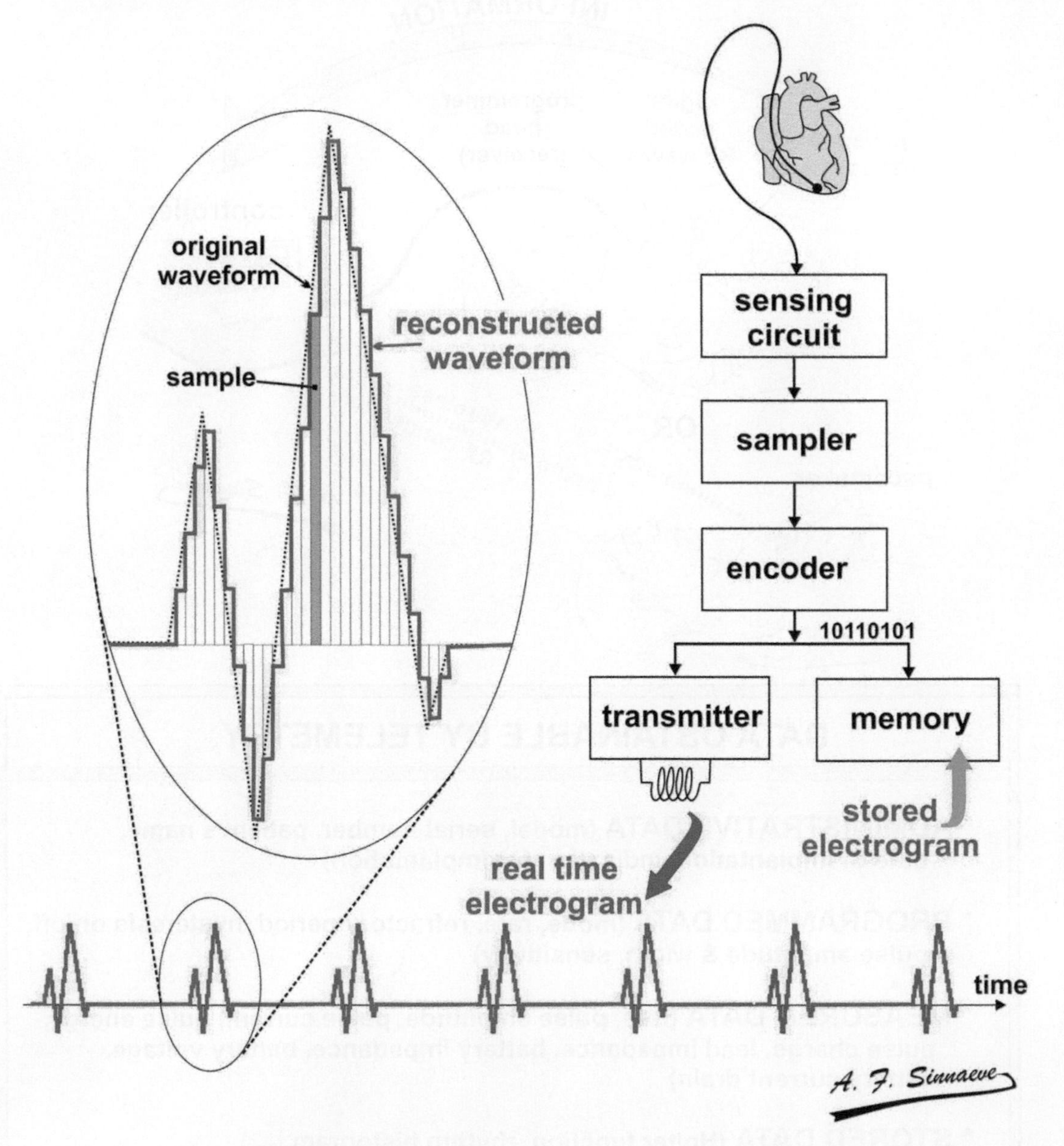

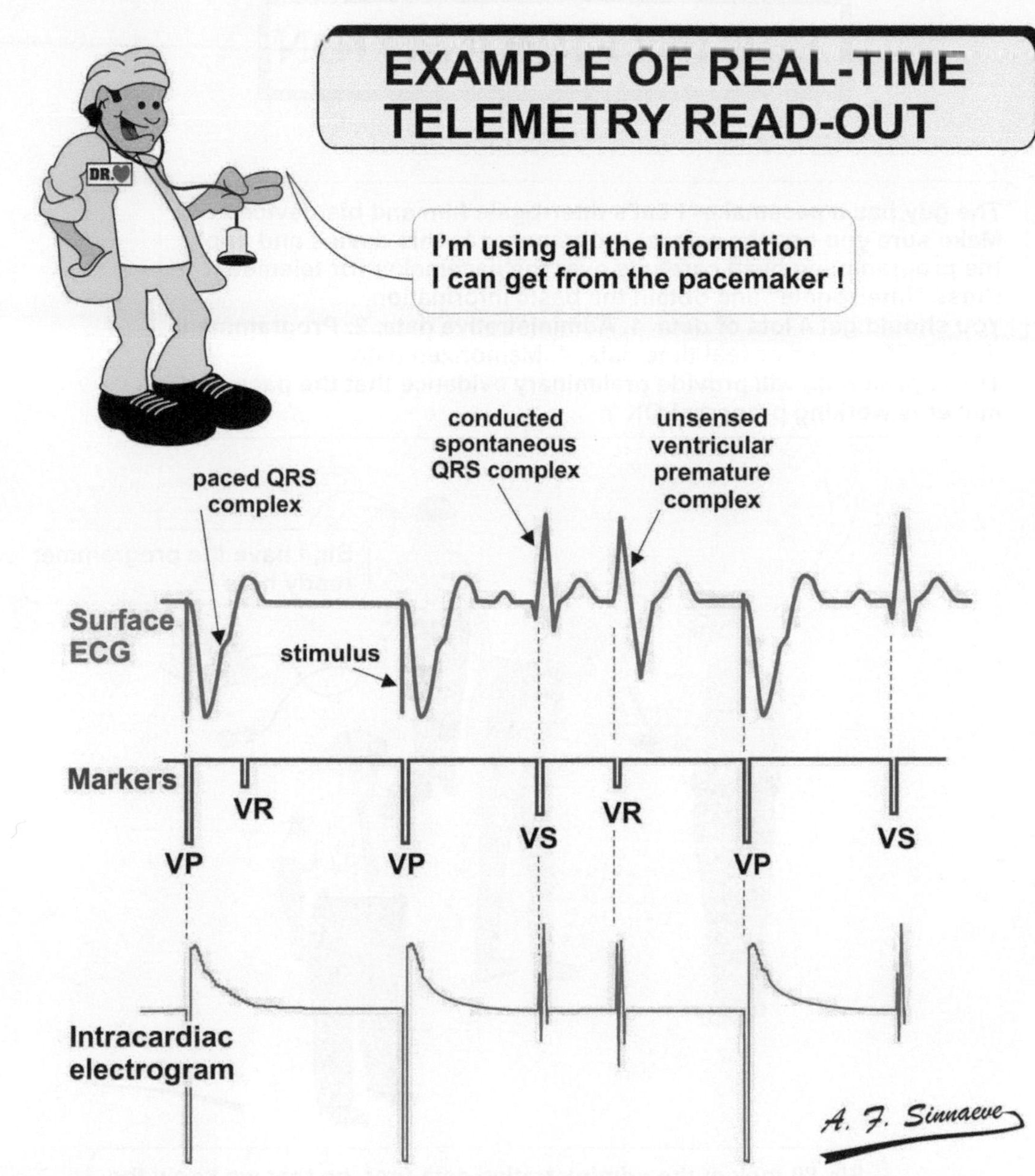

Abbreviations : VP = ventricular pace ; VS = ventricular sense ; VR = ventricular sense in the refractory period

THE INTERROGATION

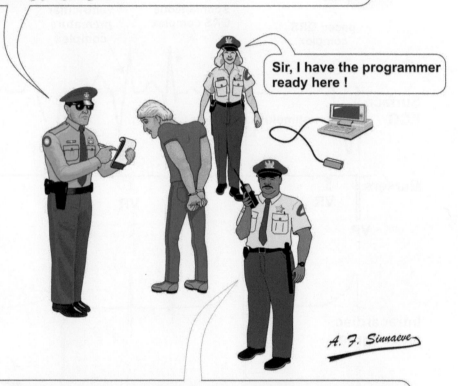

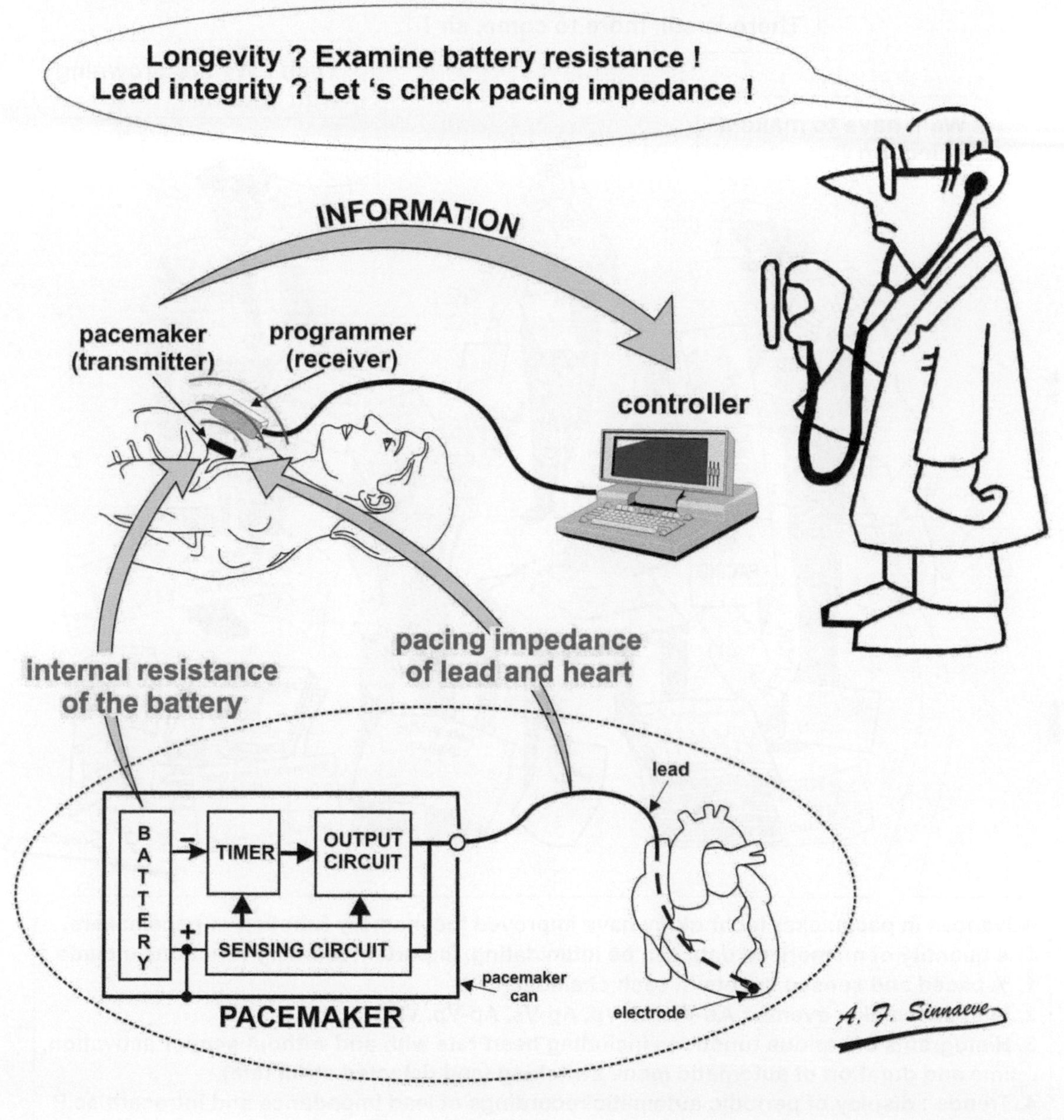
MEASUREMENT OF RESISTANCE & IMPEDANCE BY TELEMETRY
Longevity ? Examine battery resistance !
Lead integrity ? Let 's check pacing impedance !
INFORMATION
pacemaker (transmitter)
programmer (receiver)
controller
internal resistance of the battery
pacing impedance of lead and heart
lead
BATTERY
TIMER
OUTPUT CIRCUIT
SENSING CIRCUIT
pacemaker can
PACEMAKER
electrode
A. F. Sinnaeve

THE MEMORIZED DATA

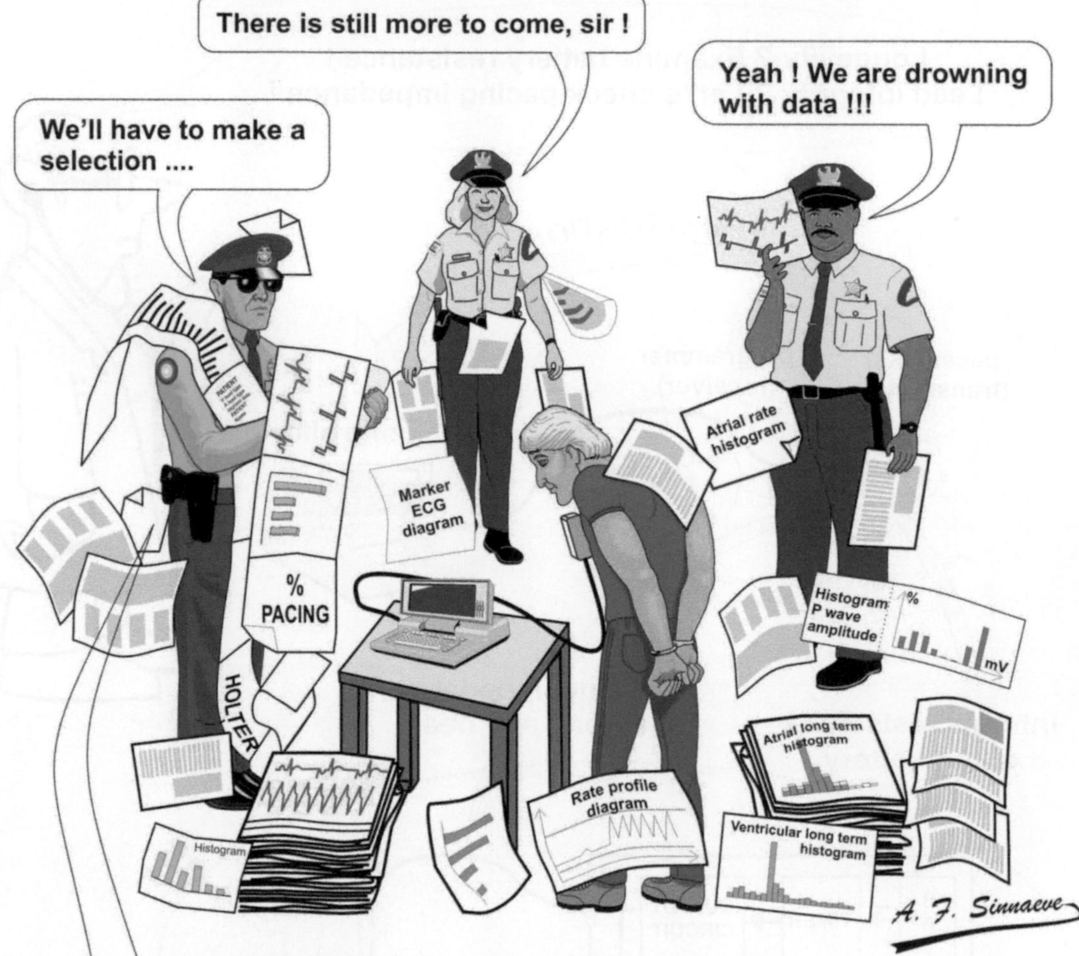

Advances in pacemaker technology have improved the memory function of pacemakers. The quantity of memorized data can be intimidating. Important memory functions include :

1. **% paced and sensed events in each chamber.**
2. **% of pacemaker events : As-Vs, As-Vp, Ap-Vs, Ap-Vp, VPC.**
3. **Histograms of various functions including heart rate with and without sensor activation, time and duration of automatic mode switching (and detected atrial rate).**
4. **Trends : display of periodic automatic recordings of lead impedance and intracardiac P and QRS amplitude.**
5. **Diagnosis of arrhythmias with marker chains and/or stored atrial and ventricular electrograms. This function can be automatic or patient-activated by placing a magnet or activator over the pacemaker.**

Abbreviatons : Ap = atrial paced event, As = atrial sensed event, Vp = ventricular paced event, Vs = ventricular sensed event, VPC = ventricular premature complex

THE MEASURED DATA

The measured data is real-time ! And the data of 2 channels (A and V) is displayed simultaneously. We have here information about :

1. The output - pacing rate in beats per minute (bpm)
   - pulse voltage amplitude in volts (V)
   - pulse duration in milliseconds (ms)
2. The battery - battery voltage in volts (V)
   - battery current drain in microamperes (μA)
   - battery impedance in ohms (Ω)
3. The leads - lead impedance in ohms (Ω)
   - lead configuration (bipolar/unipolar)

Why look at the battery current drain ?

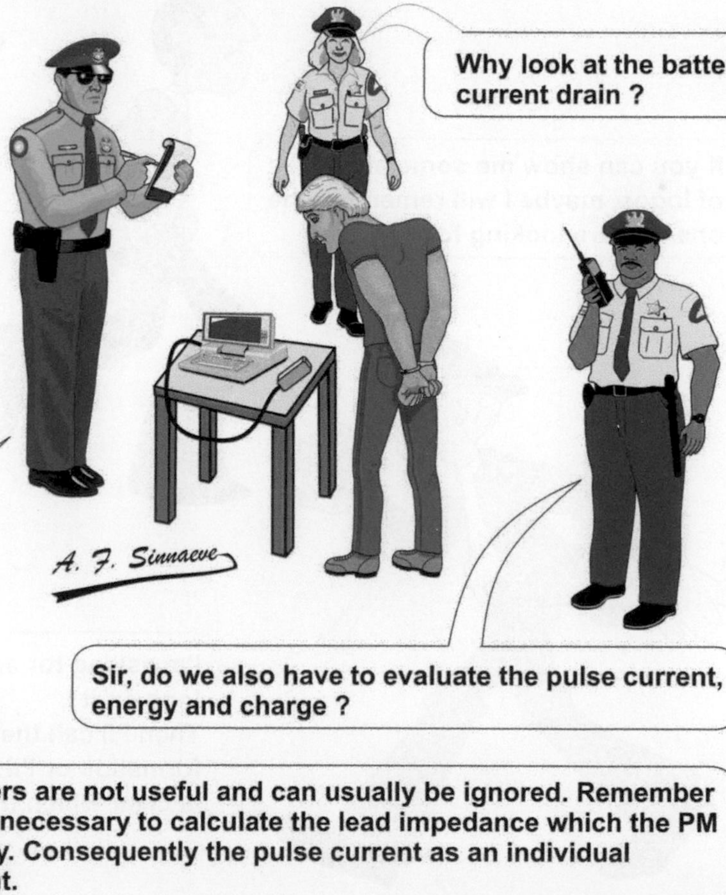

Remember that the current drain is in μA and not in mA !!! The current drain is the most important determinant of battery life.

Sir, do we also have to evaluate the pulse current, energy and charge ?

Actually, these parameters are not useful and can usually be ignored. Remember that the pulse current is necessary to calculate the lead impedance which the PM determines automatically. Consequently the pulse current as an individual parameter is unimportant.

THE UNIDENTIFIED PACEMAKER

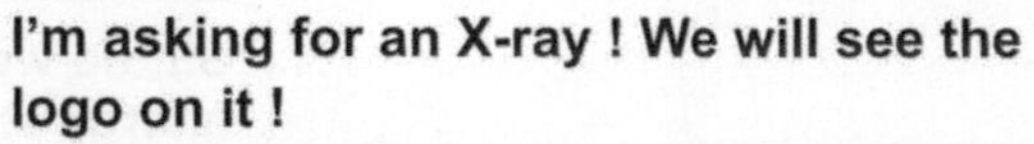

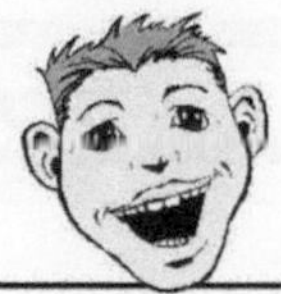

THE PACEMAKER AS A HOLTER RECORDER

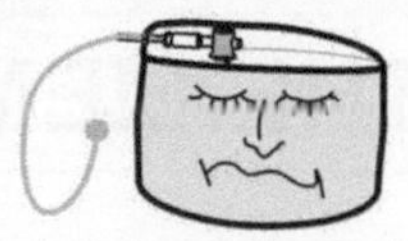

DECIMAL COUNTING FOR HUMANS Ten digits : 0, 1, 2, 3, 4, 5, 6, 7, 8, 9	BINARY COUNTING FOR MACHINES Only two digits : 0 and 1 called "bits"
$14 = 1.10^1 + 4.10^0$ $= 10 + 4$	$1110 = 1.2^3 + 1.2^2 + 1.2^1 + 0.2^0$ $= 8 + 4 + 2 + 0$

EQUIVALENT

A sequence of eight adjacent bits forms a "byte".

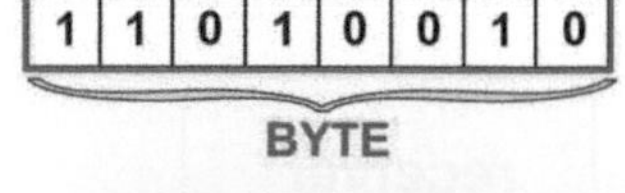

When information is read by the pacemaker and stored in its electronic memory, it is done byte-by-byte. Memory is usually measured in "kilobytes" (kB). One kilobyte = 1024 bytes.

RAM STORAGE
Address
Data byte

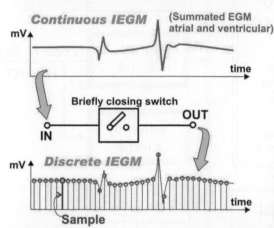

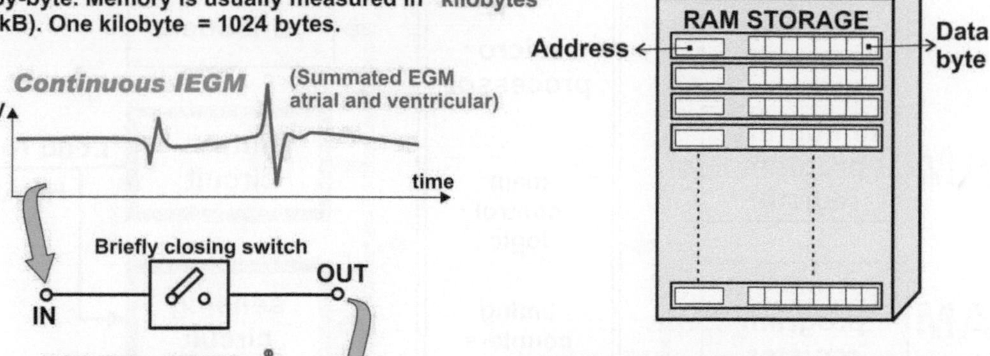

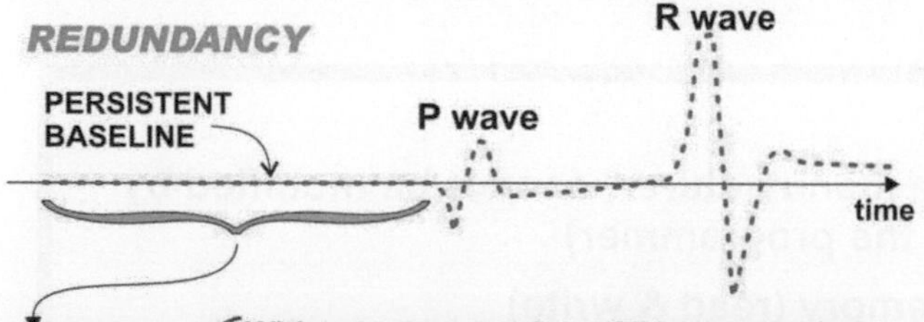

The microprocessor cannot handle continuous signals. Hence, "sampling" is used to measure the signal repeatedly during a very brief instant, creating a set of discrete values or "samples". Sampling is usually performed at 128 or 256 samples per second.

The intracardiac electrogram (IEGM) is immediately stored in the RAM of the pacemaker. Each sample corresponds with one byte of data storage. Each byte is stored at a specific memory address for retrieval at a later time. A 128kB RAM includes 128 x 1024 = 131 072 bytes. When sampling at 256 samples/s, this RAM is sufficient for 131,072 / 256 = 512 s = 8.5 minutes of IEGM.

REDUNDANCY

PERSISTENT BASELINE
P wave
R wave
time

Compression algorithms reduce the number of bytes and increase the amount of IEGM that can be stored in the RAM of the pacemaker

25 samples
- Without compression : 25 bytes needed
- After compression : only 2 bytes needed (value & number of identical samples)

REQUIREMENTS FOR 24-h RECORDING OF IEGM :
24 h/day x 60 min/h x 60 s/min = 86,400 s/day
128 samples/s x 1 byte/sample x 86,400 s/day = 11million bytes/day
Sampling at 128 samples/s requires a RAM of 11,000 kB

THE FUTURE : within 3 - 5 years ??

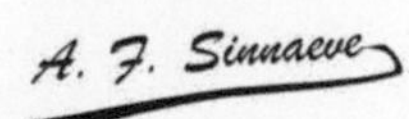

THE MEMORY OF A VVI PACEMAKER

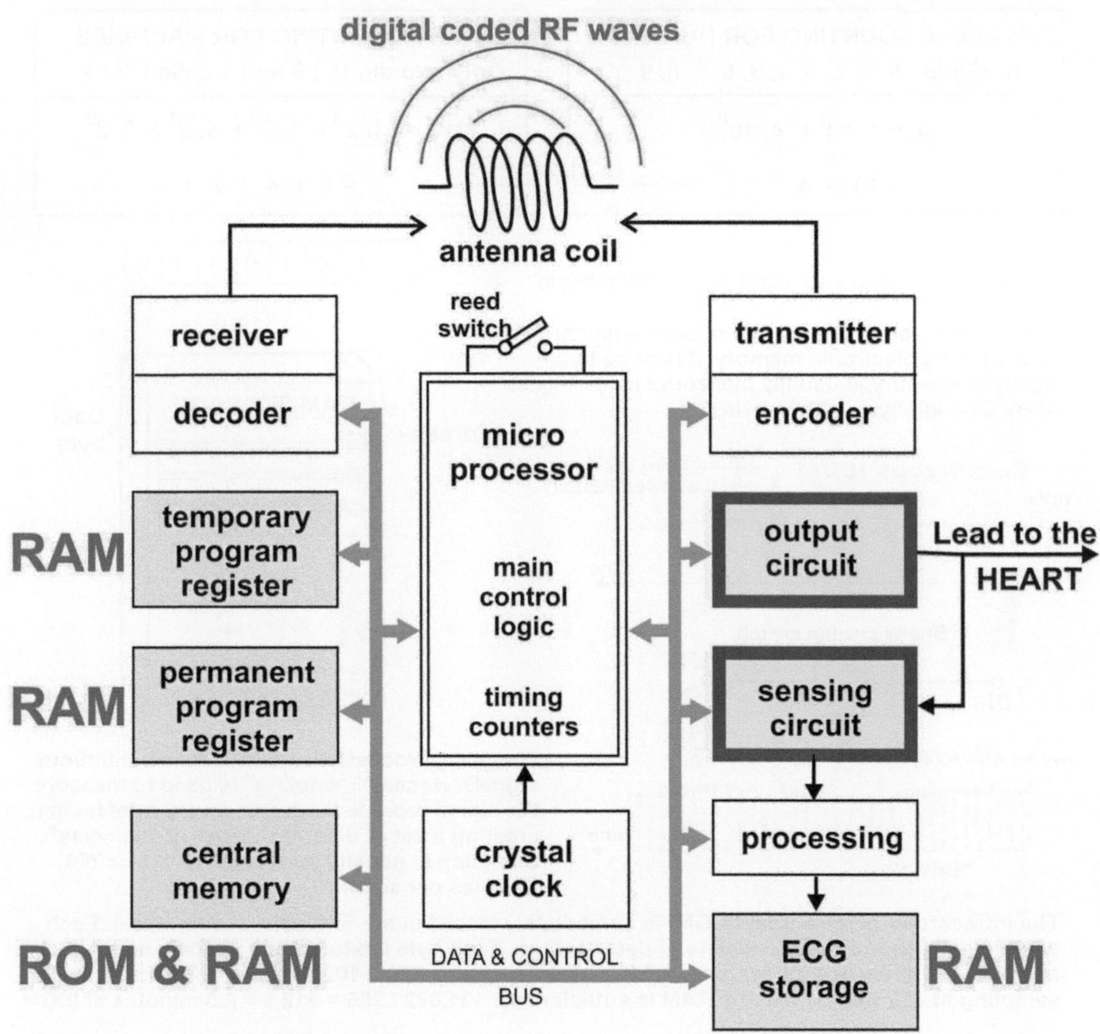

ROM = read only memory
(is installed by the manufacturer; cannot be modified by the physician via the programmer)

RAM = random access memory (read & write)
(content can be changed by measurements of the pacemaker or by the physician via the programmer)

A. F. Sinnaeve

PACEMAKER DIAGNOSTICS

* Device information
* Device-Patient interface Information
* Patient information

Device Information

Program settings. This data can be viewed in this format or in more detail on another screen.

Device identification / implant date. This data can be very important, especially in patients who are not geographically stable and who are not maintained in consistent follow-up.

Device longevity estimate appears on the initial and on another screen (based on remaining battery voltage / impedance and percent pacing).

The "Elective replacement indicator" warning automatically appears in the "Significant Events" window on the screen.

Lead Monitoring

Amplitude and pulse width

Sensitivity

Measured impedance

Lead status

Quick Look™ Follow-Up

Automatic Measurements are displayed upon Initial Interogation

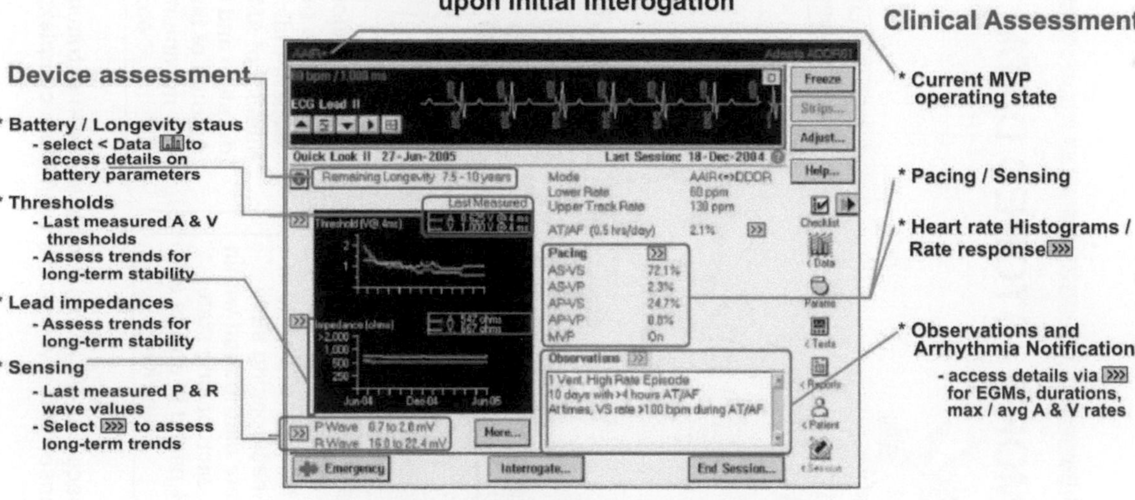
Clinical Assessment
Device assessment
* Battery / Longevity staus
- select < Data to access details on battery parameters
* Thresholds
- Last measured A & V thresholds
- Assess trends for long-term stability
* Lead impedances
- Assess trends for long-term stability
* Sensing
- Last measured P & R wave values
- Select >>> to assess long-term trends
* Current MVP operating state
* Pacing / Sensing
* Heart rate Histograms / Rate response >>>
* Observations and Arrhythmia Notifications
- access details via >>> for EGMs, durations, max / avg A & V rates
Freeze
Strips...
Adjust...
Help...
ECG Lead II
Quick Look II 27-Jun-2005
Last Session: 18-Dec-2004
Remaining Longevity 7.5 - 10 years
Mode AAIR<=>DDDR
Lower Rate 60 ppm
Upper Track Rate 130 ppm
AT/AF (0.5 hrs/day) 2.1%
Pacing
AS-VS 72.1%
AS-VP 2.3%
AP-VS 24.7%
AP-VP 0.8%
MVP On
Observations
1 Vent. High Rate Episode
10 days with >4 hours AT/AF
At times, VS rate >100 bpm during AT/AF
Emergency
Interrogate...
End Session...
More...

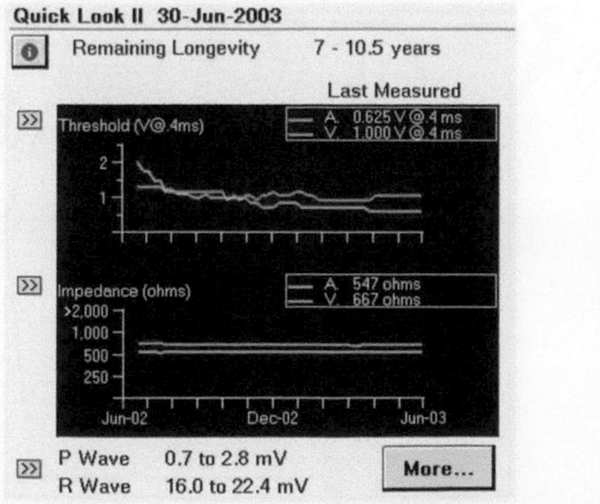
Quick Look II 30-Jun-2003
Remaining Longevity 7 - 10.5 years
Last Measured
Threshold (V@.4ms)
A 0.625 V @ .4 ms
V 1.000 V @ .4 ms
2
1
Impedance (ohms)
A 547 ohms
V 667 ohms
>2,000
1,000
500
250
Jun-02
Dec-02
Jun-03
P Wave 0.7 to 2.8 mV
R Wave 16.0 to 22.4 mV
More...

A. F. Sinnaeve

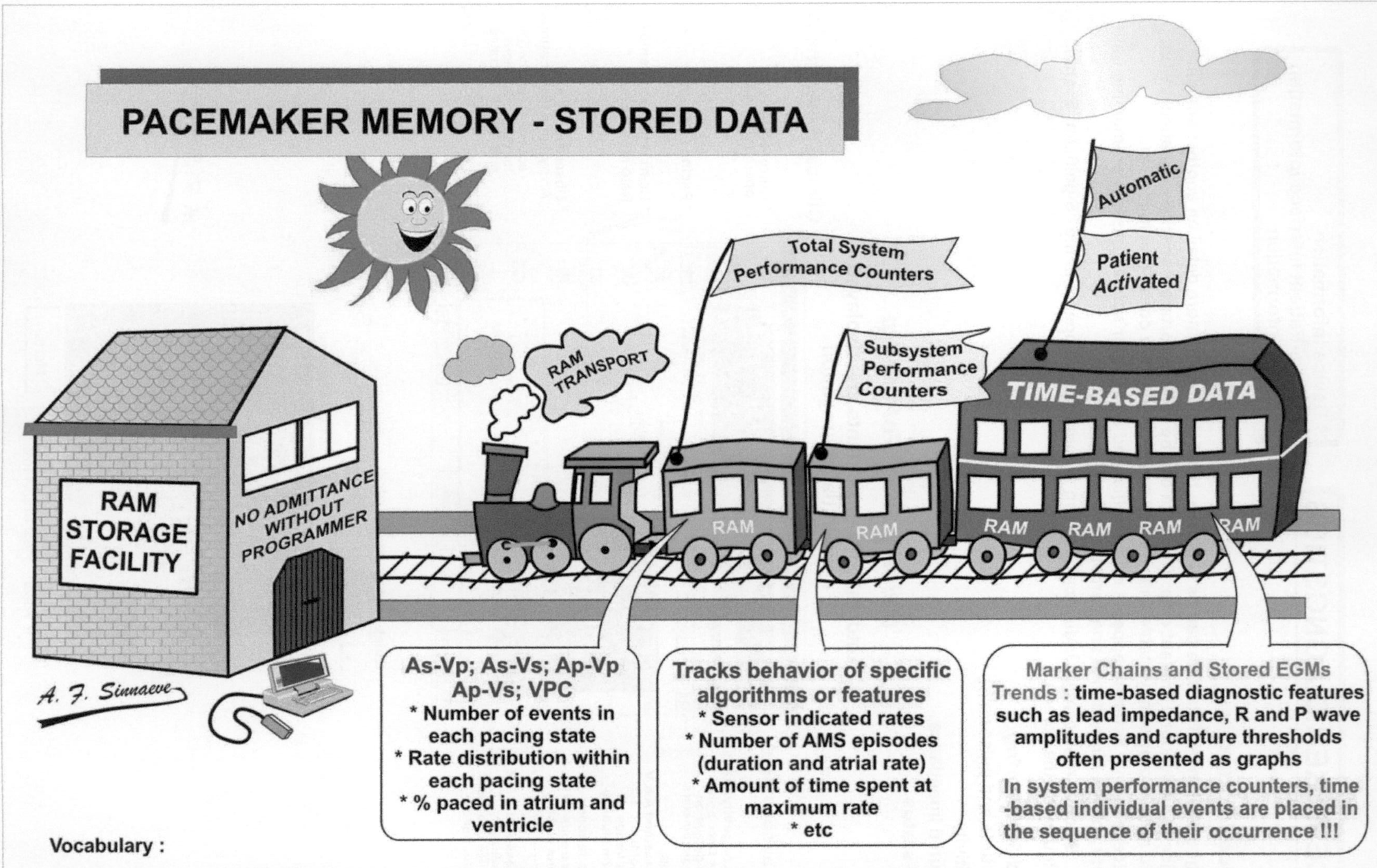
PACEMAKER MEMORY - STORED DATA
RAM STORAGE FACILITY
NO ADMITTANCE WITHOUT PROGRAMMER
RAM TRANSPORT
Total System Performance Counters
Subsystem Performance Counters
Automatic
Patient Activated
TIME-BASED DATA
RAM
RAM
RAM
RAM
RAM
RAM
As-Vp; As-Vs; Ap-Vp Ap-Vs; VPC
* Number of events in each pacing state
* Rate distribution within each pacing state
* % paced in atrium and ventricle
Tracks behavior of specific algorithms or features
* Sensor indicated rates
* Number of AMS episodes (duration and atrial rate)
* Amount of time spent at maximum rate
* etc
Marker Chains and Stored EGMs
Trends : time-based diagnostic features such as lead impedance, R and P wave amplitudes and capture thresholds often presented as graphs
In system performance counters, time -based individual events are placed in the sequence of their occurrence !!!
A. F. Sinnaeve
Vocabulary :
As-Vp (= PV) = atrial sense-ventricular pace ; As-Vs (= PR) = atrial sense - ventricular sense; Ap-Vp (= AV) = atrial pace-ventricular pace; Ap-Vs (= AR) = atrial pace-ventricular sense; VPC = ventricular premature complex; EGM = electrogram; RAM = random access memory; AMS = automatic mode switching

STORAGE OF PACING STATES

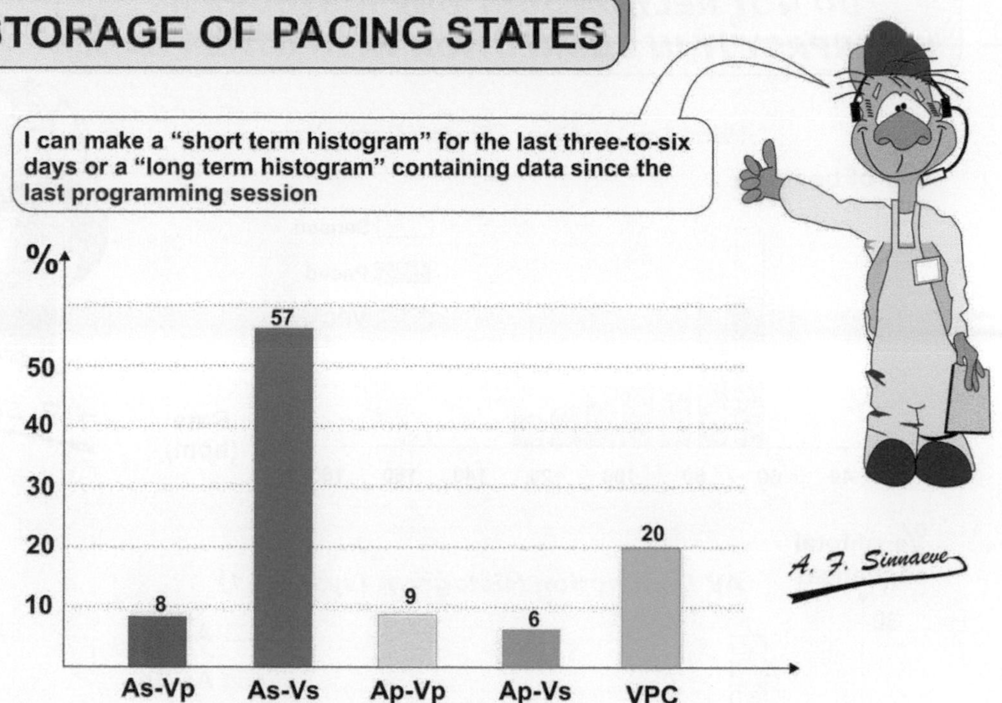
I can make a "short term histogram" for the last three-to-six days or a "long term histogram" containing data since the last programming session
%
57
50
40
30
20
10
8
9
6
20
As-Vp
As-Vs
Ap-Vp
Ap-Vs
VPC
A. F. Sinnaeve

 **(Ap-Vp) + (Ap-Vs) : total % of atrial paced events ;**

- *** if this total is large, there is a lot of pacing at the basic rate**
- *** if this total is large, it suggests sick sinus syndrome and atrial incompetence**

 **(As-Vp) + (As-Vs) : total % of atrial sensed events ;**

- *** if As-Vp is very large there is an AV block or the AV delay (AVI) is programmed too short**
- *** if As-Vs is large, the pacemaker functions on stand-by basis most of the time**

 **(As-Vs) + (Ap-Vs) : total % of sensed ventricular events**

- *** if this total is large, there is a good spontaneous AV conduction**

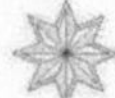 **(As-Vp) + (Ap-Vp) : total % of paced ventricular events**

 **VPC : note that a VPC according to the pacemaker is not necessarily equal to a clinical PVC**

Abbreviations :
As-Vp (= PV) = atrial sense-ventricular pace; As-Vs (= PR) = atrial sense-ventricular sense; Ap-Vp (= AV) = atrial pace-ventricular pace; Ap-Vs (= AR) = atrial pace-ventricular sense; VPC = ventricular premature complex; PVC = premature ventricular complex

**DO NOT RELY ON JUST ONE HISTOGRAM !
INTERPRET IT IN CONNECTION WITH OTHER DATA.**

A. F. Sinnaeve

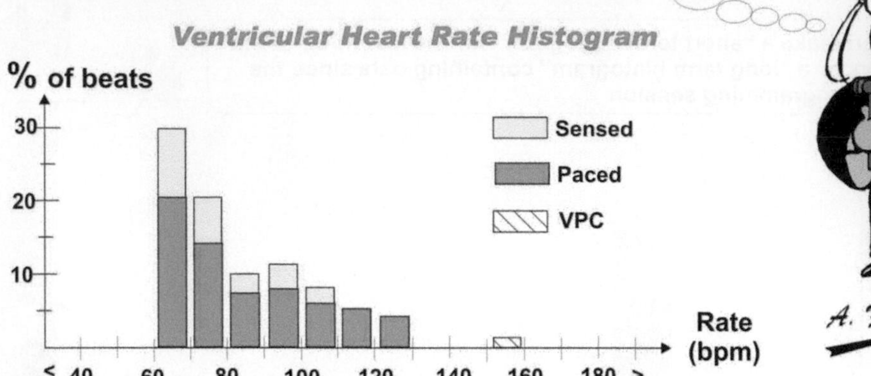

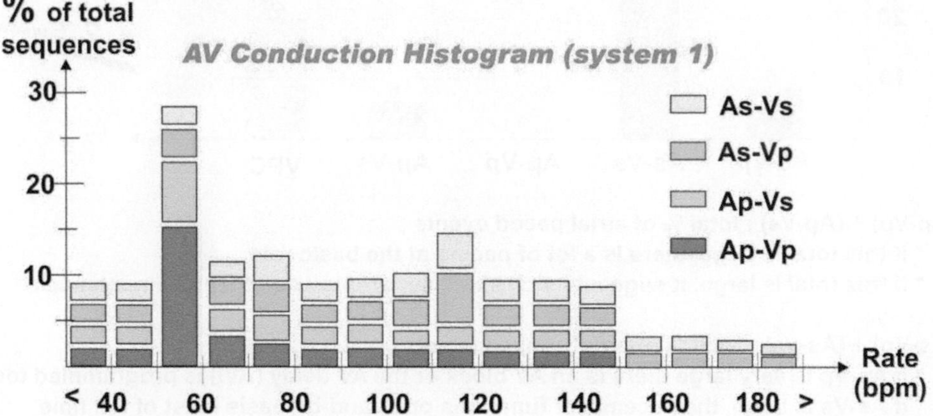

AV Conduction Table (system 2)

Rate (bpm)	As-Vp	As-Vs	Ap-Vp	Ap-Vs	VPC
30 - 54	45	0	9 546	0	0
55 - 69	308 978	79	2 974 366	1 322	0
70 - 89	298 459	1 504	621 788	1 908	6 968
90 - 109	11 693	989	608	398	84 241
110 - 129	100	315	0	0	7 173
130 - 149	0	152	0	0	447
150 - 179	0	409	0	0	2 235
180 - 224	0	205	0	0	625
225 - 249	0	0	0	0	1
> 250	0	0	0	0	0
Total :	619 275	3 653	3 606 308	3 628	101 690

Abbreviations :
As-Vs (= PR) = atrial sense - ventricular sense; As-Vp (=PV)= atrial sense - ventricular pace; Ap-Vs (=AR) = atrial pace - ventricular sense; Ap-Vp (=AV) = atrial pace - ventricular pace; bpm = beats per minute; VPC = ventricular premature complex

P WAVE AMPLITUDE HISTOGRAM

The P wave histogram can be helpful for :
* Evaluation of the safety margin for atrial sensing
* Detection of lead displacement
* Detection of atrial arrhythmias
* Detection of interference
* Detection of near-field & far-field sensing

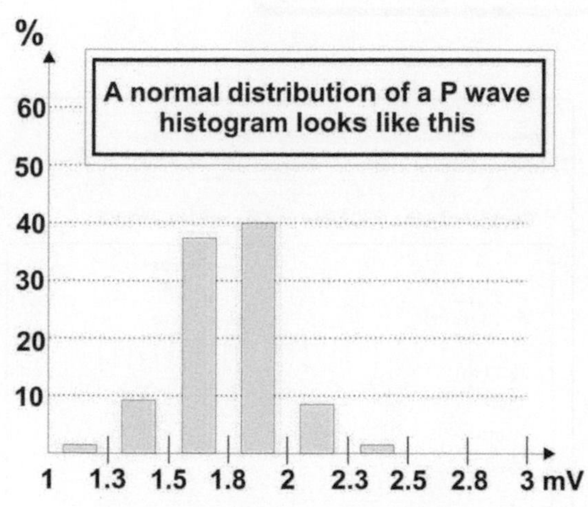

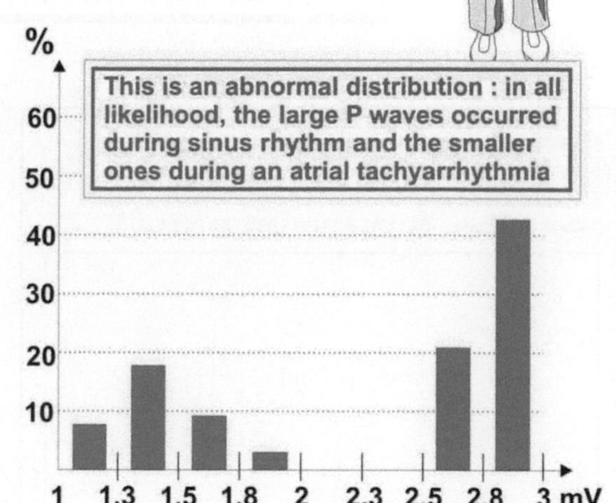

Evaluation of the safety margin for atrial sensing. Signal vs. programmed sensitivity.

The histogram is limited on its lower side by the programmed sensitivity !!!
Programming different sensitivities may unmask undersensing

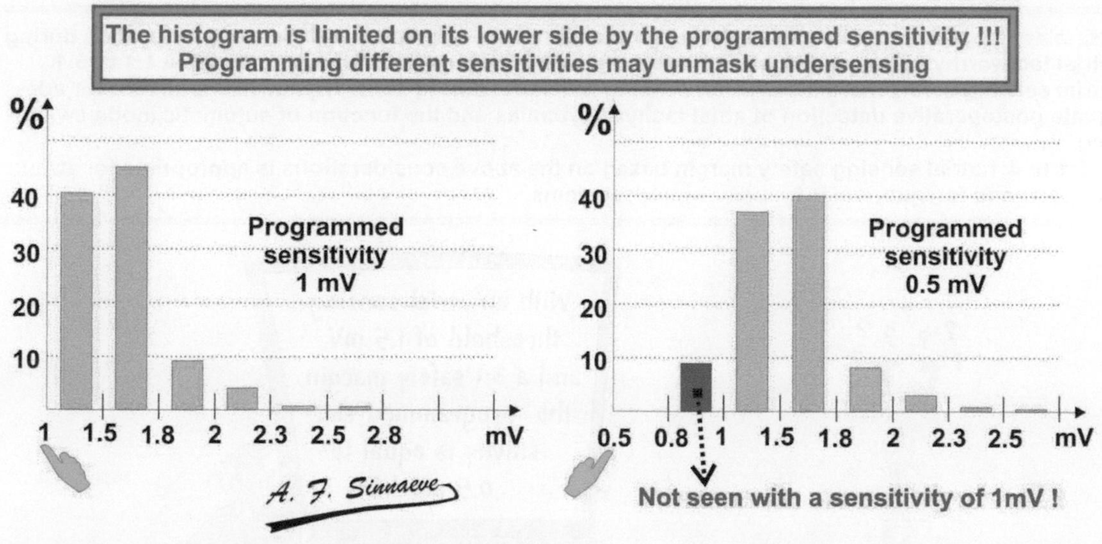

PACEMAKER DIAGNOSTICS - SENSING THRESHOLDS

While sensing can be evaluated at the time of follow-up, current devices can do this automatically and adapt sensitivity accordingly. Data are usually recorded every 7 days (can be set to as often as every 2 hours). Diagnostic information includes atrial and ventricular sensitivity.

A pacemaker can perform the following functions :

- **Measures intrinsic P and R wave endocardial signals**
- **Adapts sensitivity based on target safety margins (x3 or x4)**
- **Automatically provides safe sensing margins**
- **Increases detection sensitivity for automatic mode switching**

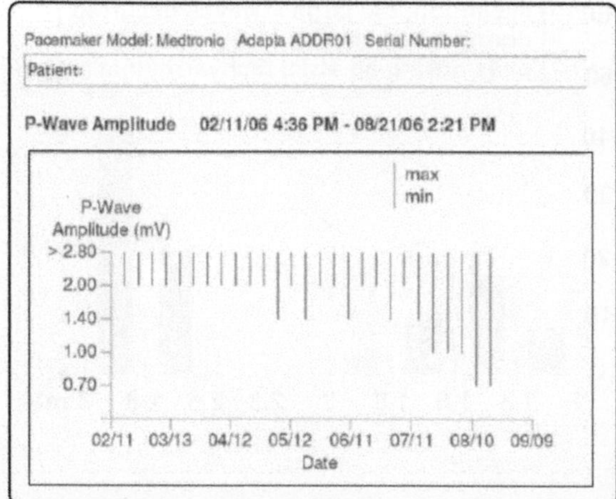

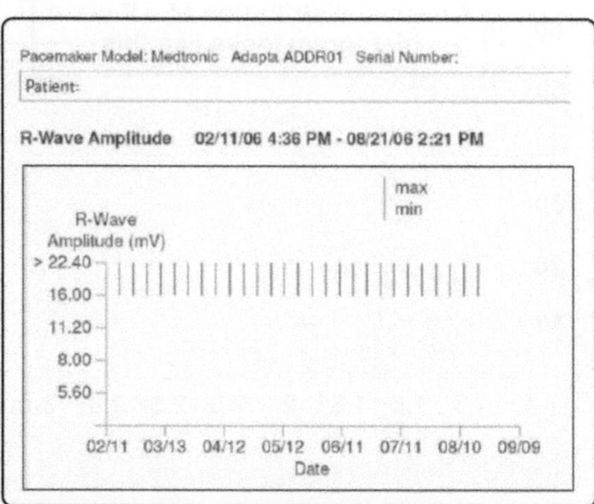

Bipolar atrial sensing thresholds during sinus rhythm are correlated with sensing thresholds during atrial tachyarrhythmias, but there is a large degree of variance in individual patients. A 4:1 to 5:1 atrial sensing safety margin based on sensing threshold during sinus rhythm is a predictor for adequate postoperative detection of atrial tachyarrhythmias and the function of automatic mode switching.

A 3:1 to 4:1 atrial sensing safety margin based on the above considerations is appropriate for atrial unipolar and for ventricular unipolar/bipolar systems

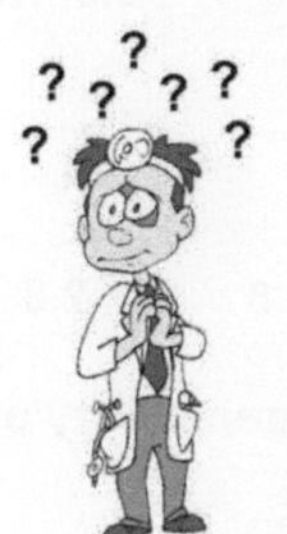

With an atrial sensing threshold of 1.5 mV, and a 3:1 safety margin, the programmed sensitivity is equal to 0.5 mV ! ! !

A. F. Sinnaeve

The pacemaker automatically collects the data !
These histograms are very useful for the evaluation of the condition of the patient, the performance of the total system and the adjustment of the sensor characteristics.

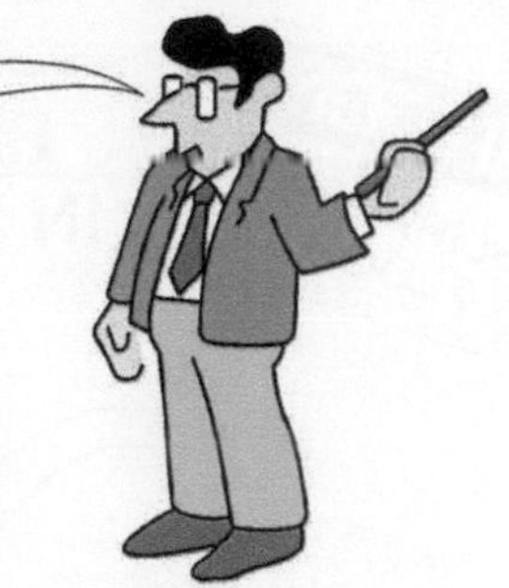

HEART RATE HISTOGRAM

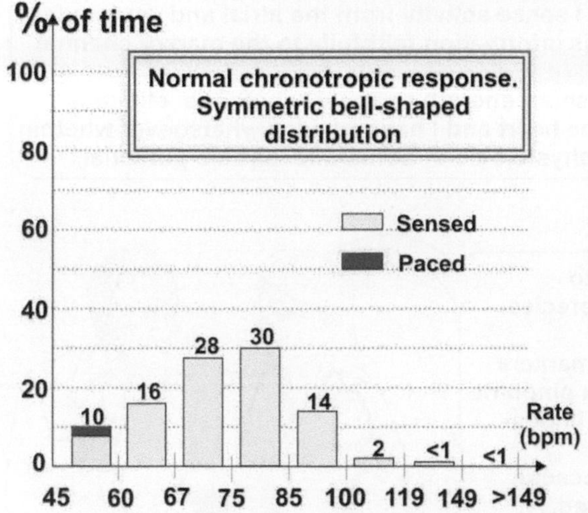

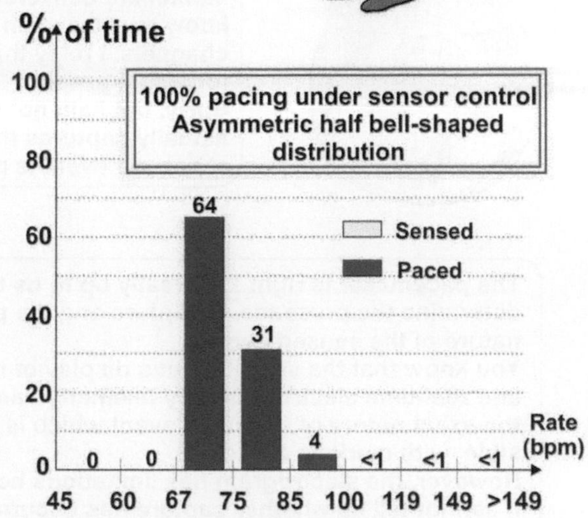

SENSOR INDICATED RATE HISTOGRAM

Such histograms are useful to determine whether the sensor is adjusted properly !
The histogram indicates the rate the pacemaker would be pacing if the patient were 100% paced.
If the spontaneous rate is faster than the sensor indicated rate and inhibits the pacemaker, this histogram is an underestimation of the actual heart rate.

A. F. Sinnaeve

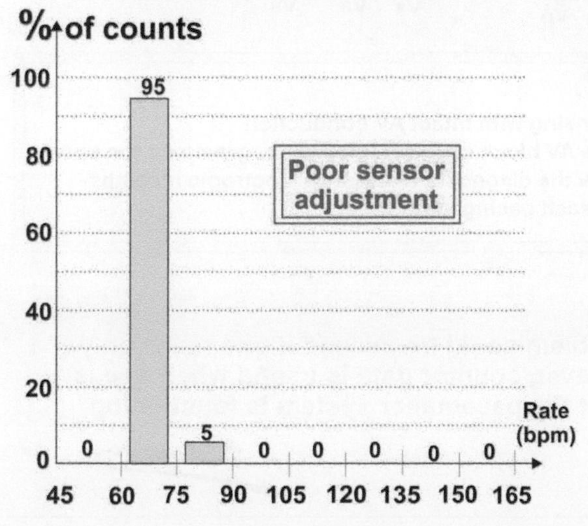

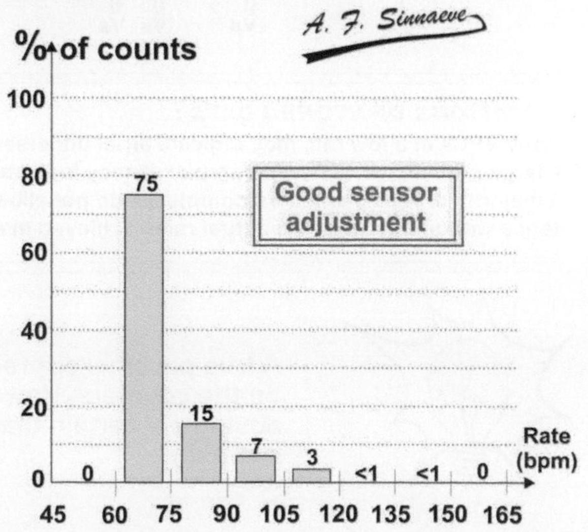

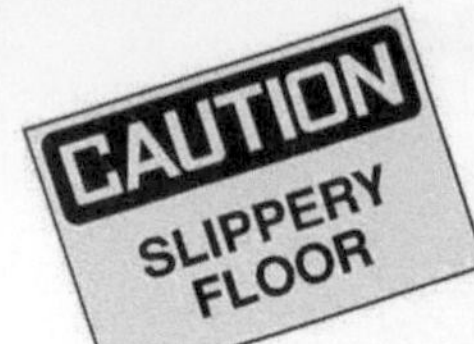

BEWARE OF STORED DATA IN THE PACEMAKER MEMORY

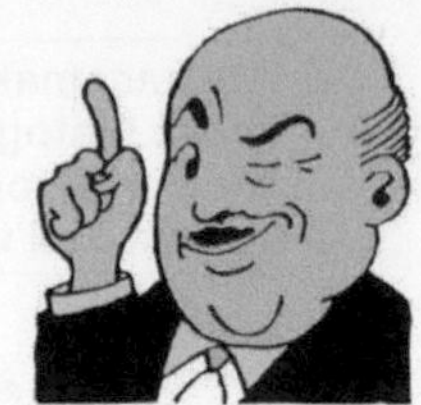

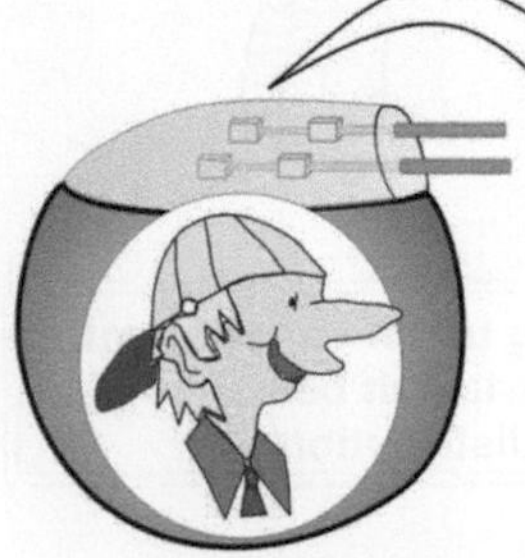

I am a very smart pacemaker because I can tell precisely when stimuli are delivered to the atrial and ventricular channels. I also know exactly when I sense activity from the atrial and ventricular channels. I relay this information faithfully to the marker channel for visual proof.
Sorry, but I am not smart enough to know whether a stimulus actually captures the heart and I have no idea whatsoever whether a sensed event is physiologic or some undesirable potential.

The pacemaker is right ! It's really up to us to determine the presence of capture and the precise nature of the sensed events.
You know that the simultaneous display of markers and real-time electrograms by telemetry can pinpoint the exact nature of a sensed event which is impossible with markers alone.
However, the electrogram has limitations because it cannot tell us whether capture has occurred.

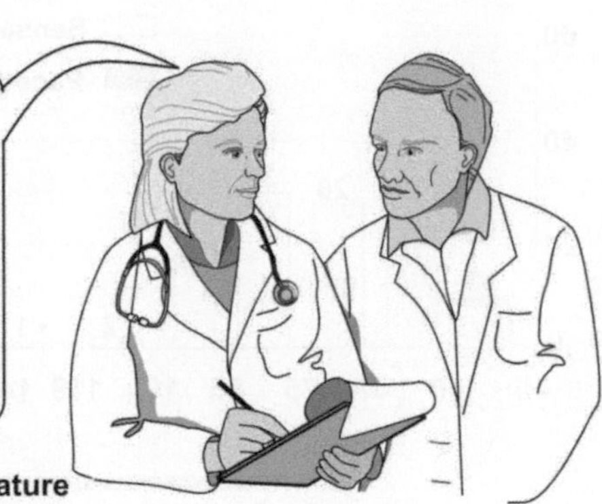

A simultaneously recorded electrogram might reveal the true nature of the oversensed signals : false signals from a defective lead? myopotentials? electromagnetic interference? etc.

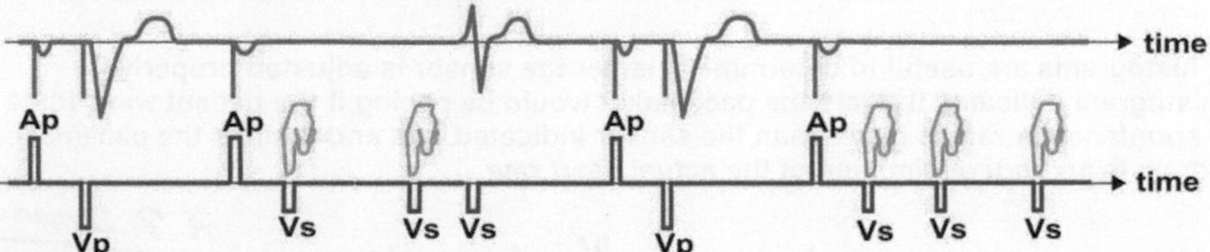

LIMITATIONS OF STORED DATA :

* Many VPCs at a low rate may indicate atrial undersensing with intact AV conduction
* A large percentage of As-Vp complexes may indicate AV block or an AV interval programmed too short
* A majority of Ap-Vp or Ap-Vs complexes do not allow the diagnosis of atrial chronotropic incompetence without knowing the actual rates achieved in each pacing state

A true pacemaker problem could be missed if one relies only on the counters. However, counter data is useful when one is absolutely certain that the pacemaker system is functioning normally.

A. F. Sinnaeve

PACEMAKER MEMORY : ARRHYTHMIAS & AUTOMATIC MODE SWITCHING - part 1

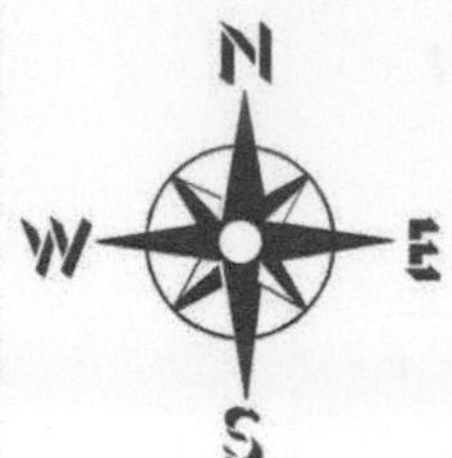

The *Medtronic Cardiac Compass* report provides up to 14 months of clinically significant significant data including AT/AF total hrs/day, ventricular rate during AT/AF (maximum/day and average/day), % atrial and ventricular pacing/day, ventricular rate (day and night separately), physical activity, and heart rate variability.
The examples below display only the relevant AT/AF data.

Asymptomatic AT/AF escaping - ECG documentation

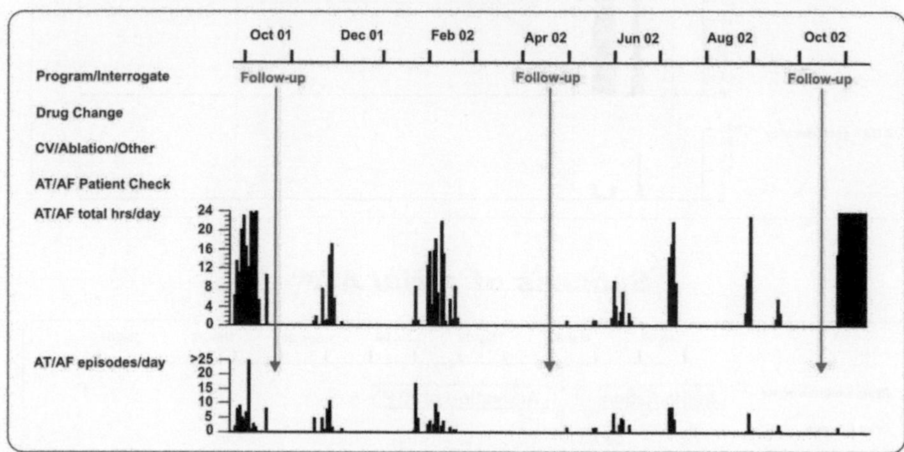

Antiarrhythmic drug efficacy

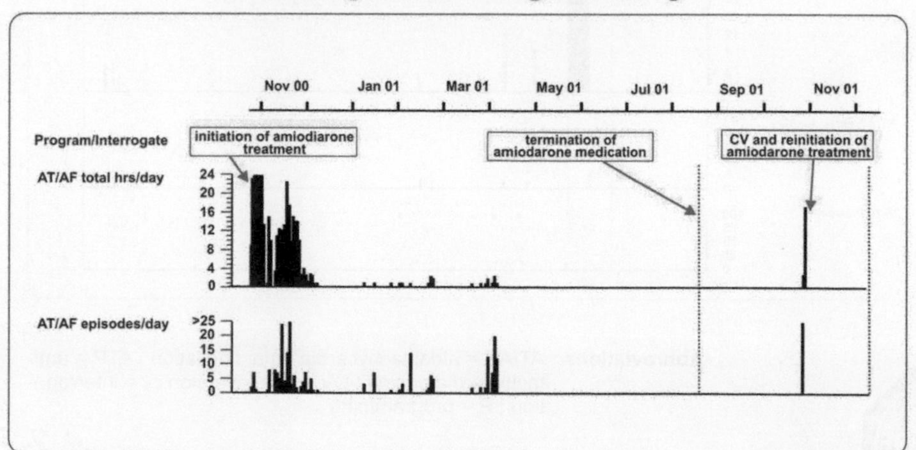

A. F. Sinnaeve

PACEMAKER MEMORY : ARRHYTHMIAS & AUTOMATIC MODE SWITCHING - part 2

Effect of isthmus ablation for the treatment of atrial flutter precipitating atrial fibrillation

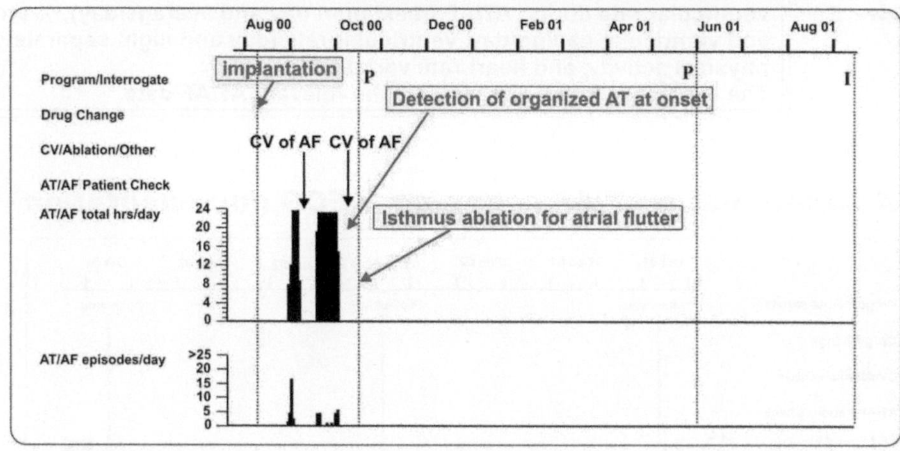

Success of atrial ATP

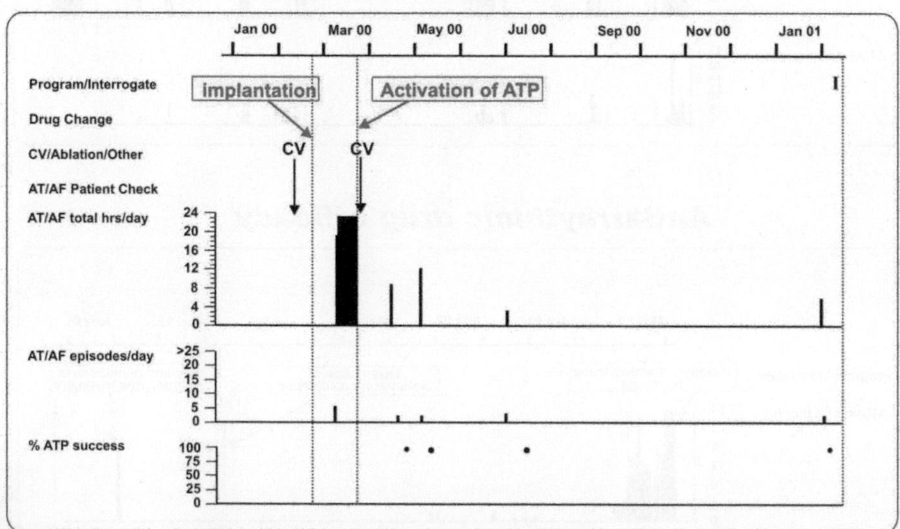

Abbreviations : AT/AF = atrial tachycardia/atrial fibrillation ; ATP = anti-tachycardia pacing ; CV = cardioversion ; I = interrogation ; P = programming ;

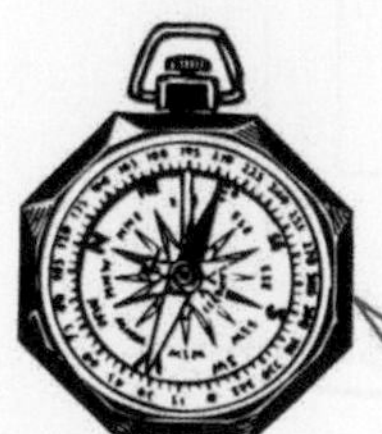

A. F. Sinnaeve

For good navigation, a good compass is needed !

PACEMAKER MEMORY : ARRHYTHMIAS & AUTOMATIC MODE SWITCHING - part 3

Medtronic arrhythmia report

Arrhythmia Summary : 02/11/06 to 08/21/06

Mode Switch Count	251 (0.5 hrs/day - 2.1%)	VHR Episodes	1
AHR Episode Trigger	Mode Switch > 30 sec	VHR Detection	180 ppm for 5 beats
AHR Episodes	204	VHR Termination	180 ppm for 5 beats
AHR Detection	175 bpm - No Delay	SVT Filter	On

Type		Date/Time	Duration hh:mm:ss	Rates (bpm) : Max A	Max V	Avg V	Sensor	EGM
VHR	Longest	08/15/06 5:32 PM	:11	87	256	180	60	Yes
AHR	First	07/08/06 10:04 AM	:16:28	400	90	87	77	No
AHR	Longest	08/15/06 2:39 PM	6:11:38	>400	87	83	80	No
AHR	Fastest	08/18/06 11:48 AM	3:06:40	>400	98	88	64	No
AHR		08/21/06 3:26 AM	:11:42	380	83	82	60	Yes
AHR		08/21/06 7:18 AM	2:36:51	>400	84	81	84	Yes
AHR	Last	08/21/06 1:25 PM	:31:07	400	93	85	81	Yes

V. Rate during Atrial Arrhythmias

VS □ VP ■

% of V. Beats: 50, 40, 30, 20, 10, 0

< 80 100 120 140 160 180 200 >

Ventricular Rate (bpm)

Atrial Arrhythmias

Duration	Count
=>72hr	0
24hr - <72hr	0
12hr - <24hr	0
4hr - <12hr	3
1hr - < 4hr	55
10min - < 1hr	84
1min - <10min	71
<1min	38
	251

Histograms showing data about automatic mode switching (St Jude)

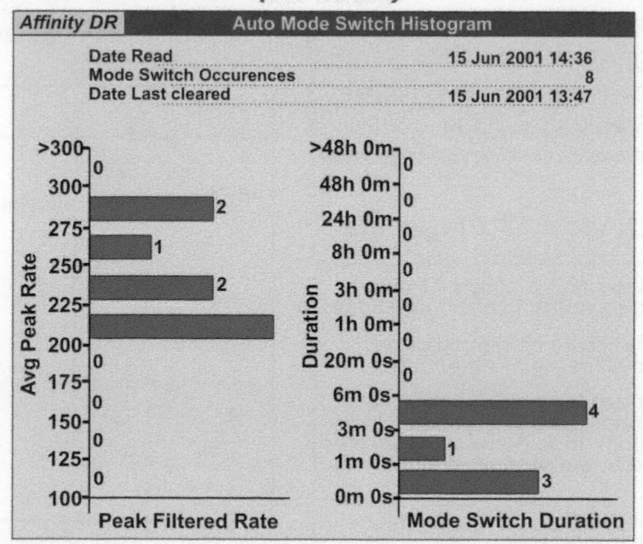

A. F. Sinnaeve

Abbreviations : AHR = atrial high rate ; EGM = electrogram ; SVT = supraventricular tachycardia ; V = ventricular ; VHR = ventricular high rate ; VP = ventricular paced event ; VS = ventricular sensed event ;

CLINICAL APPLICATION OF STORED ATRIAL EGMs

* Evaluation of pacemaker function
* Insights into the mechanisms and onset mechanisms of arrhythmias
* Prevention and termination of arrhythmias
* Patient triggered recordings
* Evaluation of treatment success (drugs, ablation, preventive & antitachycardia pacing)

Visual inspection of EGMs and markers gives rise to diagnosis in almost 100% of cases in contrast to the many misinterpretations by a device !

Pre- and Post-Trigger EGM storage **(Guidant Pulsar Max ™II Pulse Generator)**

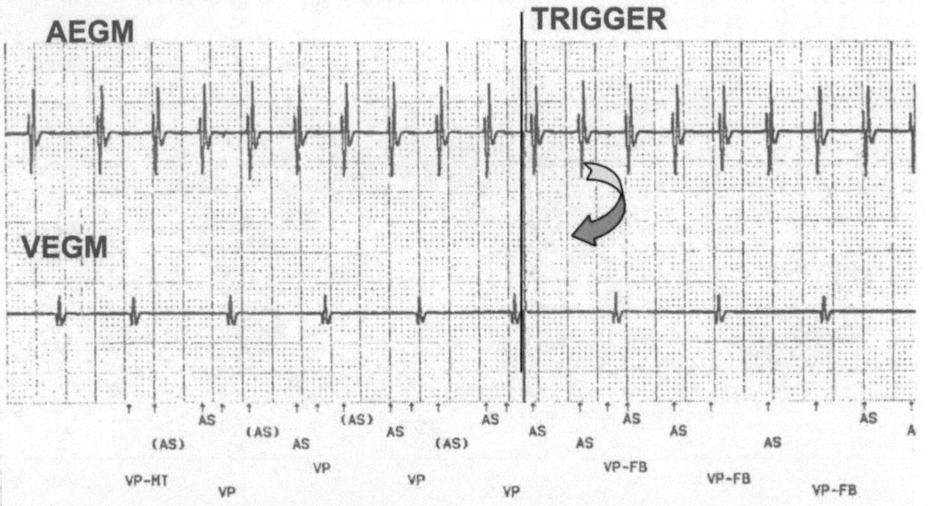

Factors influencing AT DETECTION

* The detection algorithm of the PM
* The signal and the programmed sensitivity
* Timing cycles : Blanking periods

Limitations of device AT Diagnosis

* Intermittent atrial sensing : a single AT episode will be stored as multiple short episodes
* Long postventricular atrial blanking period will cause 2:1 undersensing of atrial flutter
* AV nodal and reentrant tachycardias will be missed even with short blanking periods because A is too close to V. Atrial tachycardias can also be missed in the setting of a relatively long PR interval.
* Far-field sensing of the R wave. Better rejection algorithms are important

Undetected AV Nodal tachycardia

AEGM is in the postventricular atrial blanking period

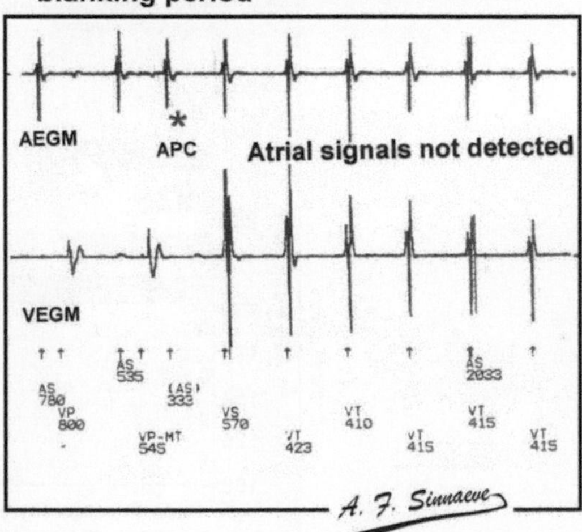

Abbreviations : AEGM = atrial electrogram ; APC = atrial premature complex ; AS = atrial sensed event ; AT = atrial tachycardia ; PM = pacemaker ; VEGM = ventricular electrogram ; VP = ventricular paced event ;

CLINICAL APPLICATION OF STORED ATRIAL EGMs part 2

Differential Diagnosis of device-detection of AT

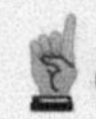 ***Correct AT detection***

 ***Inappropriate AT detection***

a) ventricular far-field oversensing
b) myopotential oversensing
c) EMI oversensing and lead fracture
d) P wave double counting
e) sinus tachycardia
f) runs of APCs
g) AT detection algorithm idiosyncrasies

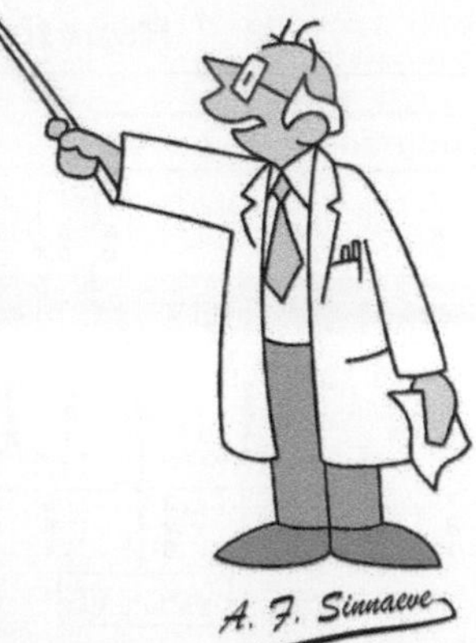

Atrial flutter with varying degree of AV block

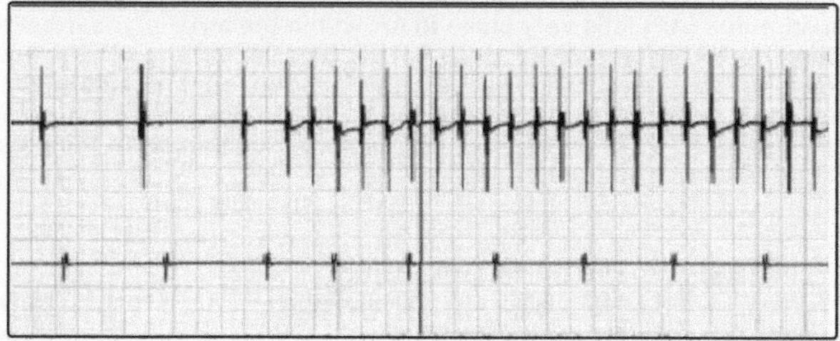

Rapid ventricular tachycardia

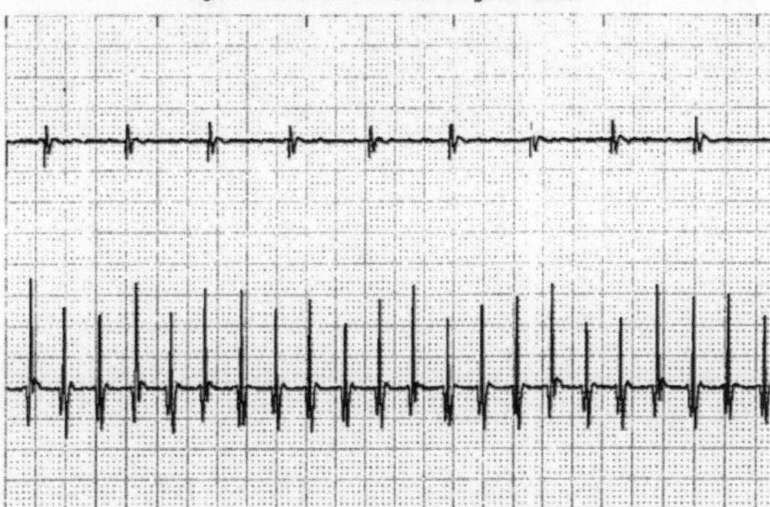

Abbreviations : AEGM = atrial electrogram; APC = atrial premature complex; AT = atrial tachycardia; EMI = electromagnetic interference; VEGM = ventricular electrogram;

THE VALUE OF STORED ELECTROGRAMS EXAMPLES - part 1

Repetitive nonreentrant VA synchrony

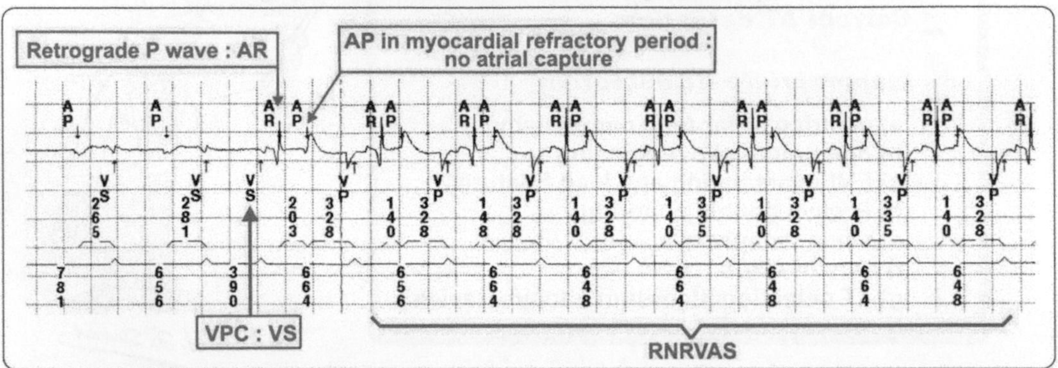

A VPC generates a retrograde P wave which falls in the PVARP and is labeled AR. The succeeding atrial stimulus (AP) falls very close to AR within the atrial myocardial refractory period generated by AR. Therefore, AP does not capture the atrium. AP is followed by VP which also gives rise to a retrograde P wave with a conduction time similar to that linked to the first retrograde P wave. AP is again delivered early and does not capture the atrium because it falls within the atrial myocardial refractory period related to the preceding AR. The process then becomes self-perpetuating.

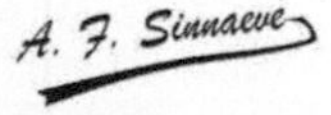

Termination of RNRVAS

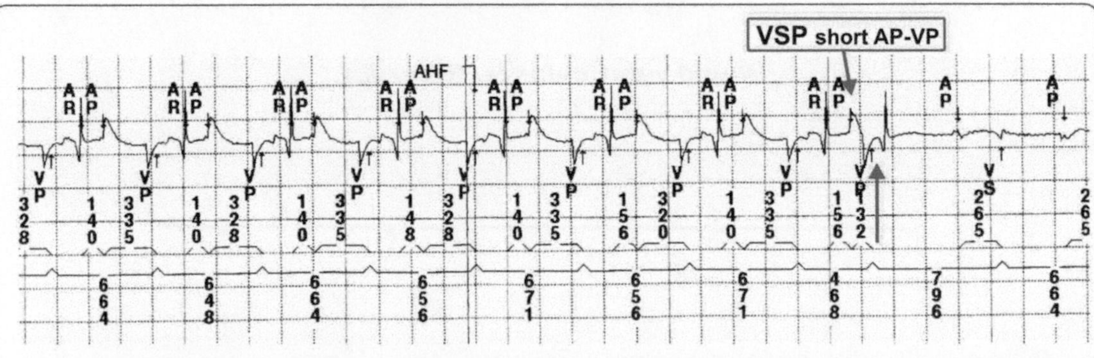

Abbreviated AP-VP from ventricular safety pacing (VSP) causes earlier emission of VP. This early VP also initiates a retrograde P wave. This retrograde P wave does not generate a marker as it seems to be in the postventricular atrial blanking period. The early timing of the retrograde P wave permits the following AP to capture the atrium and RNRVAS terminates.

Abbreviations : AP = atrial paced event ; AR = atrial event detected in the unblanked part of the refractory period ; VS = ventricular sensed event ; VP = ventricular paced event ; RNRVAS = repetitive nonreentrant VA synchrony ; VPC = ventricular premature complex ;

THE VALUE OF STORED ELECTROGRAMS EXAMPLES - part 2

Oversensing detected by inappropriate mode switching

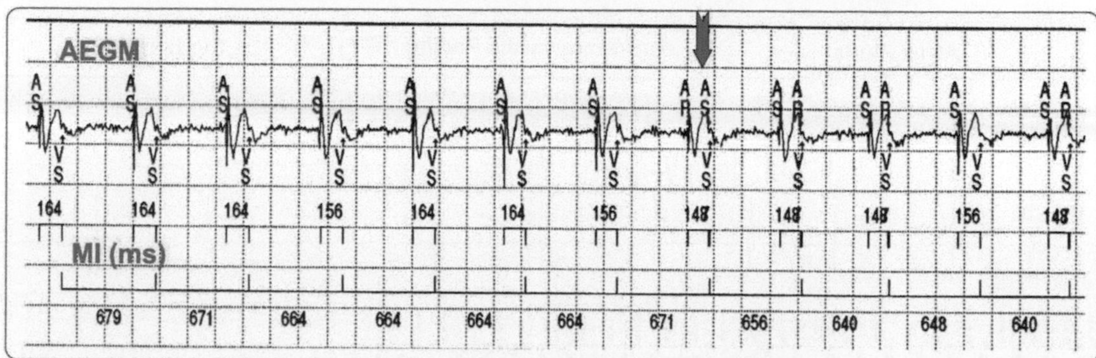

Inappropriate mode switching due to FFRW oversensing triggered by high atrial sensitivity. This is an example of pre-ventricular far-field sensing by the atrial channel. Automatic mode switching will occur in devices that respond to long-short cycle sequences for AMS activation. Note that the atrial channel sensed the far-field R wave before the ventricular channel sensed the R wave as a near-field signal.

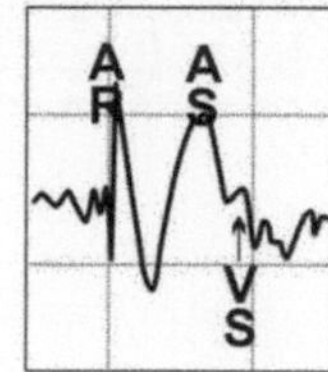

Far-field oversensing causing AMS in a St Jude pacemaker

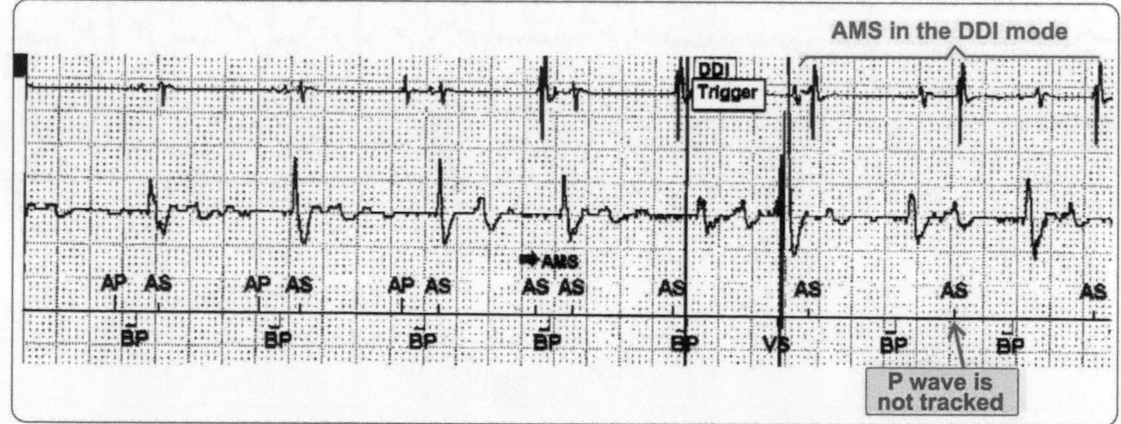

In this annotation, atrial signals sensed in the PVARP are labeled AS. The atrial channel senses the far-field R wave. The sequences of long-short cycles induce AMS in this device.

A. F. Sinnaeve

Abbreviations : AMS = automatic mode switching ; AP = atrial paced event ; AR = atrial refractory sensed signals within the unblanked terminal portion of the AV delay ; AS = atrial sensed event ; BP = biventricular pacing ; FFRW = far-field R wave ; VS = ventricular sensed event ;

THE VALUE OF STORED ELECTROGRAMS EXAMPLES - part 3

Successful atrial ATP

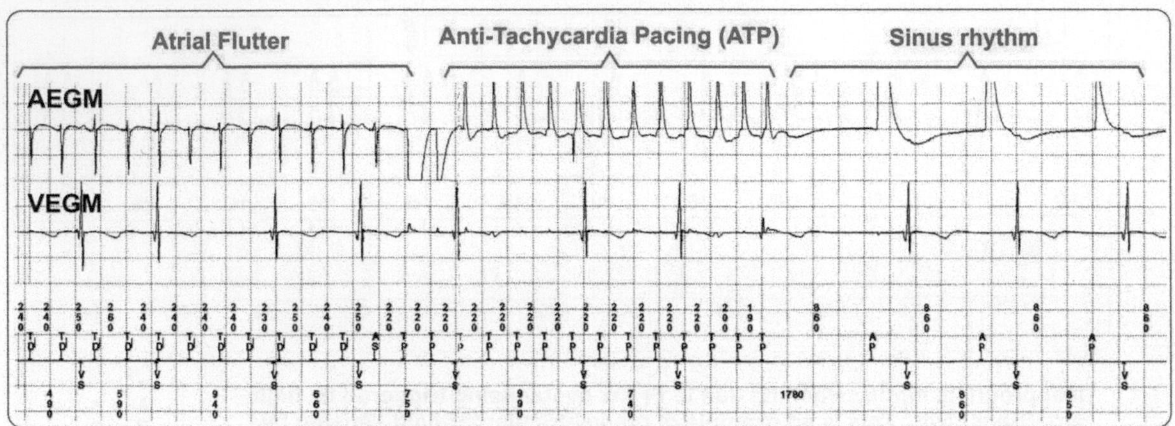

Inappropriate VT detection due to ventricular oversensing by myopotentials

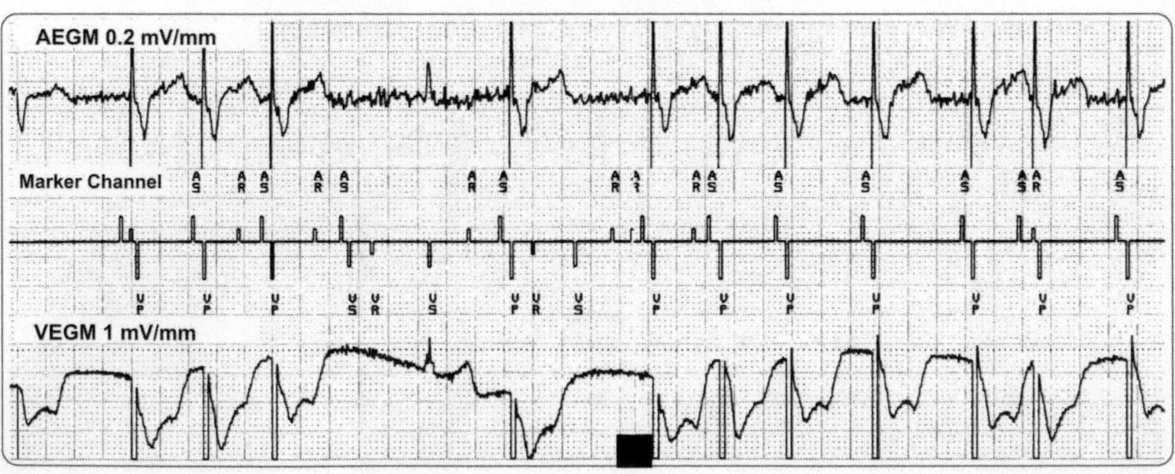

A. F. Sinnaeve

Abbreviations : AP = atrial paced event ; AR = atrial event detected during the unblanked part of the refractory period ; AS = atrial sensed event ; TD = tachycardia detected ; TP = tachycardia pacing ; VF = ICD ventricular fibrillation cycle ; VP = ventricular paced event ; VS = ventricular sensed event ;

AUTOMATIC CAPTURE VERIFICATION - part 1

Capture verification systems promote safety by increasing the pacemaker output during unexpected rises in pacing threshoild

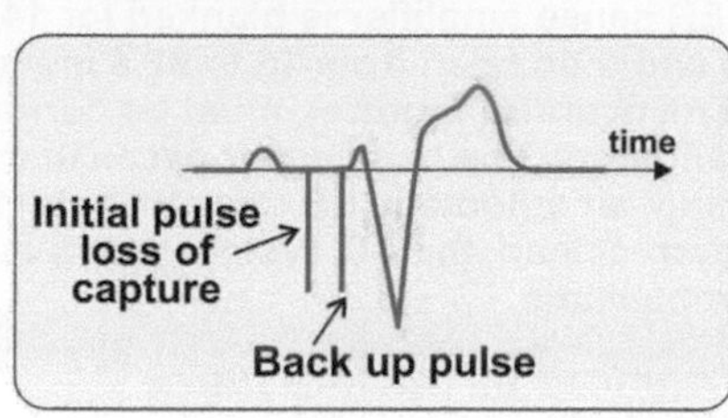

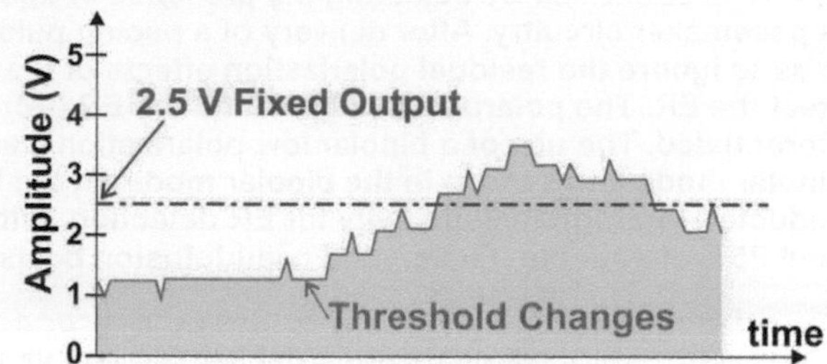

Capture is confirmed by detecting the presence or absence of an evoked reponse potential by the pacemaker circuitry. Systems with automatic capture recognition increase safety, reduce current drain from the battery and increase device longevity.

Detection of evoked potential indicating capture

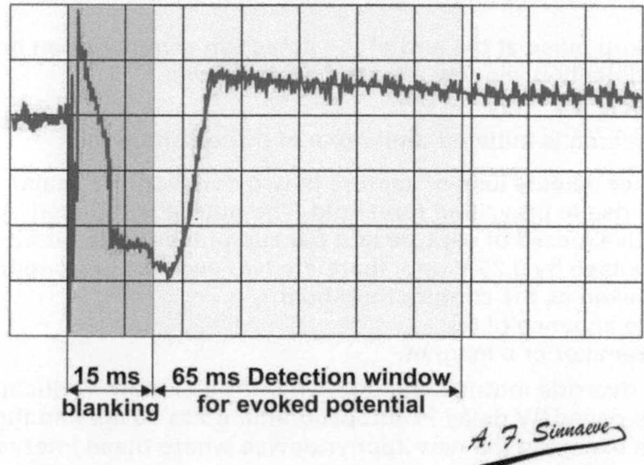

If capture is not confirmed, a backup pulse is delivered at the end of the detection window

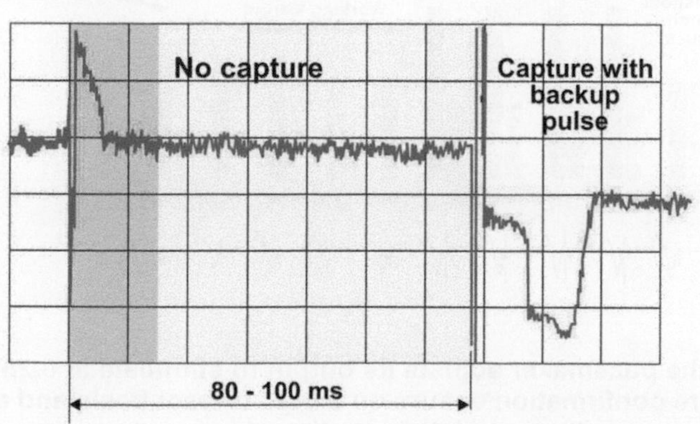

Evoked response sensing can be affected by :

*** Lead - tissue interface (acute vs. chronic lead).**
*** Lead polarization responsible for the use of low polarization leads in the traditional "Autocapture" function of St Jude pacemakers which was the first system released commercially.**
*** Tip-to-ring spacing.**
*** Lead tip design.**
*** Other factor.**

Traditional St Jude Autocapture

"Autocapture" (AC) is a proprietary algorithm developed by St Jude Medical, Sylmar, CA, USA, that was the first to commercially provide these automatic functions in a single chamber pacemaker.
It requires a bipolar low polarization lead.
The AC algorithm comprises four fully automatic pacemaker functions:

1. **Capture confirmation.**
2. **Backup high voltage pulse in case of loss of capture.**
3. **Threshold search and documentation.**
4. **Output regulation**

AUTOMATIC CAPTURE VERIFICATION - part 2

St Jude Traditional Autocapture - Continued

Capture Confirmation

Capture is confirmed by detecting the presence or absence of an evoked response (ER) potential by the pacemaker circuitry. After delivery of a pacing pulse, the ER sense amplifier is blanked for 14 ms (so as to ignore the residual polarization effects of the pulse) and then open from 15 to 62.5 ms to detect the ER. The polarization signal, and the ER (from local myocardial capture), must be correctly differentiated. The use of a bipolar low polarization lead is mandatory. The pacemaker paces in the unipolar mode and senses in the bipolar mode. At the beginning, an automatic ER sensitivity test is conducted to program sensitivity for ER detection. With the correct lead, the AC system works in about 95% of patients. Fusion and pseudofusion beats are problematic.

Unsuccessful stimulus followed by successful capture by backup pulse
(all beats are atrial sensed and ventricular paced)

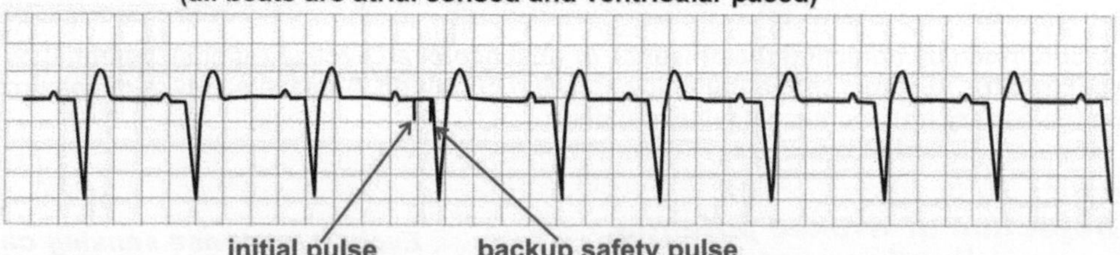

Backup pulse after loss of capture

The pacemaker delivers a 4.5 V / 0.49 ms backup pulse at the end of the detection window when no ER signal is detected within the 15 - 62.5 ms detection window after the pacing pulse.

Threshold search

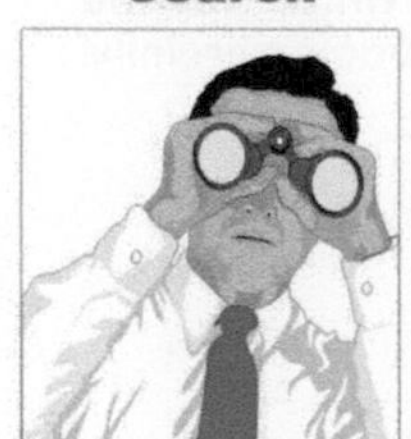

An automatic threshold search is initiated under one of three conditions :

a. Whenever the pacemaker detects loss of capture in two consecutive beats, which it interprets as a rise in prevailing threshold. The output is reduced by 0.25 V till two consecutive losses of capture and backup pulses are emitted. The output is then increased by 0.25 V until there are two consecutive capture confirmations. This is taken as the capture threshold.
b. Every eight hours in the absence of (a).
c. Manually using a programmer or a magnet.

Fusion management : To override intrinsic conduction during capture verification and threshold search, the paced AV delay is autoprogrammed to 50 ms and the sensed AV delay to 25 ms except in the new Zephyr device where these intervals are programmable (50/25, 100/70, 120/100). The programmed settings are restored after the search is complete.

Function of the St Jude algorithm

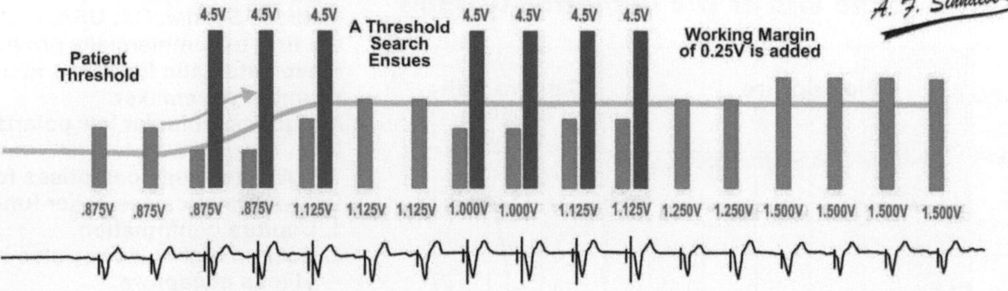

Output Regulation

After determination of the threshold, the pacemaker adjusts its output to stimulate at 0.25V above the prevailing threshold. Capture confirmation occurs on a beat-to-beat basis and a backup pulse, threshold determination and output regulation continue to operate.

AUTOMATIC CAPTURE VERIFICATION with unipolar or bipolar non-low polarization leads

New technology now permits ventricular detection of the evoked potential for automatic capture verification without the need for special leads.
This technology is available in devices from Medtronic, St Jude and Boston Scientific. In the case of St Jude the pacemaker offers a choice between the traditional Autocapture system (with a long track record of reliability) which requires a special lead, and the new system which offers this function with a choice of a large variety of leads.
The Boston Scientific and St Jude systems both work on a beat-to-beat basis, but the Medtronic system does not.

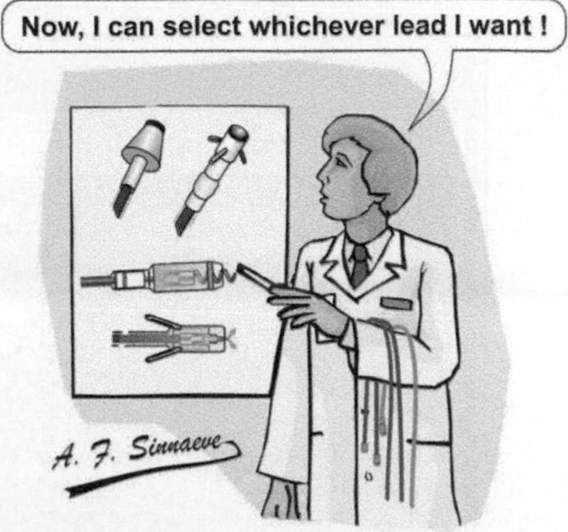

Now, I can select whichever lead I want !
A. F. Sinnaeve

Medtronic Capture

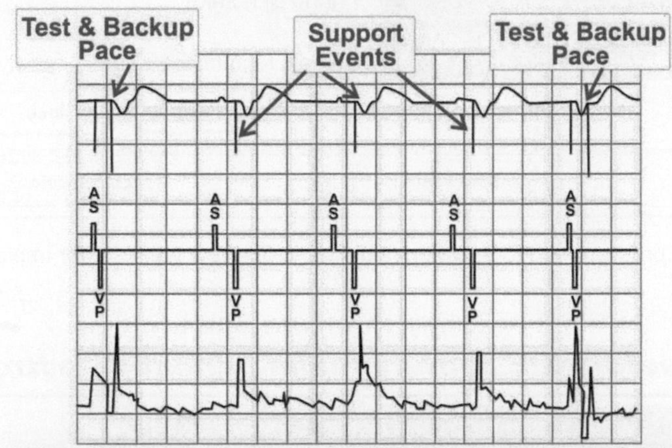

The test pulse is associated with shortening of the AV delay *A. F. Sinnaeve*

The Medtronic Capture verification system does not require a special lead or polarity. It automatically monitors pacing thresholds only at periodic intervals such as once a day. Once the threshold is determined, the pacemaker determines a target output based on a programmable safety margin (usually 2:1 in terms of voltage) and a programmable minimum amplitude.

* The *support cycles* are pacing cycles at the programmed amplitude and pulse width that may or may not include ventricular paced events. The pacing threshold search begins with the support cycles.
* A *test pace* follows each set of support cycles and is delivered at a test amplitude or pulse width.
* A *backup pace* automatically follows each test pace regardless of capture or loss-of-capture for that pace. It is delivered 110 ms after the test pace at the programmed amplitude and a 1.0 ms pulse width setting.
  The pacemaker may use one to three of the test paces in a series to determine if a particular amplitude or pulse width is above or below the patient's stimulation threshold.
* When the first of the three test paces indicates capture, or the last two test paces indicate capture following loss-of-capture on the first pace, the series is determined to be above the threshold.
* When two of the three test paces indicate loss-of-capture, the series is determined to be below the threshold.

AUTOMATIC CAPTURE VERIFICATION with unipolar or bipolar non-low polarization leads - 2

Capture management trend : Medtronic

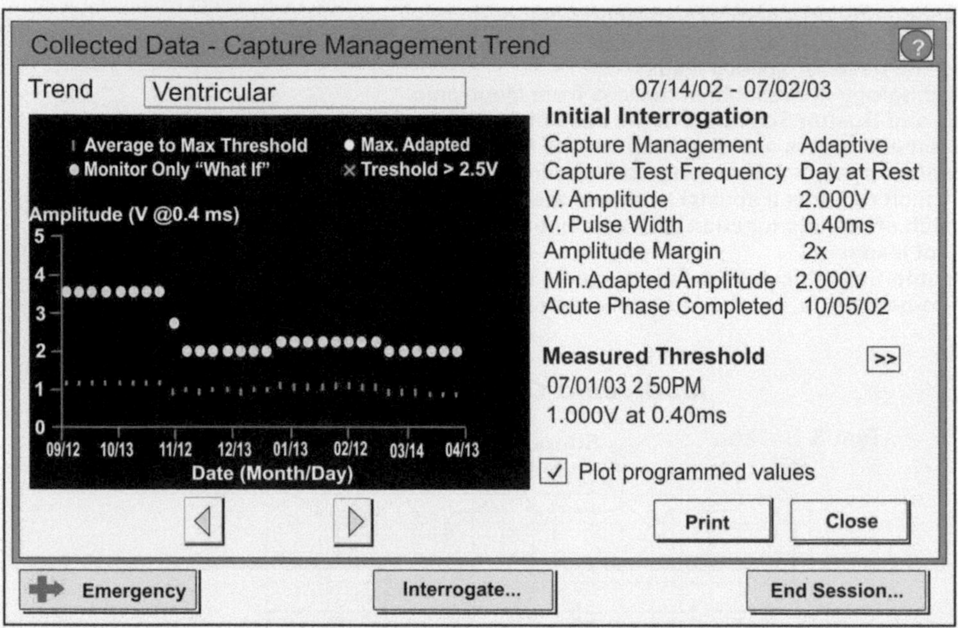

The adapted voltage was programmed to a higher value in the first few weeks after implantation

A. F. Sinnaeve

Programming automatic capture management : Medtronic

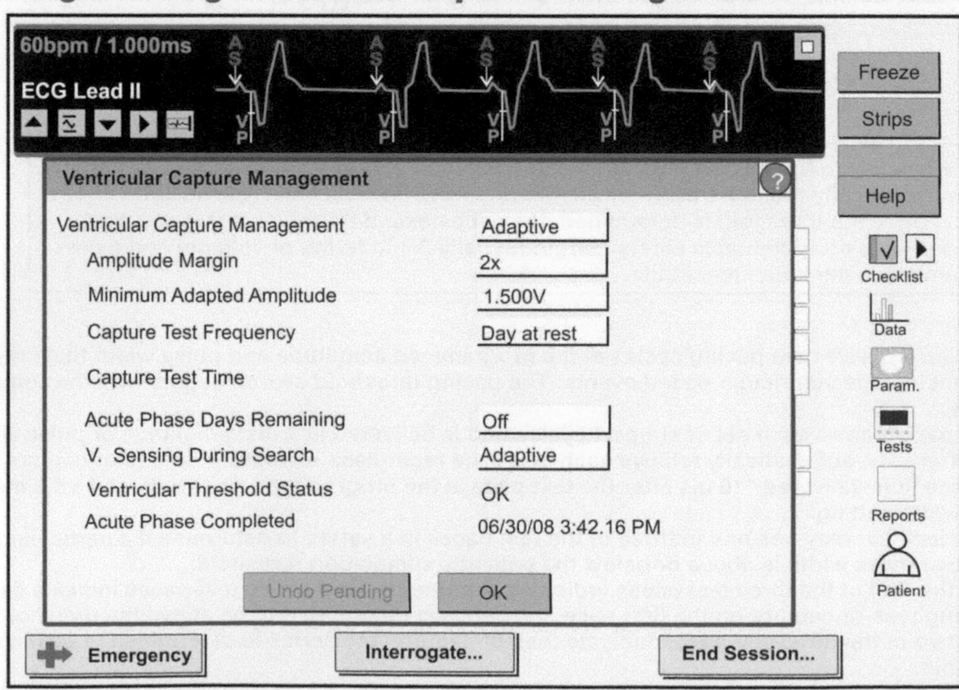

ATRIAL CAPTURE MANAGEMENT : MEDTRONIC

The Medtronic Atrial Capture Management does not use sensing of the evoked response to determine capture. The pacemaker determines the threshold by monitoring the effect of test pacing pulses in the atrium in one of two ways :

1. **Observing whether the captured atrial test paces reset the sinus node and the timing of P-P interval of the underlying sinus rhythm (Atrial Chamber Reset Method).**
2. **Observing the ventricular response to determine if the test paced events are conducted via the AV node (AV Conduction Method)**

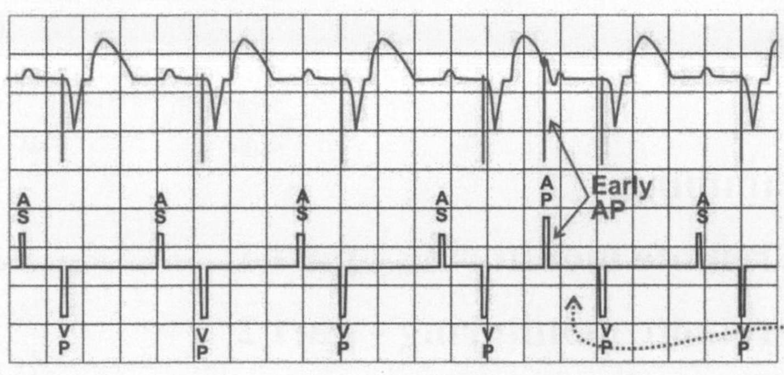

Atrial Chamber Reset Method

Capture occurs when the sinus node is reset by a test pacing pulse.

There is no AR in the AP-VP interval. The sinus node is reset. This indicates successful atrial capture by AP.

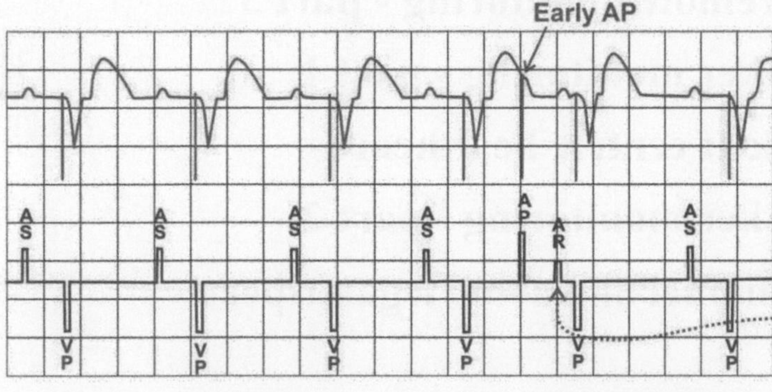

Atrial Chamber Reset Method

There is an AR marker in the AP-VP interval. The sinus node is not reset. This indicates unsuccessful atrial capture by AP.

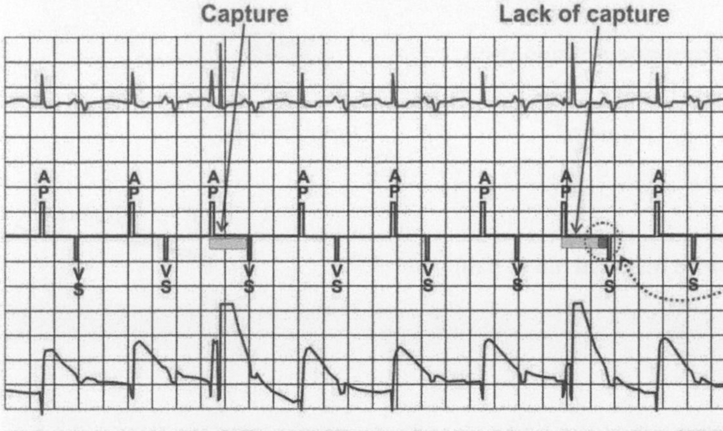

Ventricular Conduction method

This method relies on intrinsic AV conduction

prolongation of 70 ms indicating loss of capture

A. F. Sinnaeve

A backup pulse is delivered 70 ms after a test pacing pulse. With loss of atrial capture on the right, only the backup pulse is effectual so that conducted VS is delayed by 70 ms from the test pulse compared to the test on the left where the AP-VS interval with successful capture by AP is 70 ms less than on the right.

Abbreviations : AP = atrial paced event ; AR = atrial event sensed during refractory period ; AS = atrial sensed event ; VP = ventricular paced event ; VS = ventricular sensed event ;

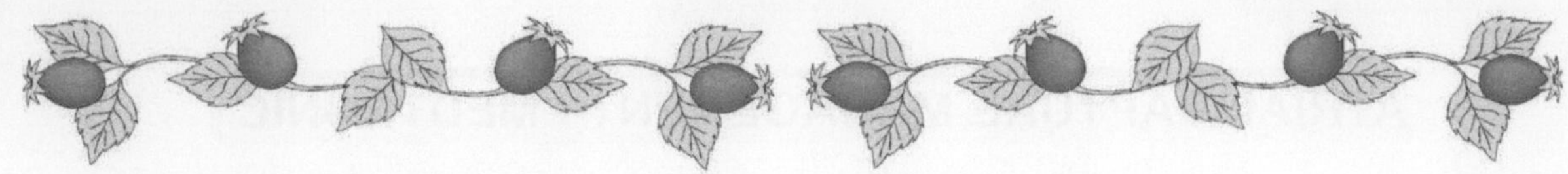

REMOTE PACEMAKER MONITORING

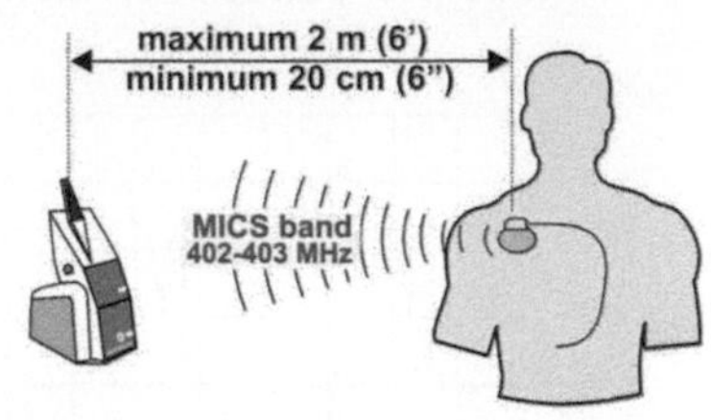

* Wireless programming
* Internet-based remote monitoring - part 1
* Internet-based remote monitoring - part 2
* Internet-based remote monitoring - part 3
* Remote pacemaker monitoring - part 1
  benefits of patient centric healthcare
* Remote pacemaker monitoring - part 2
  organizational model and some legal aspects

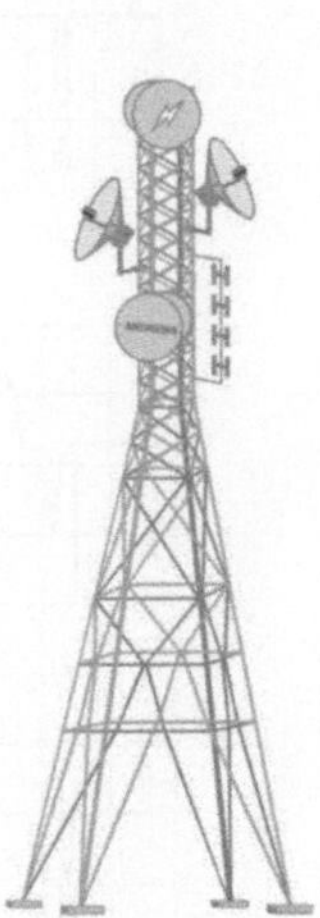

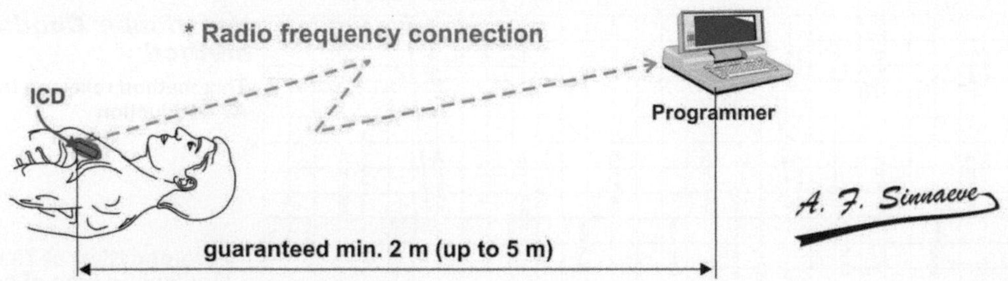

A. F. Sinnaeve

WIRELESS PROGRAMMING

A wireless programmer is easier to handle and less cumbersome. It gives greater speed and even added security and safety !

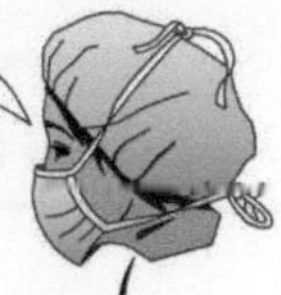

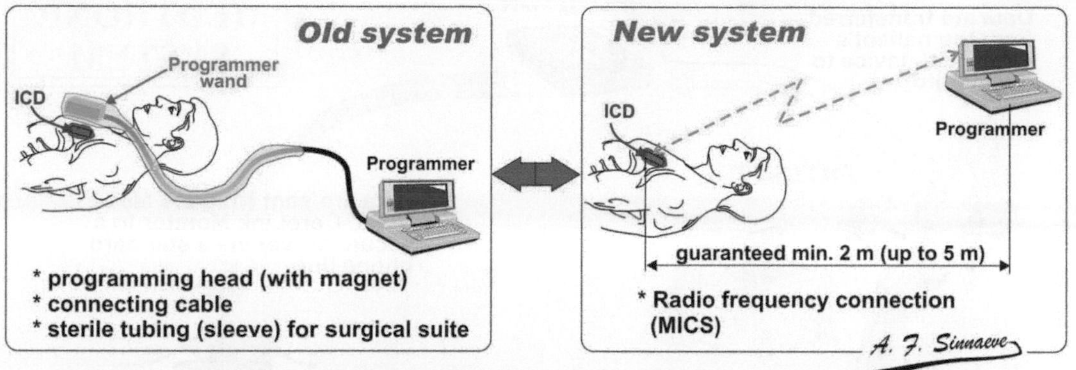

Advantages : * More convenient (less infections, no more sterile sleeves, physician can close wound while the device is being programmed at a distance)
* Faster retrieval of data
* Device optimization during follow-up (treadmill testing, etc.)

MICS (Medical Implant Communications System)

★ Special frequency band approved by FCC (Federal Communications Commission); also known as "Medical Device Radiocommunications Service" or as "MedRadio".

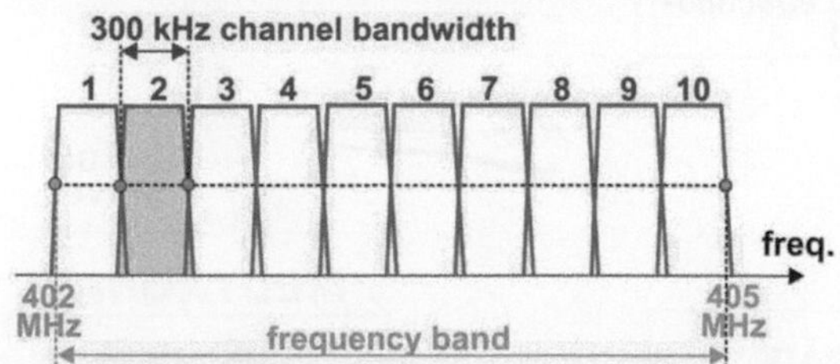

* the MICS frequency band operates from 402 MHz to 405 MHz and is conducive to transmitting radio signals in the human body
* effective isotropic radiated power max. 25 μW
* 10 channels are available with a max. bandwidth of 300 kHz
* no voice transmission is allowed
* the *Medtronic* application of MICS is called *"Conexus Wireless Telemetry"* and works with the latest devices

★ To extend the operating life of the battery, an ultra low-power RF transceiver is applied and a wake-up mode of operation is used.

* the transceiver inside the ICD is normally "asleep" and its current drain from the battery is extremely small (less than 1 μA)
* a handheld *activator* is used to "wake-up" the circuit and to enable the communication with the programmer

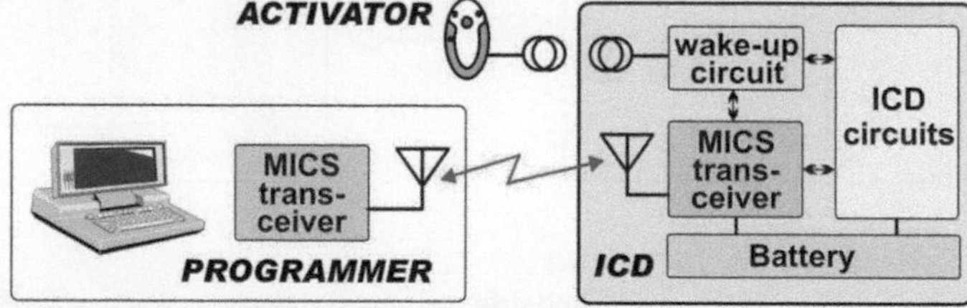

★ To avoid interference, the system scans all 10 channels in the MICS band prior to establishing a telemetry session. The channel with the lowest ambient signal level (i.e. the least noisy channel) or the first channel with an ambient level below a certain threshold, will be chosen for the telemetry session (LBT = Listen Before Talk).
Medtronic uses *"Smart Radio"*, a protocol that chooses the least interfered channel for its "Conexus Wireless Telemetry". This protocol allows multiple simultaneous programming sessions to be collected without interference.

NOTE :
1. An initial handshake with the programmer wand is needed to activate the telemetry.
2. The "Invisi-Link" Wireless Telemetry (St Jude Medical) also uses the 402-405 MHz frequency band.
3. Boston Scientific (Guidant) has a similar system called "ZIP wandless telemetry", working in the ISM band at 914 MHz (USA) or 869.85 MHz (Europe). (ISM : Industrial-Scientific-Medical).

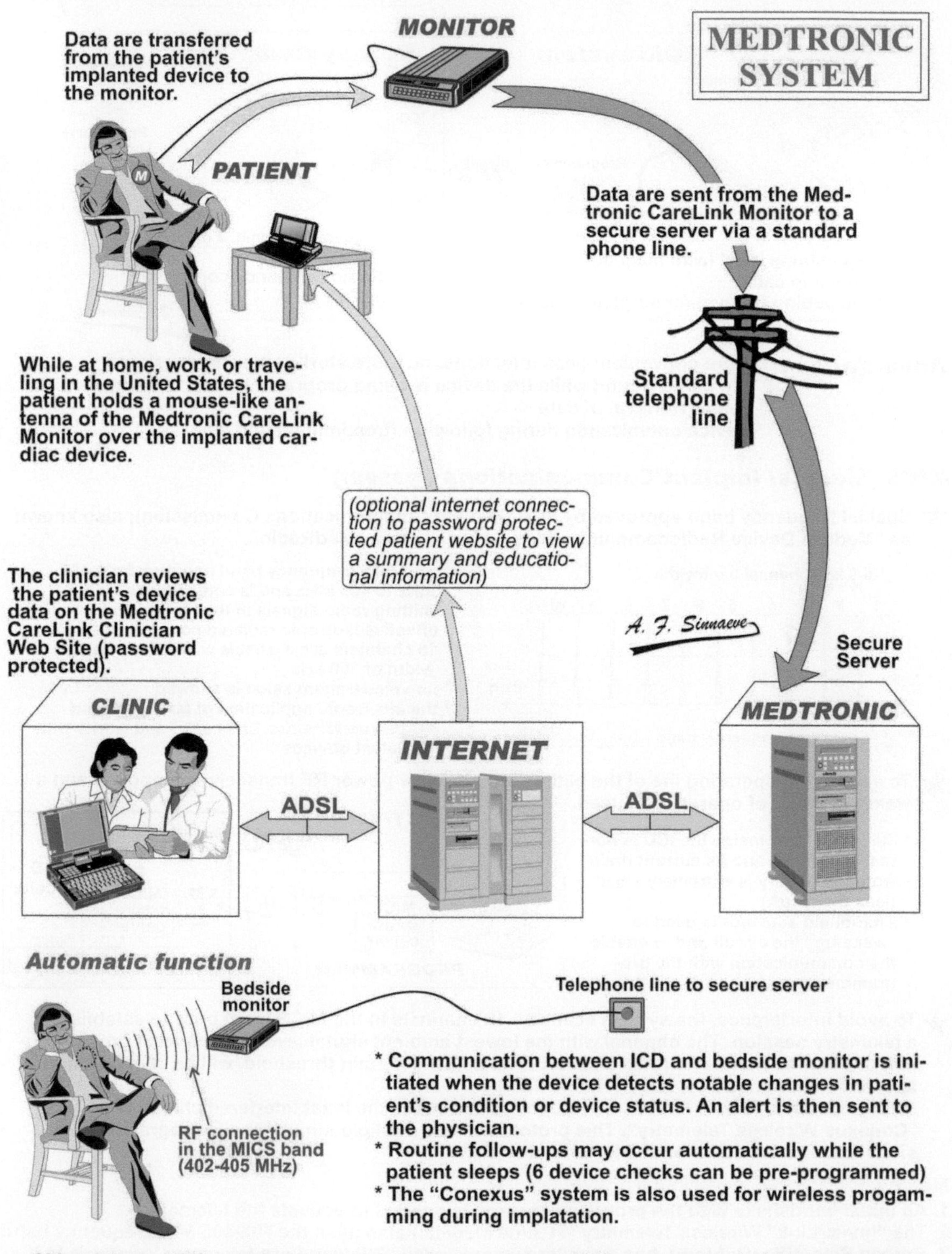
INTERNET-BASED REMOTE MONITORING OF ICDs - 1
MEDTRONIC SYSTEM
MONITOR
Data are transferred from the patient's implanted device to the monitor.
PATIENT
Data are sent from the Medtronic CareLink Monitor to a secure server via a standard phone line.
While at home, work, or traveling in the United States, the patient holds a mouse-like antenna of the Medtronic CareLink Monitor over the implanted cardiac device.
Standard telephone line
(optional internet connection to password protected patient website to view a summary and educational information)
The clinician reviews the patient's device data on the Medtronic CareLink Clinician Web Site (password protected).
A. F. Sinnaeve
Secure Server
CLINIC
INTERNET
MEDTRONIC
ADSL
ADSL
Automatic function
Bedside monitor
Telephone line to secure server
* Communication between ICD and bedside monitor is initiated when the device detects notable changes in patient's condition or device status. An alert is then sent to the physician.
* Routine follow-ups may occur automatically while the patient sleeps (6 device checks can be pre-programmed)
* The "Conexus" system is also used for wireless progamming during implatation.
RF connection in the MICS band (402-405 MHz)
Abbreviatons : MICS = medical implant communications system ; ADSL = asymmetric digital subscriber line

INTERNET-BASED REMOTE MONITORING OF ICDs - 2

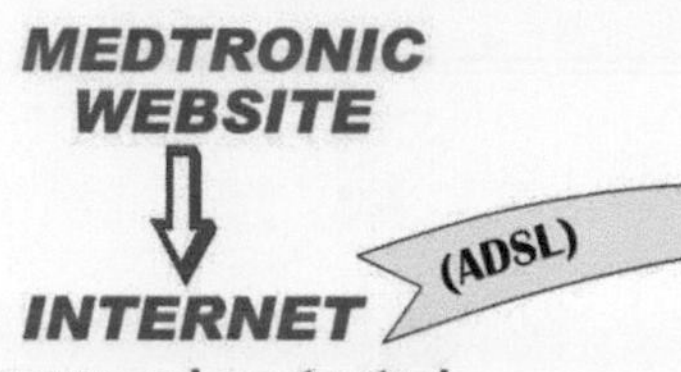

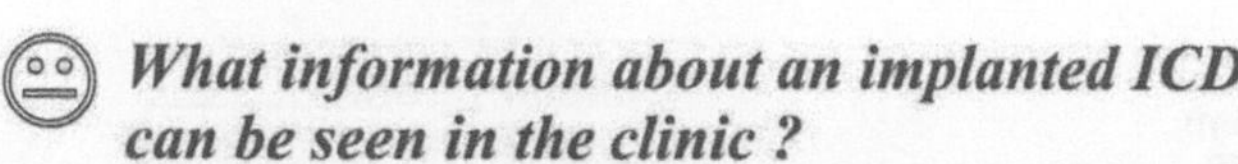

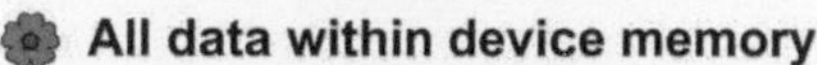

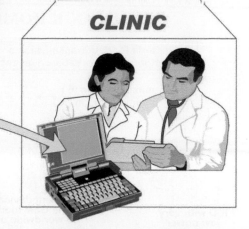

A. F. Sinnaeve

What information about an implanted ICD can be seen in the clinic ?

- **All data within device memory**
  - * **patient parameters**
  - * **device parameters (ICD status, lead information, ...)**
  - * **stored episodes (VF - FVT - VT - SVT - NST - mode switch - % pacing - ...)**
- **All diagnostics**
  - * **stored intracardiac electrograms**
  - * **10 seconds real-time electrogram of presenting rhythm**

What cannot be done by the remote monitoring ?

- **Direct communication with and interrogation of the ICD is impossible.**
- **Transtelephonic reprogramming of the device is not a present reality.**

What are the advantages ?

- **Remote follow-up is easy to use and convenient for the patient as it may reduce the frequency of clinic visits.**
- **The remote follow-up provides the clinician with the same information that is available at an office visit used to assess the appropriateness of device therapies and operation.**
- **Internet-based follow-up may serve as a triage tool to determine which patients need further medical attention.**
- **The tremendous wealth of physiological data collected by implanted devices may also be important in the discovery of undocumented and asymptomatic arrhythmias, new disease processes, and the management of chronic diseases including drug initiation and titration.**
- **Remote follow-up offers an alternative for the overcrowded and overwhelmed clinics.**

INTERNET-BASED REMOTE MONITORING OF ICDs - 3

BIOTRONIK HOME MONITORING SYSTEM

The criteria for data transmission are entirely programmable by the clinician, allowing for customized reports based on each patients needs.

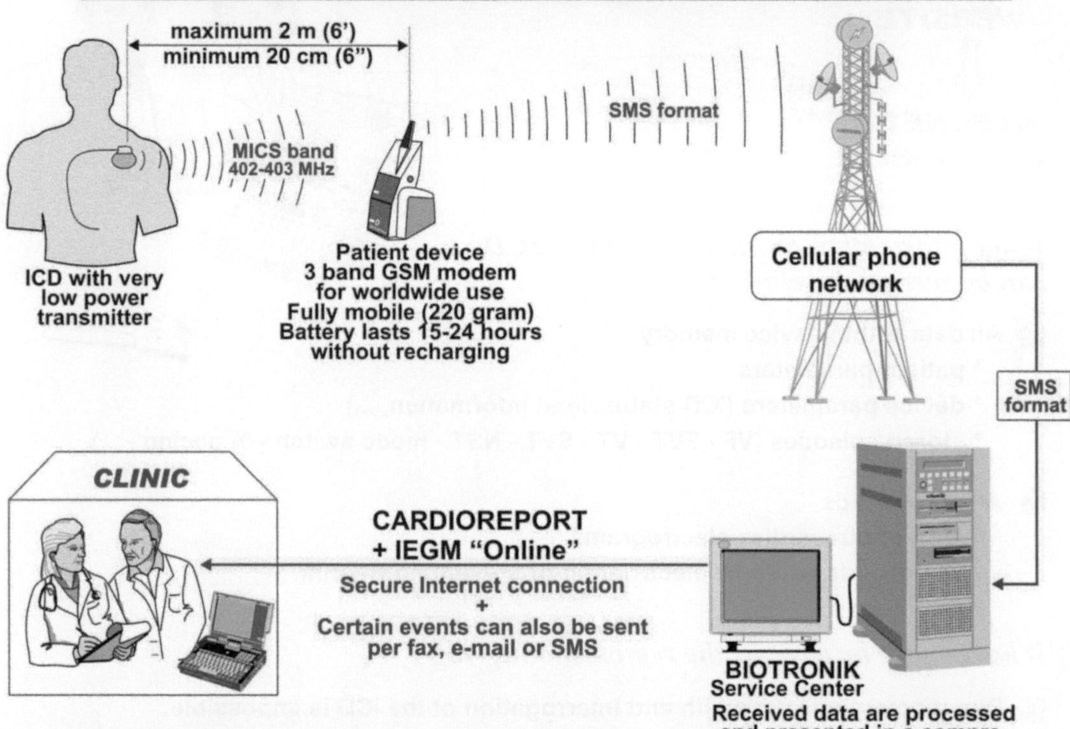

The use of daily "Home Monitoring" communication may shorten the device battery life for max. 2 months (conservative estimate assuming daily transmission through "Cardio Messenger", occasional event reports and 12 IEGMs per year)

Trend Reports

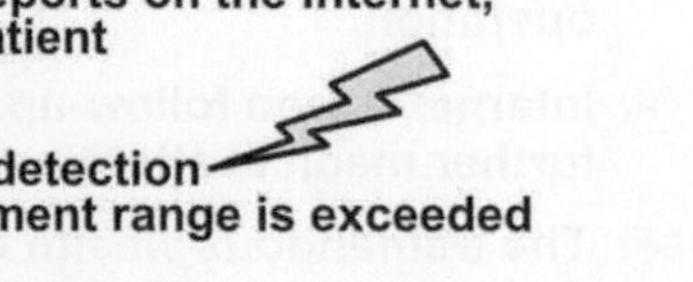

* **Time controlled transmission (any time between 0:00 and 23:50) (recommended between 0:00 and 4:00 while the patient is asleep)**
* **Monitoring interval : 1 day**
* **Data are presented in graphs and tables. When viewing reports on the internet, Cardio Reports can be individually configured for each patient**

Event Reports

* **Event controlled messages are sent upon termination of detection**
* **Event triggered messages are also sent when a measurement range is exceeded**

Home Monitoring Scope of Functions

* **Monitoring system integrity**
  - **Battery status, battery voltage**
  - **Detection and therapy activation**
* **Monitoring lead integrity**
  - **Atrial and ventricular pacing impedances**
  - **Shock impedance**
* **Bradycardia & tachycardia rhythm and therapy monitoring**
  - **Sensing/pacing counters**
  - **Detected episodes**
  - **SVT frequency**
  - **Delivered therapies**
  - **Success of ATPs & shocks**

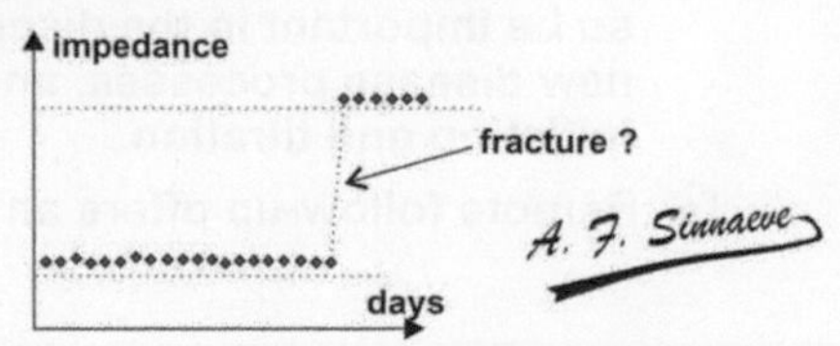

Abbreviations : ATP = antitachycardia pacing; GSM = global system for mobile communications; IEGM = internal electrogram; MICS = medical implant communications system; SMS = short message service; SVT = supraventricular tachycardia

REMOTE PACEMAKER MONITORING - 1

Healthcare is changing to patient centric

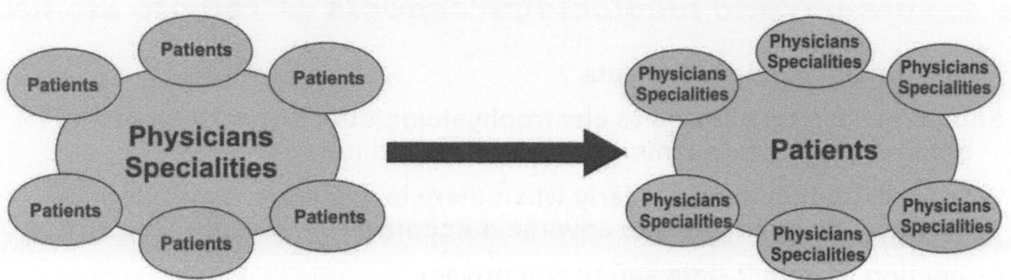

Physicians could be anywhere

Remote patient monitoring and body sensor networks will be key drivers of patient centric healthcare

Why is remote monitoring of pacemakers important ?

- **Large and growing number of patients can no longer be accommodated in an outpatient setting.**
- **Better and more efficient patient care at lower costs.**

Benefits of remote pacemaker monitoring

- **Ability to obtain an earlier diagnosis (and management) of abnormal events.**
- **Increased safety.**
- **Lower costs.**
- **Reduced follow-up costs (by saving on transportation cost, particularly when the distance between home and medical facility is >75 miles).**
- **Patients have expressed a high degree of satisfaction with the convenience and ease of use of remote monitoring.**
- **Emergency room visits : data can be relayed to a remotely located cardiologist or electrophysiologist.**
- **Proactive device and medical therapy : this eliminates the need for unwarranted trips to the emergency room and device clinic, which alleviates anxiety because of prompt response to patients concerns**

Other benefits of remote pacemaker monitoring

- **Frequent clinician visits have a negative impact on some patients' ability to hold down a job, go on holiday, and even spend time with their family.**
- **The facilitation of a remote service will free up time to improve the patient's quality of life, and provide more choice and flexibility.**
- **Peace of mind that comes from knowing that expert care is only a "(cellular) phone call" away. However, some systems only work with a land line.**

Pacemaker remote monitoring :
Very high patient acceptance !

A win-win situation for patients
(and healthcare providers)

Great ! We now have a digital doctor who makes electronic housecalls !

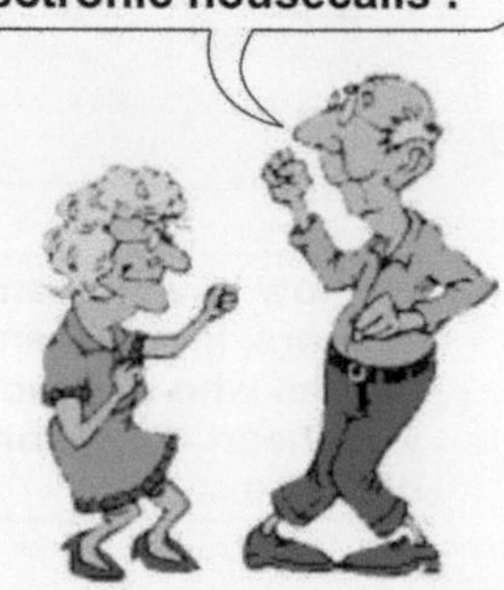

A. F. Sinnaeve

REMOTE PACEMAKER MONITORING - 2

Quality assurance and medicolegal aspects of remote monitoring

- **Who is qualified to access data ?**
- **Should access be allowed to electrophysiologists only, cardiologists, other physicians, technician or a specialized nurse ?**
- **Who is responsible, particularly when there is a delay in observing events, which may lead to adverse outcome ?**
- **Protection of data ? Data safety and privacy ?**
- **Always inform patients of the availability of remote monitoring !**

Organizational model for remote monitoring

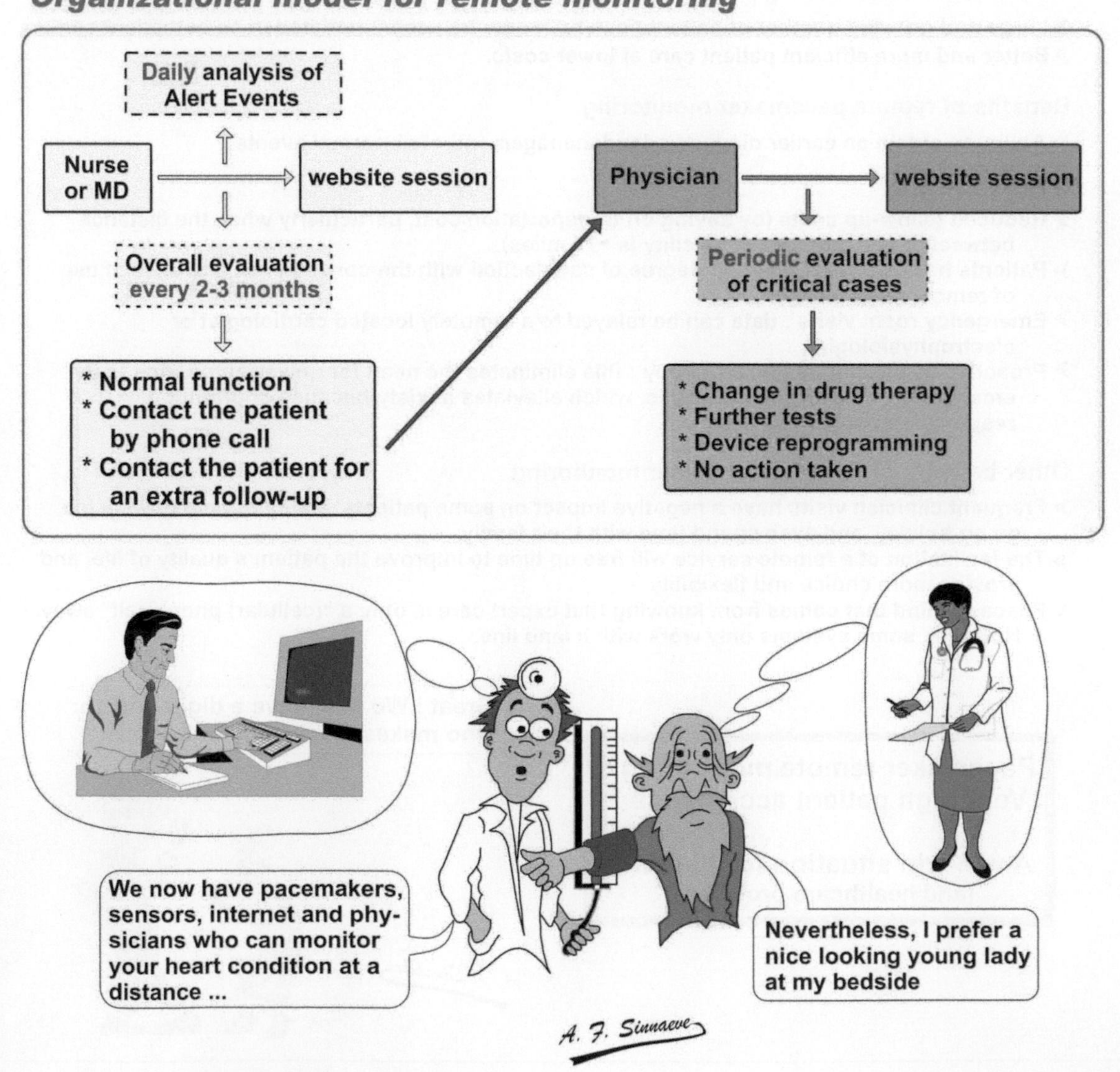

Daily analysis of Alert Events
Nurse or MD
website session
Overall evaluation every 2-3 months
* Normal function
* Contact the patient by phone call
* Contact the patient for an extra follow-up
Physician
website session
Periodic evaluation of critical cases
* Change in drug therapy
* Further tests
* Device reprogramming
* No action taken
We now have pacemakers, sensors, internet and physicians who can monitor your heart condition at a distance ...
Nevertheless, I prefer a nice looking young lady at my bedside
A. F. Sinnaeve

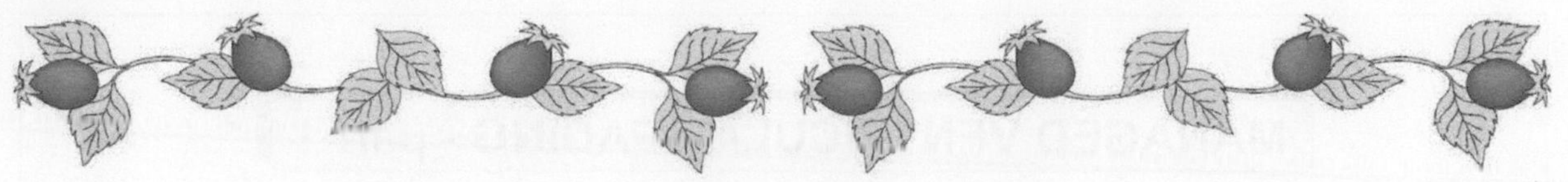

SPECIAL FUNCTIONS

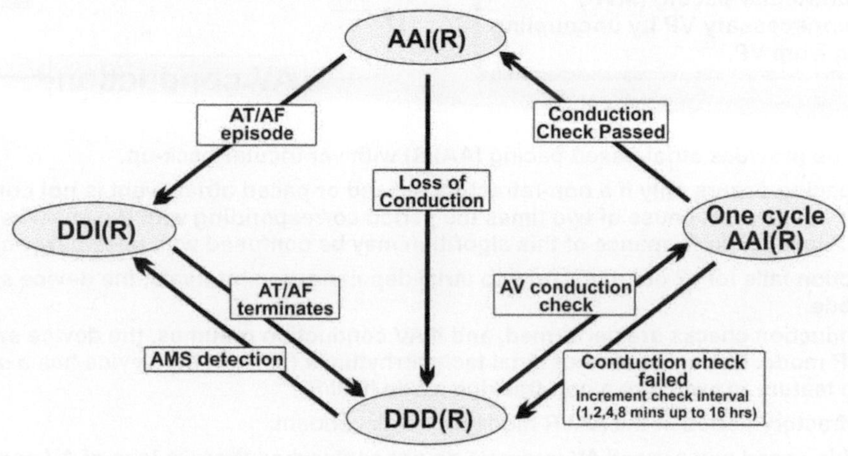

* **Managed ventricular pacing - part 1**
  basic principles
* **Managed ventricular pacing - part 2**
  AAI(R) mode and ventricular back-up
* **Managed ventricular pacing - part 3**
  A-V conduction check and DDD(R) switch
* **Rate drop response**

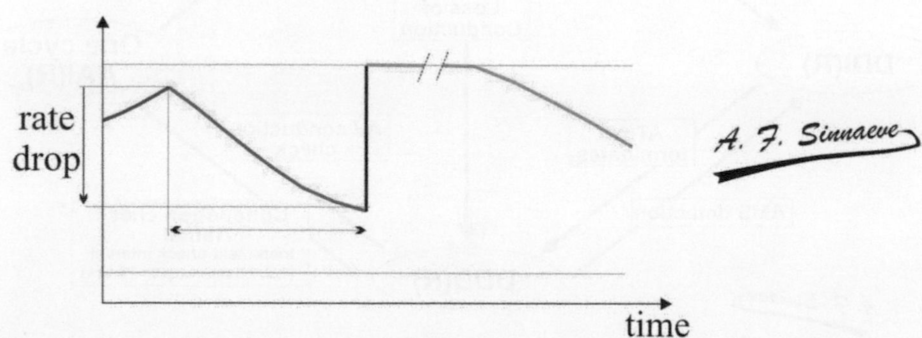

MANAGED VENTRICULAR PACING - part 1

The detrimental effects of right ventricular pacing (VP) are directly related to the cumulative percentage of VP (Cum%VP). Managed ventricular pacing (MVP) minimizes unnecessary VP by uncoupling atrial pacing from VP.

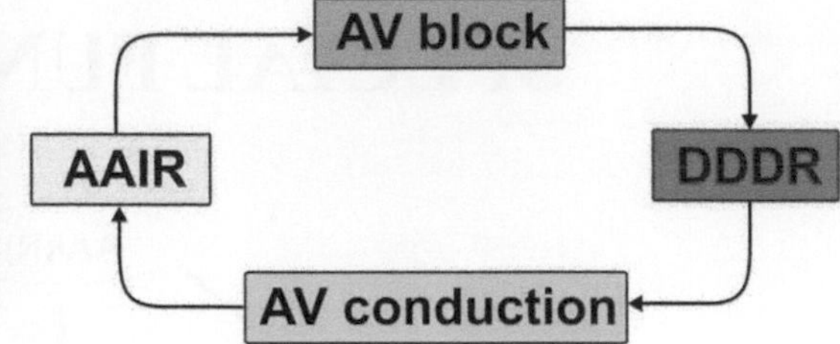

*** The MVP mode provides atrial-based pacing (AAI/R) with ventricular back-up.**

*** Ventricular pacing occurs only if a non-refractory sensed or paced atrial event is not conducted (allowing for a maximum pause of two times the period corresponding with the lower rate limit plus 80 ms). Nominal performance of this algorithm may be confused with pacemaker malfunction.**

*** If AV conduction fails for "2 out of 4" atrial to atrial depolarization intervals, the device switches to DDD/R mode.**

*** Periodic conduction checks are performed, and if AV conduction resumes, the device switches back to AAI/R mode. During periods of atrial tachyarrhythmia (AT/AF), the device has a standard mode switch feature to switch to a non-tracking mode (DDI/R).**

*** The atrial refractory period in the AAI/R mode is rate-dependent**

*** Programmable paced and sensed AV intervals do not apply when there is loss of AV conduction. In the AAI/R there is no AV interval restriction. No maximum AV interval is imposed.**

Safety

*** MVP is safe but there is the potential risk of ventricular proarrhythmia caused by pause-dependent VT especially in the setting of hypokalemia or a long QT interval.**

*** Patients with marked 1st degree AV block may develop pacemaker syndrome.**

*** MVP pacing is inappropriate in chronic fixed complete AV block**

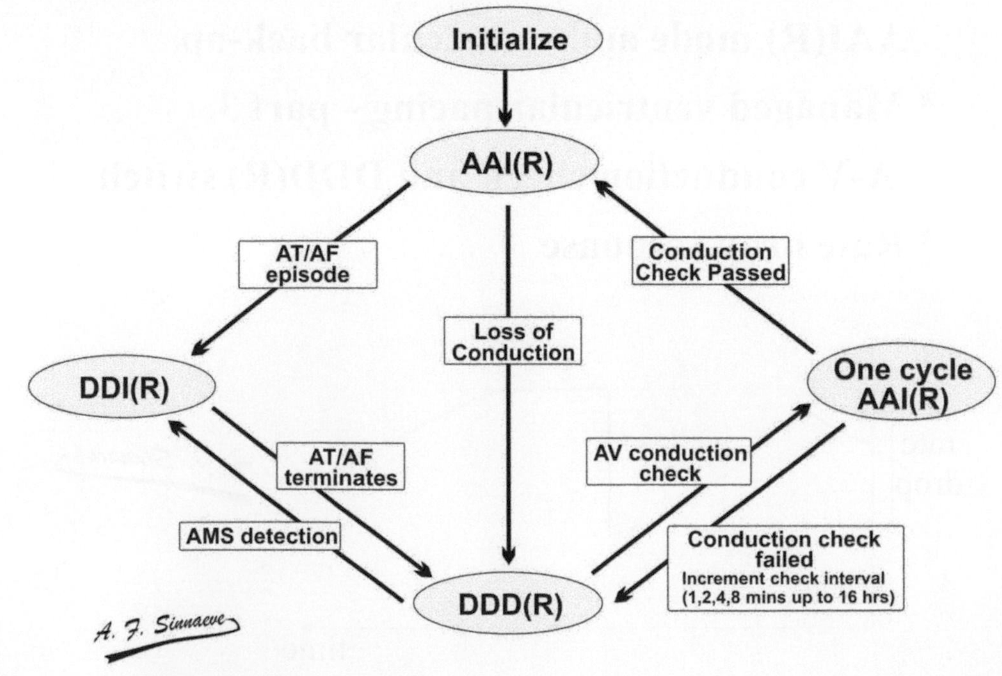

MANAGED VENTRICULAR PACING - part 2

* ***Reduces unnecessary RV pacing***
* ***Promotes intrinsic AV conduction***
* ***Provides back-up dual chamber pacing***
* ***Provides AAI - AAIR pacing while the system monitors for AV conduction***
* ***Reduces the risk of atrial fibrillation as Cum%RV pacing is decreased***

AAI(R) mode :

Atrial based pacing allowing intrinsic AV conduction

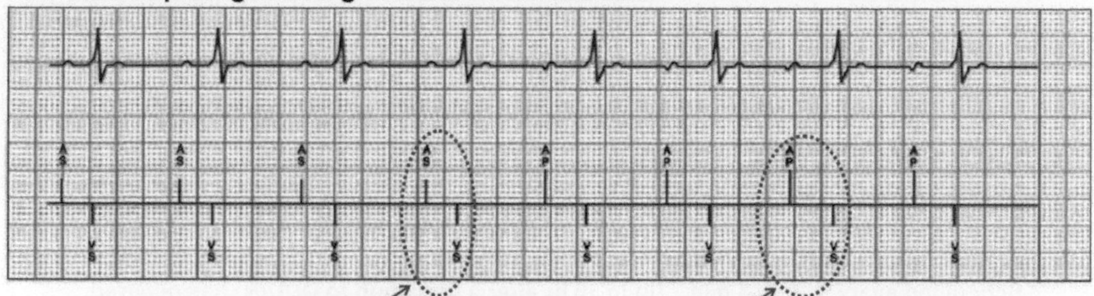

PR intervals are only restricted by the underlying atrial rate or sensor rate; VS events simply need to occur prior to the next AS or AP.

Ventricular Back-Up :

Ventricular pacing only as needed in the presence of transient loss of conduction

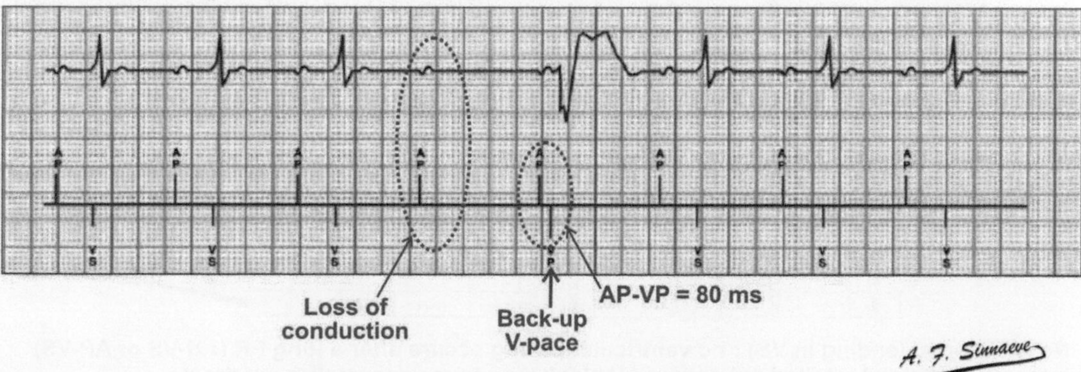

A. F. Sinnaeve

MANAGED VENTRICULAR PACING - part 3

DDD(R) Switch

Ventricular support if loss of A-V conduction is persistent

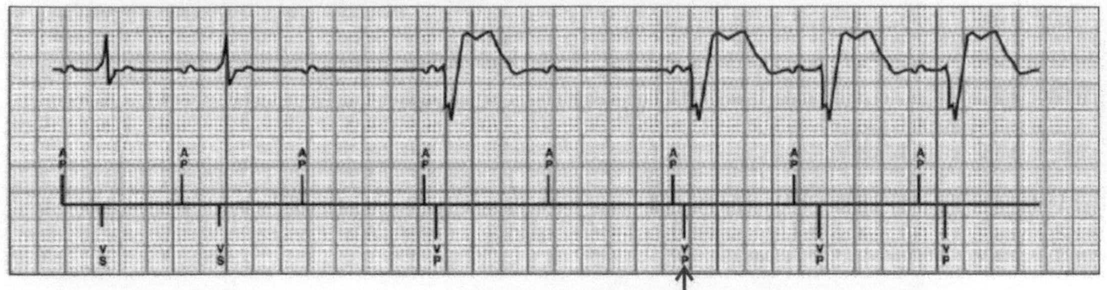

Switch to DDD(R) occurs after back-up VP ; programmed PAV/SAV are used during this mode of operation

DDD(R) to AAI(R) : **AV conduction check (1 beat)**

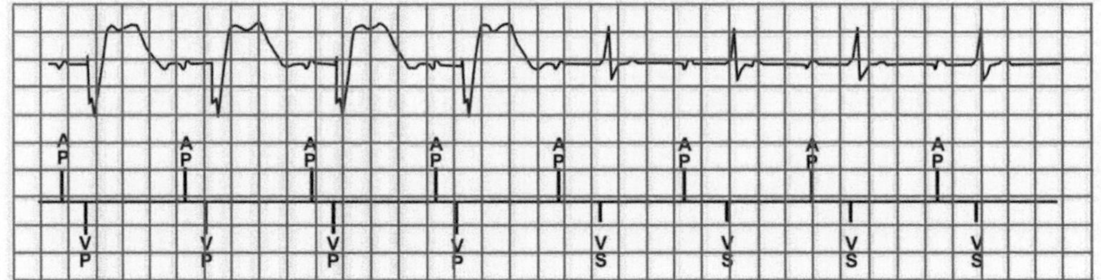

- **Scheduled every 1, 2, 4, 8 min... up to 16 hr after a transition to DDD(R) has occured.**
- **Temporarily uses AAI(R) timing to monitor for a conducted VS during one A-A interval.**
- **If VS occurs, conduction check passes.**
- **Mode switches from DDD(R) to AAI(R).**

MVP

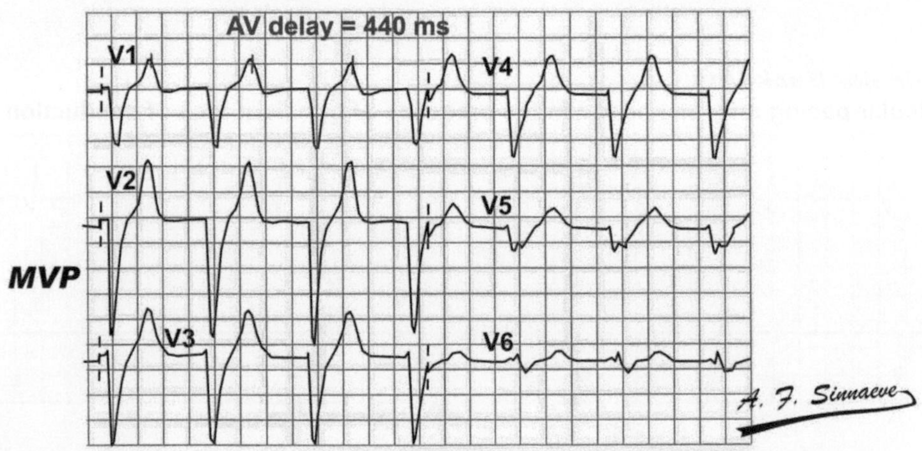

No AV interval (ending in VS) : no ventricular pacing occurs after a long PR (AS-VS or AP-VS) interval. Sustained marked 1st degree AV block may cause pacemaker syndrome.

RATE DROP RESPONSE

The rate drop response (RDR) shown below for Medtronic devices (in the DDD and DDDR modes) is intended to provide backup pacing and prevent associated symptoms in patients who experience occasional episodes of significant drop in heart rate (e.g. syncope from cardio-inhibitory and mixed forms of carotid sinus syndrome). When a rate drop episode is detected, the pacemaker intervenes with an elevated rate for a brief period of time. When the "Intervention Duration" expires, the pacemaker slowly reduces the pacing rate by approximately 5 ppm steps per minute until the intrinsic rate is sensed or the "Lower Rate" is reached, whichever is higher.
RDR can be set to intervene following a drop in heart rate which meets programmed criteria. RDR can also be set to intervene when the rate drops below the Lower Rate by programming RDR. Both responses can also be programmed.

DROP DETECTION in the DDD mode

Pacing starts when heart rate drops by 25 bpm (programmed drop size) within a programmed duration (detection window) to a value equal to the programmed drop rate (not the lower rate !). The detection window is the maximum time used to determine drop size. Both drop size and drop rate criteria must be met for intervention pacing to occur. High-rate pacing intervention (100 ppm) is programmable for a given duration in the example below.

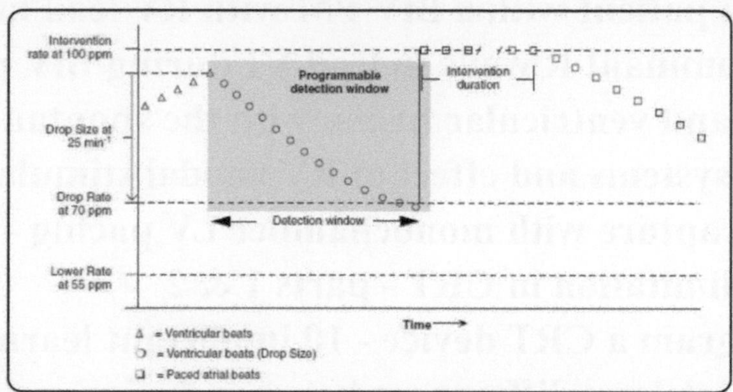

LOWER RATE DETECTION

A pacemaker-defined RDR episode at the Lower Rate occurs when the heart rate drops to the Lower Rate and the atrium or ventricle is paced at the Lower Rate for a consecutive number of Detection Beats. The number of Detection Paced Beats (at the Lower Rate) to confirm the low rate episode must be programmed (1,2, or 3)

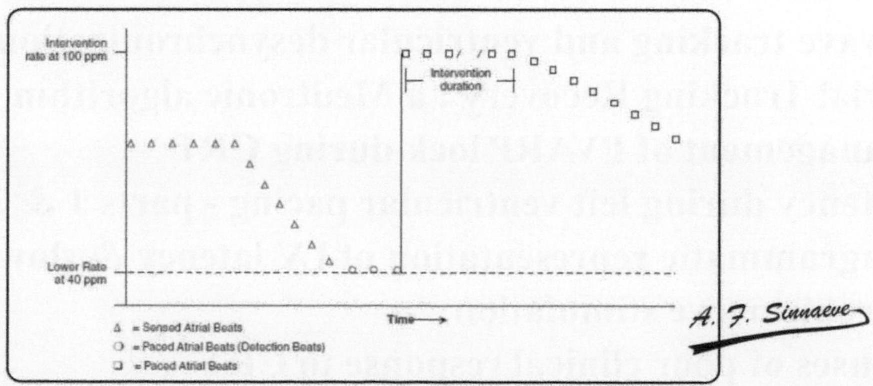

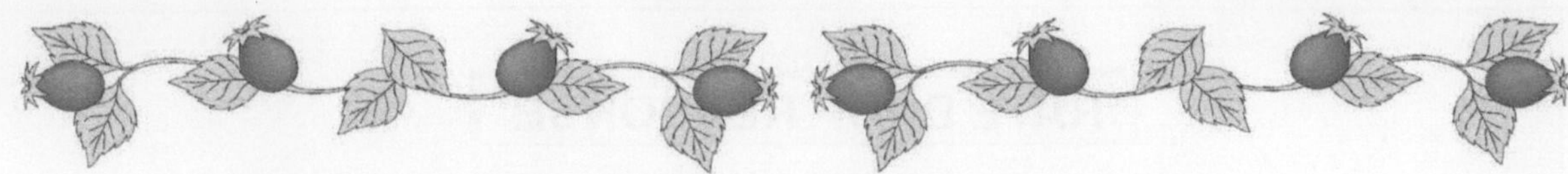

BIVENTRICULAR PACING & CARDIAC RESYNCHRONIZATION

* Left ventricular dyssynchrony
* Leads & electrodes for BiV pacing
* BiV pacing - ventricular lead polarity
* Frontal plane axis during single chamber & BiV pacing
* Monochamber LV pacing in a patient with a BiV pacemaker
* ECG from a patient with a BiV PM with RV lead in the apex
* ECG from a patient with a BiV PM with RV lead in the RVOT
* Lack of a dominant R wave in lead V1 during BiV pacing
* BiV pacing and ventricular fusion with the spontaneous QRS
* BiV pacing systems and effect of RV anodal stimulation
* RV anodal capture with monochamber LV pacing - 1 & 2
* Upper rate limitation in CRT - parts 1 & 2
* How to program a CRT device - 10 important learning points
* Effective AV delay - differences between device manufacturers
* Inter-atrial conduction delay (IACD) - parts 1 & 2
* Late atrial sensing & right IACD - impact on CRT parts 1, 2 & 3
* The PVARP lock during CRT
* Electrical desynchronization in BiV pacemakers
* P wave tracking and ventricular desynchronization
* Atrial Tracking Recovery : a Medtronic algorithm
* Management of PVARP lock during CRT
* Latency during left ventricular pacing - parts 1 & 2
* Diagrammatic representation of LV latency & slow conduction
* Phrenic nerve stimulation
* Causes of poor clinical response to CRT
* Device monitoring of lung fluid

A. F. Sinnaeve

LEFT VENTRICULAR DYSSYNCHRONY AND RESPONSE TO CRT

CRT has become increasingly accepted as a treatment modality for patients with heart failure (HF), low ejection fraction (EF) and LV wall contraction dyssynchrony. However, it has become clear that up to 30% of patients do not respond to CRT. Hence, identification of potential responders to CRT before implantation of an ICD is extremely important !

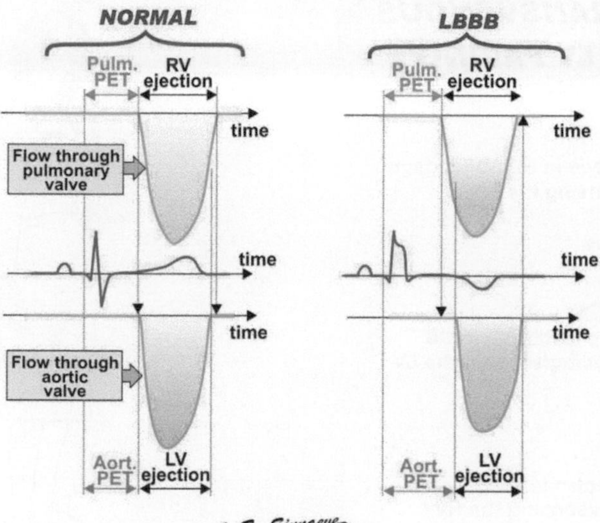

Interventricular dyssynchrony due to left bundle branch block (LBBB). The LV is delayed with respect to the RV.

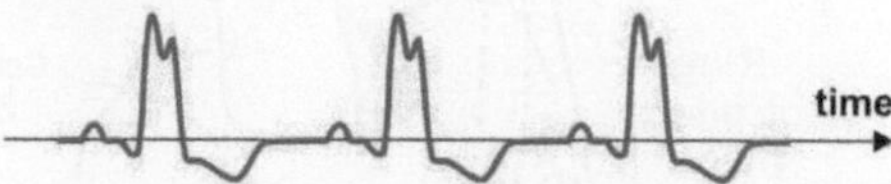

Normally, the pre-ejection time (PET) of the pulmonary artery and the aortic artery are almost equal. With complete LBBB, there a distinct prolonging of the aortic pre-ejection time is noted.

A. F. Sinnaeve

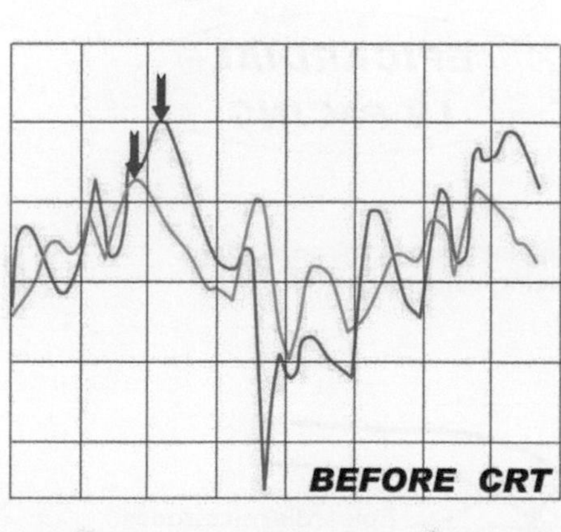

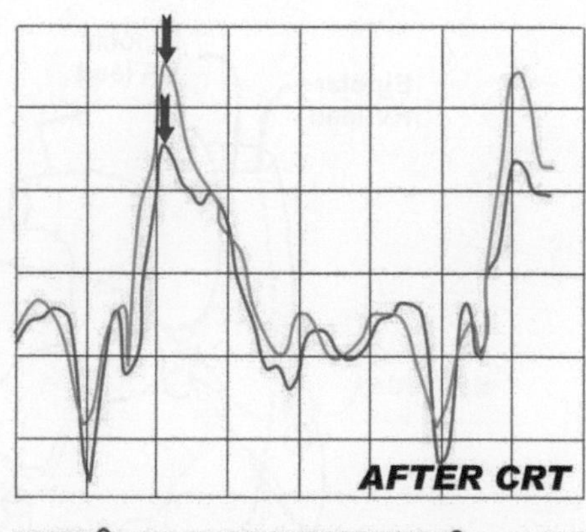

Intraventricular or LV mechanical dyssynchrony : in the example Tissue Doppler Imaging (TDI) shows a patient with the basal posterior wall delayed with respect to the basal anteroseptal wall of 90 ms; the delay was totally abolished after CRT. The peak systolic velocity during ejection phase in each view is shown by arrows.

Studies showed that patients with extensive LV dyssynchrony respond well to CRT.

LEADS AND ELECTRODES FOR BIVENTRICULAR PACING

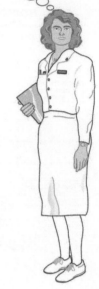

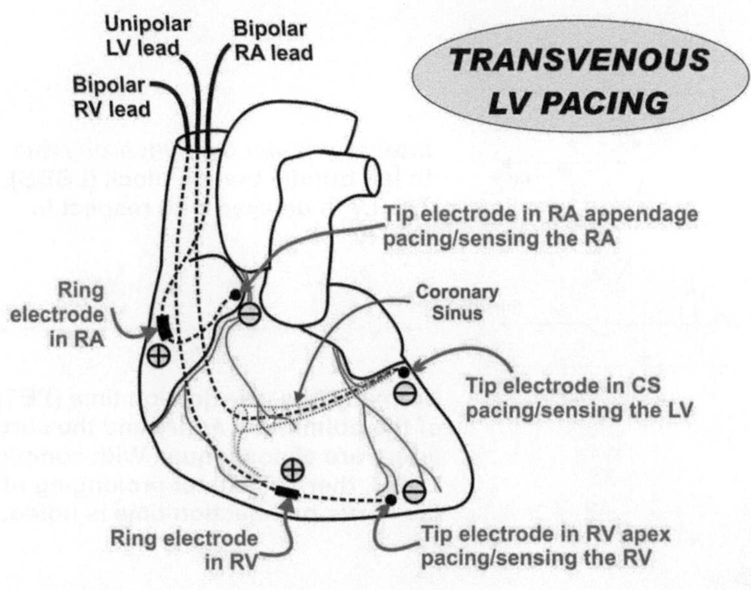

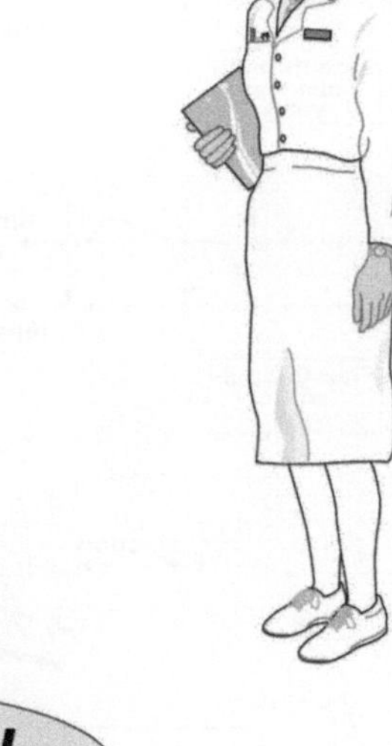

A 3 chamber pacemaker
for congestive heart
failure ! What will they
think of next ?

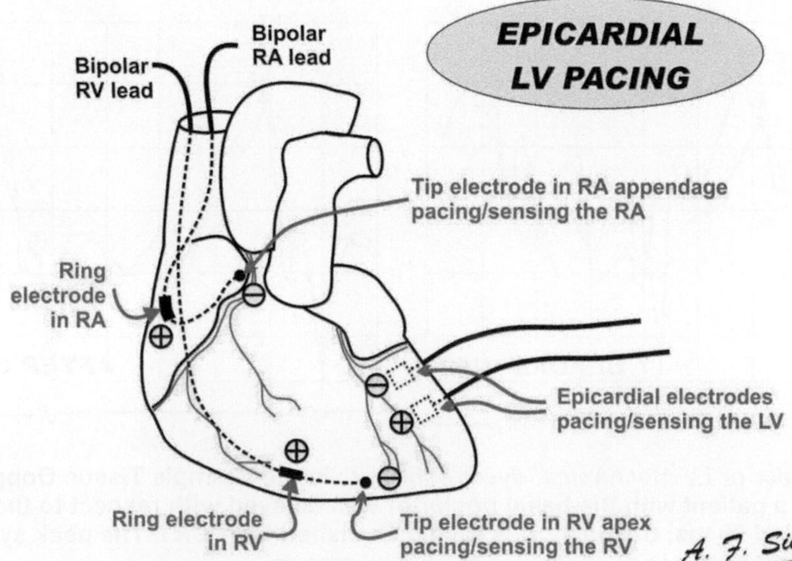

Abbreviations : CS =coronary sinus; LV = left ventricle; RA = right atrium; RV = right ventricle;

BIVENTRICULAR PACING SYSTEMS VENTRICULAR LEAD POLARITY

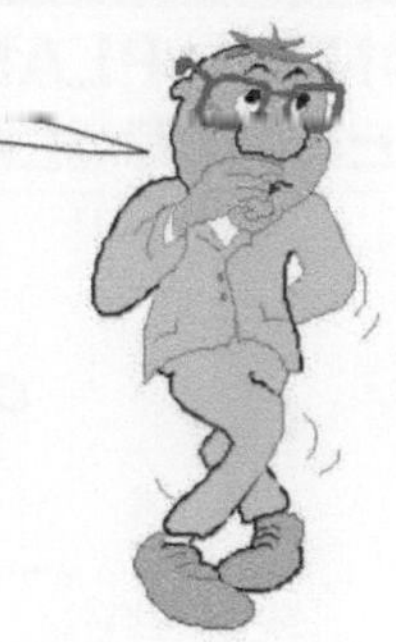

Both RV and LV leads may be unipolar as well as bipolar in BiV pacing systems ! Moreover, unipolar systems may use the can or a shared common ring ! It is confusing !? And when is RV anodal stimulation possible in a BiV system ?

Dual Ventricular Bipolar

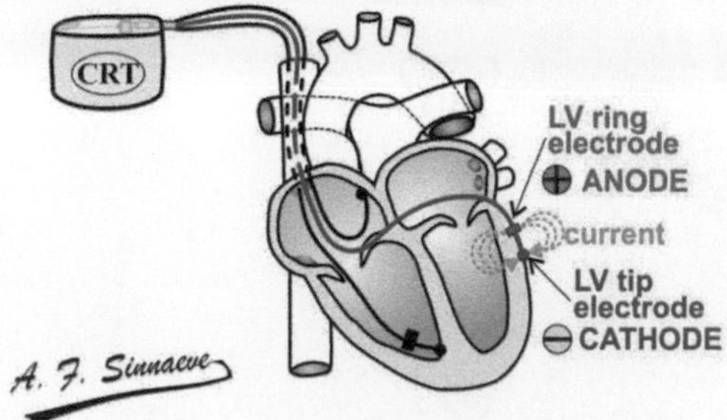

* both leads are bipolar
* during LV pacing there is an electric current between LV tip electrode and the LV ring electrode
* NO RV ANODAL capture possible

Shared Common Ring Bipolar

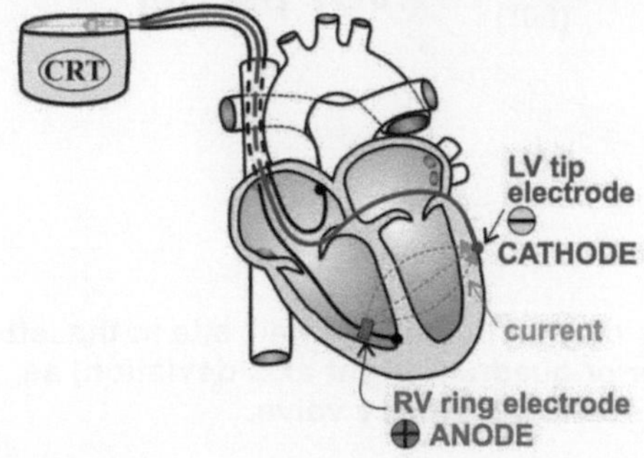

* LV lead is unipolar ; RV lead is bipolar and the RV ring is shared
* during LV pacing there is an electric current between LV tip electrode and the shared RV ring electrode
* RV ANODAL CAPTURE POSSIBLE if the LV pulse amplitude is large enough

Note :

1. the normal RV threshold is lower than the LV threshold (due to better contact)
2. anodal capture is caused by the high current density generated at the RV anode by the high LV output. The threshold for RV anodal stimulation is variable and it may be higher or lower than the LV pacing threshold.

Triangular CRT with the addition of an RV lead

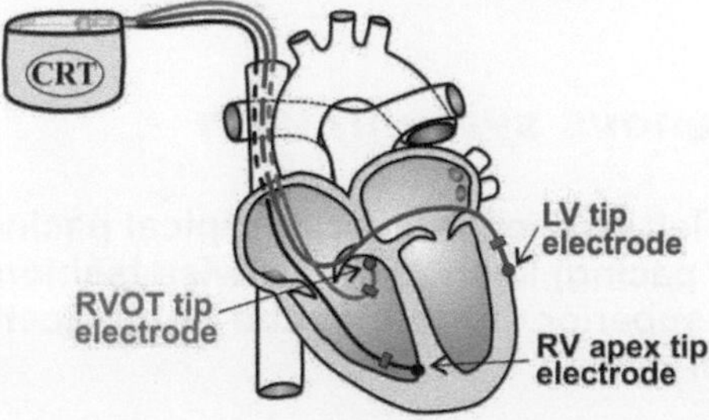

3 ventricular leads (2RV & 1LV)
The arrangement can be useful in patients refractory to conventional chronic CRT.

Two leads in different LV veins with some separation

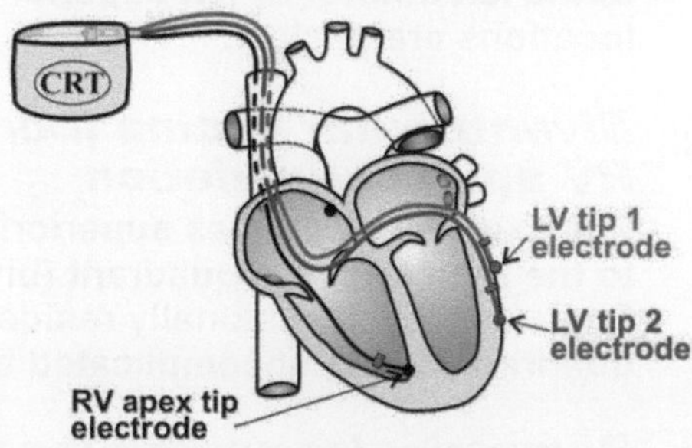

The value of this arrangement remains to be determined.

Abbreviations : CRT = cardiac resynchronization therapy ; BiV = biventricular ; LV = left ventricle ; RV = right ventricle ; RVOT = right ventricular outflow tract ;

FRONTAL PLANE AXIS DURING SINGLE CHAMBER VENTRICULAR AND BIVENTRICULAR PACING

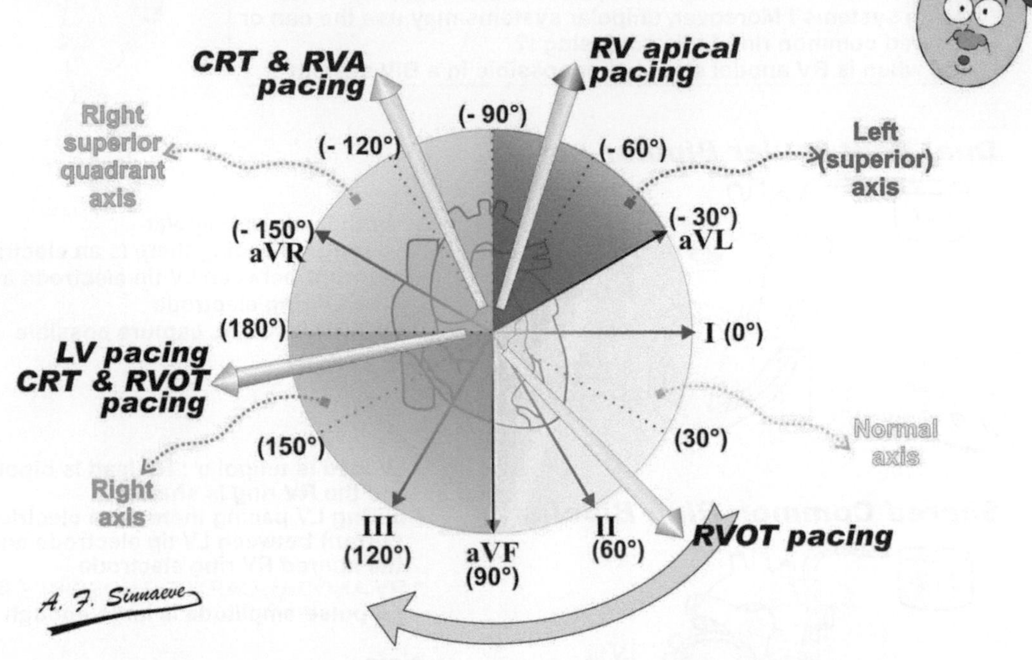

1 *Monochamber RV pacing*

During RV outflow tract/septal pacing, the axis may be in the "normal" site in the left inferior quadrant and it moves to the right inferior quadrant (right axis deviation) as the site of stimulation moves superiorly towards the pulmonary valve.

2 *Monochamber LV pacing from target site in the coronary venous system*

The axis points to the right inferior quadrant (right axis deviation) and less commonly to the right superior quadrant. In an occasional patient the axis may point to the left inferior or left superior quadrant. The reasons for these unusual axis locations are unclear.

3 *Biventricular pacing (coronary venous system) with RV apical stimulation*

The axis usually moves superiorly from the left (monochamber RV apical pacing) to the right superior quadrant (biventricular pacing) in an anticlockwise fashion. The axis may occasionally reside in the left superior rather than the right superior quadrant during uncomplicated biventricular pacing.

4 *Biventricular pacing (coronary venous system) with RV outflow tract/septal stimulation*

The axis is often directed to the right inferior quadrant (right axis deviation).

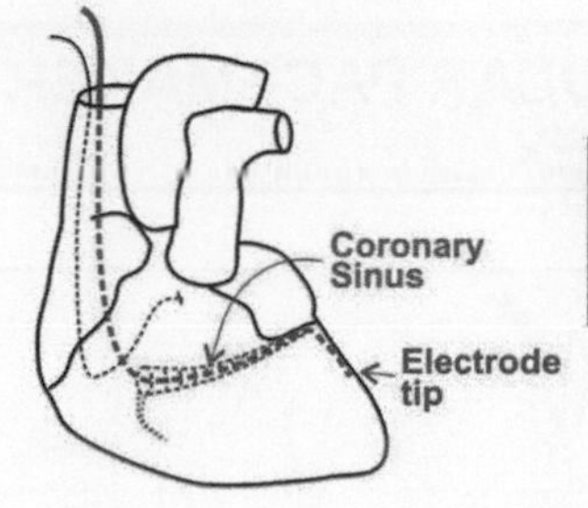

MONOCHAMBER LV PACING IN A PATIENT WITH A BiV PACEMAKER

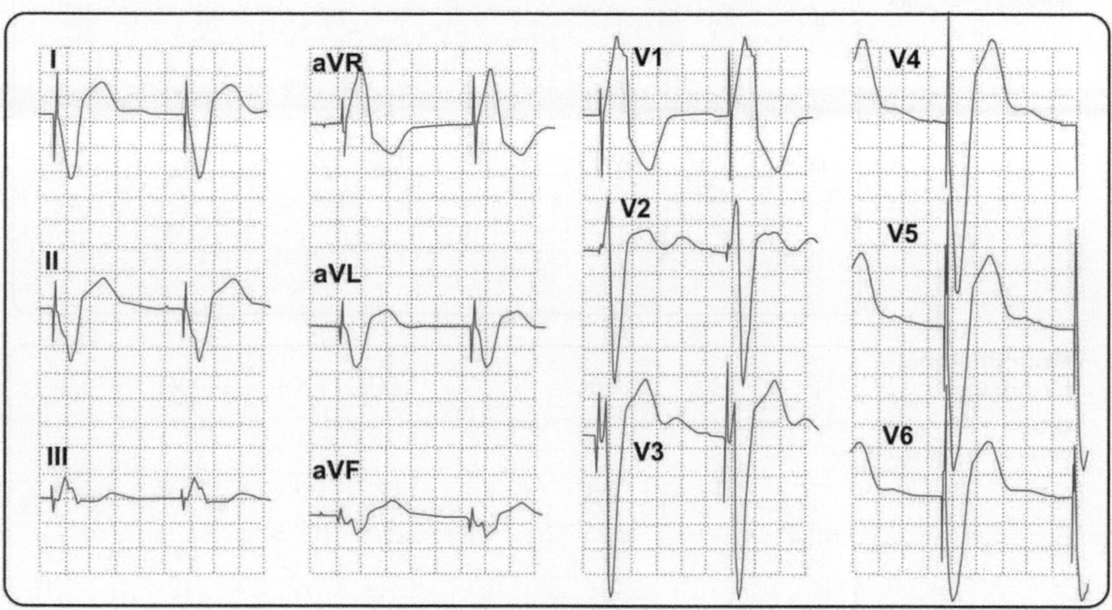

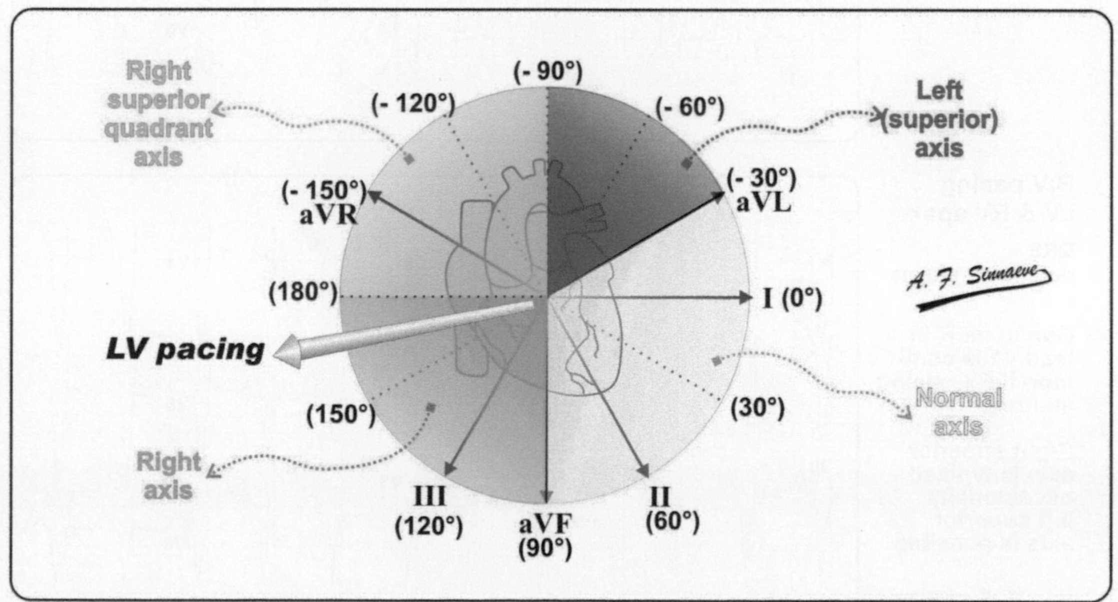

Abbreviations : BiV = biventricular ; LV = left ventricle ; RVOT = right ventricular outflow tract ;

ECG FROM A PATIENT WITH A BIVENTRICULAR PACEMAKER WITH RV LEAD IN THE APEX

Monochamber RV apical pacing

QRS duration = 243 ms

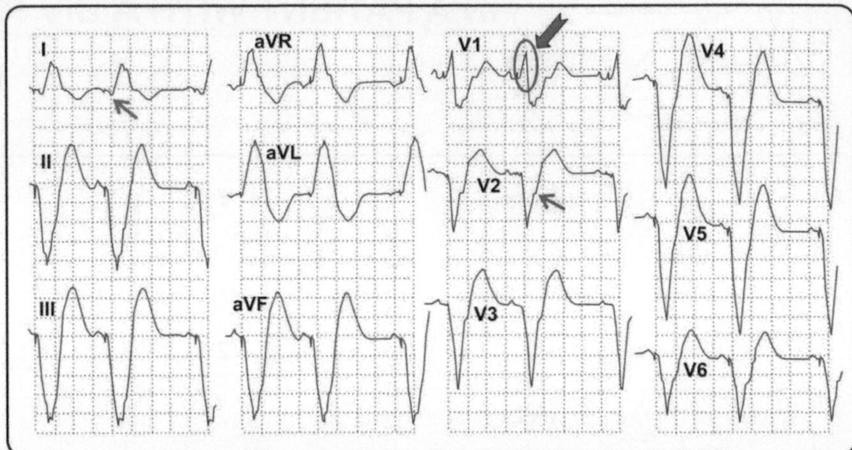

Monochamber LV pacing

QRS duration = 240 ms

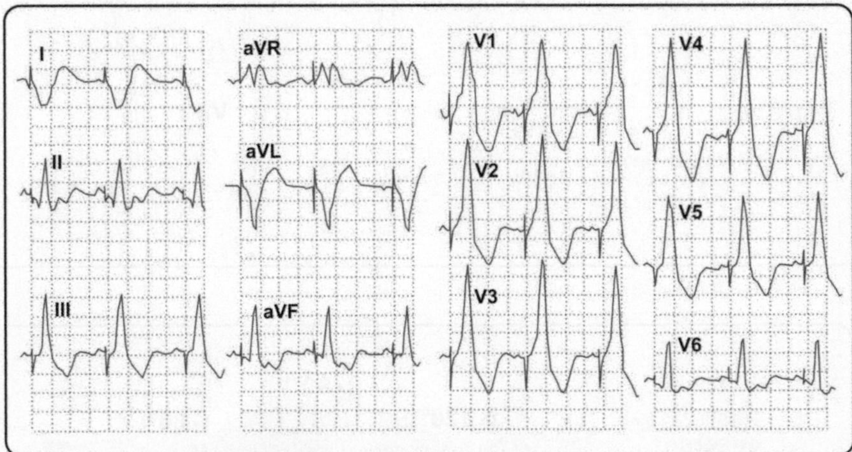

BiV pacing LV & RV apex

QRS duration = 170 ms

Dominant R in lead V1 is common if RV pacing at apex.

Right superior axis is typical; occasionally left superior axis is possible.

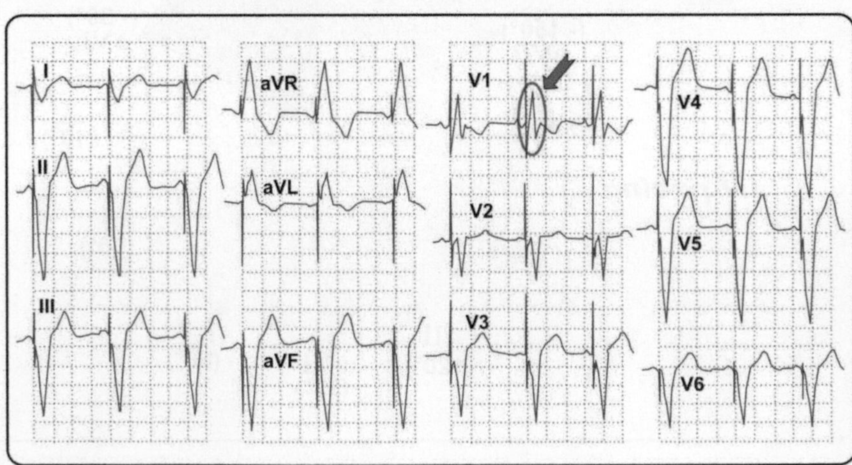

A. F. Sinnaeve

Abbreviations : BiV = biventricular ; LV = left ventricle ; RV = right ventricle ;

ECG FROM A PATIENT WITH A BIVENTRICULAR PACEMAKER WITH RV LEAD IN THE RVOT

Monochamber RVOT Pacing

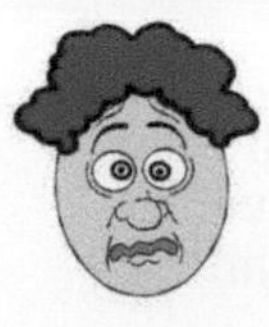

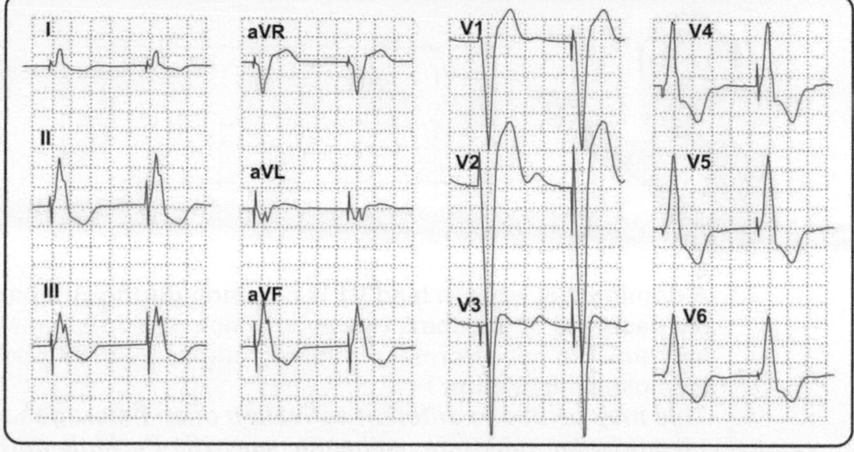

Monochamber LV Pacing (RVOT Off)

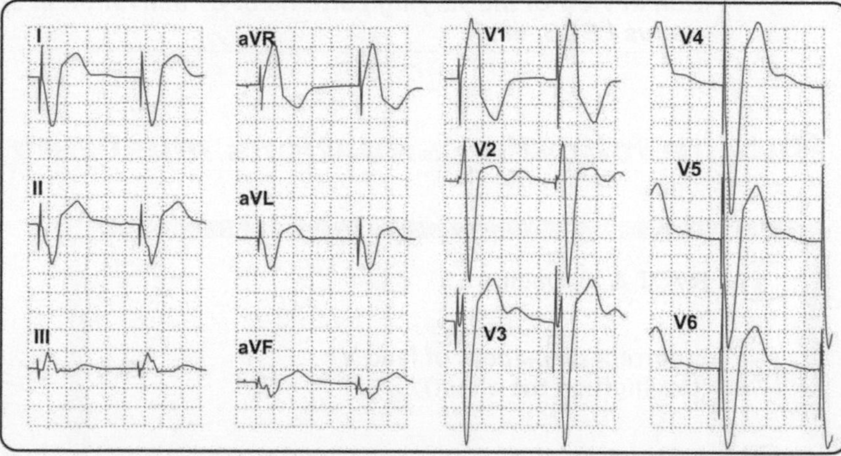

Biventricular Pacing LV & RVOT

Note right axis in frontal plane and LBBB in lead V1

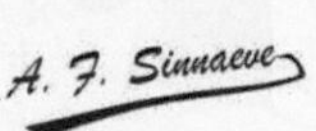

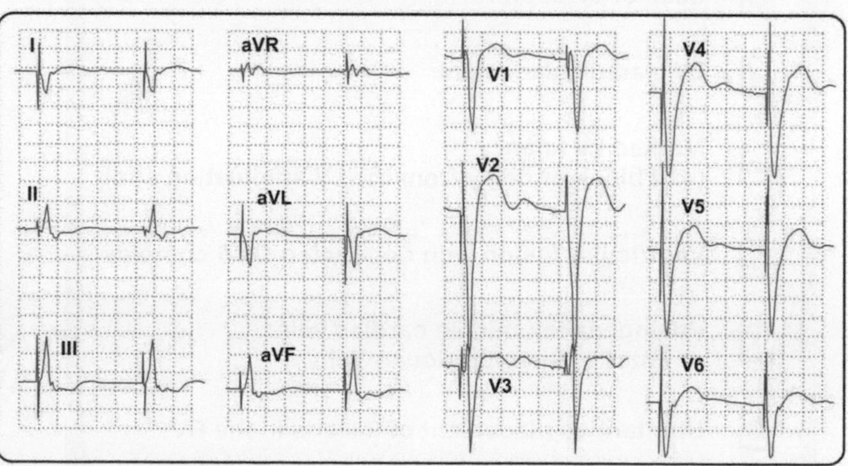

Abbreviations : BiV = biventricular ; LBBB = left bundle branch block ; LV = left ventricle ; RV = right ventricle ; RVOT = right ventricular outflow tract ;

LACK OF A DOMINANT R WAVE IN LEAD V1 DURING BiV PACING

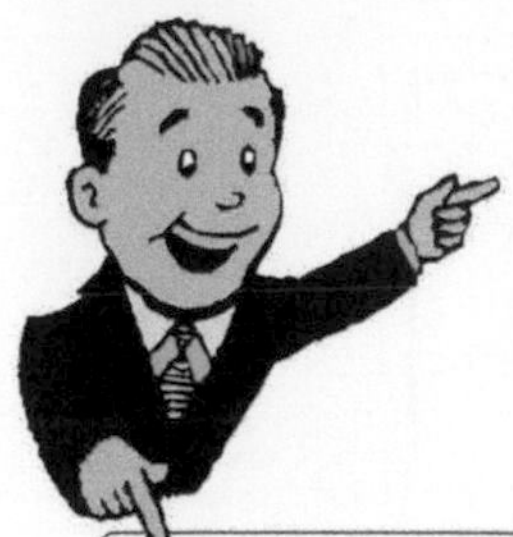

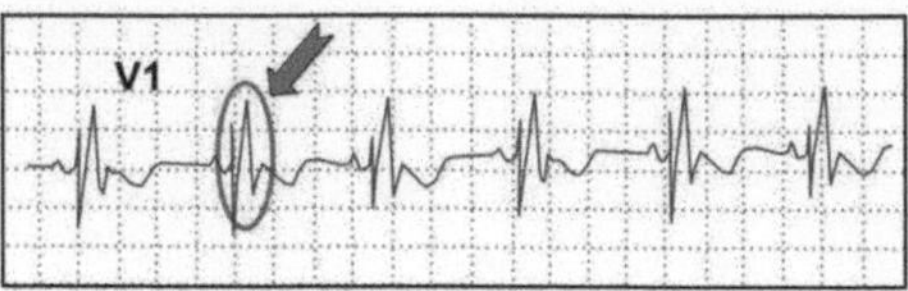

A dominant R wave in lead V1 is common during BiV pacing if RV pacing is at the apex. However, a lack of a dominant R wave in lead V1 may be normal during uncomplicated BiV pacing with RV apical stimulation !
This may be due to different activation of an heterogeneous biventricular substrate (ischemia, scar, His-Purkinje participation in view of the varying patterns of LV activation in spontaneous LBBB, etc.)

But the following situations must be ruled out :

1. **RVOT & LV pacing**
2. **Incorrect placement of lead V1 (too high on the chest)**
3. **Lack of LV capture**
4. **LV lead displacement**
5. **Marked LV latency (exit block or delay from the LV stimulation site)**
6. **Ventricular fusion with conducted QRS complex**
7. **Pacing via the middle cardiac vein or anterior interventricular vein**
8. **Unintended placement of 2 leads in the RV**

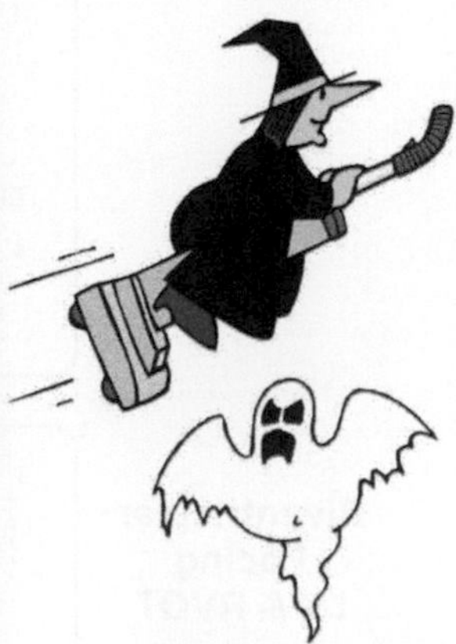

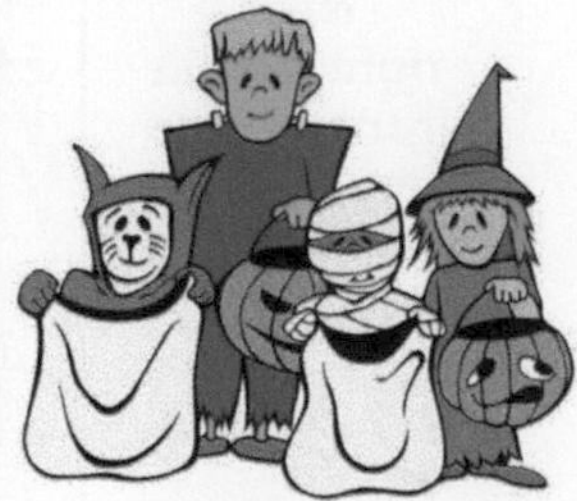

A. F. Sinnaeve

Abbreviations : BiV = biventricular ; LBBB = left bundle branch block ; LV = left ventricle ; RV = right ventricle ; RVOT = right ventricular outflow tract ;

BiV Pacing and Ventricular Fusion with the Spontaneous QRS

BiV pacing with Fusion
Initial ECG ; As-Vp = 100ms
QRS narrowing too good to be true

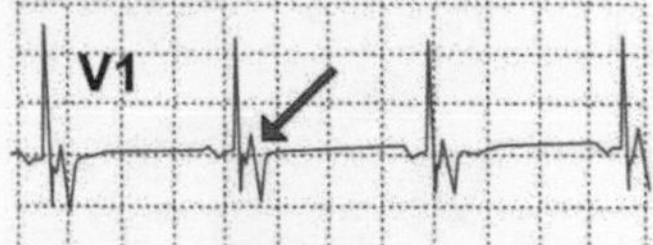

BiV pacing ; As-Vp = 100ms
Recorded some time later
Now a tall R

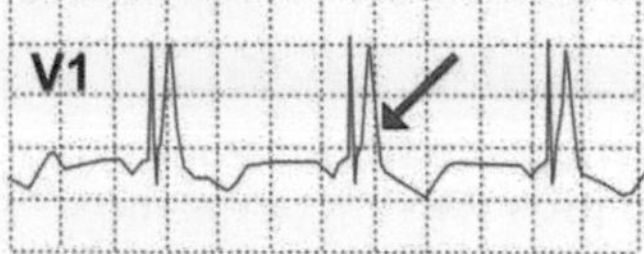

BiV pacing ; As-Vp = 130ms
Fusion again !

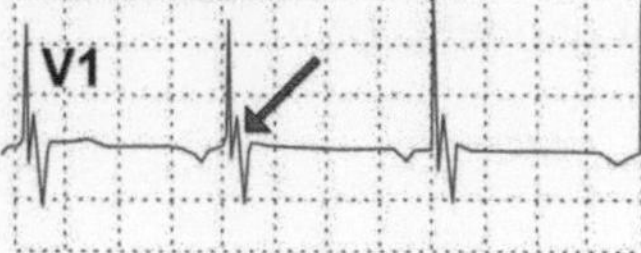

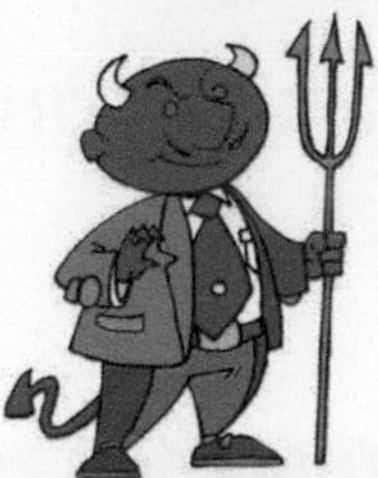

* In patients with sinus rhythm and a relatively short PR interval, a ventricular fusion phenomenon may lead to misinterpretation of the ECG. This is a frequent pitfall with BiV pacing in the presence of a relatively short PR interval and a more narrow paced QRS complex

* Ventricular fusion may be intermittent and present only in situations associated with enhanced AV conduction (increased catecholamines) !

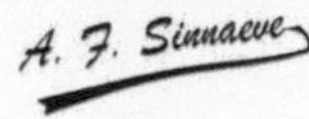

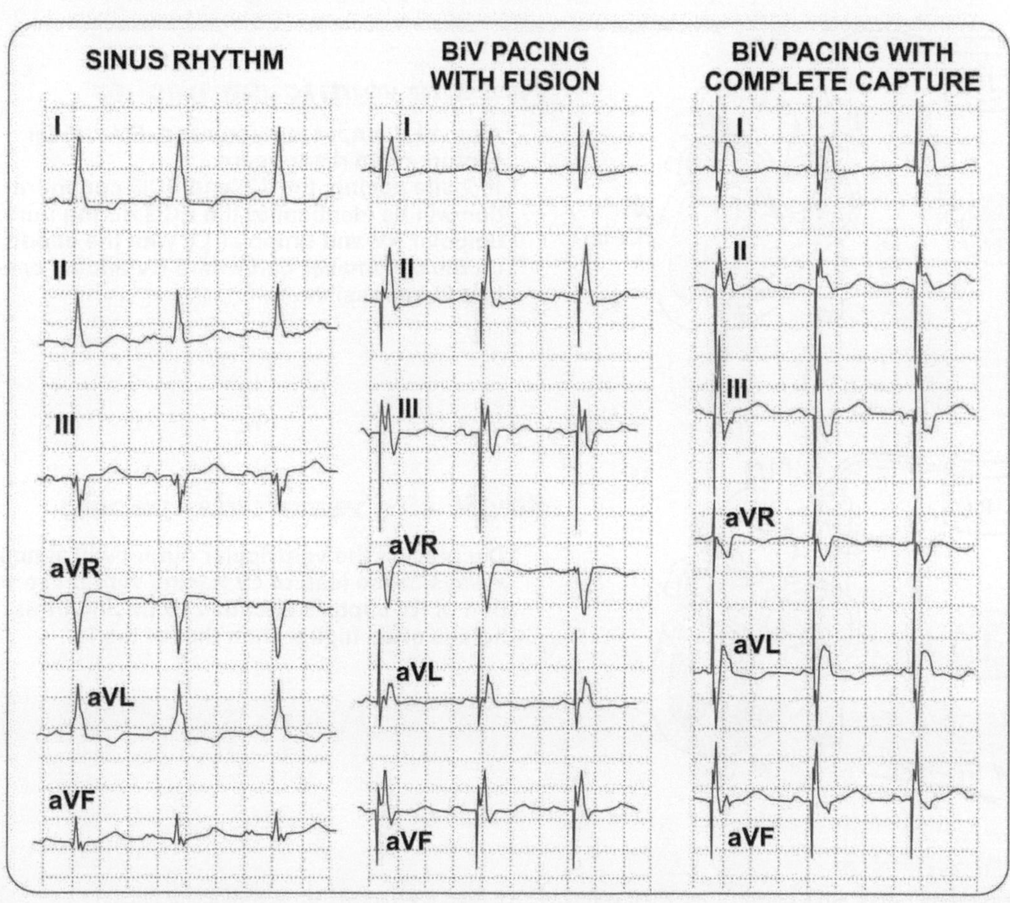

Abbreviations : BiV = biventricular ; As = atrial sense ; Vp = ventricular pace ;

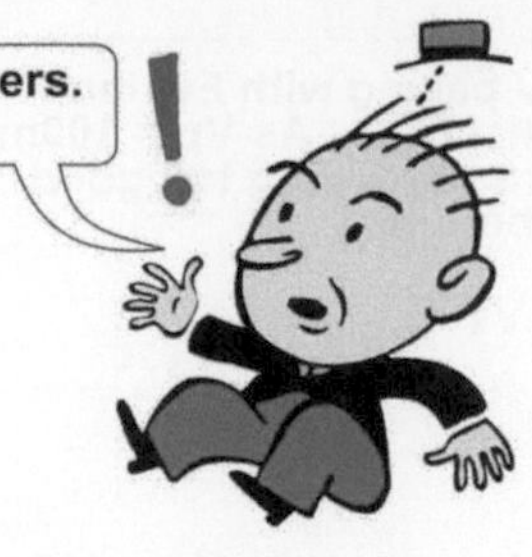
We never saw anodal pacing with conventional RV pacemakers.
Why does it occur with biventricular pacing ?

BiV PACING SYSTEMS
EFFECT OF RV ANODAL STIMULATION

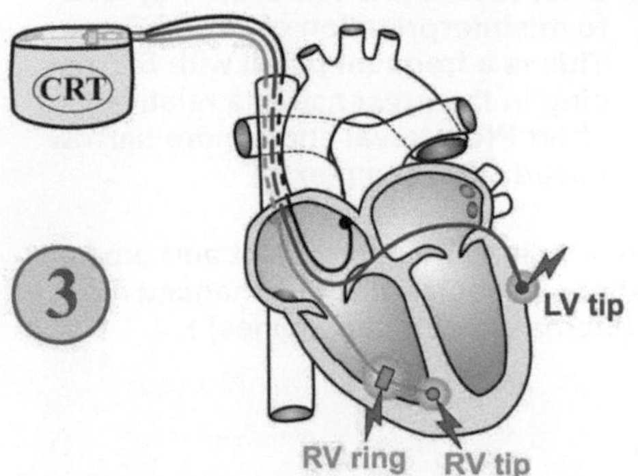

Triple site ventricular pacing

* Simultaneous ventricular capture from both LV and RV tip plus RV ring *(RV anodal capture at the ring).*
* Triple pacing produces a 12-lead ECG configuration somewhat different from the pure 2 site pacing without anodal capture.

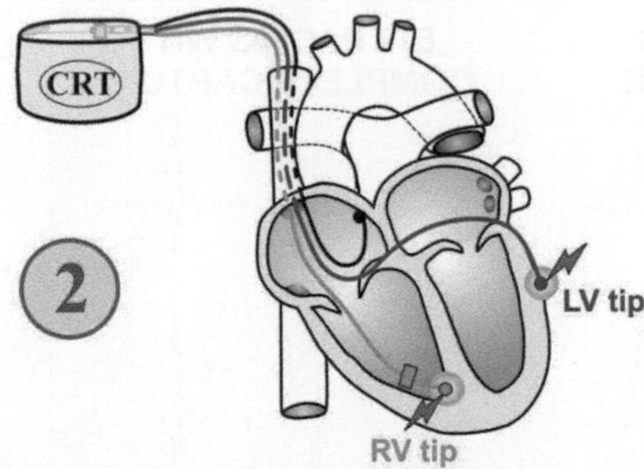

Two site ventricular pacing

* As the LV output is decreased, RV anodal capture often disappears.
* In 2 site pacing, the 12-lead ECG configuration will be identical to the ECG during pure unipolar RV and unipolar LV with the anode on the pacemaker can where RV anodal capture is impossible.

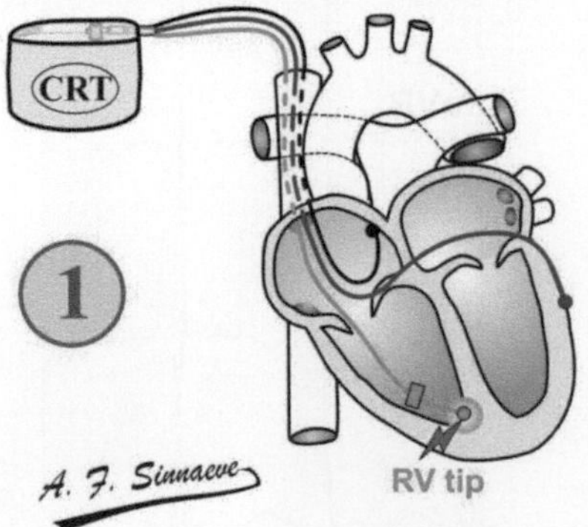

Single site ventricular pacing

* Decreasing the ventricular output will almost always cause loss of LV pacing with preservation of RV capture because LV pacing threshold is often higher than that of the RV.

A. F. Sinnaeve

Abbreviations : Ap = atrial pacing ; LV = left ventricle ; RV = right ventricle ; Vp = ventricular pacing ;

RV ANODAL CAPTURE WITH MONOCHAMBER LV PACING - 1

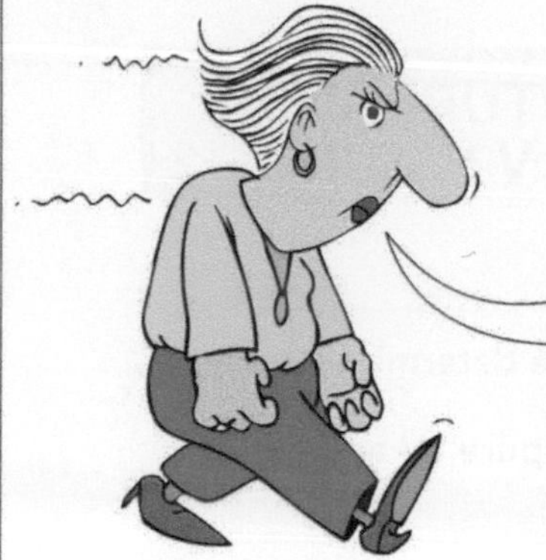

It's a mad world !
Monochamber LV pacing (i.e. from LV tip to RV ring) mimics the standard BiV pacing !
The pattern of LV depolarization cannot be ascertained if the LV threshold is high because RV anodal stimulation (via the RV ring electrode) prevents pure LV activation.

BiV pacing

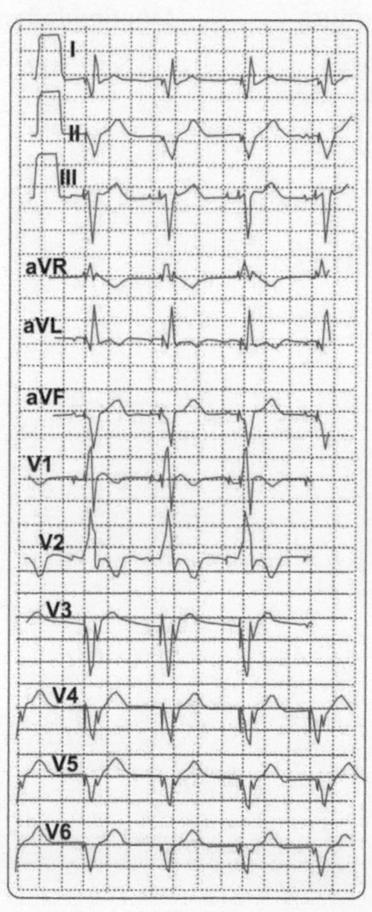

High output monochamber LV pacing (RV output off) RV anodal capture. AV = 90 ms

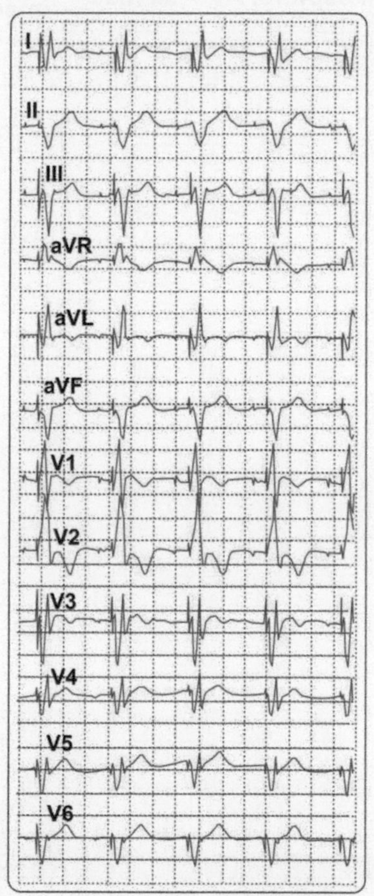

A. F. Sinnaeve

Abbreviations : AV = atrioventricular ; BiV = biventricular ; LV = left ventricle ; RV = right ventricle ;

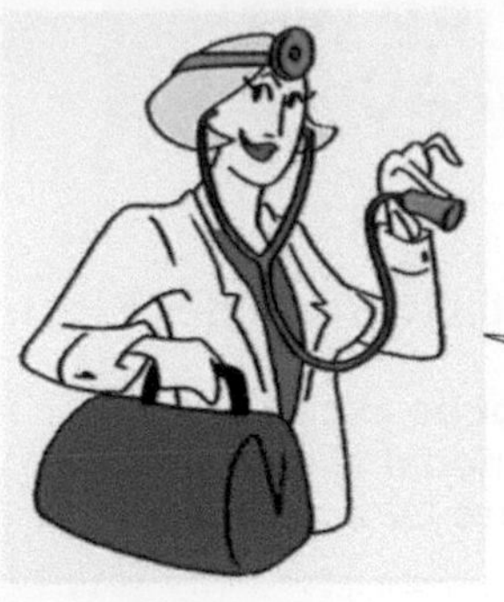

RV ANODAL CAPTURE WITH MONOCHAMBER LV PACING - 2

* The RV anodal threshold can be determined by lowering the LV output.
* Pacing from LV to can to show pure LV activation is not available in BiV ICDs.

High output monochamber LV pacing (RV output off) RV anodal capture. AV = 90 ms

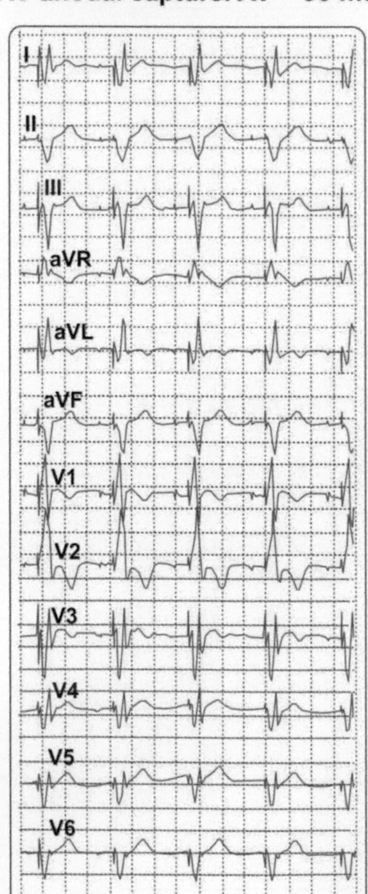

LV output at 3.5 V (RV output off) 2:1 anodal RV stimulation intermittent RV capture

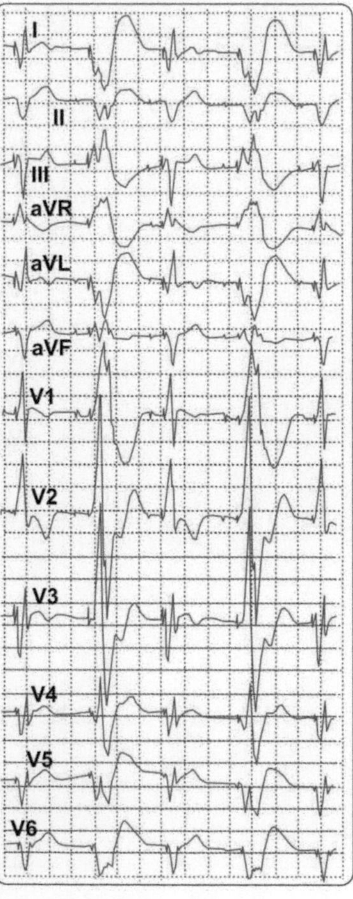

LV output at 2.8 V (RV output off) Pure LV pacing LV stimulation only

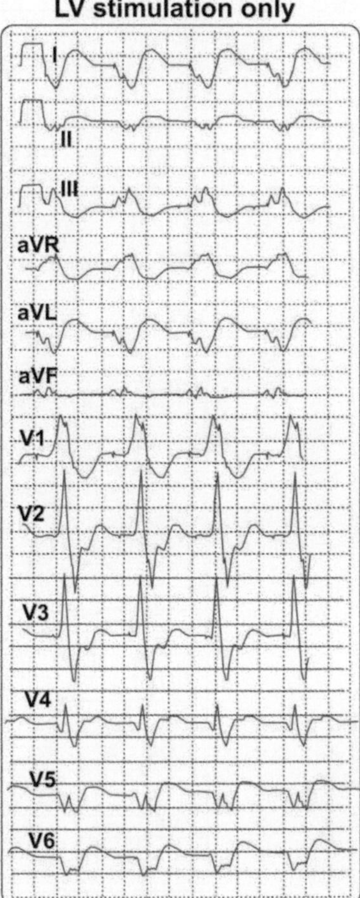

A. F. Sinnaeve

Abbreviations : AV = atrioventricular ; BiV = biventricular ; LV = left ventricle ; RV = right ventricle ;

UPPER RATE LIMITATION IN CRT - part 1

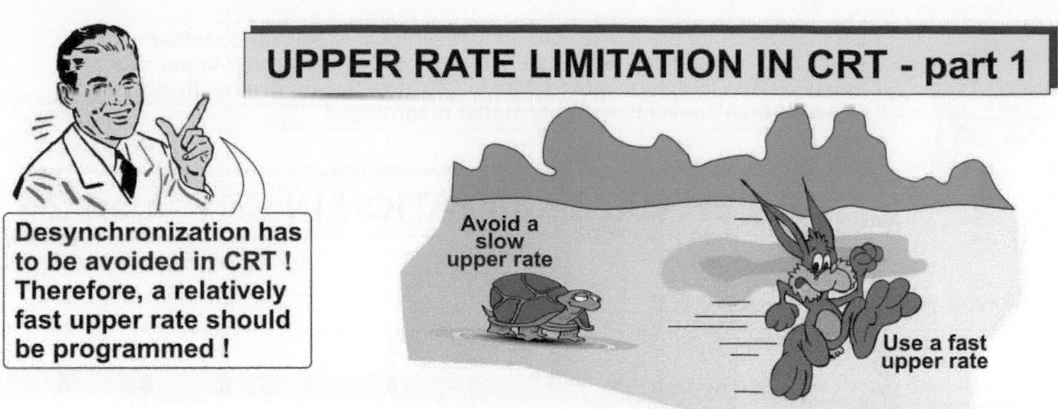

Normal upper rate response of the Wenckebach type

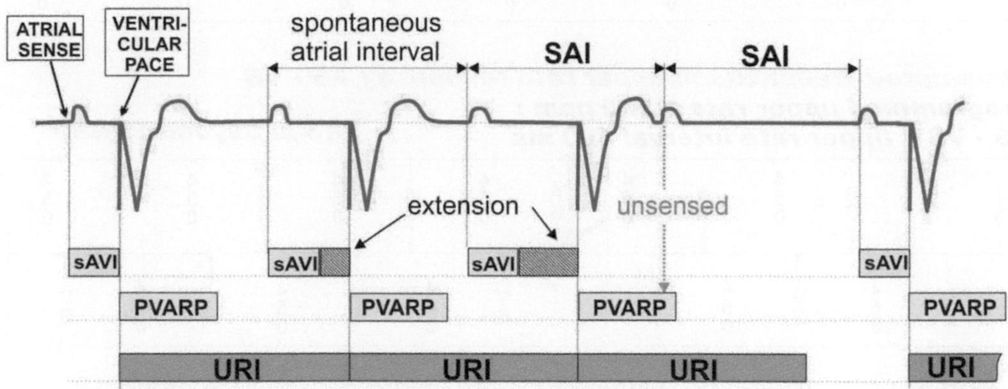

The pre-empted Wenckebach behavior with short sAVI

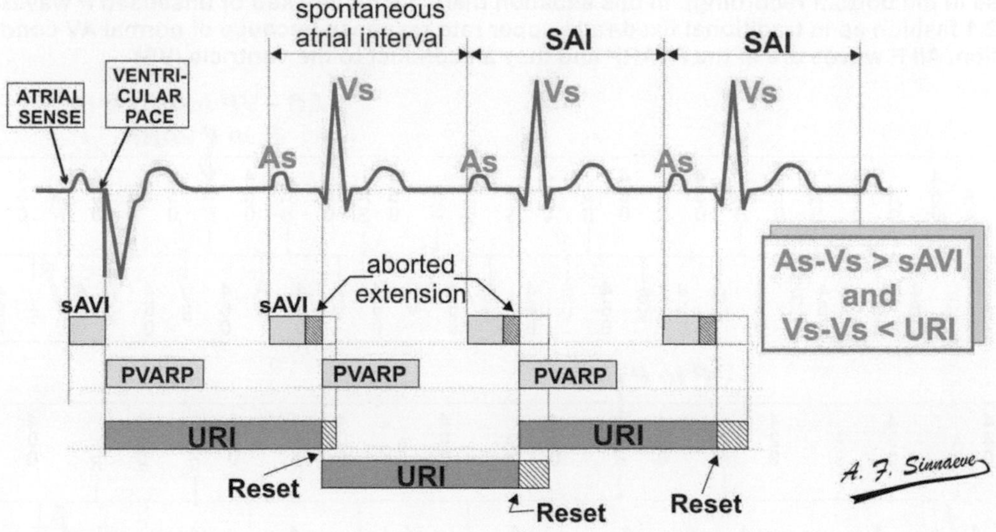

Abbreviations : As = atrial sense, Vs = ventricular sense, CRT = cardiac resynchronization therapy ; sAVI = AV delay after sensing, PVARP = postventricular atrial refractory period, URI = upper rate interval ; SAI = spontaneous atrial interval

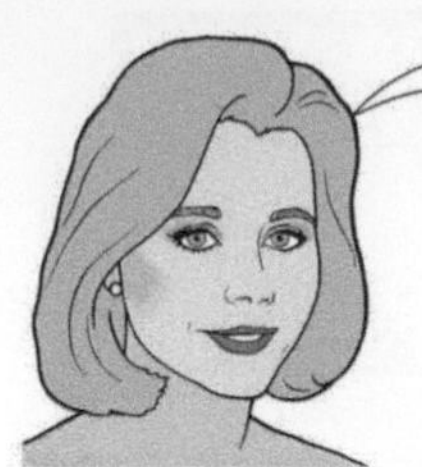

CRT devices that memorize episodes of ventricular sensing together with preceding events have facilitated the diagnosis of pacemaker upper rate behavior. The long-term stored data in CRT devices are diagnostically far superior than conventional 24 hr Holter recordings !

UPPER RATE LIMITATION IN CRT - part 2

Normal BiV pacing : AS - BV

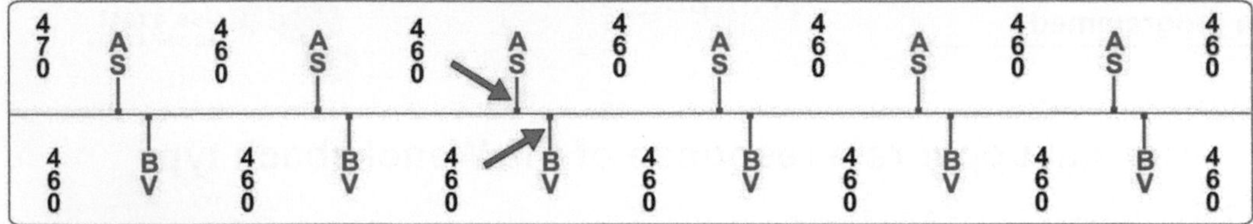

Pre-empted Wenckebach upper rate response : AS - VS
Programmed upper rate = 130 ppm :
VS - VS < upper rate interval 460 ms

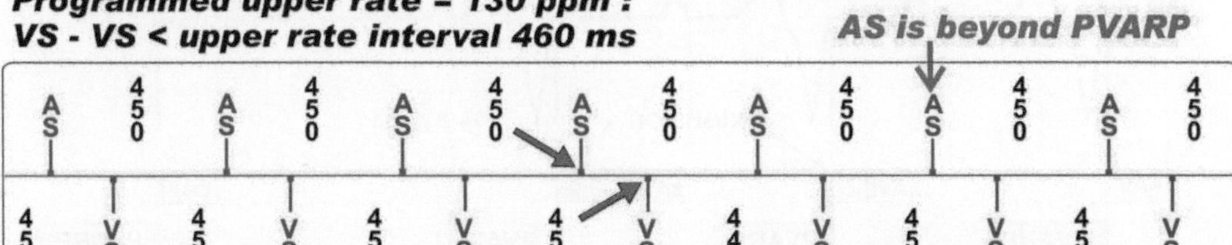

Cardiac Resynchronization Therapy : Wenckebach upper rate response

A standard Wenckebach upper rate response terminates with uiniform AR-VS sequences with every P in the PVARP. Note that the sequence with AR-VS combinations occurs when the spontaneous AR-AR or VS-VS intervals are shorter than the TARP (see a similar response in the bottom recording). In this situation there are no blocked or unsensed P waves in a 2:1 fashion as in traditional fixed-ratio upper rate response because of normal AV conduction. All P waves are in the PVARP and they all conduct to the ventricle (VS)

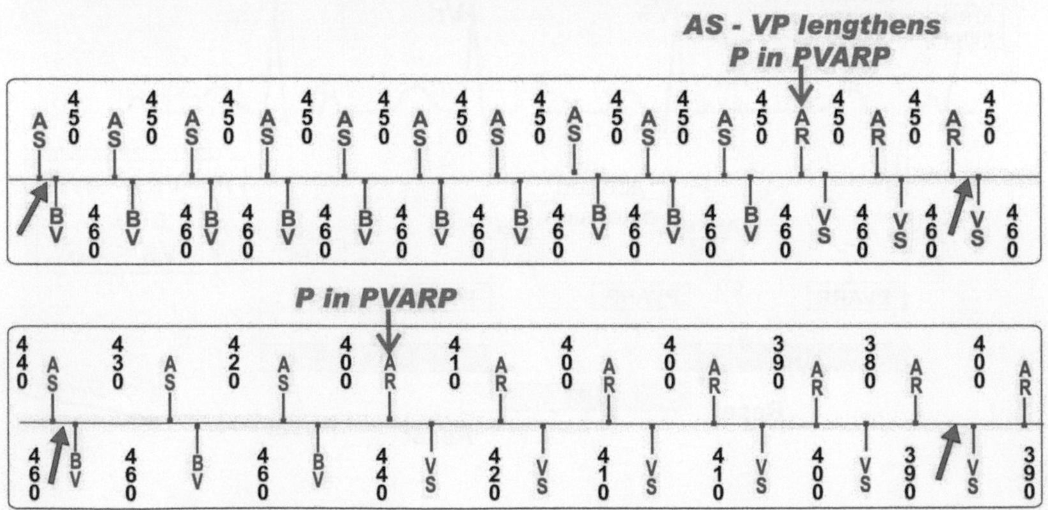

Abbreviations : AS = atrial sense ; AR = atrial sense during refractory period ; BV = biventricular pace ; PVARP = postventricular atrial refractory period ; VP = ventricular pace ; VS = ventricular sense ; TARP = total atrial refractory period.

A. F. Sinnaeve

HOW TO PROGRAM A CRT DEVICE

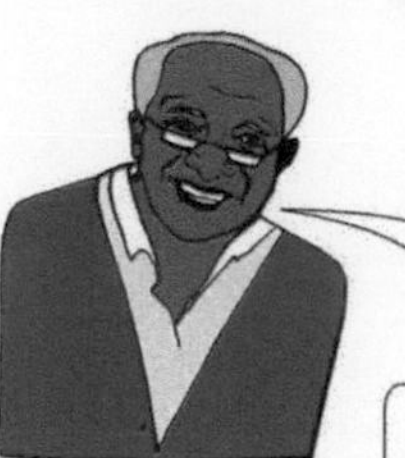

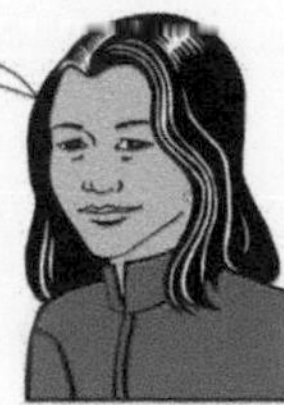

Programming CRT devices is difficult and quite different from conventional pacemakers. Could you please explain the most important aspects.

Ten points come to mind !

IMPORTANT LEARNING POINTS

1. The lower rate of CRT devices should be programmed to permit atrial sensing because atrial pacing produces a lesser hemodynamic benefit and may predispose to atrial fibrillation. The upper rate should be relatively fast (≥ 140 ppm) to prevent loss of atrial tracking with resultant inhibition of ventricular synchronization during sinus tachycardia and during exercise.

2. The postventricular atrial refractory period (PVARP) should be relatively short (≤ 250 ms). It is important to turn off PVARP extension after a pacemaker-defined premature ventricular complex (PVC) and algorithms that use PVARP prolongation for the automatic termination of pacemaker-mediated tachycardia (PMT). A short PVARP is safe because endless loop tachycardia is rare in CRT patients.

3. Electrical desynchronization can occur as an upper rate response but also occurs at atrial rates below the programmed upper rate when P waves are continually trapped in the PVARP. A relatively slow upper rate, a long PVARP and a long PR interval predispose for the latter. A special pacemaker function can detect this form of electrical desynchronization below the upper rate and can restore P wave tracking by automatic PVARP abbreviation for one cycle.

4. In selected patients the left ventricular output can be programmed to x 1.5 the threshold voltage at the same pulse duration to conserve battery life because CRT devices require a much higher current drain from the battery than conventional devices.

5. Atrial fibrillation and atrial tachyarrhythmias should be treated aggressively and AV junctional ablation should be performed. With conservative therapy, the presence of CRT should be confirmed with Holter recordings and an exercise stress test.

6. In the presence of a bipolar left ventricular lead, some devices provide "electrical repositioning" whereby the 2 electrodes in each ventricle can be configured in a variety of combinations. This function can be useful in eliminating phrenic nerve stimulation and in lowering the LV output for pacing.

A.F. SINNAEVE

A. F. Sinnaeve

HOW TO PROGRAM A CRT DEVICE

7. Availability of the 12-lead ECG during programming is essential !

8. Optimizing the AV delay should be done in most, if not in all patients. The optimal AV delay changes with the passage of time. Methodology varies and there is no gold standard. A degree of fusion with spontaneous right ventricular activity may be acceptable in some patients provided there is no hemodynamic deterioration.

9. Intra- and interatrial conduction delay complicate AV optimization and may occasionally require AV junctional ablation to provide effective CRT. Interatrial conduction delay should be recognized before CRT implantation whereupon the atrial lead can be placed on the interatrial septum to prevent programming difficulties.

10. V-V interval optimization is beneficial only in selected patients with a suboptimal CRT response. Patients likely to benefit usually have slowed intraventricular conduction in the area of myocardial scar, LV latency or less than satisfactory lead position that may benefit from V-V interval optimization. Most commonly, the LV is pre-excited. Anodal stimulation cancels the V-V delay to zero.

A.F. SINNAEVE

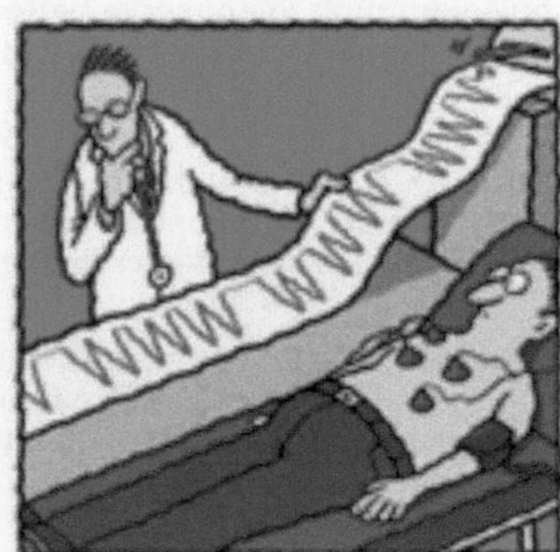

A. F. Sinnaeve

IMPACT OF V-V INTERVAL PROGRAMMING ON THE EFFECTIVE AV DELAY : *DIFFERENCES BETWEEN DEVICE MANUFACTURERS*

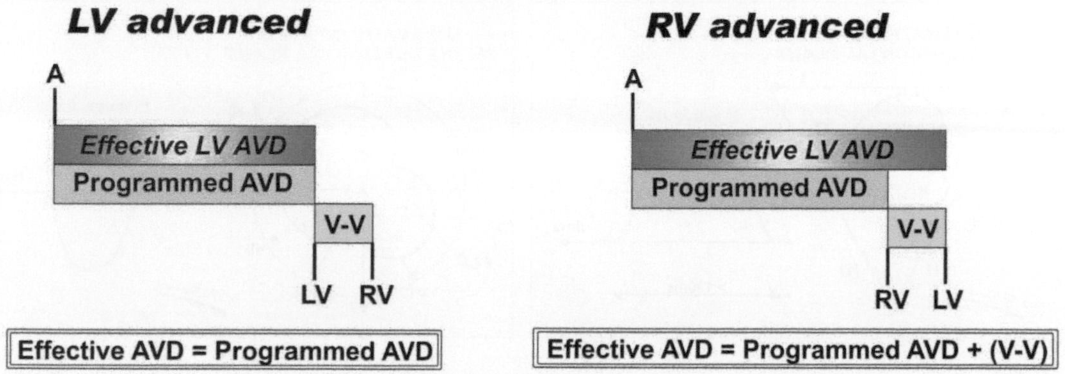

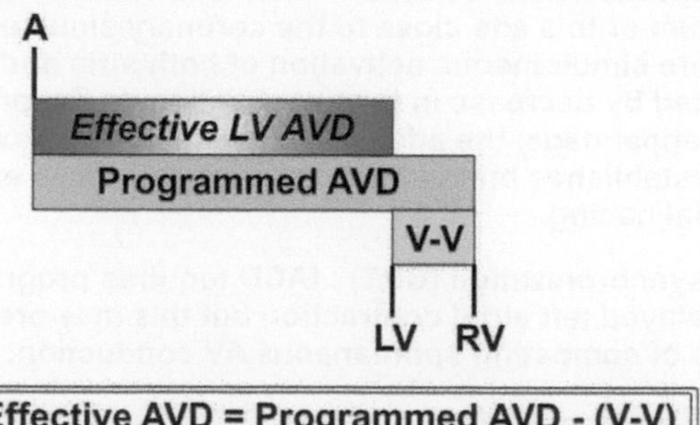

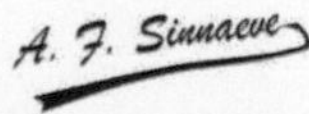

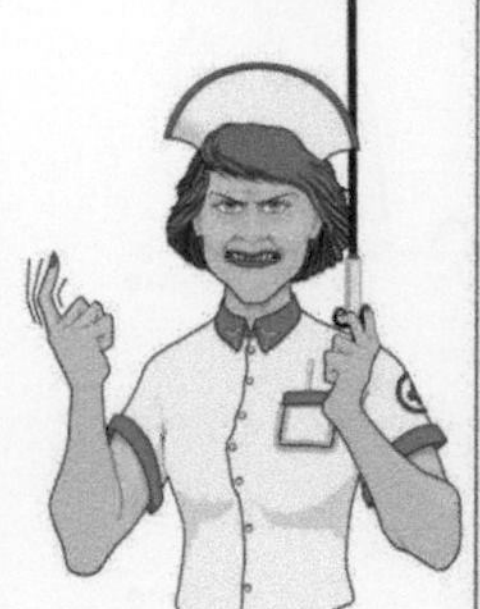

Effective V-V interval programming allows us to separately program the RV and LV AV delays. Depending on the device manufacturer, V-V interval programming will have different impact on the effective AV delay and it is crucial to understand these differences.
In most devices (all manufacturers but Guidant) the channel that is advanced by V-V interval programming will be placed at the programmed PV/AV delay.
In Guidant devices PV/AV timing applies to the RV channel (RV based) so that when LV activation is advanced by V-V interval programming, the LV AV delay can be calculated by subtracting the V-V interval from the PV/AV delay. In the Guidant system, RV cannot be advanced.

Abbreviations : AVD = atrioventricular delay ; LV = left ventricle ; RV = right ventricle ; PV = ventricular paced event ;

INTER-ATRIAL CONDUCTION DELAY (IACD) - 1

IACD is characterized by a wide and notched P wave (>120 ms) traditionally in ECG lead II, associated with a wide terminal negativity of the P wave in lead V1.

IACD as seen in the frontal plane

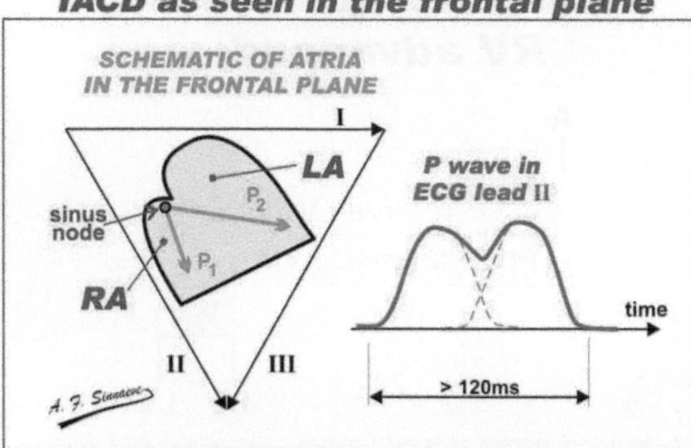

IACD as seen in the horizontal plane

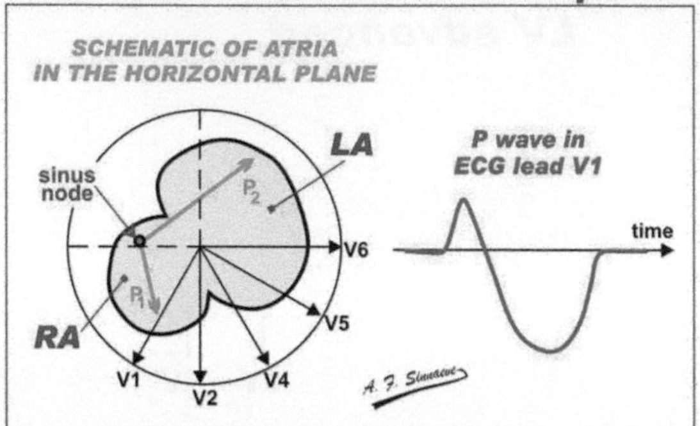

- **When the ECG suggests IACD, confirmation should be done with intracardiac recordings at the time of implantation.**
- **With inter-atrial conduction delay, the atrial lead should be placed on the high- or mid-atrial septum or to a site close to the coronary sinus os. Pacing from these sites produces a more simultaneous activation of both atria and abbreviation of total atrial activation judged by decrease in P wave duration. In the presence of long-term pacing from the right appendage, the addition of a lead in the proximal coronary sinus (left atrial pacing) establishes biatrial pacing which produces essentially the same effect as single lead atrial pacing.**
- **For cardiac resynchronization (CRT) : IACD requires programming a long AV delay to adjust for delayed left atrial contraction but this may preclude CRT because of the emergence of competing spontaneous AV conduction.**

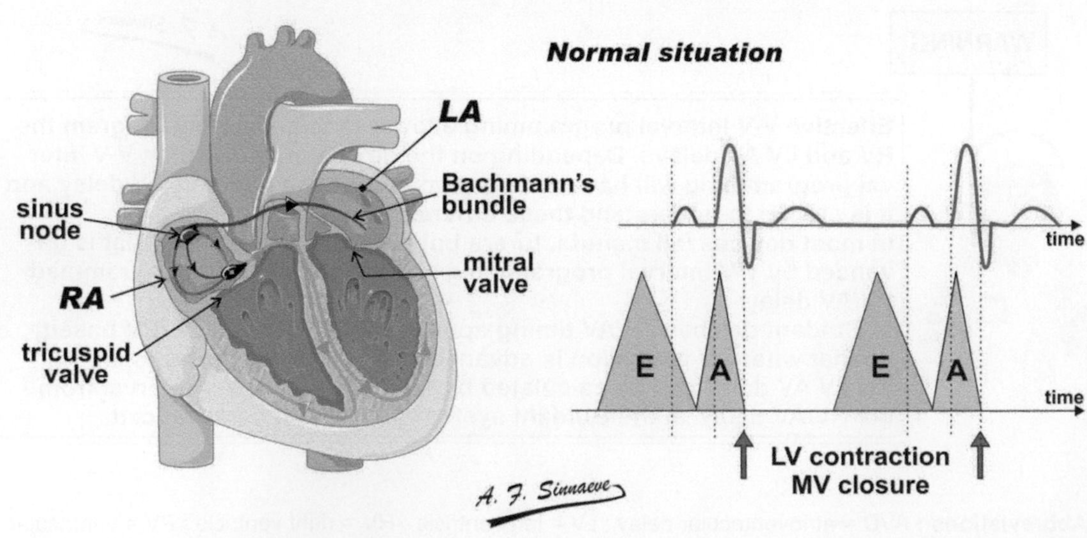

INTER-ATRIAL CONDUCTION DELAY (IACD) - 2

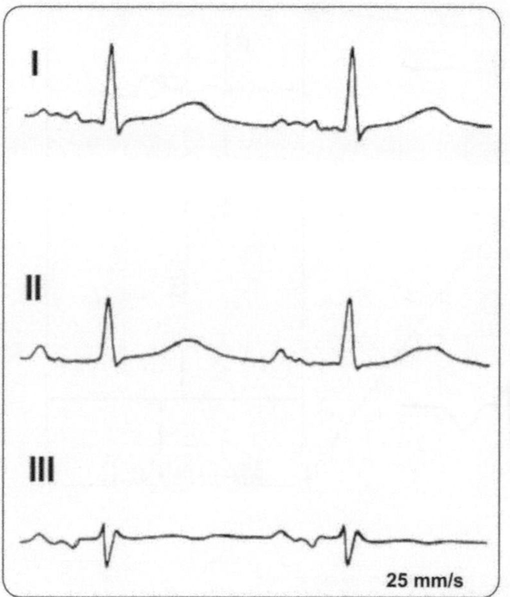

In IACD the delay measured between the beginning of the P wave (or the first deflection as detected in the RA) and the atrial deflection recorded in in the distal CS is typically > 120 ms

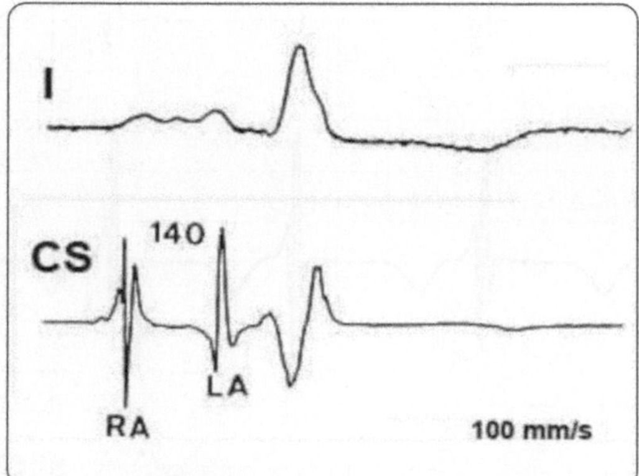

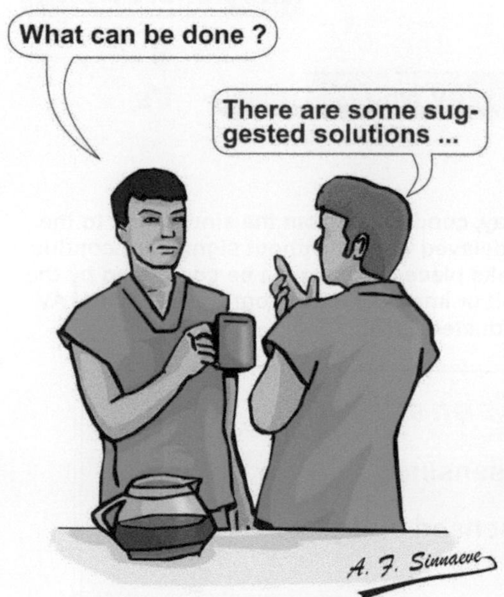

The solutions are :

* AV delay needs to be extended
* Individual Doppler echo AV optimization
* Pharmacologic AV blocking agents
* Position atrial lead in mid-septum or proximal coronary sinus or vicinity of coronary sinus os
* Biatrial or dual site right atrial pacing (2 sites may be used if there is already a lead in the right atrial appendage)
* AV Junctional ablation especially with CRT

LATE ATRIAL SENSING DUE TO RIGHT INTRAATRIAL CONDUCTION DELAY
IMPACT ON CARDIAC RESYNCHRONIZATION

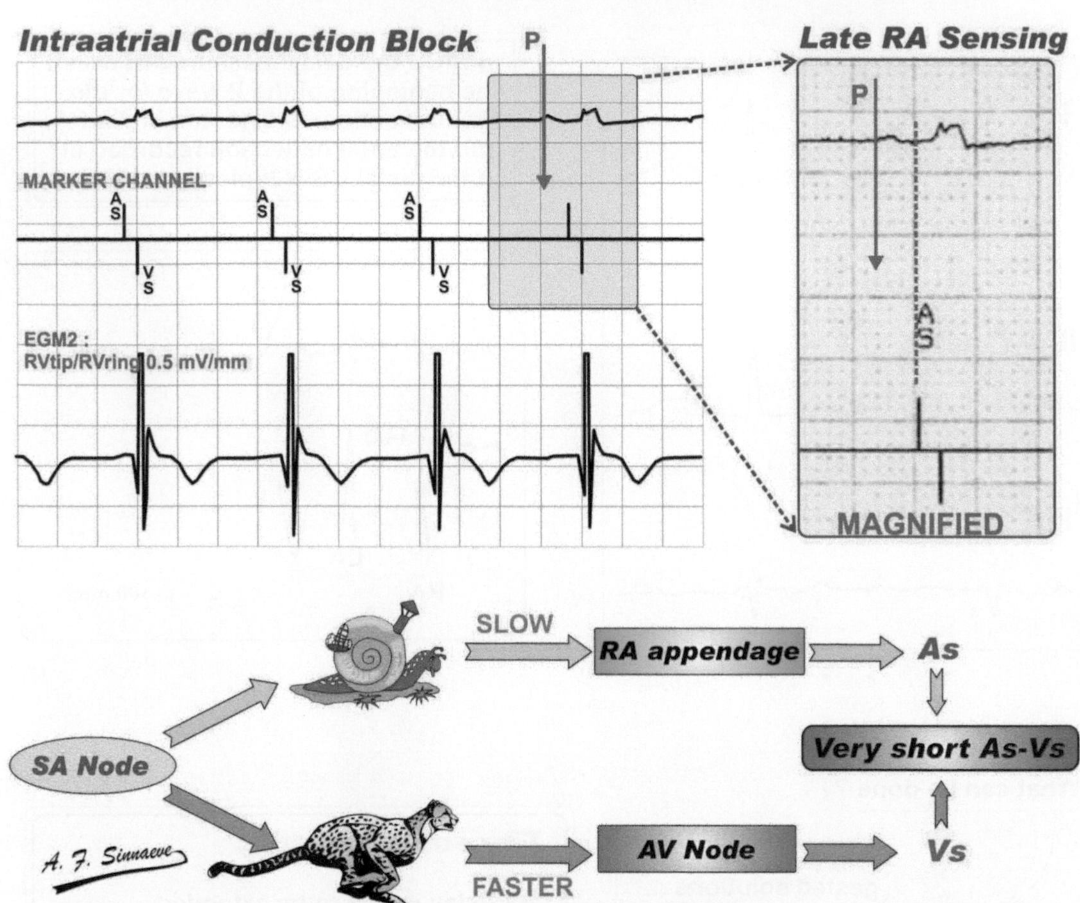

In some patients with right intraatrial conduction delay, conduction from the sinus node to the right atrial (RA) appendage (site of atrial sensing) is delayed with or without significant conduction delay to the left atrium (LA). LA activation may take place or may even be completed by the time the device senses the RA EGM. It may be difficult or impossible to program an optimal AV delay with CRT in the absence of fusion with the conducted QRS.

Treatment of late atrial sensing :

1. **Triggered mode (BiV) upon RV sensing**
2. **Programming widely different sensed and paced AV delays**
3. **Ablation of the AV junction**

Abbreviations : As = atrial sensed event ; BiV = biventricular ; CRT = cardiac resynchronization therapy ; EGM = electrogram ; LA = left atrium ; RA = right atrium ; SA = sinoatrial ; Vs = ventricular sensed event ;

LATE ATRIAL SENSING DUE TO RIGHT INTRAATRIAL CONDUCTION DELAY - part 2
IMPACT ON CARDIAC RESYNCHRONIZATION

Triggered biventricular pacing

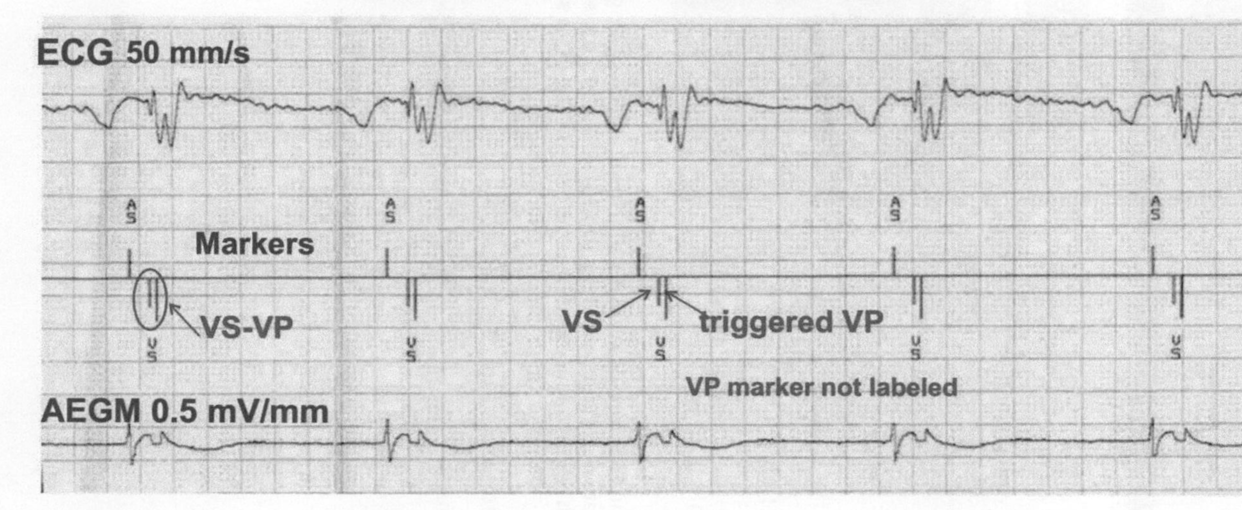

Ventricular triggering attempts CRT by triggering a biventricular output immediately when the device senses (RV channel) a QRS complex within the programmed AV delay or it senses a pacemaker-defined ventricular premature complex. The delivered triggered stimulus may occur too late for effective electrical resynchronization. There are a minimal data about the efficacy of this feature and the question arises as to whether pacing-induced LV depolarization actually occurs and if it does, to what degree. The beneficial effect, if any, should be assessed by Doppler echocardiography.

A. F. Sinnaeve

LATE ATRIAL SENSING DUE TO RIGHT INTRAATRIAL CONDUCTION DELAY - part 3
IMPACT ON CARDIAC RESYNCHRONIZATION

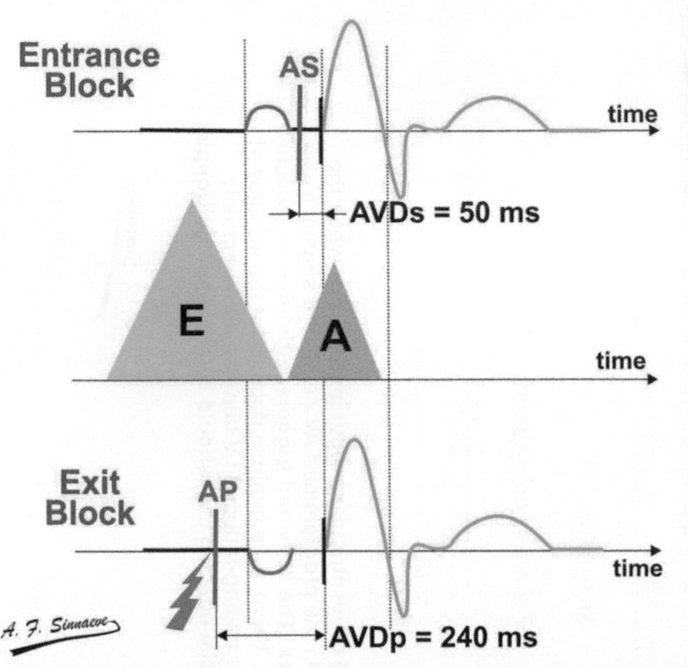

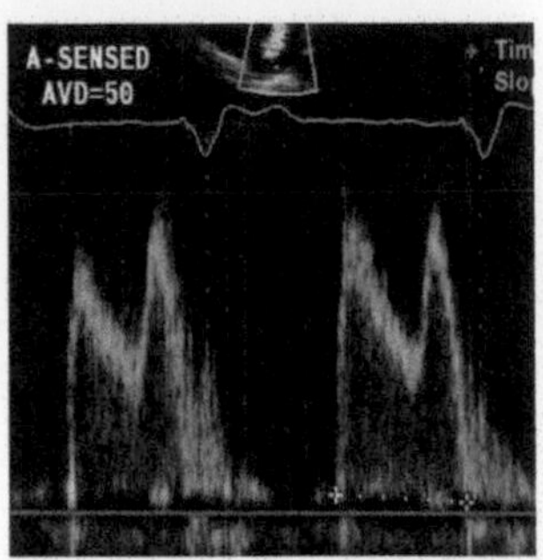

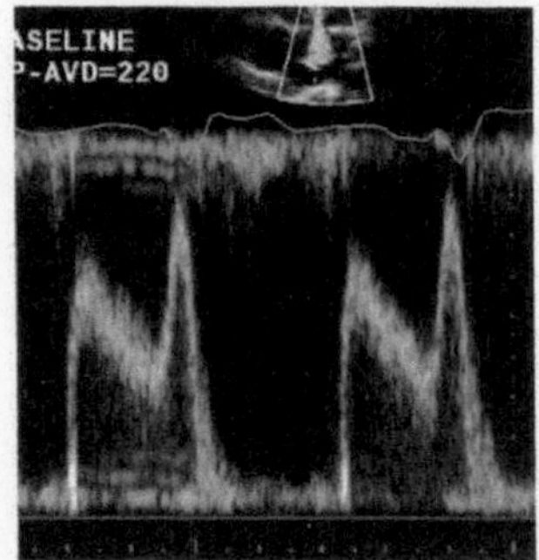

There is a short sensed AV delay in sinus rhythm (late sensing). During atrial pacing there is a prolonged atrial latency interval and intraatrial conduction delay (bottom). A short sensed AV delay and long paced AV delay achieved similar hemodynamic results as shown on the right side.

Marked late atrial sensing

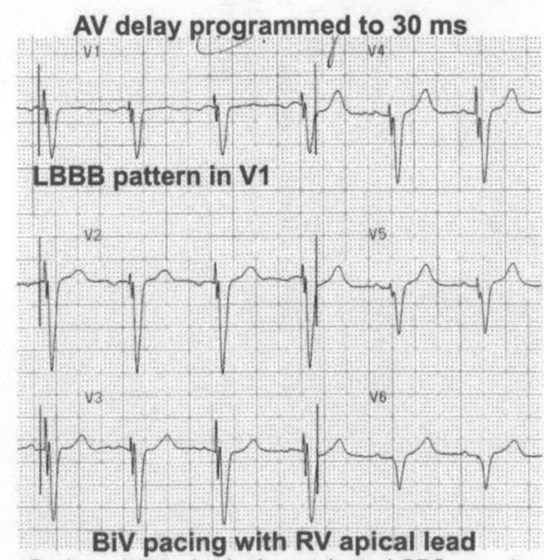

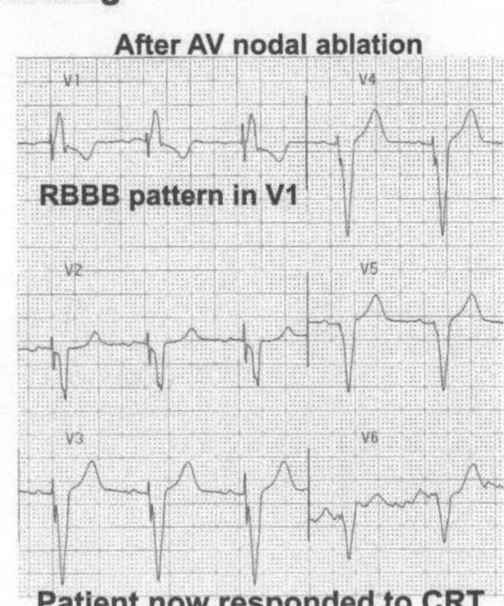

Abbreviations : AP = atrial pacing ; AS = atrial sensing ; AVDs = AV delay sensed ; AVDp = AV delay paced ; CRT = cardiac resynchronization therapy ; LBBB = left bundle branch block ; RA = right atrium ; RBBB = right bundle branch block ;

THE PVARP LOCK DURING CRT

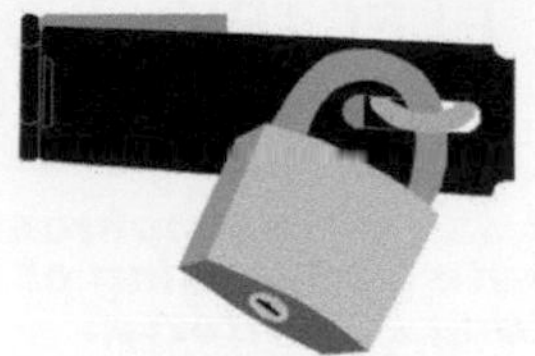

Beware : Loss of CRT !

P wave is locked in PVARP below the programmed upper rate **(150 ppm or 400 ms interval here)**

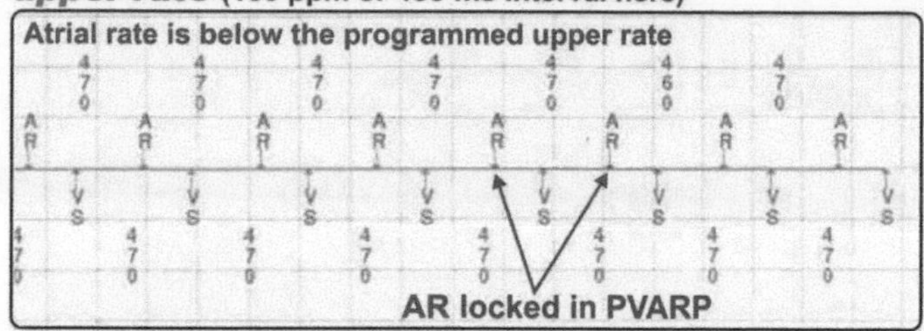

* **Program algorithm that shortens PVARP for one cycle. This does not work if P wave is in the postventricular atrial *blanking* period.**
* **Shorten PVARP**
* **Drugs to slow sinus rate**
* **Ablation of AV junction in refractory cases which usually involve patients with a long PR interval**

Loss of resynchronization below the programmed upper rate

* **The native PR interval (AR-VS) must be longer than the programmed sensed AV delay (AS-VP)**
* **Total atrial refractory period (TARP) = AV delay + PVARP**
* **Because AR-AS > AS-VP, TARP controlled by AR-AS interval must be longer as the PVARP remains constant.**
* **Resynchronization will occur when P-P interval > (AR-VS) + PVARP or when the special algorithm abbreviates the PVARP.**

Loss of resynchronization caused by T wave sensing

P in PVARP below the upper rate with loss of CRT.

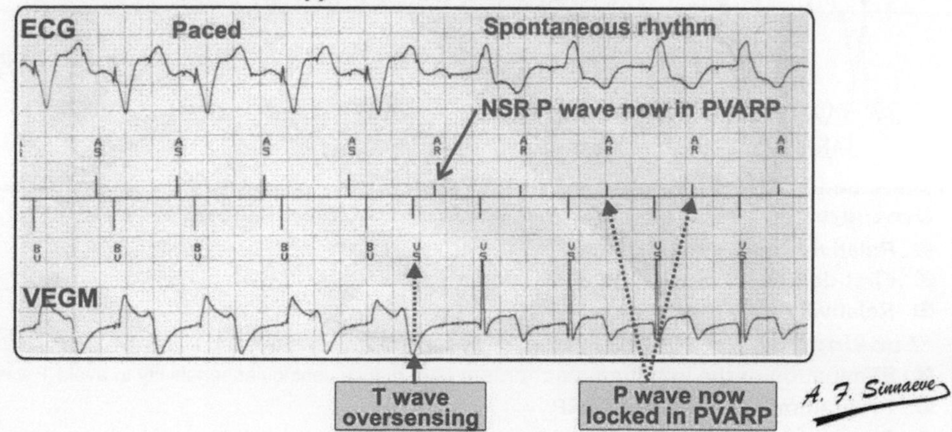

A. F. Sinnaeve

A single VPC can produce the same effect.

Abbreviations : AR = atrial refractory sensed event ; AS = sensed atrial event ; CRT = cardiac resynchronization therapy ; PVARP = postventricular atrial refractory period ; VP = paced ventricular event ; VS = sensed ventricular event ;

ELECTRICAL DESYNCHRONIZATION IN BIVENTRICULAR PACEMAKERS

CRT is another example where one must know the timing cycles of the device to understand its function

1 Loss of resynchronization below the programmed upper rate and locking of P waves inside the PVARP due to a long P-R interval

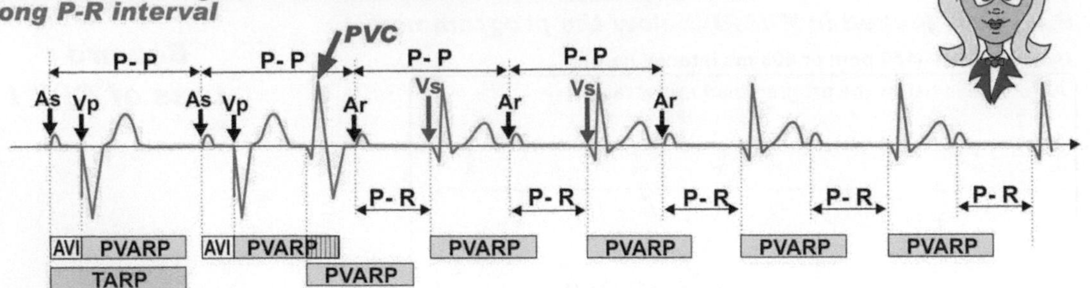

NOTE :
The same locking of P waves inside the PVARP can be caused by T wave oversensing

2 No locking of P waves inside the PVARP if the P-R interval is shorter

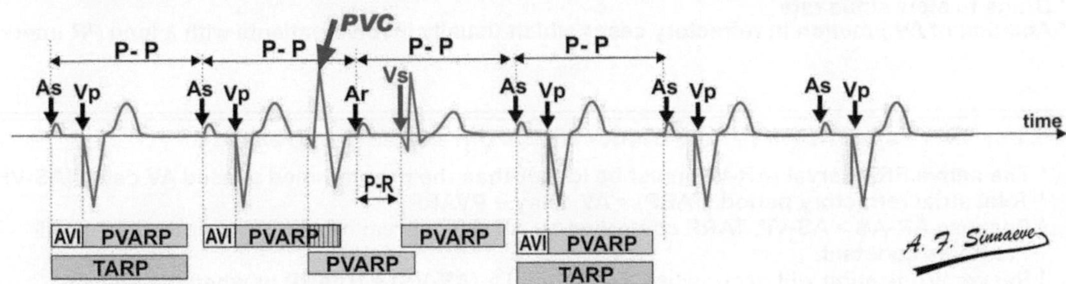

3 Sinus tachycardia can produce desynchronization even when the P-R interval is relatively short

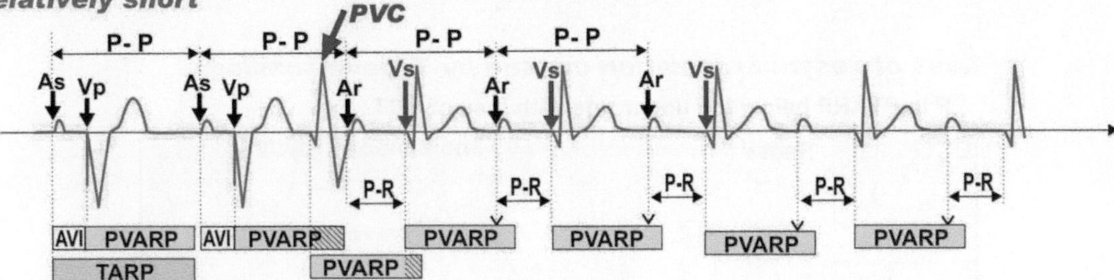

Development of electrical desynchronization may be favored by :

- **Relatively fast sinus rhythms**
- **First-degree AV block (long P- R interval)**
- **Relatively long programmed PVARP**

"Locking" of the P waves can often be prevented by :

- **Elimination of the initiating mechanism** (e.g. reduce ventricular sensitivity to avoid T wave sensing)
- **Programming a shorter PVARP**
- **Slowing the sinus rate with drugs**
- **Refractory cases (marked 1st degree AV block) can be treated by AV junctional ablation**

Abbreviations : AVI = programmed AV interval ; As = sensed atrial event ; Ar = sensed atrial event during refractory period ; P-P = period between two consecutive P waves ; P-R = period between a P wave and its following R wave ; PVARP = post-ventricular atrial refractory period ; PVC = premature ventricular complex ; TARP = total atrial refractory period ; Vp = paced ventricular event ; Vs sensed ventricular event .

P WAVE TRACKING AND VENTRICULAR DESYNCHRONIZATION

If I'm exercising too hard, my CRT- ICD device cannot follow !

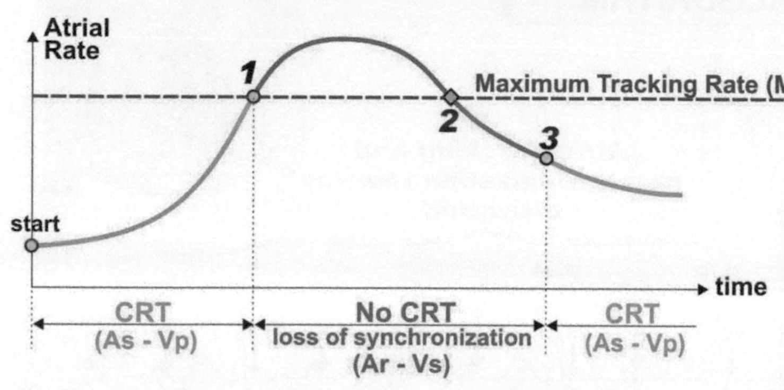

Total atrial refractory period :

TARP = AVI + PVARP

Maximum tracking rate :

$$MTR = \frac{60{,}000}{TARP}$$

From start to point 1 : As - Vp sequence

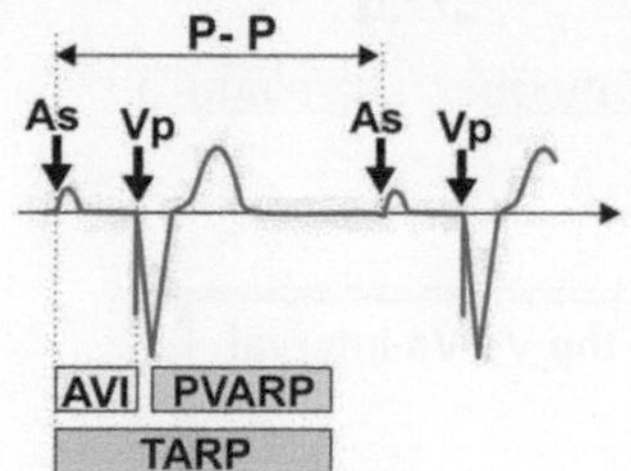

P-P > TARP ⟶ atrial rate < MTR

The spontaneous atrial rate is lower than the maximum tracking rate. Since both ventricles are paced, adequate CRT is delivered.

From point 1 to point 2 : Ar - Vs sequence

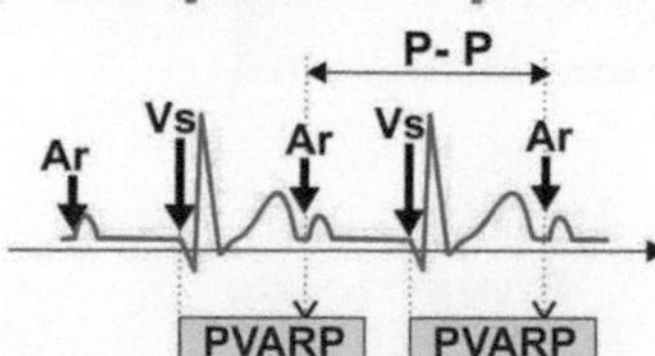

P-P < TARP ⟶ atrial rate > MTR

As soon as the atrial rate exceeds the MTR, the P wave falls within the PVARP and ventricular resynchronization is lost.

Note : (Ar - Vs) > AVI (= As - Vp)

From point 2 to point 3 : Ar - Vs sequence

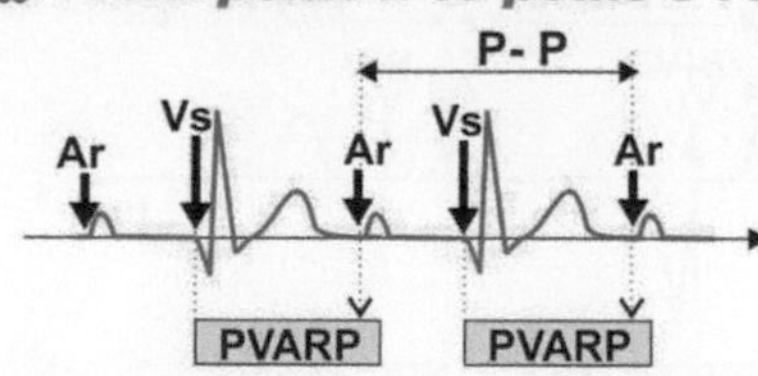

P-P > TARP ⟶ atrial rate < MTR

The timing cycles of the device force the continuation of the Ar - Vs sequences as long as P-P < [(Ar - Vs) + PVARP]

At point 3 the atrial rate is decreased far enough as to make P-P = [(Ar - Vs) + PVARP]

From point 3 to the end : As - Vp sequence

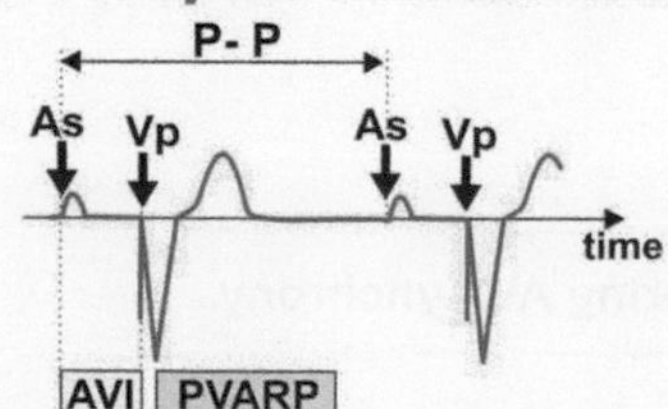

P-P > [(Ar - Vs) + PVARP] and ventricular synchronized pacing restarts

P-P > TARP ⟶ atrial rate < MTR

Same ECG as between points 1 and 2

A. F. Sinnaeve

Note : The actual "Total atrial refractory period" generated by Ar-Vs sequences is longer than the programmed TARP because Ar-Vs > programmed As-Vp (=AVI) !

Abbreviations : As = atrial sensed event ; Ar = atrial event sensed in the atrial refractory period where tracking cannot occur ; AVI = programmed AV interval ; CRT = cardiac resynchronization therapy ; MTR = maximum tracking rate ; P-P = interval between to consecutive P waves ; PVARP = postventricular atrial refractory period ; TARP = total atrial refractory period ; Vp = biventricular paced event ; Vs = ventricular sensed event.

At last !
The end of the tunnel !

ATRIAL TRACKING RECOVERY : A MEDTRONIC ALGORITHM

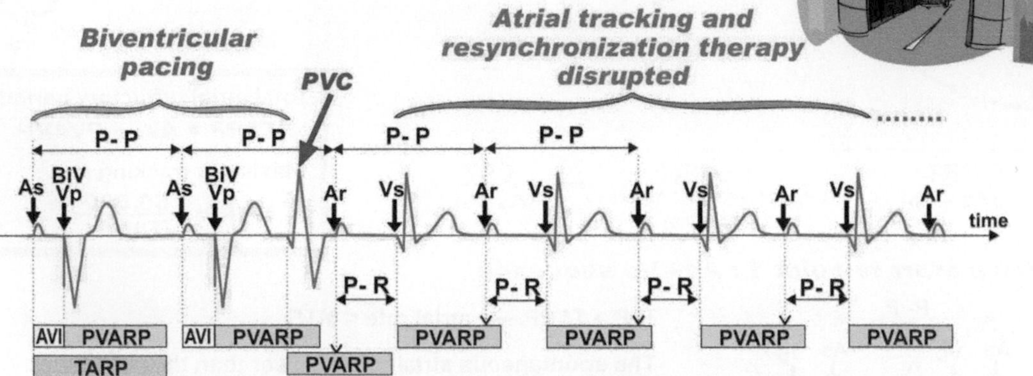

- ☑ The algorithm recognizes Vs-Ar sequences only when the Vs-Vs interval is longer than the programmed upper rate interval.
- ☑ Atrial events must occur during PVARP.
- ☑ After eight Ar-Vs cycles, the device intervenes by shortening the PVARP.
- ☑ If the attempt fails, the process continues until As-BiV Vp intervals are restored at their programmed value.

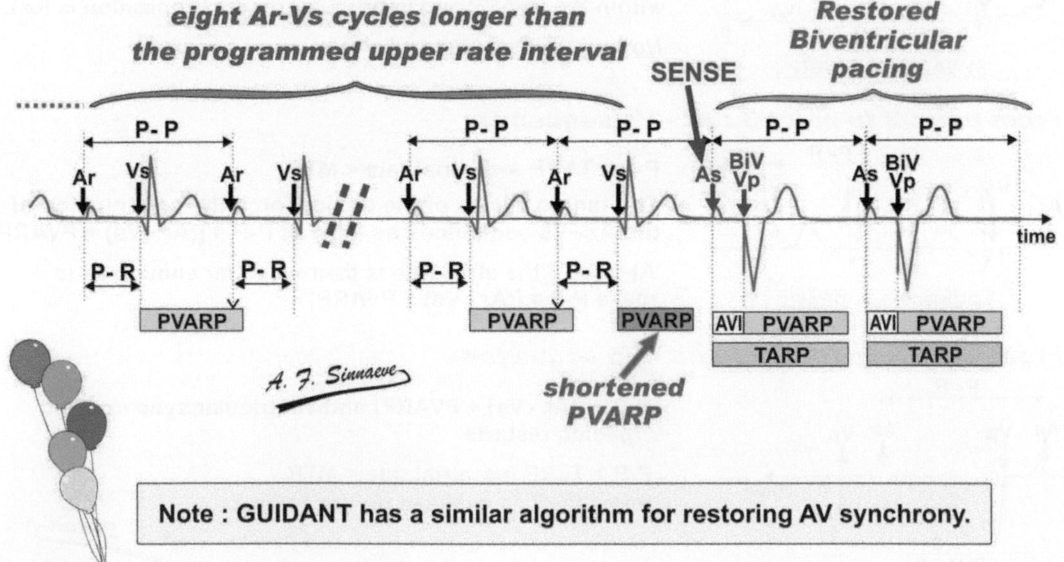

Note : GUIDANT has a similar algorithm for restoring AV synchrony.

Abbreviations : AVI = programmed AV interval ; As = sensed atrial event ; Ar = sensed atrial event during refractory period ; P-P = period between two consecutive P waves ; P-R = period between a P wave and its following R wave ; PVARP = post-ventricular atrial refractory period ; PVC = premature ventricular complex ; TARP = total atrial refractory period ; BiV Vp = biventricular paced event ; Vs sensed ventricular event .

MANAGEMENT OF PVARP LOCK DURING CRT

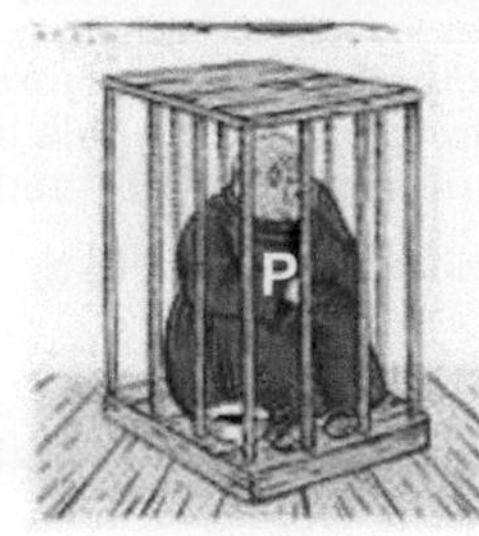

AUTOMATICITY in CRT

No CRT is possible with a trapped P wave in the PVARP !

Release the trapped P wave in the PVARP

Automatic restoration of CRT by PVARP abbreviation for 1 cycle

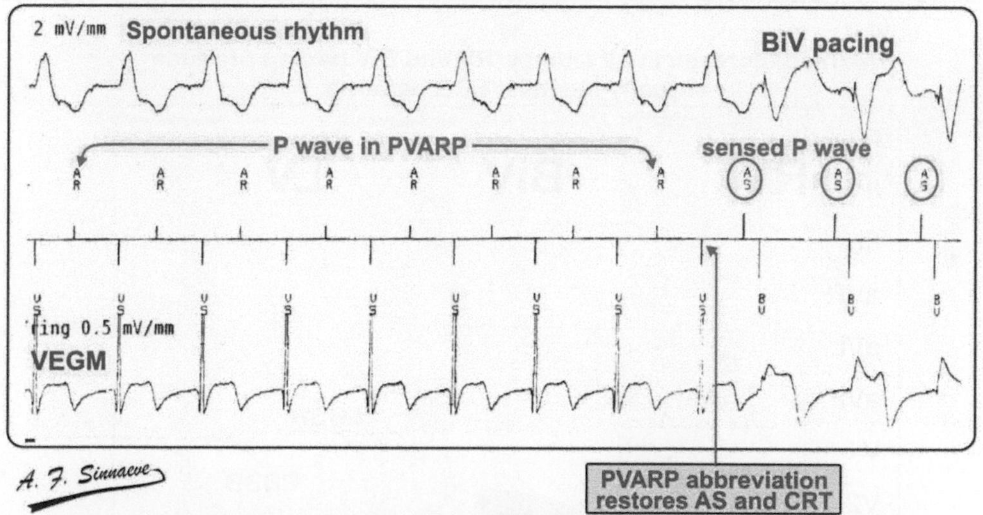

CRT and PVARP programmability

* Keep PVARP short if possible
* Do not use PMT termination algorithm using PVARP extension in most patients.
* Do not use post VPC + PVARP in most patients.
* Remember to program a fast upper rate which needs a short PVARP ! PMT is rare in CRT patients.

Take home message for CRT

Short PVARP ⟷ High upper rate interval

Abbreviations : AR = atrial refractory sense ; AS = sensed atrial event ; BV and BiV = biventricular ; CRT = cardiac resynchronization therapy ; PVARP = postventricular atrial refractory period ; PMT = pacemaker mediated tachycardia ; VP = paced ventricular event ; VPC = ventricular premature complex ; VS = sensed ventricular event ;

LATENCY DURING LEFT VENTRICULAR PACING

Electrical latency :
interval from the pacemaker stimulus to the onset of the paced QRS complex.

At physiologic rates pronounced latency is uncommon during RV pacing but may be more prevalent during LV pacing because of LV pathology including scars. During RV pacing this interval normally measures < 40 ms. The normal value for LV pacing has not yet been determined.

Prolonged LV latency delays LV depolarization during simultaneous biventricular pacing, producing an ECG pattern dominated by RV pacing.

Latency may be related to non-homogeneous impulse propagation from the paced site, conduction block in proximity to the electrode or prolonged refractoriness. It is often rate and output dependent.
The conventional surface ECG cannot differentiate failure of excitation from delayed propagation in the myocardium around the electrode.

Marked increase in LV latency. RV and BiV pacing produce virtually identical ECG patterns.

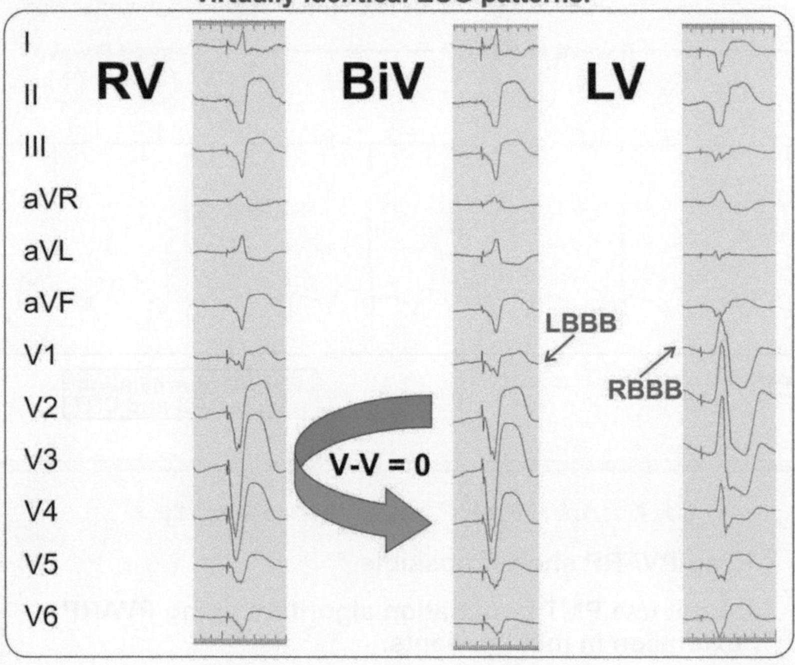

Impact of prolonged LV latency interval on the ECG.

The latency interval during LV pacing is shown in the figure on the next page. The above recordings compare QRS morphology in 12-lead ECGs during RV, BiV, and LV pacing in the VVI mode at 80 ppm. The patient was in atrial fibrillation with complete AV block (excluding fusion with the spontaneous QRS complex). RV and LV outputs were each at twice the threshold voltage. During BiV pacing (V-V delay = 0) the QRS morphology is identical to that of RV pacing !

Abbreviations : AV = atrioventriculair ; BiV = biventricular ; LV = left ventricle ; RV = right ventricle ; V-V = interventricular interval between RV and LV stimuli ;

LATENCY DURING LEFT VENTRICULAR PACING
part 2

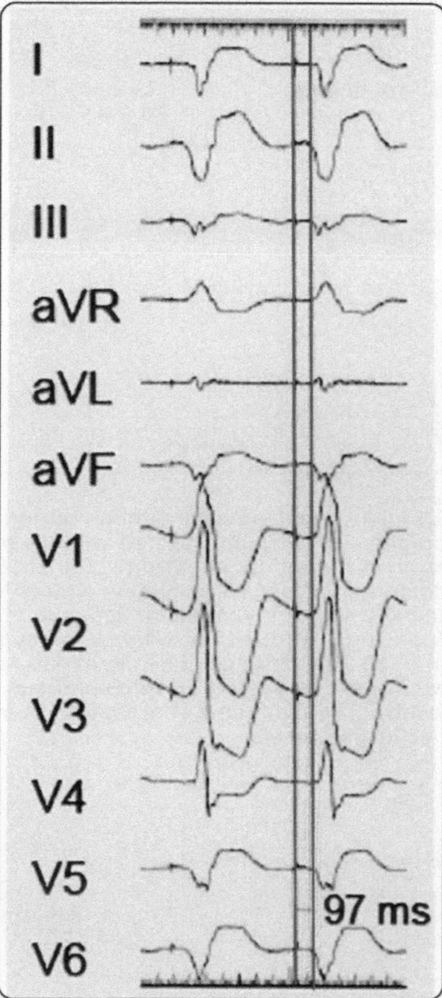

Latency interval.
Same patient and setting of LV output as in the preceding figure.
During LV pacing the stimulus to QRS latency interval measures 97 ms.

An isoelectric onset of the QRS complex in one or only a few leads can mimic latency. Consequently the demonstration of latency requires a 12-lead ECG taken at fast speed for diagnosis !

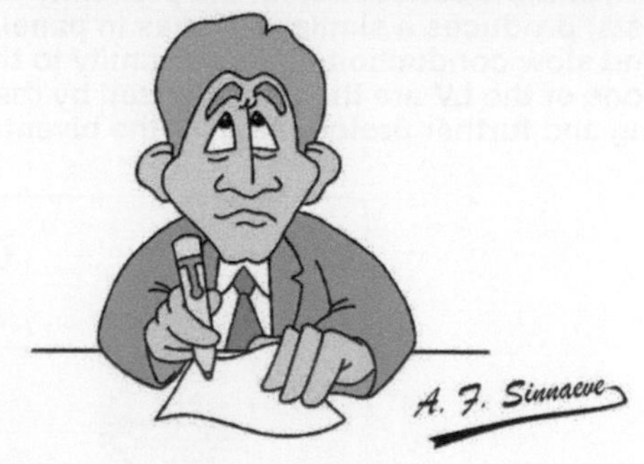

Correction of delayed LV activation

In patients with a biventricular system using the RV apex and abnormal LV latency, programming of incremental left to right V-V delays can unmask a dominant R wave in lead V1.
When the largest offset is insufficient (> 80 ms), the RV channel should be turned off to provide better hemodynamics.
When attempting to provide better electrocardiographic electrical synchrony by programming the V-V interval, it is important to appreciate that the relationship between the presence and/or amplitude of the paced R wave in lead V1 has not yet been correlated with the best mechanical or hemodynamic response in individual patients.

DIAGRAMMATIC REPRESENTATION OF LV LATENCY AND SLOW CONDUCTION

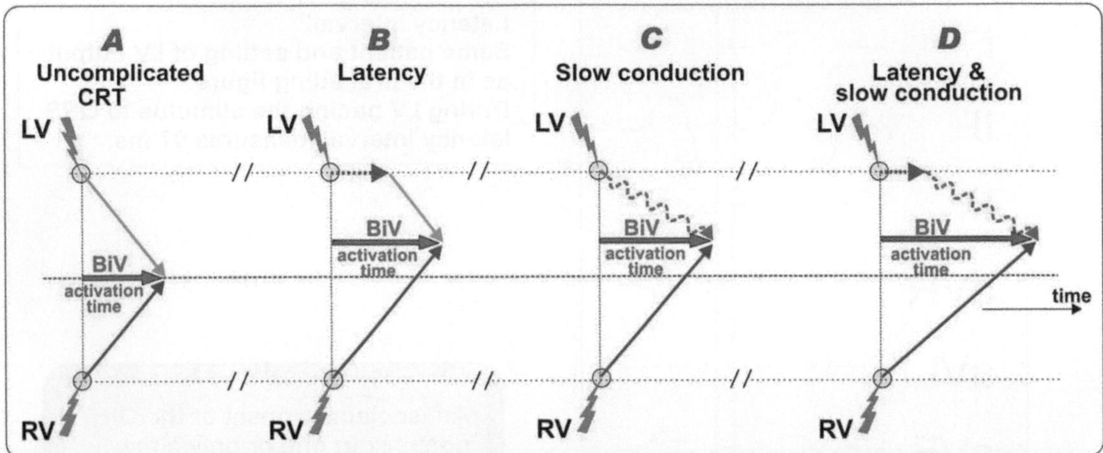

Diagrammatic representation of the significance of LV latency and slow conduction during simultaneous biventricular pacing. Panel 1A. During uncomplicated CRT, undisturbed impulse propagation from both pacing sites produces balanced fusion of RV and LV wavefronts. Panel 1B. In the presence of a prolonged LV latency interval (dashed dark-red arrow) LV activation occurs late and the RV wavefront depolarizes more myocardium causing a longer biventricular activation time. Panel 1C. Slow conduction in the proximity to the LV pacing site (due to scar tissue or myocardial fibrosis) produces a similar effect as in panel 1B. Panel 1D. Coexistence of a long LV latency interval and slow conduction in the proximity to the LV pacing site may occur in some patients. Major portions of the LV are then depolarized by the RV wavefront with minimal contribution from LV pacing and further prolongation of the biventricular activation time.

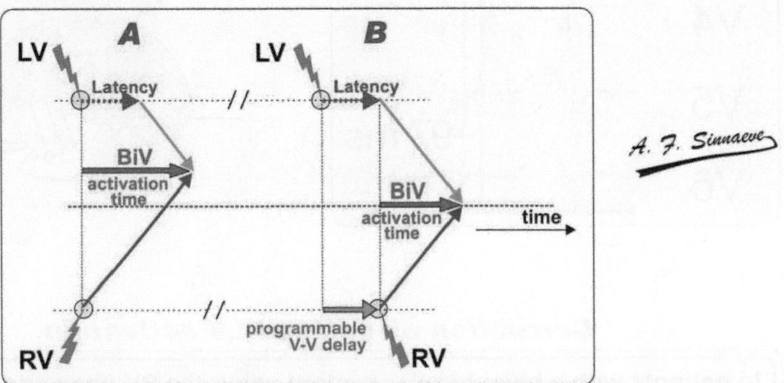

A. F. Sinnaeve

Panel 2. Compensatory programming for LV latency. Panel 2A. Simultaneous activation of both ventricles (on the left), results in late LV activation and more myocardium depolarized by the RV wavefront. Panel 2B. V-V programming permits LV pre-exitation to compensate for the prolonged LV latency interval. Both ventricles are activated synchronously resulting in a shorter biventricular activation time.
Pacing the LV only may result in some degree of fusion with native conduction on the right side depending on the programmed AV delay. This approach may yield satisfactory hemodynamic results in patients with a markedly prolonged LV latency interval

Abbreviations : AV = atrioventricular ; BiV = biventricular ; CRT = cardiac resynchronization therapy ; LVp = left ventricular pace ; RVp = right ventricular pace ; V-V = time interval between LVp and RVp ;

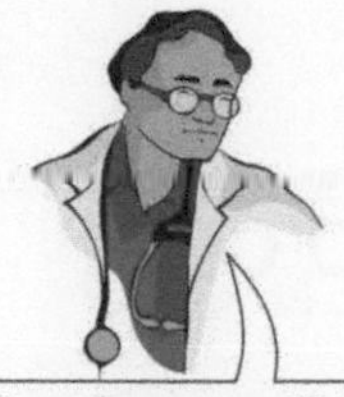

PHRENIC NERVE STIMULATION

Phrenic nerve stimulation is not uncommon (5-10% of patients) in LV pacing due to :

* close vicinity of the epicardial coronary venous lead to the left phrenic nerve when the LV lead is implanted in a posterior or posterolateral coronary vein. It may also be caused by lead dislodgment
* constraints of coronary venous anatomy

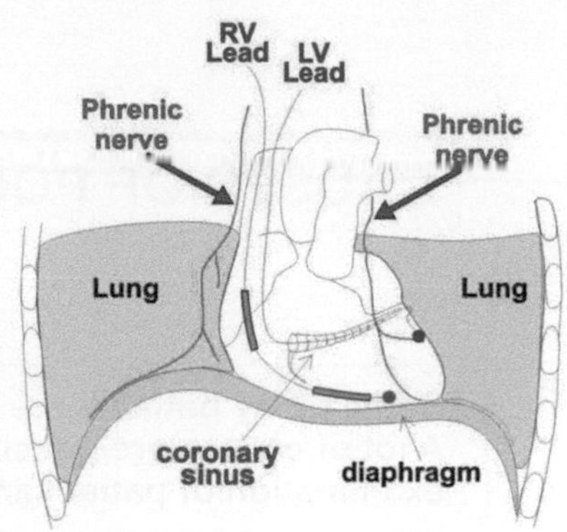

HOW TO AVOID DIAPHRAGMATIC STIMULATION

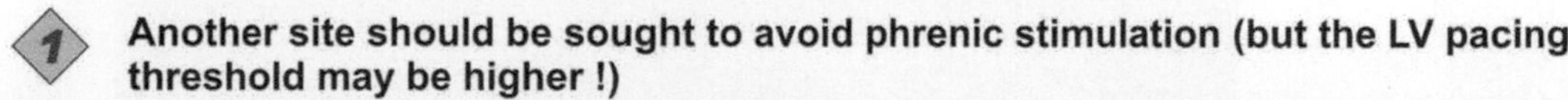

1. Another site should be sought to avoid phrenic stimulation (but the LV pacing threshold may be higher !)

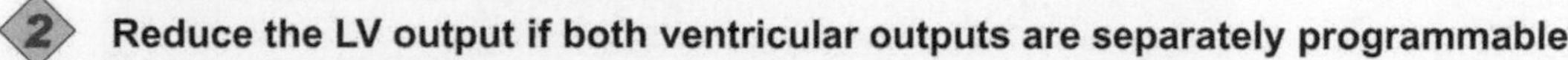

2. Reduce the LV output if both ventricular outputs are separately programmable

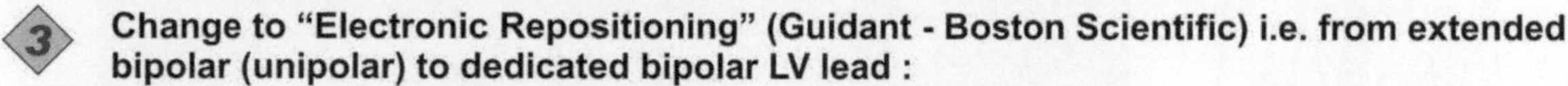

3. Change to "Electronic Repositioning" (Guidant - Boston Scientific) i.e. from extended bipolar (unipolar) to dedicated bipolar LV lead :

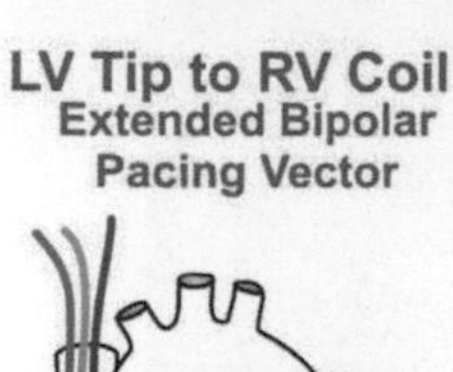

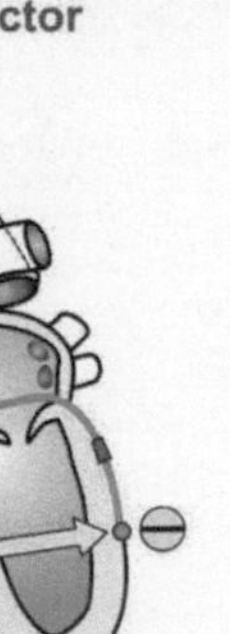

LV Tip to RV Coil
Extended Bipolar Pacing Vector

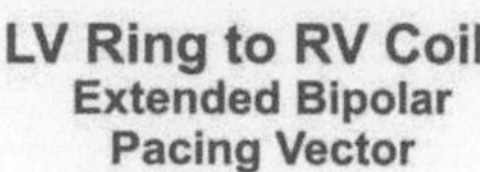

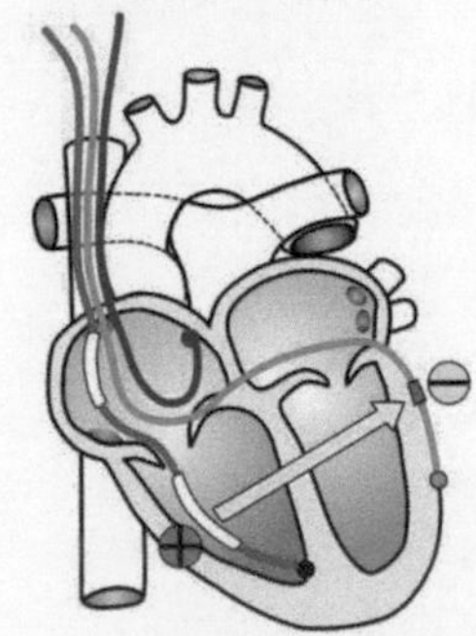

LV Ring to RV Coil
Extended Bipolar Pacing Vector

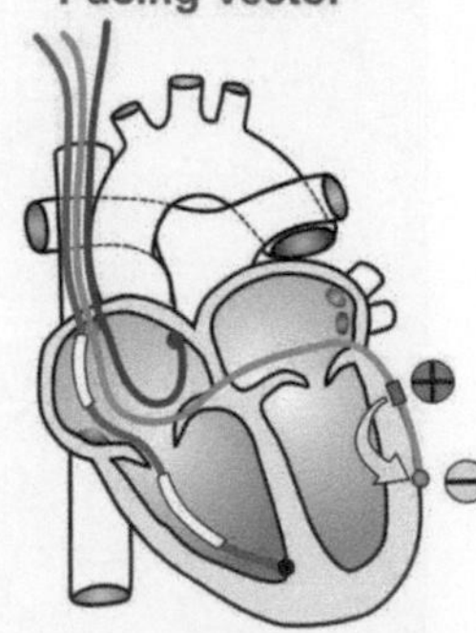

LV Tip to LV Ring
Dedicated Bipolar Pacing Vector

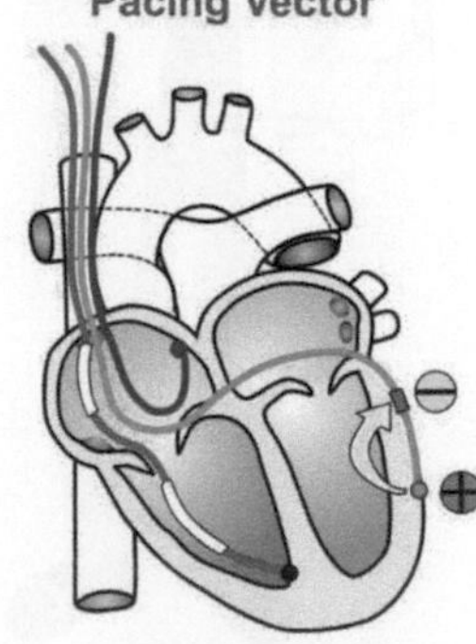

LV Ring to LV Tip
Dedicated Bipolar Pacing Vector

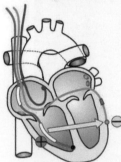

A. F. Sinnaeve

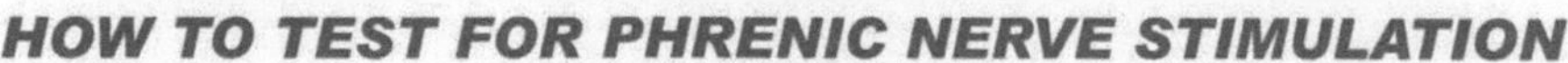

HOW TO TEST FOR PHRENIC NERVE STIMULATION

1. *AT IMPLANTATION :*
Phrenic nerve stimulation at implantation is assessed with a high voltage output at 10 volts and deep breathing maneuvers.

2. *AFTER IMPLANTATION :*
The occurence of phrenic nerve stimulation early after LV lead implantation may be due to LV lead displacement even if inapparent on the chest X-ray.
If the LV capture threshold is far below that of the phrenic nerve stimulation threshold, a reduction of LV pacing amplitude (volts) below the phrenic nerve stimulation threshold may simply solve the problem. This approach runs the risk of loss of LV capture so that lead repositioning is often necessary. Increasing the pulse duration to maintain LV capture with a low voltage output rarely works.
Recently, some bipolar pacing LV leads and devices (Guidant - Boston Scientific) allow reprogramming of the LV lead pacing configuration that may decrease phrenic nerve stimulation without the need of an invasive procedure for correction.

Abbreviations : LV = left ventricle ; RV = right ventricle

CAUSES OF POOR CLINICAL RESPONSE TO CRT

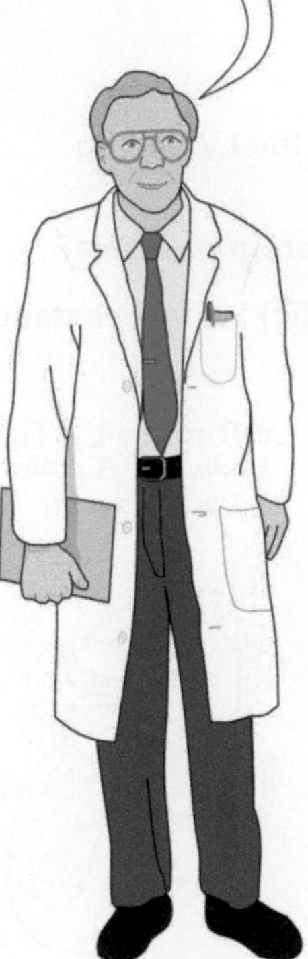
Some of my patients are nonresponders to CRT !
A lot of causes are possible and therefore a careful examination of patient and system is necessary !

- LV lead dislodgment or high threshold
- LV lead in the anterior or middle cardiac vein
- LV lead on nonviable myocardium
- No LV dyssynchrony despite wide QRS
- Irreversible mitral regurgitation
- Long AV delay
- Suboptimal AV delay and/or VV delay
- Atrial tachyarrhythmias with fast ventricular rate
- Frequent VPCs
- ??? Severely impaired myocardial function
- Comorbidities
- Delayed LV activation : Increased LV latency or severe local intramyocardial conduction delay or both
- Too strict definition of positive response

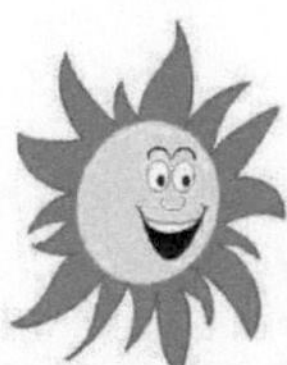

Contrast-enhanced MRI has promising potential for identifying scar and potentially viable tissue !

A. F. Sinnaeve

Abbreviatons : AV = atrioventricular ; CRT = cardiac resynchronisation therapy ; LV = left ventricle ; MRI = magnetic resonance imaging ; VPC = ventricular premature complex ; VV delay = interventricular delay ;

DEVICE MONITORING OF LUNG FLUID

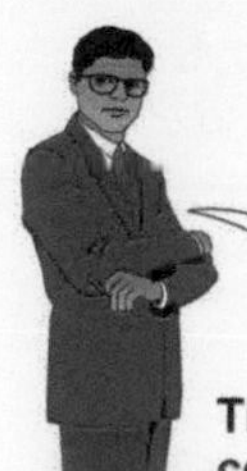

Volume overload is a major complication in patients with moderate-to-severe heart failure and is a frequent cause of hospitalizations

The *OptiVol Fluid Status Monitoring (Medtronic)* works by measuring intrathoracic impedance many times a day. A small subthreshold electrical impulse travels between the RV coil and the can of the ICD and the impedance is calculated according Ohm's law. Since body fluids are good conductors, the impedance decreases when fluid accumulates in the lungs.

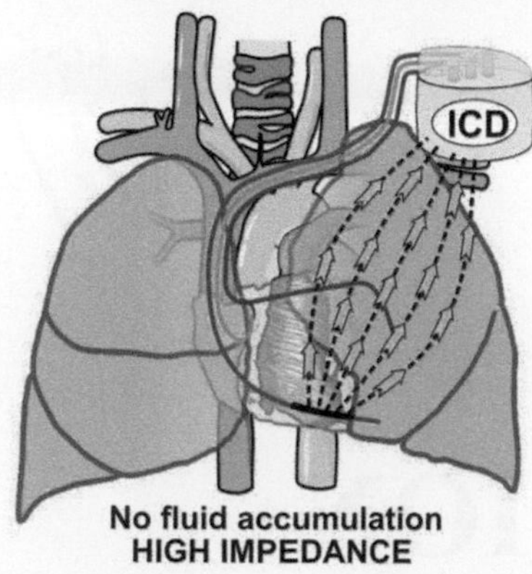

No fluid accumulation
HIGH IMPEDANCE

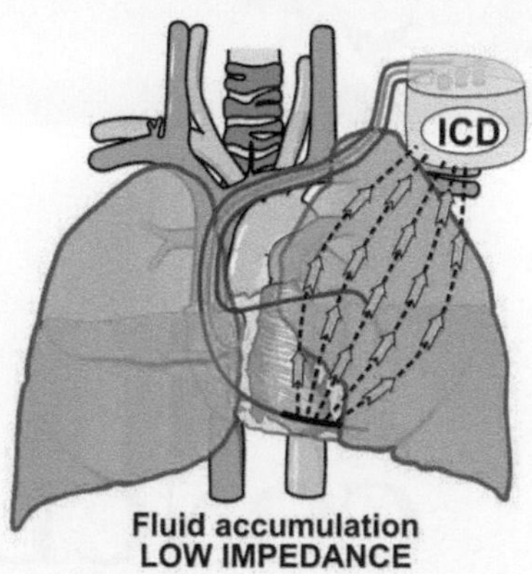

Fluid accumulation
LOW IMPEDANCE

The *"Thoracic Impedance Trend"* is a plot of daily average impedance values. The data are stored on a 14-month basis and can be viewed in the reports.

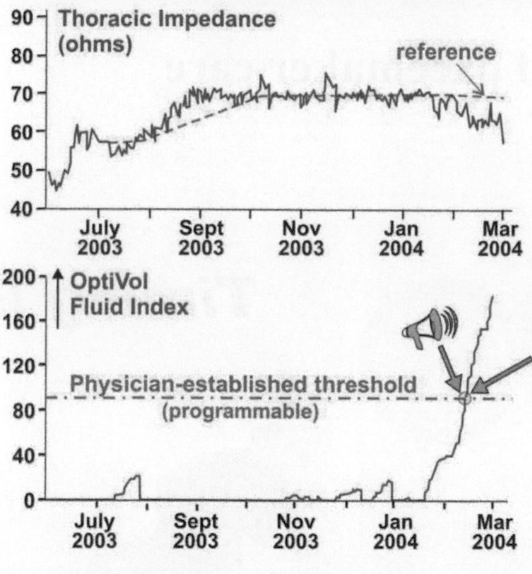

An *"OptiVol Fluid Index"* is calculated based on the intrathoracic impedance. As the fluid accumulates in the lungs the impedance decreases below the reference and fluid index increases. If the condition is not resolved and the fluid index crosses a threshold, an observation will be triggered. When the fluid buildup has been resolved and the daily impedance value is trending at or above the reference impedance, the fluid index will return to zero.

An *audible warning* will sound from the implanted device once per day for 30 seconds at a time specified by the physician. The alert will continue to sound daily until the fluid index drops below the threshold.
(the audible tone may be turned off)

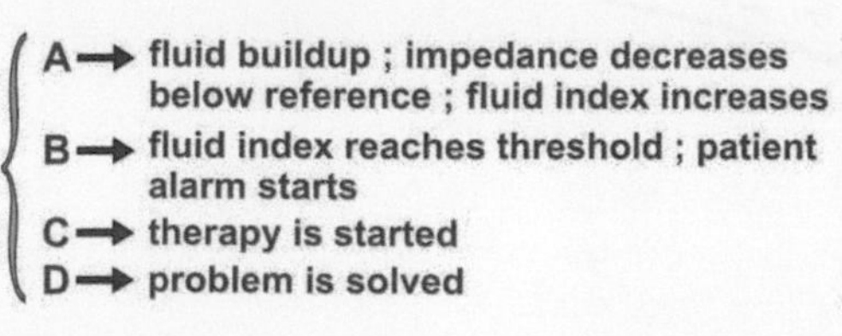

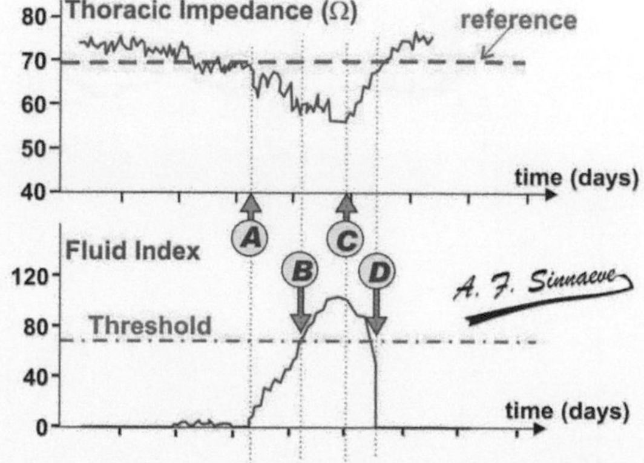

Abbreviations : CHF = congestive heart failure ;
RV = right ventricle

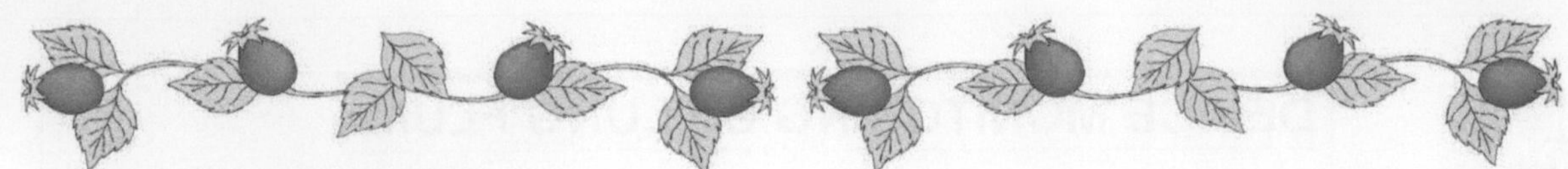

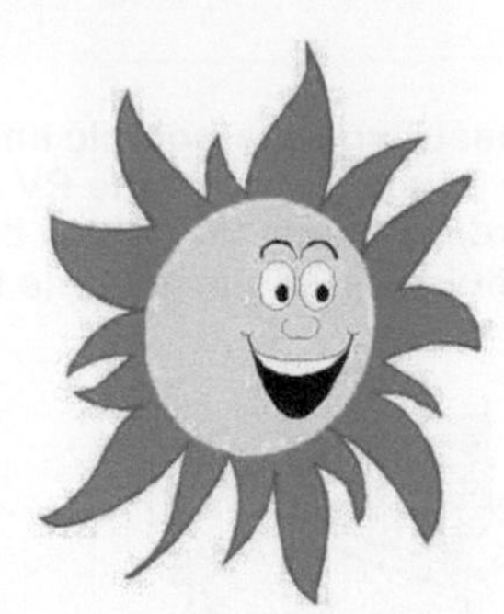

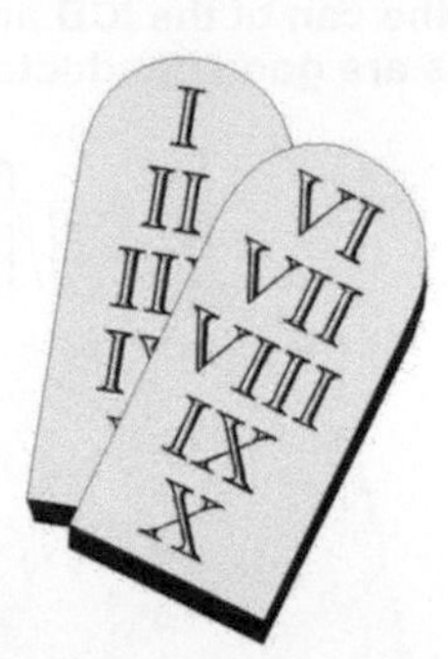

CONCLUSION

* **Professional success**
* **Ten commandments of pacemaker care**

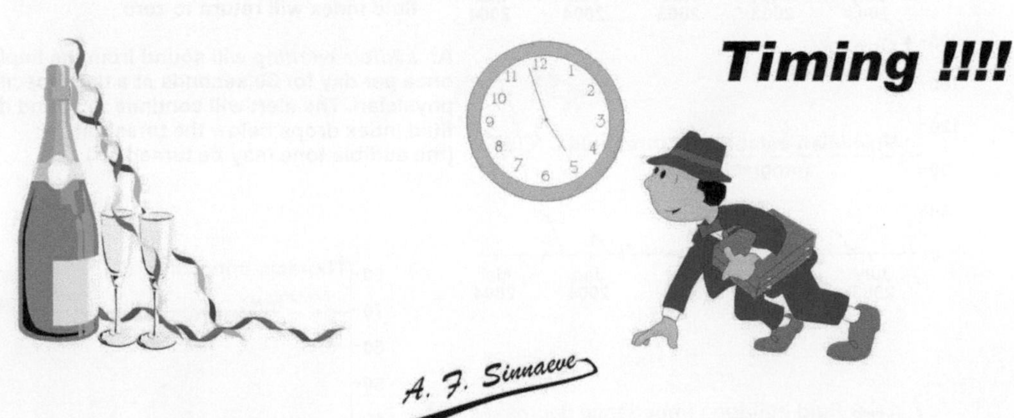

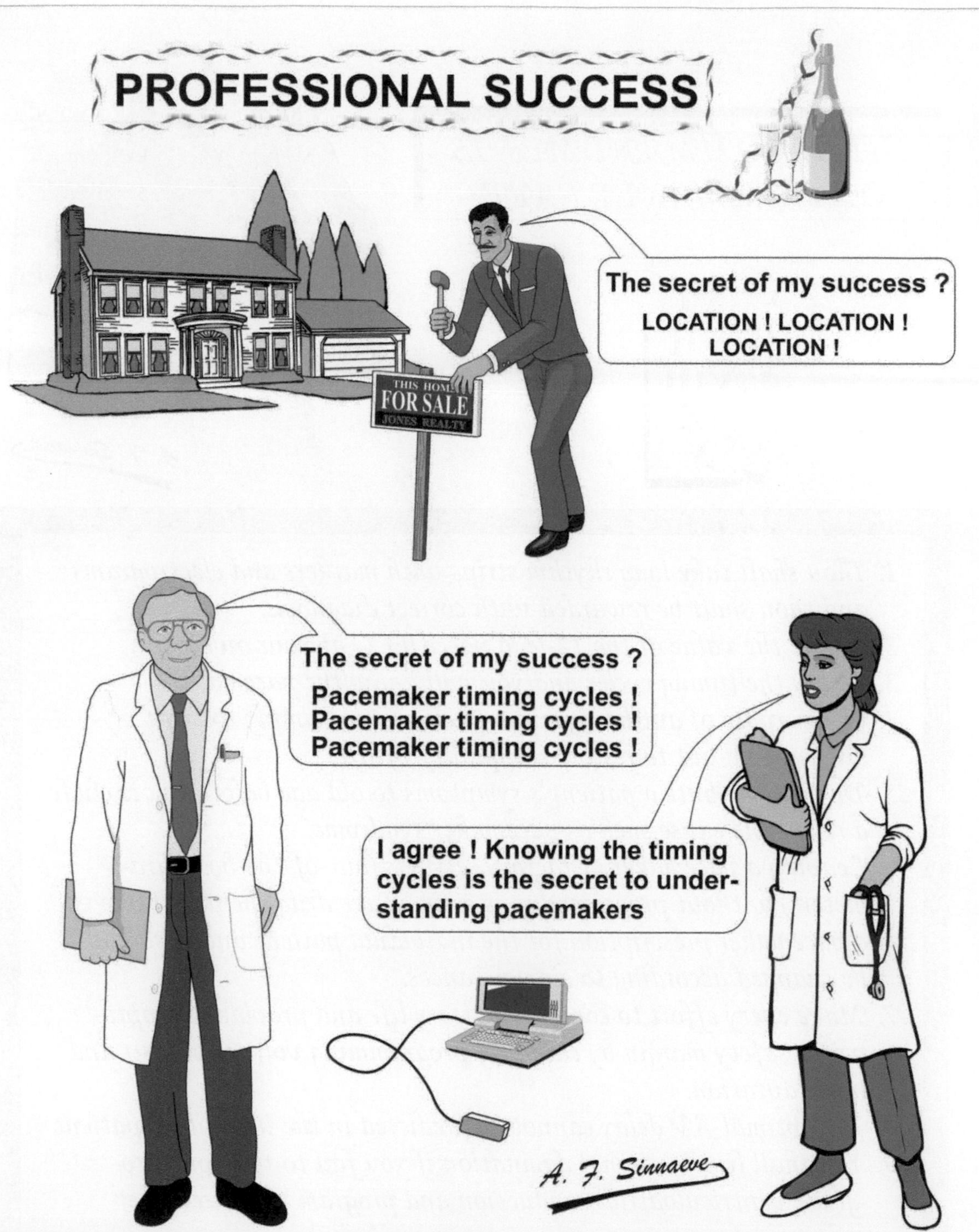

"All comprehension of pacemaker electrocardiography depends on the interpretation of pacemaker timing cycles"

SEYMOUR FURMAN MD, pioneer in cardiac pacing

THE 10 COMMANDMENTS OF PACEMAKER CARE

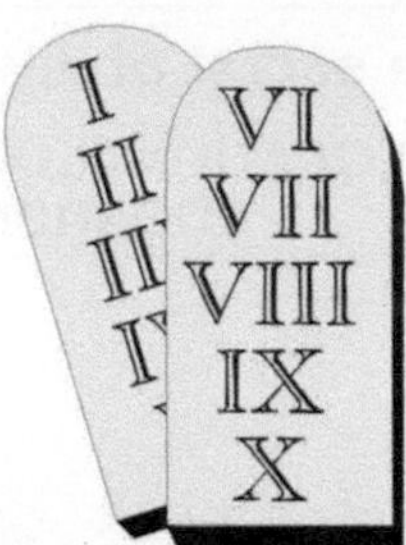

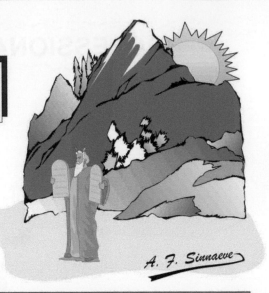

1. Thou shalt take long rhythm strips with markers and electrograms and thou shalt be rewarded with correct diagnosis.
2. Ignore the value of the 12-lead paced ECG at your own peril.
3. Know the timing cycles and you will know the pacemaker.
4. The purpose of antibradycardia pacing is not simply to treat bradycardia but to restore the quality-of-life.
5. Do not attribute a patient's symptoms to old age before you exclude a reversible cause such as pacemaker syndrome.
6. Leaving a pacemaker at factory settings (out-of-the-box parameters) without programming is a sin ! Like drug therapy, there is a pacemaker prescription for the individual patient and it should be changed according to circumstances.
7. Make every effort to conserve battery life and provide an appropriate safety margin by carefully programming voltage output and pulse duration.
8. The optimal AV delay cannot be predicted in the individual patient
9. You shall live in eternal damnation if you fail to test for retrograde ventriculoatrial conduction and program the pacemaker accordingly.
10. You will be banished into the wilderness for ever, if you fail to keep meticulous records of pacemaker follow-up.

Cardiac pacing

Implantation

A pacemaker (also known as a pulse generator) is a device that delivers electrical stimuli over leads with electrodes in contact with the heart. The lithium-iodine battery is sealed in a titanium can and provides electricity out of a chemical reaction. The pacemaker is like a little computer. The epoxy connector block on top of the pacemaker makes the connection from lead to pacemaker. The lead is an insulated wire. There are two types of leads: *bipolar*, with the two electrodes embedded inside the heart, and *unipolar*, where only one electrode is inside the heart, and the pacemaker can acts as the other electrode. Both types are widely used. In both types, the tip electrode is virtually always the negative pole or cathode. Virtually all pacemakers are implanted transvenously under local anesthesia using either the cephalic vein exposed by cutdown or percutaneous puncture of the subclavian vein. The leads are passed to the right side of the heart under x-ray vision (fluoroscopy). More recently, for the treatment of heart failure, the left ventricle may be paced by insertion of a lead into a tributary of the coronary sinus, a venous structure on the epicardial surface of the left ventricle. The pacemaker pocket is fashioned over the pectoralis major muscle below the collarbone. True epicardial leads require thoracic surgery and are used only when there is no venous access.

Basic function

The pacing lead functions as a "two-way street" for the transmission of electricity to the heart for pacing as well as for the sensing of spontaneous cardiac electric activity from the heart to the pacemaker. The operative techniques and intraoperative measurements are straightforward compared to the technical knowledge required to understand the electrophysiology of pacing and follow-up of patients for the best use of the important programmable functions. The function of an implanted pacemaker can be altered by means of a programmer, which is a kind of a dedicated desktop computer. A modern pacemaker lasts 7–10 years. When the battery is depleted, the entire pacemaker (excluding the leads) is replaced.

Power source

The lithium–iodine battery is the gold standard of pacemaker power sources, and the only one presently used in pacemakers. The battery has a long shelf life and is hermetically sealed to protect the electronic components of the pacemaker. In lithium–iodine batteries, lithium is the anode and iodine the cathode. When delivering electric current, this battery progressively develops a slow rise in internal resistance that can be measured by telemetry. The rising battery impedance causes a fairly linear drop in cell voltage, translated by design into a gradual decline in the pacing rate reflecting the status of the battery. The battery retains a satisfactory voltage for 90% of its life. Battery capacity (expressed in amperehours, Ah) is the quantity that expresses the longevity of a lithium–iodine battery. A pacemaker generally holds a capacity between 0.8 and 2.5 Ah.

The current drain from the battery (expressed in μA) is utilized to produce the stimulus and to feed the various sensing, detection, and "housekeeping" electronic circuits. The output voltage of a fresh cell is 2.8 volts (V). The cell voltage at the elective replacement point is 2.2–2.4 V. The pacemaker replacement time can be determined by measuring the pacemaker rate upon application of a magnet or the battery voltage and/or impedance by telemetry with the programmer.

Reminder: The pacemaker (or pacing) stimulus is also known as a spike, an artifact, or an output pulse.

Caveat: Do not confuse cathode with anode! The terminology of the battery terminals appears different from that of the load. For the battery the anode is the negative electrode where electrons are freed from lithium atoms and *positive* lithium ions are produced. In the battery the cathode is the positive terminal where free electrons rebind with iodine to form *negative* iodide ions. At the load, the cathode is the negative terminal and the anode is the positive one. The connection of battery to circuit is simple: positive-to-positive and negative-to-negative. Remember that the anode of the battery or load is where the electrons leave. The cathode of both battery and load is where the electrons enter. It is as simple as that! These are the universal definitions found in all good books about electricity and/or electronics. It is not true that the anode and cathode of the battery are reversed by convention. The only convention is that the electric current flows from positive to negative.

Rate or interval?

The pacemaker, design engineers, and the medical staff all "think" in terms of intervals rather than rate. We should do away with rate when defining timing cycles. Rate is a relatively simple designation during continuous pacing or continuous inhibition but it is of little value and confusing if pacing and sensing alternate. Yet, for ease of programming, manufacturers have expressed parameters in terms of rate rather than interval. Programmed rates may also be useful when communicating with the patient or anyone with little knowledge of pacing. The abbreviation *bpm* refers to beats per minute of the intrinsic heart rate and *ppm* refers to the paced rate. However, these abbreviations are often used interchangeably.

Caveat: Peculiar rhythms are created by ECG machines and Holter recorders functioning at an incorrect speed. In a Holter recording, intermittent slowing of the recording will cause a pseudotachycardia. The diagnosis is evident when the QRS and T waves are too narrow when compared to those recorded at normal speed. Conversely, a faster speed will cause pseudobradycardia, with excessively long AV delays or PR intervals as well as QRS complexes.

Single chamber pacemakers

VOO mode

A VOO pacemaker generates stimuli with no relationship to the spontaneous rhythm. The VOO mode is labeled "fixed-rate" or asynchronous. The competitive stimuli will capture the ventricle only when they fall outside the absolute refractory period of the ventricle that follows spontaneous beats. The VOO mode is now obsolete, and it is used only for testing purposes by applying a magnet over the pacemaker. Ventricular fibrillation induced by a competitive pacemaker stimulus falling in the ventricular vulnerable period (the R-on-T phenomenon) is very rare outside of circumstances such as myocardial ischemia or infarction, electrolyte abnormalities, or autonomic imbalance. Indeed, transtelephonic transmission of the electrocardiogram with a magnet over a pacemaker is quite safe.

VVI mode

A VVI pacemaker senses the intracardiac ventricular depolarization or electrogram which is recorded by measuring the potential (voltage) difference between the two electrodes (anode and cathode) used for pacing. A VVI pacemaker has an internal clock or lower rate timing cycle that begins with a paced (VP) or sensed ventricular event (VS). The initial portion of the cycle (after VP or VS) consists of the ventricular refractory period (VRP, usually 200–350 ms), during which the pacemaker cannot sense any signals. More specifically, any signal during the refractory period cannot initiate a new lower rate interval (LRI). Beyond the VRP, a sensed ventricular event inhibits the pacemaker and resets the LRI, so that the timing clock returns to baseline. A new pacing cycle is reinitiated, and if no event is sensed the timing cycle ends with the release of a ventricular stimulus according to the LRI. The sensing function prevents the competition between pacemaker and intrinsic rhythm seen with VOO pacing. Hence the old term "demand pacemaker" for a VVI pacemaker, to describe the delivery of a stimulus when the spontaneous rate is less than the lower rate of the pacemaker.

Caveats:

1. When a patient presents with an ECG showing no pacemaker stimuli, the pacing function should be tested by the application of a pacemaker magnet, which converts any pacemaker to the fixed-rate or asynchronous mode (VVI to VOO). One should refrain from performing carotid sinus massage (a vagal reflex producing sinus node slowing and AV block) in this situation, because it may cause prolonged bradycardia resulting in the delivery of pacemaker stimuli that may or may not be capable of capture. It is safer to first establish effective pacing with magnet application.
2. The stimulus-to-stimulus interval (automatic interval) is usually equal to the escape interval, which is measured electronically from the time of intracardiac sensing to the succeeding stimulus. In practice, the escape interval is measured from the onset of the sensed QRS complex in the surface ECG. The escape interval measured in this way must necessarily be longer than the electronic escape interval, because intracardiac sensing takes place a finite time after the onset

of the surface ECG. Thus, if the QRS complex is wide and intracardiac sensing occurs 90 ms from the beginning of the surface ECG, the measured escape interval (with calipers) will be 90 ms longer than the programmed automatic interval.

Hysteresis

In hysteresis the electronic escape interval is longer than the automatic interval. Its purpose is to maintain sinus rhythm and atrioventricular (AV) synchrony for as long as possible at a spontaneous rate lower (e.g. 50 bpm) than the automatic rate of the pacemaker (e.g. 70 ppm). Thus when the spontaneous rate drops below 50 bpm, the pacemaker will take over at 70 ppm. It will continue to pace at 70 ppm until the spontaneous rate exceeds the automatic rate, i.e., when the spontaneous QRS complex occurs within the 857 ms automatic interval.

If the search hysteresis feature is enabled, the pacemaker will periodically reduce the lower pacing rate for a few cycles by a programmable value in order to reveal potential intrinsic activity below the programmed lower rate or sensor rate. Hysteresis will remain active when intrinsic activity is sensed during the search period. If there is no intrinsic activity during the search, pacing resumes at the lower rate, or the sensor-indicated rate.

Caveat: Do not misinterpet hysteresis for oversensing with pauses.

Symbolic representation of pacemaker events and basic measurements

AS (P) = atrial sensed event
AP (A) = atrial paced event
VS (R) = ventricular sensed event
VP (V) = ventricular paced event
AR = atrial event sensed in the pacemaker refractory period
VR = ventricular event sensed in the ventricular refractory period.

Some devices depict a ventricular premature complex as a VPC or PVC. The refractory period is defined below. The intervals between events are measured by electronic calipers.

Timing cycles are expressed in milliseconds (ms):

One second = 1000 milliseconds

The 60,000 rule is useful in converting rate to intervals:

60,000/heart rate = interval in milliseconds
60,000/interval in milliseconds = heart rate

A pacemaker rate of 70 ppm gives an interval of 857 ms

bpm = beats per minute, which refers to the rate of a spontaneous rhythm. ppm = pulses per minute, which refers to the rate of a pacemaker. These designations are often used interchangeably.

Other single chamber pacemakers

A **VVT** pacemaker releases a ventricular stimulus immediately upon sensing, which is the opposite of inhibition with the VVI mode. The VVT mode requires three timing intervals: LRI and VRP, like the VVI mode, but additionally an upper rate interval (URI) to limit the maximum paced ventricular rate in response to ventricular sensing of rapidly occurring potentials. Upon sensing a QRS complex the pacemaker immediately discharges a stimulus (within the QRS) in the absolute refractory period of the ventricular myocardium. The VVT mode ensures stimulation rather than inhibition whenever the pacemaker senses signals other than the QRS complex. The triggered VVT mode is now rarely used as a primary pacing mode, but it was useful in the early days when VVI pacemakers were highly susceptible to external interference and the VVT mode was used to prevent inhibition.

An **AAI** pacemaker is identical to the VVI mode except that it paces and senses in the atrium. It requires a higher sensitivity because the atrial electrogram is smaller than the ventricular one. The pacemaker refractory period (during which the LRI cannot be initiated) should be longer than 400 ms to prevent sensing of the conducted QRS complex as a far-field event in the atrial electrogram. Sensing of the far-field QRS complex by an AAI pacemaker (especially a more sensitive unipolar system) will cause slowing of the pacing rate because the sensed event (though not originating from the atrium itself) resets the LRI. An AAI pacemaker may be considered in patients with sick sinus syndrome with normal AV conduction. The subsequent development of AV block in carefully selected patients is less than 2% per year. The advantages of AAI pacing are related to the preservation of normal ventricular depolarization and cost-effectiveness. This is in contrast to modes with pacing-induced ventricular depolarization, which tend to produce long-term LV dysfunction related to the cumulative duration of RV pacing.

Reminders:

1. Many ventricular premature complexes are not sensed by the atrial lead as far-field signals in the AAI mode.
2. The AOO and AAT modes work in the atrium and are functionally similar to their ventricular counterparts.

Basic electricity

Electrons flow from the negative terminal to the positive terminal of an electric circuit. In the early days, the concept of electron flow was not fully understood so scientists randomly decided that current in a conductor flowed from the positive terminal to the negative terminal. It is still convention (and confusing to some) today to show current flowing in this direction (i.e., opposite to electron flow).

Current is the amount of charge (electrons or other charged particles) that flows through an electric circuit within a unit of time. Its unit is the ampere (A). The flow of water is a good analogy for electricity. Water flows through a pipe because of water pressure. Voltage is the potential difference that controls the flow of electrons through an electric circuit. Current flows from a site of high potential to a low one. The basic unit of electric potential difference (voltage) is the volt (V). The electrons in a pacemaker circuit come from the battery. Thus, voltage is the force behind the electrons and current is a measure of how many electrons are flowing per unit of time. Resistance or impedance is a measure of the opposition to the flow of electrons. Resistance limits the current that flows through a circuit for a particular applied voltage. The unit of resistance is the ohm (Ω).

Current (I), voltage (V) and resistance (R) are related by Ohm's law:

$$V = I \times R$$

According to Ohm's law an increase in the pressure (voltage) must cause an increase in the flow (current) if the resistance remains the same. Increasing the resistance while keeping the voltage the same decreases the current (flow).

The battery supplies the voltage that creates the flow (current) in a circuit with a given load or resistance. The battery capacity denotes how long the battery will last while providing a current of 1 ampere. It is measured in ampere hours (Ah). So a battery with a capacity of 1000 mAh (1 Ah) would last for one hour in a one-amp circuit (1000 mAh is 1A for 1 hour). A lithium-iodine battery with a capacity of 2 Ah in a pacemaker circuit with a current drain of 25 μA (= 0.000025A) will last for 2 Ah/0.000 025 A = 80,000 hours or approximately 3333 days = approximately 9 years.

Chronic pacing threshold and safety margin

The pacing threshold is the minimum "electrical activity" that causes consistent pacing outside the myocardial refractory period of the heart. In practice the pacing threshold is determined in terms of volts (V) and pulse duration. All effort should be made at the time of implantation to obtain a pacing threshold as low as possible, because its initial value may ultimately determine the threshold at maturity and hence the voltage and pulse duration required for safe long-term pacing. Local steroid elution attenuates the increase of pacing threshold during lead maturation and maintains low pacing thresholds during follow-up. Steroid elution made the implantation of high-efficiency pacing leads with a small surface of 1.2 mm^2 feasible. Steroid-eluting leads are associated with remarkably low pacing threshold by virtue of their effect on the electrode–myocardial interface and tissue reaction. About eight weeks after implantation in most cases, the pacing threshold has stabilized and attained its chronic value. Then, the output voltage and pulse duration of the pacemaker should be programmed to maintain consistent long-term capture with an adequate margin of safety and maximal conservation of battery capacity. The capture threshold can vary during the course of a normal day and according to metabolic and pharmacological factors. Consequently it is important to provide protection for threshold fluctuations by a safety margin in terms of the pacemaker output.

In practice, the safety margin is determined in terms of volts, not pulse duration. The general recommendation is a voltage safety margin of 2 (or 100%). The output voltage of the pacemaker should be double the chronic voltage threshold at the same pulse duration. Voltage safety margin = output voltage/threshold voltage = 2 : 1 at an identical pulse duration. This value is acceptable in pacemakers without automatic adjustment of the output. However, the concept of a 2 : 1 safety margin has been challenged in view of data gathered by systems capable of automatic determination of the pacing threshold and adjustment of the output pulse. This experience has shown that a safety margin of 2 : 1 may not be sufficient in the occasional patient. Indeed, some physicians program a larger safety margin in pacemaker-dependent patients.

The relationship of voltage and pulse duration at threshold and at any time afterwards is not linear, and is represented by the *strength–duration curve.* A shorter pulse duration requires a higher voltage to attain the pacing threshold. The strength–duration curve is steep with a short pulse duration, and becomes essentially flat at a pulse duration greater than 2 ms, a point which is called the *rheobase*. The curve shifts to the right as the chronic pacing threshold becomes established. Although the terms *rheobase* and *chronaxie* are used to describe the strength–duration curve, they are rarely used in the routine follow-up of pacemaker patients.

Important reminders:

1. At a fixed voltage, increasing the pulse duration from 0.1 to 0.2 ms may not necessarily yield a voltage safety margin of 2, or 100%, despite the steepness of the strength–duration curve (on the left) for short pulse durations.
2. At a fixed voltage, tripling the pulse duration (not starting beyond 0.2 ms) will provide an adequate voltage safety margin based on the configuration of the strength–duration curve. Thus, a threshold of 2.5 V at 0.2 ms permits a programmed "chronic" output of 2.5 V at 0.6 ms, for a voltage safety margin of 2.
3. When the pulse duration is $\geq$ 0.3 ms, tripling the pulse duration while keeping the voltage constant may not provide a voltage safety margin of 2 because of the less steep and eventually straight configuration of the strength–duration curve (on the right) at longer pulse durations.
4. The relatively flat configuration of the strength–duration curve from 0.5 to 1.5 ms indicates that an increase in pulse duration in this range (keeping the voltage constant) will certainly not provide a voltage safety margin of 2.
5. Try to pace at a voltage lower than the traditional output of 5 V for greater efficiency and less wasted battery output.

The pacing threshold is lowest during a short period called the supernormal phase which corresponds with the second half of the T wave. Consistent ventricular capture during this period and failure at other times, suggests that the pacemaker output is near threshold.

Let us consider some examples:

(a) Threshold 2.5 V at 0.1 ms: program 2.5 V at 0.3 ms.
(b) Threshold 2.5 V at 0.2 ms: program 2.5 V at 0.6 ms.
(c) Threshold 2.5 V at 0.3 ms: program 5 V at 0.3 ms.
(d) Threshold 0.5 V at 0.2 ms. This is a very low pacing threshold. The pacemaker can be programmed at 0.5 V at 0.6 ms, but many would prefer going to 1 V at 0.4 or 0.5 ms, a setting that would still provide substantial battery conservation.
(e) Threshold 5 V at 0.3 ms. Increasing the pulse duration when the voltage is fixed at 5 V may not provide an adequate voltage margin. Increase the voltage output above 5 V if available in the pacemaker. If not, watch the patient carefully for bradycardia and asystole and decide whether to reposition the lead or implant a high-output pulse generator providing a 10 V output.

Reminder: The pacing thresholds are less than 2.5 V at 0.5 ms pulse duration in more than 95% of patients with steroid-eluting leads. Patients with such leads rarely have a significant pacing threshold increase compared to those with non-steroid leads. Consequently it does not make sense to leave the output (voltage and pulse duration) at nominal values. Appropriate programming of the pacemaker output can increase battery longevity. Furthermore, as the voltage of the lithium-iodine battery is 2.8 V, pacing is more efficient when performed close to that voltage.

Caveats:

1. Always test the pacing threshold on deep respiration and coughing to detect an unstable electrode.
2. In the presence of left bundle branch block (LBBB) with a QRS complex resembling a paced ventricular beat, pseudocapture will be seen when the rate of the pacemaker stimulus is very close to that of the spontaneous rhythm and the stimulus falls just before the spontaneous QRS complex. This may resemble capture with latency (delayed interval from stimulus to ventricular activation). Long rhythm strips are needed for the diagnosis, which will be obvious when the ventricular stimulus moves away from the QRS complex.
3. Beware of isoelectric paced QRS complexes that can mimic lack of capture. Look for the T wave, because the presence of repolarization means that depolarization must have occurred.

Automatic determination of the pacing threshold

Some pacemakers have algorithms that periodically and automatically measure the ventricular capture threshold. The pacemaker recognizes the presence of capture, provides a stronger backup pulse if there is loss of capture, and then adjusts the output automatically at a given value over the pacing threshold. Such periodic threshold measurements are memorized by the device, and the threshold graph during the preceding follow-up period can be retrieved by interrogation of the pacemaker.

Capture verification has increased patient safety, and it probably increases battery longevity.

Some programmers are also designed to perform a pacing threshold test automatically at the time of follow-up, and a printout of the procedure can be filed in the pacemaker chart.

Sensing

A pacemaker senses the potential difference between the two electrodes (anode and cathode) used for pacing. A bipolar system senses the potential difference between the two electrodes in the heart and requires recording of the bipolar electrogram to determine the characteristics of the signal available for sensing. The final bipolar electrogram depends on the electrograms registered at the two sites and the travel time of depolarization between the two electrodes. The bipolar electrogram can be easily recorded at the time of implantation with an ECG machine (leads applied to the two legs), by connecting the tip and proximal electrodes of the pacing lead to the free or loose right-arm and left-arm electrodes and recording lead I (which provides the potential difference between the two arms and therefore the potential difference between the two intracardiac electrodes).

For a unipolar system (one electrode in the heart and the other on the pacemaker can), the unipolar electrogram from the tip electrode closely resembles the available voltage for sensing, because the contribution from the unipolar plate is usually negligible. The unipolar electrogram can be easily recorded by connecting the unipolar V lead of the ECG to the tip electrode, with the other ECG electrodes on the limbs in the usual fashion. The amplitude of the electrogram (in the setting of an adequate slew rate) must exceed the sensitivity of the pacemaker for reliable sensing. The ventricular signal often measures 6–15 mV, a range that exceeds the commonly programmed ventricular sensitivity of 2–3 mV. Occasionally a pacemaker senses the supraventricular QRS complex normally, but does not detect some ventricular extrasystoles because their electrogram (originating from a different site) is smaller, a situation not always correctible by reprogramming ventricular sensitivity. This is an accepted limitation of the sensing function of pacemakers. The atrial signal is smaller, and should ideally exceed 2 mV.

A signal with a gradual slope (low slew rate) is more difficult to sense than one with a sharp upstroke (high slew rate). If the signal amplitude is large enough, the slew rate will always be sufficient and need not be measured. Determination of the slew rate is most useful when a signal is low or borderline (3–5 mV in the ventricle). On a long-term basis, the amplitude of the signal diminishes slightly but the slew rate may diminish further. These changes are usually of no clinical importance for sensing except in the case of smaller signals.

The sensing circuit contains a bandpass filter that transmits some electrical frequencies more freely than others. A pacemaker filter is designed to pass all the signals of interest and attenuate unwanted signals such as T waves or external interference. A typical bandpass filter favors the passage of signals with a frequency of 20–80 Hz in order to sense the wide range of QRS complexes, and attenuates signals outside this range.

Caveat: The escape interval in a VVI pacemaker is measured from the onset of the surface QRS complex. In pacemakers with identical automatic and electronic escape intervals, the measured escape interval must of necessity be longer than the automatic interval by a value ranging from a few milliseconds to almost the entire duration of the QRS complex (with "late" sensing), depending on the temporal relationship of the intracardiac electrogram and the surface ECG. Do not confuse this with hysteresis.

Sensitivity

Programmability of sensitivity is important because the ideal electrode for sensing does not exist. Sensitivity is a measure of the minimal potential difference required between the terminals of a pacemaker to suppress its output. Looking above a wall is a good analogy of the numeral representation of sensitivity. The higher the wall, the less one will see above it. The lower the wall, the more one will see above it. The higher the numerical value of sensitivity, the less sensitive the pacemaker becomes. Thus, a setting of 6 mV can only sense a signal of 6 mV or greater and cannot sense signals smaller than 6 mV. On the other hand, a "higher" sensitivity of 1 mV will allow sensing of all signals of 1 mV or larger. The sensing threshold is determined by programming the pacing rate lower than the intrinsic rate while the sensitivity is gradually reduced (larger numerical value in mV) until failure to sense is observed. The sensing threshold is the largest possible numeric sensitivity value associated with regular sensing. As a rule, sensitivity should be programmed at a numerical value at least half the threshold value: e.g., from a sensing threshold of 8 mV one can program a sensitivity of 4 mV. Oversensing requires a decrease in sensitivity (increase in the numerical value). Most programmers now permit a fully automatic assessment of the signal amplitude at the time of follow-up. These measurements are taken from the sense amplifier, and represent the signal amplitude after it has been processed.

Caveats:

1. Always test appropriate sensing, especially atrial sensing, with deep respiration, to unmask significant fluctuations of the signal with respiration.
2. The absolute amplitude of the signal measured from the electrogram is only a rough approximation of the signal utilized for sensing. This is because the sensing circuit filters and processes the signal for sensing.

Polarity: unipolar versus bipolar pacing and sensing

New lead technology and design have eliminated the previous advantage of unipolar leads. In practice, the long-term performance of unipolar and bipolar systems is similar. Bipolar leads, by virtue of their greater signal-to-noise ratio (promoting greater protection against extraneous interference), allow the use of higher sensitivities. A high sensitivity is especially useful for atrial sensing, an important requirement of contemporary dual chamber pacemakers with the capability of diagnosing supraventricular tachyarrhythmias. This diagnosis permits a change in the pacing mode automatically to avoid rapid ventricular pacing. Bipolar leads are also associated with less crosstalk in dual chamber pacemakers (ventricular sensing of the atrial stimulus). Bipolar leads are less sensitive than unipolar systems to external interference (myopotentials etc.). The configuration of many pacemakers is programmable to either the unipolar or the bipolar mode (provided they have bipolar leads) to correct certain pacemaker problems. In some devices, when the circuit detects a high impedance (resistance) from a fracture in one of the electrodes, the pacemaker can automatically change from the bipolar to the unipolar mode of pacing using the intact electrode.

Reminders:

1. The tip electrode is almost always the cathode, because the cathodal pacing threshold is lower. In a bipolar system the proximal (ring) electrode is the anode, while in a unipolar system the pacemaker can is the anode.
2. Contemporary pacemakers allow programming of unipolar or bipolar function in a variety of ways in individual channels: pacing only, sensing only, or both. A bipolar lead can be unipolarized by using either the tip or the ring electrode as the only intracardiac electrode for sensing and/or pacing.

Ventricular fusion and pseudofusion beats

Ventricular fusion beats occur when the ventricles are depolarized simultaneously by spontaneous and pacemaker-induced activity. A ventricular fusion beat can exhibit various configurations depending on the relative contributions of the two foci involved in ventricular activation. A ventricular fusion beat is often narrower than a pure ventricular paced beat. Fusion therefore occurs in the heart itself.

Ventricular pseudofusion beats consist of the superimposition of an ineffectual ventricular stimulus on a surface QRS complex originating from a single focus, and they represent a normal manifestation of VVI pacing. A VVI pacemaker obviously does not sense the surface QRS complex. Rather, it senses the intracardiac ventricular electrogram registered between the two pacing electrodes. A substantial portion of the *surface* QRS complex can be inscribed before the *intracardiac* electrogram generates the required voltage (according to the programmed sensitivity) to inhibit the ventricular channel of a VVI pacemaker. Thus a VVI pacemaker can deliver a ventricular stimulus within the spontaneous QRS complex before the device has the opportunity to sense the "delayed" electrogram generated in the right ventricle as the depolarization reaches the recording site(s). The stimulus thus falls in the absolute refractory period of the ventricular myocardium. The stimulus does not depolarize any portion of the ventricles, and true fusion does not occur. The "fusion" occurs on the ECG recording and not in the heart itself as in ventricular fusion. True sensing failure must always be excluded with long ECG recordings. Pacemaker stimuli falling beyond the surface ECG always indicate undersensing. A pseudopseudofusion beat (discussed later) is a variant of a pseudofusion beat seen in patients with dual chamber pacemakers.

Operational characteristics of a simple DDD pacemaker

Ventricular channel

As in a standard VVI pacemaker, the ventricular channel of a DDD pacemaker requires two basic timing intervals: the lower rate interval (corresponding to the programmed lower rate) and the ventricular refractory period.

The **lower rate interval** (LRI) of a DDD pacemaker is the longest interval between consecutive ventricular stimuli without an intervening sensed P wave, or from a sensed ventricular event to the succeeding ventricular stimulus without an intervening sensed P wave.

The **ventricular refractory period** (VRP) is traditionally defined as the period during which the pacemaker is insensitive to incoming signals. The function of the ventricular refractory period in a DDD pacemaker is similar to that in a VVI pacemaker. Yet many pacemakers can now actually sense within part of the refractory period to perform pacemaker functions (and influence certain timing intervals) other than resetting the lower rate interval. The pacemaker VRP now focuses only on the lower rate interval, which cannot be reset or reinitiated by a ventricular signal falling within the refractory interval. The VRP starts with either a sensed or a paced ventricular event, and is usually equal after pacing and sensing. The lower rate (interval) of many DDD pacemakers is ventricular-based in that it is initiated by a paced or sensed ventricular event. Atrial-based lower rate timing is more complex, and is discussed later.

DDD pacing or VVI pacing with an atrial channel

Now the pacemaker acquires an atrioventricular interval and an upper rate interval.

The **AV interval** (AVI) is the electronic analog of the PR interval and is designed to maintain AV synchrony between the atria and the ventricles. The AV interval starts from the atrial stimulus and extends to the following ventricular stimulus, or it starts from the point when the P wave is sensed and also terminates with the release of the ventricular stimulus. *Atrial tracking* is a term used to describe the response of a dual chamber pacemaker to a sensed atrial event which leads to the emission of a ventricular output pulse. Let us assume for now that the AV delay in our simple DDD pacemaker after atrial sensing is equal to that after atrial pacing, though they may be different in more complex pacemakers.

The **upper rate interval** (URI) is the speed limit to control the response of the ventricular channel to sensed atrial activity. For example, if the upper rate interval is 500 ms (upper rate = 120 ppm), a P wave occurring earlier than 500 ms from the previous atrial event (atrial rate faster than 120 ppm) will not be followed by a ventricular stimulus. Such an arrangement allows atrial sensing with 1:1 AV synchrony between the lower rate and the upper rate. The upper rate interval of any DDD pacemaker is a ventricular interval, and it is defined as the shortest interval between two consecutive ventricular stimuli or from a sensed ventricular event to the succeeding ventricular stimulus while maintaining 1:1 AV synchrony with sensed atrial events. In a simple DDD pacemaker the upper rate interval is intimately related to the electronic refractory period of the atrial channel, as discussed later.

Derived timing intervals

The four basic timing intervals of a simple DDD pacemaker, as already explained, consist of lower rate interval (LRI), ventricular refractory period (VRP), AV interval (AVI), and upper rate interval (URI). Additional timing intervals can be derived from these four basic intervals. Let us assume that the lower rate of our simple DDD pacemaker is ventricular-based. The **atrial escape interval** (AEI) is the LRI minus the AVI. This is sometimes called the VA interval. The atrial escape interval starts with either a ventricular paced or a sensed event, and terminates with the release of the atrial stimulus. Although derived from two other intervals, the atrial escape interval is crucial in the analysis of DDD pacemaker function because it represents the interval the pacemaker uses to determine when the next atrial stimulus should occur after a sensed or paced ventricular event. In our DDD pacemaker with ventricular-based lower rate timing, the atrial escape interval always remains constant after programming the lower rate interval and AV delay.

At this point our simple DDD pacemaker has four basic intervals and one derived one. As the DDD pacemaker grows in complexity, we shall see how a basic upper rate interval is best equated with in terms of the total atrial refractory period (TARP). The latter had been considered initially a fundamental interval for the sake of simplicity in the construction of a simple DDD pacemaker. It is actually a derived interval as discussed later.

Influence of events in one chamber upon the other

The operation of the two channels of a DDD pacemaker are intimately linked, and an event detected by one channel generally influences the function of the other.

Atrial channel. As in the normal heart, an atrial event must always be followed by a ventricular event after some delay. A sensed atrial event alters pacemaker function in two ways: (a) it *triggers* a ventricular stimulus (after a delay equal to the AVI) provided the ventricular channel senses no signal during the AVI; (b) it *inhibits* the release of the atrial stimulus that would have occurred at the completion of the atrial escape interval. In other words, it aborts the atrial escape interval, which therefore does not time out in its entirety. This is self-evident, because the atrial cycle starts with a sensed P wave and there is no need for atrial stimulation immediately after a spontaneous atrial event. Therefore the atrial channel functions simultaneously in the triggered mode (to deliver the ventricular stimulus for AV synchrony) and in the inhibited mode to prevent competitive release of an atrial stimulus after sensing a P wave. The function of the atrial channel can thus be depicted by "TI" in the third position of the standard pacemaker code. Because the ventricular channel functions only in the inhibited mode, a DDD pacemaker can be coded as a DDTI/I device, which would be more awkward but more correct than the traditional DDD designation.

Ventricular channel. A sensed ventricular event *outside the AV delay*, such as a ventricular extrasystole (or premature ventricular complex) will inhibit the atrial and ventricular channels. The atrial escape interval in progress is immediately terminated, and release of the atrial stimulus is inhibited. The sensed ventricular event also inhibits the ventricular channel and initiates a new atrial escape interval. Thus both the atrial and ventricular channels are inhibited simultaneously. When a ventricular event is sensed *within the AV delay* there is no need for the pacemaker to release a ventricular stimulus at the completion of the AV delay because spontaneous ventricular activity is already in progress. Therefore the pacemaker aborts the AV delay by virtue of the sensed ventricular event. The AV delay is thus abbreviated. The sensed ventricular event immediately starts a new atrial escape interval.

Atrial refractory period

It is axiomatic that the atrial channel of a DDD pacemaker must be refractory during the *AV delay* to prevent initiation of a new AV delay before completion of an AV delay already in progress.

The **postventricular atrial refractory period** (PVARP) begins immediately after the emission of a ventricular event and is the same after a ventricular stimulus or a sensed ventricular signal. An atrial signal falling within the PVARP cannot initiate a programmed AV interval. The PVARP is designed to prevent the atrial channel from sensing the ventricular stimulus, the far-field QRS complex (a voltage that can be seen by the atrial channel), very premature atrial ectopic beats, and retrograde P waves. In the normal heart, an isolated ventricular event may occasionally be followed by a retrograde P wave because of retrograde ventriculoatrial (VA) conduction (the AV junction being a two-way street). Although this is a physiological phenomenon, it may be hemodynamically unfavorable if it becomes sustained. The PVARP should be programmed to a duration longer than the retrograde VA conduction time, to prevent the atrial channel from sensing retrograde P waves.

The **total atrial refractory period** (TARP) is the sum of the AVI and the PVARP. The duration of the TARP always defines the shortest upper rate interval or the fastest paced ventricular rate. The AVI, PVARP, and URI are interrelated in a simple DDD pacemaker without a separately programmable URI. In such a system, the URI is controlled solely by the duration of the TARP according to the formula: upper rate (ppm) = 60,000/TARP (ms). So far, in the simple DDD pacemaker, the TARP is the upper rate interval, and it is constructed by means of a few timing cycles.

Sensing in the refractory period: true or false?

The first part of any refractory period consists of a blanking period during which the pacemaker cannot sense at all. The second part of the refractory period permits sensing, and each detected event is often represented symbolically by a "refractory sense marker." In the atrium refractory sensed events cannot initiate an AV delay, and in the ventricle they cannot start an atrial escape interval or lower rate interval. In one designation, AR and VR depict an atrial refractory sensed event and ventricular refractory sensed event respectively. The rapid and irregular atrial rates in atrial fibrillation, if sensed by the atrial channel, will inscribe many AR events within the AV delay beyond the initial blanking period (initiated by atrial sensing or pacing) and multiple AR events in the PVARP beyond the initial postventricular atrial blanking period initiated by ventricular pacing or sensing.

Upper rate interval versus PVARP

Now that the function of the PVARP is clear, it makes sense to consider the PVARP itself as a basic interval controlling the upper rate. In this way the upper rate interval can be demoted to a derived interval. This manipulation converts the upper rate interval of our evolving DDD pacemaker or the TARP (AVI + PVARP) to a derived function.

The six intervals of a simple DDD pacemaker

According to the above concepts, we now have a DDD pacemaker working with four basic intervals (LRI, VRP, AVI, and PVARP) and two derived intervals (AEI, and TARP = URI). Such a pacemaker can function quite well provided the atrial stimulus does not interfere with the function of the ventricular channel. If it does, the disturbance is called AV *crosstalk*, because the atrial stimulus, if sensed by the ventricular channel, can cause ventricular inhibition.

The fifth basic timing interval

Prevention of crosstalk is mandatory, and it requires the addition of a brief ventricular blanking period beginning coincidentally with the release of the atrial stimulus. This is known as the postatrial ventricular blanking period (PAVB). No signal can be detected during this blanking period. The ventricular channel then "opens" after this short blanking period so that ventricular sensing (with reset of the atrial escape interval and lower rate interval) can occur during the remainder of the AV delay. Obviously a long postatrial ventricular blanking period will predispose to ventricular undersensing. The addition of this important blanking interval yields a DDD pacemaker with five basic cycles and two derived cycles. This format was the basis of the first-generation DDD pacemakers that were clinically used and accepted. Even a sophisticated contemporary DDD pacemaker reduced to having only these seven intervals would function satisfactorily if appropriately programmed. The addition of further timing intervals represents refinements rather than essential elements of DDD pacing.

Do we need more than seven timing intervals in our evolving DDD pacemaker?

Further refinements of DDD pacemaker function have introduced two other timing intervals:

(a) Ventricular safety pacing (VSP) to complement the blanking period in dealing with crosstalk. This function does not prevent crosstalk but merely offsets its consequences.

(b) Upper rate interval programmable independently of the TARP for a smoother upper rate response than the rather abrupt slowing provided by the TARP when it is the only interval controlling the upper rate (interval).

Refractory periods

In a DDD pacemaker, how does an event in one channel affect the refractory period of the other? Four possible events may be considered: AS, AP, VS, and VP.

(a) VS and VP both initiate the VRP and PVARP, starting simultaneously.

(b) AP initiates the AV delay and an atrial refractory period extending through the entire duration of the AV delay. The AV delay is therefore the first part of the TARP, the second part being the PVARP. Release of AP initiates an important interval (postatrial ventricular blanking period) to prevent crosstalk, which is a pacemaker disturbance where the ventricular channel senses the atrial stimulus (discussed later).

(c) AS generates an atrial refractory period in the AV delay like AP, but it is not associated with a ventricular blanking because AS cannot induce crosstalk (discussed later).

The faces of DDD pacing

A DDD pacemaker with ventricular-based lower rate timing capable of dealing with four events (AS, AP, VS, VP) can behave in one of four ways, judged by the examination of a single cycle starting with VS and the way the cycle terminates:

1. DVI: VS–AP–VP
2. AAI: QRS–AP–QRS
3. VDD: VS–AS–VP
4. Totally inhibited "mode" without stimuli

In the inhibited situation the RR interval (VS–VS) is shorter than the lower rate interval, and the PR interval is shorter than the programmed AV delay. Inhibition does not always mean that the pacemaker senses both the atrial and ventricular signals. Indeed, in the presence of atrial undersensing, the ECG may show inhibition if the pacemaker (actually working in the DVI mode) emits no stimuli because the RR interval is shorter than the atrial escape interval.

Ventricular pseudopseudofusion beats

Remember that in a DDD pacemaker a sensed ventricular event inhibits both the atrial and ventricular channels. A ventricular pseudofusion beat occurs when a ventricular stimulus falls within the spontaneous QRS before the intracardiac ventricular electrogram has developed sufficient amplitude to be sensed. In the same way, an atrial stimulus can fall within the surface QRS complex before the intracardiac ventricular electrogram has developed sufficient amplitude to be sensed. In this situation, when an atrial stimulus deforms the QRS complex, the arrangement is called a *pseudopseudofusion ventricular beat*, to underscore that the process involves two chambers instead of just one, as in the case of pseudofusion beats.

Caveat: In the presence of normal atrial and ventricular sensing, a pacemaker stimulus falling within the QRS complex may be atrial (pseudopseudofusion) or ventricular (pseudofusion). In a device with a ventricular-based lower rate, the stimulus is atrial if it terminates the atrial escape interval, which is always constant. In a device with an atrial-based lower rate system (where atrial events control the lower rate), the stimulus is atrial if it terminates an interatrial interval equal to the lower rate interval.

Crosstalk and crosstalk intervals

In patients without an underlying cardiac rhythm, inhibition of the ventricular channel by crosstalk can be catastrophic. The postatrial ventricular blanking period (PAVB) starts with the atrial stimulus and is usually programmable from about 10 to 60 ms. Note again that no blanking period is in effect after atrial sensing. Some pacemakers are designed with an additional safety mechanism to counteract the inhibitory effect of crosstalk should the postatrial ventricular blanking period be unsuccessful. This special "safety period" is really a crosstalk detection window, and it is often described in pacemaker specifications as starting from the atrial stimulus. In fact, it cannot be functional until the brief postatrial ventricular blanking period has timed out. Nevertheless, the AV delay is often described as having two parts. The first part is the *ventricular safety pacing* (VSP) window, which extends from the onset of the AV delay for a duration of 100–110 ms. During the VSP interval, a sensed ventricular signal does not inhibit the DDD pacemaker. Rather, it immediately *triggers* a ventricular stimulus delivered prematurely only at the completion of the VSP interval, producing a characteristic abbreviation of the paced AV interval (AP–VP). If a QRS complex is sensed within the VSP window, it will also trigger an early ventricular stimulus. However, this triggered ventricular stimulus falls harmlessly within the QRS complex in the absolute period of the ventricular myocardium. In the second part of the AV delay beyond the VSP interval, a sensed ventricular signal inhibits the pacemaker in the usual fashion.

Manifestations of crosstalk

1. In pacemakers with a VSP interval, crosstalk will cause shortening of the paced AV delay (AP–VP). In a device with ventricular-based lower rate timing, the pacing rate will increase because the sum of the constant atrial escape interval and the abbreviated AV delay becomes less than the lower rate interval. In a device with atrial-based lower rate timing, the pacing interval remains constant as it is controlled by the interval between two consecutive atrial stimuli, which is always equal to the programmed lower rate interval.
2. In pacemakers without a VSP interval, the ECG will show: (a) prolongation of the interval between the atrial stimulus and the succeeding conducted QRS complex to a value greater than the programmed AV delay; (b) ventricular asystole, if there is no AV conduction; (c) an atrial pacing rate interval shorter than the lower rate interval (atrial pacing rate faster than the lower rate), because the interval between two consecutive atrial stimuli becomes equal to the sum of the atrial escape interval (AEI) and the short postatrial ventricular blanking period (PAVB) because sensing of the atrial stimulus can only occur after the blanking period has timed out.
3. Crosstalk tachycardia. In pacemakers with VSP and ventricular-based lower rate timing, a lower rate of 80 ppm (LRI = 750 ms) yields an atrial escape interval of 450 ms if the AV delay = 300 ms. During continual crosstalk with an abbreviated paced AV delay (AP–VP) of 100 ms, the pacing interval becomes 450 + 100 = 550 ms, corresponding to a rate of 109 ppm.

Caveat: VSP can be puzzling in the ECG without markers. When the atrial stimulus falls within a QRS complex and is invisible on the surface ECG, a single visible ventricular stimulus will fall beyond the QRS complex. This must not be interpreted as ventricular undersensing. To make the diagnosis, go back to the previous ventricular event and with calipers move to the end of the atrial escape interval when the atrial stimulus should have occurred. Then add the VSP interval, and its end should coincide with the late stimulus in question, thereby proving it is ventricular and establishing normal pacemaker function. If VSP has not occurred and the QRS complex fell in the postatrial ventricular blanking period, add the AV delay to the atrial escape interval (measured as indicated) rather than the VSP interval.

Reminders:

1. The frequent occurrence of VSP involving spontaneous QRS complexes should immediately raise the possibility of atrial undersensing.
2. The opposite of AV crosstalk is ventriculoatrial (VA) crosstalk, where the atrial channel senses ventricular activity. VA crosstalk is important in pacemakers with automatic mode switching (discussed later).
3. In pacemakers with atrial-based lower rate timing, during AV crosstalk the atrial pacing rate will remain constant in duration to conform to the atrial-based lower rate and the AEI will vary to accommodate the constancy of the atrial pacing rate.

Increasing complexity: our simple DDD pacemaker grows to nine intervals

Many pacemakers have nine timing intervals, five related to the ventricular channel and four to the atrial channel. A ventricular paced or sensed event initiates: (a) lower rate interval (LRI), (b) upper rate interval (URI; independent of TARP), (c) PVARP, (d) ventricular refractory period (VRP), and (e) atrial escape interval (AEI). An atrial paced or sensed event initiates: (a) AV interval (AVI) and (b) TARP (derived as the sum of AVI and PVARP). An atrial paced event initiates (a) postatrial ventricular blanking period (PAVB) and (b) VSP interval.

A pacemaker with the capability of programming a longer URI independently of the TARP provides two levels of upper rate response. The first level defines the onset of the Wenckebach upper rate response and occurs when the P–P interval is shorter than the upper rate interval but longer than the TARP. The second level uses the TARP itself to define the onset of block when the P–P interval becomes shorter than the TARP.

Upper rate response of DDD pacemakers

The maximum paced ventricular rate of a DDD pacemaker can be defined either by the duration of the TARP or by a separate timing circuit controlling the ventricular channel. In general, upper rate limitation by only the TARP (as in our early DDD pacemaker) is less suitable because it produces a sudden fixed-ratio block such as 2 : 1 or 3 : 1 block. In contrast, a smoother response occurs with a Wenckebach upper rate response, which requires a separate URI timing interval that must be longer than the TARP.

Fixed-ratio block

In this system the upper rate becomes a function of only the TARP (AVI + PVARP). As the atrial rate increases, any P wave falling within the PVARP is unsensed and, in effect, blocked. The AV delay always remains constant. If the programmed upper rate is 120 ppm (TARP = 500 ms) and the lower rate is 60 ppm, a 2 : 1 response will occur when the atrial rate reaches 140 ppm. One P wave is blocked (or unsensed) and the other initiates an AV delay and triggers a ventricular response. The situation is not as simple mathematically when the lower rate is 70 ppm, because the ventricular rate cannot fall below the lower rate. An upper rate response using fixed-ratio block may be inappropriate in young or physically active individuals, because the sudden reduction in the ventricular rate with activity may be poorly tolerated.

Wenckebach upper rate response

The Wenckebach upper rate response requires a separately programmable upper rate interval (URI). The purpose of the Wenckebach response is to avoid a sudden reduction of the paced ventricular rate (as occurs in fixed-ratio block) and to maintain some degree of AV synchrony at faster rates. The URI must be longer than the TARP. During the Wenckebach upper rate response, the pacemaker will synchronize its ventricular stimulus to sensed atrial activity. The pacemaker cannot violate its URI. Therefore, upon atrial sensing, the pacemaker has to wait until the URI has timed out before it can release a ventricular stimulus. For this reason the AV delay (initiated by atrial sensing) must be extended to deliver the ventricular stimulus at the completion of the URI. The sensed AV delay gradually lengthens throughout the Wenckebach sequence, but the ventricular rate remains constant at the programmed upper rate. Mathematically the AV delay must progressively lengthen in the Wenckebach progression simply because the URI cannot be violated and the atrial rate interval or P–P interval is shorter than the URI but longer than the TARP. Eventually a P wave will fall in the PVARP, where it will not be followed by a ventricular stimulus, and a pause will occur. In other words, the Wenckebach response maintains the constant URI at the expense of extension of the AV delay (AS–VP).

1. The maximum prolongation of the AV interval represents the difference between the URI and the TARP.
2. With progressive shortening of the P–P interval, the Wenckebach upper rate response eventually switches to 2 : 1 fixed-ratio block, which occurs when the P–P interval becomes shorter than the TARP.
3. There are only two ventricular paced intervals during a Wenckebach upper rate sequence: (a) repeated ventricular pacing at the upper rate interval; (b) a longer interval (pause) between two successive ventricular beats following the undetected P wave in the PVARP. The pause may terminate with AS or AP, and the ventricular event may be VS or VP, according to circumstances. Some patients feel the pause at the end of a Wenckebach sequence as an uncomfortable sensation. The pause may be abbreviated or even eliminated with appropriate programming of the sensor function of a DDDR pacemaker. This process has been called *sensor-driven rate-smoothing*.
4. Let us consider two clinical examples:
   (a) A DDD pacemaker is programmed as follows: upper rate = 100 ppm (URI = 600 ms), AV delay = 150 ms, PVARP = 250 ms. The TARP will be 250 + 150 = 400 ms. The pacemaker will therefore respond to an atrial rate faster than 100 bpm by exhibiting Wenckebach sequences, with the longest prolongation of the AV interval being 200 ms (URI minus TARP). Thus the AV delay will vary from

its programmed value of 150 ms to a maximum of 350 ms. Fixed-ratio block will occur when the P–P interval is shorter than the TARP (400 ms), or at an atrial rate of 150 bpm.

(b) When the same DDD pacemaker is programmed with AV delay = 200 ms, PVARP = 250 ms, upper rate = 125 ppm (URI = 480 ms), it would be difficult to produce an actual Wenckebach upper rate response. The maximum prolongation of the AV interval would be 30 ms (URI minus TARP) and its maximum duration 230 ms. In this case, the pacemaker will respond with a Wenckebach sequence at an atrial rate of 125 bpm, but less than 133 ppm. When the atrial rate exceeds 133 bpm, fixed-ratio block will occur (P–P shorter than TARP of 450 ms).

Remember the three important variables: URI, TARP, and the P–P interval (atrial rate)

1. URI ≤ TARP:
   - No Wenckebach response is possible.
2. URI > TARP:
   - P–P interval > URI. When the P–P interval is longer than the URI, the pacemaker maintains 1 : 1 AV synchrony.
   - P–P interval < URI. When the P–P interval becomes shorter than the URI but longer than the TARP (i.e., URI > P–P > TARP), the pacemaker responds with a Wenckebach upper rate response.
   - P–P interval < TARP. When the P–P interval is shorter than the TARP, the pacemaker can only respond with a fixed-ratio form of upper rate limitation.

Duration of the AV interval and programmability of the upper rate

The sensed AV interval (sAVI) initiated by AS (AS–VP), and not the one initiated by AP (pAVI), determines the point where fixed-ratio block occurs, i.e., when P–P interval is less than TARP or (AS–VP) + PVARP. In many pacemakers the sAVI (AS–VP) can be programmed to a shorter value than the pAVI (AP–VP) interval, thereby shortening the TARP during atrial sensing. Furthermore the sAVI (AS–VP) can decrease further with exercise according to the sensed atrial rate and/or sensor activity. This shortening on exercise mimics the physiological response of the PR interval and provides hemodynamic benefit and a more advantageous shorter TARP. (In some pacemakers the TARP can also shorten further on exercise because of an adaptive PVARP that shortens on exercise based on designed algorithms.) Therefore a shorter TARP allows programming (separately) of a shorter URI, to permit a Wenckebach upper rate response to occur at faster atrial rate.

Lower rate timing of dual chamber pacemakers

Traditional DDD pacemakers are designed with ventricular-based lower rate timing. In this system a ventricular paced (VP) or ventricular sensed (VS) event initiates the lower rate interval (LRI) and the atrial escape interval. The atrial escape interval always remains constant. The LRI is the longest VP–VP or VS–VP interval without intervening atrial and ventricular sensed events. In atrial-based lower rate timing, the LRI is initiated and therefore controlled by atrial sensed or paced (AS or AP) events rather than ventricular events. The LRI becomes the longest AP–AP or AS–AP interval. The atrial escape interval becomes variable and adapts its duration to maintain a constant AP–AP or AS–AP interval equal to the LRI. The duration of the atrial escape interval can be calculated as the LRI minus the AV interval immediately preceding the atrial escape interval in question. In an atrial-based lower rate system, ventricular premature complexes initiate either the basic atrial escape interval (as if it were ventricular-based) or a complete LRI according to design.

Caveat: In hysteresis the escape interval after sensing is longer than the pacemaker automatic interval.

Phantom programming

This describes unintended, inadvertent, or mysterious reprogramming of a pacemaker. It may be due to reprogramming by an operator who made no record of it in the patient's chart. It may also be caused by electromagnetic interference unbeknown to the patient.

Programmability of lower rate

Patients with coronary artery disease and angina pectoris tend to have their pacemaker programmed to a low rate to avoid the precipitation of angina (chest pain). This may be true for VVI pacing but not for VDD, DDD, rate-adaptive DDD (DDDR), and rate-adaptive VVI (VVIR) pacing, which such patients tolerate well because their heart responds more efficiently on exercise. However, the upper rate should be programmed cautiously. Patients with sick sinus syndrome and atrial tachyarrhythmias may benefit from overdrive suppression by increasing the pacing rate to 80 bpm, which may eliminate or reduce atrial tachyarrhythmias (Table 1).

Table 1. Basic multiprogrammability.

Rate	Increase	(a) To optimize cardiac output; (b) to overdrive or terminate tachyarrhythmias; (c) to adapt to pediatric needs; (d) to test AV conduction in AAI pacemakers; (e) to confirm atrial capture using the AAI mode by observing a concomitant increase in the ventricular rate; (f) rate-drop response for the treatment of vasovagal syncope – an abrupt fall in the spontaneous rate causes pacing at a higher rate (than the low basic pacing rate) for a given duration; (g) to prevent polymorphic ventricular tachycardia after ablation of the AV junction for refractory supraventricular tachyarrhythmias
	Decrease	(a) To assess underlying rhythm and dependency status; (b) to adjust the rate below the angina threshold; (c) to allow the emergence of sinus rhythm and preservation of atrial transport; (d) to test sensing function; (e) sleep mode to provide a lower rate during the expected sleep time. Some devices use an activity sensor to drop the rate automatically with inactivity
Output	Increase	To adapt to pacing threshold
	Decrease	(a) To test pacing threshold; (b) to program pacemaker according to chronic threshold to enhance battery longevity; (c) to reduce extracardiac stimulation (voltage rather than pulse duration) of pectoral muscles or diaphragm; (d) to assess underlying rhythm and dependency status
Sensitivity	Increase	To sense low amplitude P or QRS electrograms
	Decrease	(a) To test sensing threshold; (b) to prevent T wave or afterpotential sensing by ventricular channel; (c) to avoid sensing extracardiac signals such as myopotentials
Refractory period	Increase	(a) Atrial: to minimize sensing of the far-field QRS during AAI pacing; (b) ventricular: to minimize T wave or afterpotential sensing by the ventricular channel
	Decrease	(a) To maximize QRS sensing; (b) to detect early ventricular premature beats
Hysteresis		To delay onset of ventricular pacing and to preserve atrial transport function in the VVI mode
Polarity	Conversion to unipolar mode	(a) To amplify the signal for sensing when the bipolar electrogram is too small; (b) to compensate temporarily for a defect in the other electrode
	Conversion to bipolar mode	(a) To decrease electromagnetic or myopotential interference; (b) to evaluate oversensing; (c) to eliminate extracardiac anodal stimulation

Table 1. Basic multiprogrammability (*continued*).

AV interval (AVI)	Increase or decrease to optimize LV function	(a) Differential: to permit a longer interval after an atrial paced event than a sensed atrial event; (b) rate-adaptive: to shorten the AV delay with an increase in heart rate
Postventricular atrial refractory period (PVARP)	Increase	To prevent sensing of retrograde P waves
PVARP extension after a VPC	On/off	To prevent sensing of retrograde P wave after a VPC
Postventricular atrial blanking period (PVAB)	Increase	To prevent VA crosstalk
Postatrial ventricular blanking period (PAVB)	Increase	To prevent AV crosstalk
Ventricular safety pacing (VSP)	On/off	To guarantee ventricular stimulation in the presence of crosstalk
Separately programmable upper rate	URI > TARP	To provide a smoother (Wenckebach) upper rate response and avoid abrupt slowing of the ventricular rate when URI = TARP

Endless loop tachycardia

Endless loop tachycardia (ELT) sometimes called pacemaker-mediated tachycardia, is a well-known complication of DDD, DDDR, and VDD pacing. It represents a form of ventriculoatrial (VA) synchrony, or the reverse of AV synchrony. Any circumstance that causes AV dissociation (separation of the P wave from the paced or spontaneous QRS complex) can initiate ELT, but only in patients with retrograde VA conduction. The most common initiating mechanism is a ventricular premature complex (VPC) with retrograde VA conduction (Table 2).

When the atrial channel senses a retrograde P wave, a ventricular stimulus is issued at the completion of the AV delay, which may have to be extended to conform to the URI. The pacemaker provides the anterograde loop of a process similar to the reentrant mechanism of many spontaneous tachyarrhythmias. VA conduction following ventricular pacing provides the retrograde limb of the reentrant loop. The atrial channel of the pacemaker again senses the retrograde P wave, and the process perpetuates itself. The cycle length of ELT is often equal to the URI, but it can be longer than the URI if retrograde VA conduction is delayed. The tachycardia is called a balanced ELT when its rate is slower than the programmed upper rate. The true programmed AV delay will be seen in ELT when the rate is slower than the programmed upper rate because the AVI is not extended. When the ELT is at the upper rate, the AV delay is extended to conform to the URI.

Diagnosis and prevention of endless loop tachycardia

The presence of retrograde VA conduction and its duration must always be determined (Table 3).

Table 2. Initiating mechanisms of endless loop tachycardia (ELT).

1. Ventricular extrasystoles (most common cause)
2. Subthreshold atrial stimulation
3. Atrial extrasystole with prolongation of AV delay to conform to programmed upper rate interval > total atrial refractory period
4. Application and withdrawal of the magnet
5. Decrease in atrial sensitivity: undersensing of anterograde P waves with preserved sensing of retrograde P waves
6. Myopotential sensing, usually by the atrial channel
7. Programmer electromagnetic interference, sensed by the atrial channel only
8. Excessively long AV delay
9. Programming the VDD mode when the sinus rate is slower than the programmed lower rate
10. Treadmill exercise (rarely) and increase in sinus rate with Wenckebach upper rate response and AV delay extension
11. Sensing of a far-field signal by the atrial lead, usually the far-field R wave

The maneuvers to initiate ELT are repeated until appropriate programming of the pacemaker prevents induction of tachycardia. In general the PVARP should be programmed at least 50 ms longer than the VA conduction time. A PVARP of 300 ms offers protection against ELT in most patients with retrograde conduction (Table 4).

Reminder: Application of the magnet over the pacemaker immediately terminates ELT in virtually 100% of the cases, because it eliminates sensing.

Table 3. Situations where retrograde VA conduction can be evaluated.

1. Programming to VVI mode
2. Programming the atrial output to sub-threshold level in the DDD mode
3. Application and withdrawal of the magnet
4. Holter monitoring
5. Treadmill exercise (rarely)

Table 4. Programmability for the prevention of endless loop tachycardia.

1. Program PVARP
2. Automatic PVARP extension after VPC
3. Adaptive PVARP
4. Programmable sensitivity: 60–75 % of anterograde P waves are at least 0.5 mV larger than retrograde P waves
5. Shortening of the AV delay
6. Programming to a non-tracking mode such as DDI is no longer acceptable

Caveats:

1. The rate of ELT is not always at the programmed upper rate. In the DDI mode an endless loop with repetitive retrograde VA conduction will occur at the lower rate, and no tachycardia is possible.
2. Programming a long PVARP will limit the upper rate. This may be important in vigorous or young patients.

ELT should be considered a complication of the past, because it is almost always prevented by programming the PVARP to contain the retrograde P waves. Problems arise when the VA conduction time is very long and a long PVARP restricts programmability of the upper rate. In such cases, pacemakers utilize special automatic tachycardia-terminating algorithms.

Repetitive non-reentrant VA synchrony: the cousin of endless loop tachycardia

ELT is a form of repetitive VA synchrony, and as mentioned it is a reentrant or circus-movement tachycardia. Repetitive VA synchrony can occur in the VVI or VVIR with continual retrograde VA conduction, where it may cause hemodynamic impairment and the pacemaker syndrome. Repetitive VA synchrony can also occur in the DDD or DDDR mode when a paced ventricular beat causes retrograde VA conduction but the retrograde P wave is unsensed (unlike ELT) because it falls within the PVARP. Under certain circumstances, this form of VA synchrony can become self-perpetuating, when the pacemaker continually delivers an ineffectual atrial stimulus (despite being well above the pacing threshold under normal circumstances) in the atrial myocardial refractory period generated by the preceding retrograde P wave. The potential reentrant circuit does not close as in ELT, and this arrhythmia is often labeled as being non-reentrant. Both ELT and repetitive non-reentrant VA synchrony depend on VA conduction, and they are physiologically similar, sharing similar initiating and terminating mechanisms. Repetitive non-reentrant VA synchrony depends on a short atrial escape interval (relatively fast lower rate and/or a long AV delay) and a relatively long VA conduction time. Thus it is more likely to occur during sensor-driven faster pacing rates. The process may therefore occur when programming a very long AV delay to promote AV conduction and normal ventricular activation. Occasionally, during ELT, magnet application over the pacemaker can cause a locked arrangement similar to repetitive non-reentrant VA synchrony (with preservation of VA conduction), so that removal of the magnet reinitiates ELT.

Types of dual chamber pacemakers

Simpler pacing modes can be easily derived from the DDD mode by the removal of certain intervals and equalizing others. All retain a fundamental LRI, ventricular refractory period, and AV delay initiated by atrial pacing, except for the DOO mode, which has only an AV delay and LRI.

DVI mode

The DVI mode may be considered as the DDD mode with the PVARP lasting through the entire duration of the atrial escape interval. As the AV delay is always refractory in a DDD pacemaker, the TARP, in effect, lasts through the entire LRI. No URI can exist because atrial sensing is impossible. Therefore the LRI, TARP, and URI are all equal. Crosstalk intervals are retained. The DVI mode is rarely used, and it is obsolete as a primary pacing mode. The term "committed," and variants thereof, are therefore obsolete descriptions of the DVI mode.

DDI mode

The DDI mode may be considered as the DDD mode with equal URI and LRI. This concept facilitates understanding of complex rhythms generated by this mode, although this conceptualization is not recommended by some experts. Nevertheless, it is easy to remember and apply. Remember the DDTI/I designation for the DDD mode. The DDI mode is simply created by removing the "T" from the atrial channel. Thus atrial sensing occurs but no "T" function is possible. In other words, a sensed P wave cannot trigger a ventricular stimulus, and a programmed AV interval cannot occur after atrial sensing. The programmed AV delay can only exist as the AP–VP interval. This means that atrial tracking cannot occur. The DDI mode will therefore always exhibit a constant ventricular paced rate equal to the LRI. There is no URI (as URI = LRI). A PVARP is retained because atrial sensing occurs. Crosstalk intervals are retained. In the early days of DDD pacing, the DDI mode was useful in patients with AV block and paroxysmal atrial tachyarrhythmias because it prevented rapid ventricular pacing during tachycardia. The use of the primary continuous DDI mode for this problem has been superseded by automatic mode switching of a DDD pacemaker to the DDI mode upon the detection of an atrial tachyarrhythmia, and reversion to the DDD mode automatically upon termination of tachycardia.

During DDI pacing with atrial fibrillation and AV block, many AR markers (atrial refractory sense events) will be seen in the atrial refractory period (in the AV delay and the PVARP) and AS markers outside the atrial refractory period. AS cannot start an AV delay. The AR markers provide diagnostic representation of the underlying arrhythmia and insight as to how the pacemaker activates the automatic mode-switching function.

VDD mode

The original atrial synchronous pacemaker was the VAT system without ventricular sensing. Then ventricular sensing was added (VAT + VVI = VDD). The VDD mode functions like the DDD mode except that the atrial output is turned off. The required timing intervals include LRI, URI, AVI, and PVARP. The omitted atrial stimulus begins an implied AV delay, during which, according to traditional design, the atrial channel is refractory. In the absence of atrial activity, the VDD mode will continue to pace effectively in the VVI mode (at the LRI of its DDD parent) because the VDD keeps all the basic cycles of the DDD mode despite the missing atrial output. This is an important disadvantage of the VDD mode, because VVI pacing during sinus bradycardia may be poorly tolerated, and may cause the pacemaker syndrome. No crosstalk intervals are required, because there is no atrial stimulation in the VDD mode.

Reminder: One can easily derive the function and timing cycles of all dual chamber pacemakers starting with a thorough knowledge of the timing cycles of DDD pacemakers.

Caveat: There are two types of response to the sensed P wave in the VDD mode according to design: (1) A P wave falling in the implied AV delay is not sensed, and the LRI remains constant. (2) In some pacemakers a P wave in the implied AV interval can be sensed, and can actually reinitiate an entirely new AV delay so that the VS–VP or VP–VP interval becomes longer than the programmed (ventricular-based) LRI. This produces a form of hysteresis with the maximum extension of the LRI being equal to the AS–VP interval.

Overdrive suppression and the underlying rhythm

Continuous pacing may suppress the underlying spontaneous rhythm, a phenomenon called *overdrive suppression*. Thus the sudden interruption of pacing may cause prolonged asystole because it takes time for a dormant rhythm to "wake up." The underlying rhythm is determined by programming to the VVI and *gradually* reducing the rate, sometimes as low as 30 ppm. Often a slow rhythm "warms up" and will emerge. Most patients tolerate such a slow rate of pacing. A patient who has a poor underlying rhythm is often labeled as being "pacemaker-dependent." This is a vague term which has never been clearly defined. One meaning refers to the occurrence of severe or life-threatening symptoms with failure to pace, as may occur with lead dysfunction, battery failure, or electromagnetic interference. Pacemaker dependency may be tested by totally and abruptly inhibiting the pacemaker, but this may dangerous. The emergence of a slow rhythm during gradual reduction of the pacemaker rate to 30 ppm does not mean that the patient is not pacemaker-dependent. The presence of pacemaker dependency should be displayed prominently on the cover of the pacemaker chart, together with the list of medications the patient is taking.

Caveat: Always have two programmers on hand in case one malfunctions during induced severe bradycardia or asystole.

Pacemaker hemodynamics

The early pacemakers had little in the way of electronics, and no hemodynamic refinement. VVI pacing was basically non-physiologic and ignored the atrium. Pacemaker syndrome was relatively common. The advent of DDD pacing was hailed as the universal pacing mode. However, patients with sick sinus syndrome and poor atrial chronotropic function complained of fatigue and inability to perform exercise to a level they thought reasonable because the heart rate did not increase on exercise. The subsequent development of rate-adaptive pacemakers (with artificial sensors in addition to the natural P-wave sensor) permitted a pacemaker to respond by increasing its rate like the normal heart on effort. These pacemakers improved effort tolerance in patients with bradycardia at rest or with activity. Many older patients have little ability to increase their cardiac output by increasing left ventricular contractility and therefore stroke volume (volume of blood ejected per heart beat), so that an increase in heart rate is their only way to increase cardiac output on effort. The cardiac output may increase by as much as 300% on exercise by rate increase alone. Unfortunately the settings on rate-adaptive pacemakers are often left on factory settings unless the patient becomes symptomatic or the physician has a particular interest in the technology.

AV synchrony

The atrial contribution provides about 15–30% of the cardiac output (volume of blood in liters ejected by the heart per minute) at rest in individuals with normal LV systolic function. Although the atrial contribution plays little or no role in exercise, when heart rate is basically the only determinant of cardiac output, AV synchrony at rest is vital to prevent pacemaker syndrome and atrial tachyarrhythmias. The loss of AV synchrony can be especially detrimental in patients with LV diastolic dysfunction, where the systolic function can be normal but the ventricle is stiff and non-compliant, as in hypertrophy from hypertension. Furthermore, patients with heart failure often do not tolerate loss of AV synchrony.

Reminder: Loss of or inappropriate AV synchrony is the cause of pacemaker syndrome. The optimal AV delay for the individual patient cannot be predicted, but it can be evaluated echocardiographically.

Ventricular activation sequence

While the AV delay and rate responsiveness are essential components of pacemakers, the role of the ventricular activation sequence is presently becoming recognized. In patients with sick sinus syndrome and normal AV conduction, AAI or AAIR pacing (associated with a small risk of AV block even in highly selected patients) provides the best hemodynamics because it preserves normal ventricular activation. Long-term RV pacing, which by necessity causes abnormal LV activation (similar to left bundle branch block), may cause long-term deterioration of LV function or precipitate congestive heart failure in patients with poor LV function. This disturbance seems to be based on the cumulative duration of right ventricular pacing. For this reason, the AV delay should be programmed to promote AV conduction if possible, so that the advantage of normal ventricular depolarization offsets the depressant effect of pacing on the LV. Patients with relatively normal AV conduction who require minimal or backup pacing could be paced with a slow lower rate such as 40–50 ppm to allow a spontaneous rhythm most of the time, with the hope of preventing long-term deterioration of LV function. Patients with a long PR interval (≥ 280 ms) require ventricular pacing for optimal hemodynamic benefit. The shorter (and optimized) AV delay produces an immediate hemodynamic benefit but the negative impact of abnormal pacing-induced LV depolarization may become a long-term problem. Thus, DDD or DDDR pacing should be weighed against the long-term detrimental risks involved with continual RV pacing. For this reason, biventricular pacing may be a better option.

Biventricular pacemakers (see *Cardiac resynchronization*, below) are used to treat congestive heart failure in patients with poor LV function and left bundle branch block. The latter produces an inefficient left ventricular contramarked first-degree AV blockcation because of abnormal ventricular depolarization and contraction. Biventricular pacing produces "resynchronization" by promoting a more physiologic pattern of depolarization and a more efficient LV contraction.

Caveat: Programming a long AV delay to promote normal AV conduction may increase the risk of endless loop tachycardia and repetitive non-reentrant VA synchrony by promoting retrograde VA conduction.

Rate-adaptive pacemakers

A sensor monitors the need for a faster pacing rate according to activity and works independently of intrinsic atrial activity. A VVI pacemaker with rate-adaptive function is coded as a VVIR pacemaker. A DDDR pacemaker is thus a DDD device with rate-adaptive function or rate modulation. However, the VDDR mode is a misnomer because such a mode operates in the VDD mode except when it is sensor-driven, when the pacing mode becomes VVIR. Table 5 shows the characteristics of pacemakers with and without the "R" designation for rate-adaptive function.

Five basic parameters can be programmed in sensor-driven pacemakers: sensor threshold, lower rate, upper sensor rate, upper tracking (or atrial-driven) rate, and sensor slope. Unfortunately many pacemakers are left at their nominal settings (out of the box), which may not be optimal for some patients.

Table 5. Characteristics of commonly used pacing modes.

Characteristics	VVI	VVIR	AAI	AAIR	DDD	DDI	DDDR	DDIR
Simplicity	+++	+++	++	++	+	+	—	—
AV synchrony	—	—	+	+	+	+[a]	+	+[a]
Potential for pacemaker syndrome	+	+	—	—	—	—	—	—
Normal LV activation	—	—	+	+	—[b]	—[b]	—[b]	—[b]
Propensity to ELT	—	—	—	—	+	+[c]	+	+[c]
Tracking of SVT	—	—	—	—	+	—	+	—
Contraindicated in AV block	—	—	+	+	—	—	—	—
Increase of pacing rate in atrial chronotropic incompetence	—	+	—	+	—[d]	—	+	+
Cost	—	+	—	+	++	++	+++	+++

[a] In the DDI mode if normal sinus rhythm is faster than the programmed rate, and in the DDIR mode if normal sinus rhythm is faster than the sensor-driven rate, AV dissociation with hemodynamic disadvantage is frequent in patients with AV block.
[b] Unless AV delay is prolonged to allow for normal anterograde conduction.
[c] Endless loop without tachycardia at the lower rate or at the sensor-driven rate.
[d] Ventricular pacing rate does not increase if the sinus rate does not increase on exercise.

The sensor threshold is the minimum degree of sensor activation to initiate an increase in heart rate. In other words, it sets the lowest level of sensor activation that will be counted and used for rate control. Threshold settings may be numeric or descriptive. Sedentary patients may require a more sensitive setting. The sensor slope determines the rate of change of the heart rate in response to sensor activation. Increasing the slope will result in an increased pacing rate for the same amount of activity. The normal sinus node produces a linear increase in the heart rate during exercise. However, the slope can be variable, and it depends on the degree of conditioning. Some manufacturers have designed pacemakers with an auto-responsive slope and threshold. The pacemaker learns the appropriate settings based on the patient's activity. These automatic systems are not perfect, but are better than empiric or no programming of the rate-adaptive response.

The pause in the Wenckebach upper rate response can be attenuated or even eliminated by appropriate programming of a DDDR pacemaker. This process is called *sensor-driven rate smoothing*.

The sensor in DDDR pacemakers can also influence intervals other than the LRI. These include:

1. The AV delay, which shortens on exercise to mimic physiologic shortening of the PR interval.
2. The PVARP. Shortening of the PVARP on exercise, coupled with adaptive shortening of the AV interval, produces substantial shortening of the total atrial refractory period. This allows programming of a faster upper rate. An adaptive PVARP allows programming of a relatively long PVARP at rest when endless loop tachycardia is likely to occur. Initiation of endless loop tachycardia is quite unusual on exercise with fast atrial-driven ventricular pacing, so that a shorter PVARP is safe.

Programming the pacemaker

An easy way to program the sensor-driven response is to have the patient walk up and down the hallway and adjust the parameters accordingly. Avoid over-programming the threshold response, which will produce an excessively fast pacing rate poorly tolerated by patients.

Caveat: After the implantation of a pacemaker, fluid in the pacemaker pocket may dampen vibrations and the response of activity rate-adaptive pacemakers. If these devices are programmed too early, there may be an excessive rate response several weeks later, after the absorption of fluid. It would appear wise to leave the rate-adaptive function of activity-driven devices turned off for a time after implantation, to prevent constantly changing pacing rates when the patient turns in bed, etc. Such fluctuations may cause confusion for the personnel monitoring the patient.

The pacemaker stimulus

Contemporary digital ECG recorders distort the pacemaker stimulus, so it may become larger and show striking changes in amplitude and polarity. Digital recorders can also miss some of the pacemaker stimuli because of sampling characteristics. Diagnostic evaluation of the pacemaker stimulus is only possible with analog machines. Many inkjet recorders and ECG machines with a stylet writer are analog recorders. With such recorders, the direction and amplitude of the pacemaker stimulus may yield valuable information about lead displacement or defects. A bipolar lead with an insulation defect may pace normally but exhibit a very large stimulus artifact on the electrocardiogram (unipolar–bipolar phenomenon), in contrast to the tiny deflections with an intact bipolar lead.

Caveats

1. Static interference may generate deflections mimicking pacemaker stimuli. Careful scrutiny of the deflections often suggests they are not pacemaker stimuli. When in doubt, measure the timing cycles to and from the deflection in question and establish the lack of relationship to pacemaker function.
2. The interval from the stimulus to the onset of cardiac depolarization is called latency. The normal value for the RV is 40 ms or less. If there is a relatively long isoelectric (zero) interval from stimulus to QRS or P wave, the commonest cause is isoelectric depolarization in the ECG lead in question. Confirmation requires the recording of several ECG leads simultaneously to demonstrate the true onset of cardiac depolarization. Hyperkalemia is a common cause of increased latency. Other causes of latency include serious metabolic disorders, right ventricular infarction, and terminal situations.

Magnet mode

The magnet mode refers to the response of a pacemaker when a magnet is applied over it. The magnet closes the special reed-switch within the pulse generator, which eliminates sensing. The device then paces at the asynchronous mode at a rate specific to the manufacturer. The magnet rate is designed to reflect the degree of battery depletion. The behavior and rate of the magnet mode varies according to manufacturer. The magnet mode can be programmed "off' in some pacemakers.

Normal QRS patterns during right ventricular pacing

Pacing from the right ventricle (RV), regardless of site, virtually always produces a left bundle branch block (LBBB) pattern in the precordial leads (defined as the absence of a positive complex in lead V_1 recorded in the fourth or fifth intercostal space). Pacing from the RV apex produces negative paced QRS complexes in the inferior leads (II, III, and aVF), because depolarization begins in the inferior part of the heart and travels superiorly away from the inferior leads. The mean paced QRS frontal-plane axis is always superior, usually in the left or less commonly in the right superior quadrant.

Pacing from the right ventricular outflow tract

Primary lead placement in the right ventricular outflow tract (RVOT) or septum, or lead displacement from the RV apex towards the RVOT initially shifts the frontal-plane paced QRS axis to the left inferior quadrant, a site considered normal for spontaneous QRS complexes. The inferior leads become positive. Then the axis shifts to the right inferior quadrant as the stimulation site moves more superiorly towards the pulmonary valve. With the backdrop of dominant R waves in the inferior leads, RVOT pacing may generate qR, QR, or Qr complexes in leads I and aVL. Occasionally, with slight displacement of the pacing lead from the RV apex to the RV outflow tract, leads I and aVL may register a qR complex in conjunction with the typical negative complexes of RV apical stimulation in the inferior leads. This qR pattern in leads I and aVL must not be interpreted as a sign of myocardial infarction.

qR and Qr complexes in inferior and precordial leads

RV pacing from any site never produces qR complexes in V_5 and V_6 in the absence of myocardial infarction or ventricular fusion with a spontaneous conducted QRS complex. A qR or Qr (but not a QS deflection) complex in the precordial or inferior leads is always abnormal during RV pacing from any site in the absence of ventricular fusion. In contrast, a q wave is common in the lateral leads (I, aVL, V_5, and V_6) during uncomplicated biventricular pacing (using the RV apex), and should not be interpreted as representing myocardial infarction or RVOT displacement of an RV apical lead. Uncomplicated RV apical pacing may (rarely) display a qR complex in lead I (but not aVL).

Dominant R wave of the paced QRS complex in lead V_1 during conventional RV apical pacing

A dominant R wave in V_1 during RV pacing has been called a "right bundle branch block" (RBBB) pattern of depolarization, but this terminology is potentially misleading because this pattern may not be related to RV activation delay. In our experience a dominant R wave of a paced ventricular beat in the right precordial leads (V_1 and V_2 recorded in the fourth intercostal spaces) occurs in approximately 8–10% of patients with uncomplicated RV apical pacing. The position of precordial leads V_1 and V_2 should be checked, because a dominant R wave can be sometimes recorded at the level of the third or second intercostal space during uncomplicated RV apical pacing. The pacing lead is almost certainly in the RV (apex or distal septal site) if leads V_1 and V_2 show a negative QRS complex when recorded one space lower (fifth intercostal space). However, a dominant R wave may not be always eliminated at the level of the fifth interspace if RV pacing originates from the midseptal region. Furthermore, in the normal situation with the ventricular lead in the RV, the "RBBB" pattern from pacing RV sites results in a vector change from positive to negative by lead V_3 in the precordial sequence. Therefore a tall R wave in V_3 and V_4 signifies that a pacemaker lead is most probably not in the RV, after excluding ventricular fusion from spontaneous AV conduction. However, left ventricular (LV) pacing generating a positive complex in lead V_1 may not necessarily be accompanied by a positive complex in leads V_2 and V_3. The ECG pattern with a truly posterior RV lead has not been systematically investigated as a potential cause of a tall R wave in V_1 during RV pacing.

We have never seen a so-called "RBBB" pattern in lead V_1 during uncomplicated RV outflow tract pacing, and it has never been reported so far. Right axis deviation of the ventricular paced beats in the frontal plane with a deep S wave in leads I and aVL does not constitute an RBBB pattern without looking at lead V_1.

Significance of a small r wave in lead V_1 during uncomplicated RV pacing

A small early r wave (sometimes wide) may occasionally occur in lead V_1 during uncomplicated RV apical or outflow pacing. There is no evidence that this r wave represents a conduction abnormality at the RV exit site. Furthermore, an initial r wave during biventricular pacing does not predict initial LV activation.

Paced QRS duration during conventional right ventricular pacing

A long paced QRS duration is a significant independent predictor of heart-failure hospitalization in patients with sinus node dysfunction and AV block. On this basis, serial determinations of the paced QRS duration may be clinically useful to evaluate LV function and the risk of developing heart failure.

Left ventricular endocardial pacing

Passage of a pacing lead into the LV rather than the RV occurs usually via an atrial septal defect (patent foramen ovale), or less commonly via the subclavian artery. The diagnosis of a malpositioned endocardial LV lead will be missed in a single-lead ECG. The problem may be compounded if the radiographic malposition of the lead is not obvious, or if insufficient projections are taken. A 12-lead paced ECG will show an RBBB pattern of paced ventricular depolarization with QRS positivity commonly preserved in the right precordial leads, or at least in V_1. The positive QRS complexes are unaltered when leads V_1 and V_2 are recorded one intercostal space lower. During LV pacing the frontal-plane axis of paced beats can indicate the site of LV pacing, but as a rule with an RBBB configuration the frontal-plane axis cannot differentiate precisely an endocardial LV site from one in the coronary venous system. The diagnosis of an endocardial LV lead is easy with transesophageal echocardiography (TEE). In the usual situation, it will show the lead crossing the atrial septum then passing through the mitral valve into the LV.

An endocardial LV lead is a potential source of cerebral emboli. Most patients with neurologic manifestations do not exhibit echocardiographic evidence of thrombus on the pacing lead. In symptomatic patients, removal of the lead after a period of anticoagulation should be considered. A chronic LV lead in asymptomatic or frail elderly patients is sometimes best treated with long-term anticoagulant therapy.

A Medline search from the years 2000–2010 revealed a substantial number of reports documenting inadvertent endocardial LV lead placement (pacing and ICD leads). The true incidence of this problem is unknown, but the Medline data suggest that there are probably many unreported cases. It is disturbing that this serious but avoidable complication (avoided simply by looking at a 12-lead ECG at the time of implantation) is still being recognized at late follow-up, by which time lead extraction can be problematic.

Manifestations of myocardial infarction in the paced rhythm

Anterior myocardial infarction

Stimulus-qR pattern

Because the QRS complex during RV pacing resembles (except for the initial forces) that of spontaneous left bundle branch block (LBBB), many of the criteria for the diagnosis of myocardial infarction (MI) in LBBB also apply to MI during RV pacing. During RV pacing, as in LBBB, an extensive anteroseptal MI close to the stimulating electrode will alter the initial QRS vector, with forces pointing to the right because of unopposed RV activation. This causes (initial) q waves in leads I, aVL, V_5, and V_6, producing an St-qR pattern. The abnormal q wave is usually 30 ms or more, but a narrower one is also diagnostic. The sensitivity of the St-qR pattern varies from 10% to 50% according to the way data are analyzed. The specificity is virtually 100% (Table 6).

Late notching of the ascending S wave (Cabrera's sign)

As in LBBB, during RV pacing an extensive anterior MI may produce notching of the ascending limb of the S wave in the precordial leads, usually V_3 and V_4 (Cabrera's sign) $\geq$ 30 ms and present in two leads. Slight slurring (with a rapid upward deflection: dV/dt or slope) of the ascending limb of the S wave does not constitute a Cabrera's sign. Cabrera's sign may occur together with the St-qR pattern in anterior MI. The sensitivity varies from 25% to 50% according to the size of the MI, but the specificity is close to 100% if notching is properly defined.

Inferior myocardial infarction

The paced QRS complex is often unrevealing. During RV pacing in inferior MI, diagnostic Qr, QR, or qR complexes provide a sensitivity of 15% and specificity of 100%. Cabrera's sign in *both* leads III and aVF is very specific but even less sensitive than its counterpart in anterior MI.

Table 6. Difficulties in the diagnosis of myocardial infarction during ventricular pacing.

1. Large unipolar stimuli may obscure initial forces, cause a pseudo Q wave and false ST segment current of injury
2. Fusion beats may cause a pseudoinfarction pattern (qR/Qr complex or notching of the upstroke of the S wave)
3. QRS abnormalities have low sensitivity (many false negatives) but high specificity (few false positives). These include qR or Qr patterns and Cabrera's sign in the appropriate leads
4. Retrograde P waves may simulate Cabrera's sign
5. Diagnosis of acute MI
   - Signs in QRS complex are not useful for the diagnosis of acute MI
   - Looking at the underlying rhythm: cardiac memory. Repolarization ST–T wave abnormalities (mostly T-wave inversion) in the spontaneous rhythm may be secondary to RV pacing per se, and not related to ischemia or non-Q-wave MI
   - Differentiation of MI versus ischemia may be impossible
   - Differentiation of acute MI versus old or indeterminate-age MI may be impossible if old MI is associated with prominent chronic T-wave changes, usually indicative of an acute process
   - ST segment abnormalities may help the diagnosis of acute myocardial infarction during ventricular pacing. ST elevation $\geq$ 5 mm in predominantly negative paced QRS complexes is the best marker. ST depression $\geq$ 1 mm in V_1, V_2, and V_3 and ST elevation $\geq$ 1 mm in leads with a concordant (same direction) QRS deflection. So-called primary T-wave abnormalities where the T wave is in the same direction as the QRS complex are not diagnostically useful during RV pacing

Diagnosis of acute myocardial infarction during right ventricular pacing

The diagnosis of myocardial ischemia or infarction should be based on the new development of ST elevation, because leads V_1–V_3 sometimes show marked ST elevation during ventricular pacing in the absence of myocardial ischemia or infarction. One study reported the value of ST segment abnormalities in the diagnosis of acute MI during ventricular pacing and their high specificity. ST elevation $\geq$ 5 mm in predominantly negative QRS complexes is the best marker, with a sensitivity of 53% and specificity of 88%, and this was the only criterion of statistical significance in their study. Other less important ST changes with high specificity include ST depression $\geq$ 1 mm in V_1, V_2, and V_3 (sensitivity 29%, specificity 82%), and ST elevation $\geq$ 1 mm in leads with a concordant QRS polarity. ST depression concordant with the QRS complex may occur in leads V_3–V_6 during uncomplicated RV pacing.

Diagnosis of myocardial ischemia during right ventricular pacing

Marked discordant ST elevation (> 5 mm) during RV pacing, a marker for the diagnosis of acute MI, could also be used for the diagnosis of severe reversible transmural myocardial ischemia. ST depression in leads V_1 and V_2 is rarely normal; it should be considered abnormal and indicative of anterior or inferior MI or ischemia. So-called primary T-wave abnormalities (discordant) are not diagnostically useful during RV pacing if they are not accompanied by primary ST abnormalities.

Cardiac memory

Cardiac memory refers to T-wave abnormalities manifested on resumption of a normal ventricular activation pattern after a period of abnormal ventricular activation, such as ventricular-pacing transient LBBB, ventricular arrhythmias, or Wolf–Parkinson–White syndrome. Pacing-induced T-wave inversion is usually localized to precordial and inferior leads. The direction of the T wave of the memory effect in sinus rhythm is typically in the same direction as the QRS vector of the abnormal impulse. The marked repolarization abnormalities reach a steady state in a week with RV endocardial pacing at physiologic rates. Memory-related repolarization abnormalities persist when normal depolarization is restored, and they resolve completely in a month. The changes and their duration are associated with complex biochemical abnormalities, and they are proportional to the amount of delivered ventricular pacing.

One report indicated that cardiac memory induced by RV pacing results in a distinctive T-vector pattern that allows discrimination from ischemic precordial T-wave inversions regardless of the coronary artery involved. T-wave axis, polarity, and amplitude on a 12-lead ECG during sinus rhythm were compared between cardiac-memory and ischemic patients. The combination of (1) positive T wave in aVL, (2) positive or isoelectric T wave in lead I, and (3) maximal precordial T wave inversion > T wave inversion in lead III was 92% sensitive and 100% specific for cardiac memory, discriminating it from ischemic precordial T-wave inversion regardless of the coronary artery involved.

Pacemaker alternans

Pacemaker QRS alternans is characterized by alternate changes in paced QRS morphology. The causes include respiratory fluctuation, pericardial effusion, mechanical pulsus alternans leading to electrical alternans from varying depolarization, and true alternating intraventricular alternans from the pacing site. Alternans can only be diagnosed after ventricular bigeminy or alternate fusion beats are ruled out by changing the pacing rate. True alternans represents a form of exit block (persisting over a range of rates) seen only in severe myocardial disease under circumstances that also cause latency and second-degree Wenckebach exit block from the pacing site.

Complications of pacemakers

Two major groups of complications are associated with pacemaker implantation: (a) non-electrical complications, including acute complications at the time of implantation such as pneumothorax and complications of lead placement and pocket formation, and (b) electrical complications and arrhythmias.

Non-electrical complications

Table 7 lists the principal non-electrical/arrhythmic complications.

Complications due to venous access

The risks of a complication related to subclavian vein puncture technique depend on operator skill and the difficulty of the subclavian puncture due to the patient's anatomy. The use of the cephalic cut-down technique almost eliminates these complications. The use of the axillary vein is safer than subclavian puncture. The incidence of pneumothorax is virtually zero with the cephalic or axillary vein approach.

Pneumothorax from subclavian puncture is uncommon but may occasionally occur in patients with emphysema or anatomic abnormalities. Pneumothorax may be asymptomatic and noted on routine follow-up chest x-ray, or it may be associated with pleuritic pain, respiratory distress, or hypotension. A pneumothorax that involves less than 10% of the pleural space is mostly benign and resolves without intervention. A pneumothorax > 10% or a tension pneumothorax requires the immediate placement of a chest tube.

Hemoptysis may occur if the lung is punctured, and it may be associated with a pneumothorax. Hemoptysis is usually self-limiting.

Hemothorax is a rare complication of subclavian puncture. It can be caused by laceration of the subclavian artery or by inadvertently introducing a large dilator or sheath into the artery. It is not caused by trauma to the lungs. In the absence of pneumothorax, bleeding is usually controlled by lung pressure. However, if the ipsilateral lung is also collapsed, blood may escape freely into the pleural space (hemopneumothorax), and this may result in substantial hemorrhage-associated hypotension and hemodynamic compromise necessitating draining.

Air embolism is a rare complication of subclavian vein puncture and mostly occurs when the lead is advanced through the introducer sheath, because of the development of physiologic negative pressure. This complication can be avoided by using the deep Trendelenburg position during advancement of the introducer sheath or leads, by pinching the sheath when the trocar is withdrawn, or by using sheaths with a hemostatic valve. The diagnosis of air embolism is obvious on fluoroscopy. Patients are mostly tolerant of this complication. However, respiratory distress, hypotension, and arterial oxygen desaturation may occur with a large embolus. Therapy consists of 100% O_2 with inotropic support. Usually no therapy is required, as the air is eventually absorbed into the lungs.

Venous thrombosis or occlusion of the subclavian and innominate veins is common but frequently asymptomatic. Acute symptomatic thrombosis is relatively uncommon and may cause unilateral arm swelling, usually several weeks after implantation. Superior vena cava syndrome (from occlusion) is more serious but rare, and causes facial

Table 7. Non-electrical/arrhythmic complications.

Venous access	Pneumothorax, subcutaneous emphysema Hemothorax Air embolism Brachial plexus injury Thoracic duct injury Trauma to the subclavian artery with occasional AV fistula (subclavian or innominate vein) Aortic perforation by atrial lead Injury to internal mammary artery Hematoma
Pacemaker pocket	Infection, septicemia, etc. Conservative therapy is often unsuccessful and removal of the entire system may be required Hematoma/seroma Erosion Pacemaker migration Twiddler's syndrome Muscle stimulation from a flipped but normally functioning unipolar or extravascular insulation defect Chronic pain, including subcuticular malposition of the pulse generator
Intravascular	Subclavian or innominate vein thrombosis Thrombosis of superior vena cava Coronary sinus dissection or perforation during implantation of a left ventricular lead Large right atrial thrombus Endocarditis with vegetations Manifest pulmonary embolism (rare) Cardiac perforation Cardiac tamponade Entanglement of lead in the tricuspid valve and ruptured chordae Tricuspid insufficiency Pericardial rub Post-pericardiotomy syndrome Severe mitral insufficiency and heart failure from abnormal depolarization of the papillary muscles Late reduction of left ventricular function from dyssynchrony with the development of heart failure
Lead problems	Displacement Malposition in the coronary venous system Endocardial left ventricular malposition across a patent foramen ovale or via subclavian arterial puncture (or via atrial or ventricular septum defect). Lead may then cause mitral valve perforation Right ventricular perforation or lead perforation of the interventricular septum Right atrial perforation with risk of lung penetration and right-sided pneumothorax and/or pneumopericardium Diaphragmatic pacing: left side with or without right ventricular perforation and right side by phrenic nerve stimulation by atrial pacing Intercostal muscle stimulation due to perforation Post-pericardiotomy syndrome (pericarditis, etc.) with or without lead perforation Intracardiac rupture of lead during attempt to remove old or broken lead

edema and cyanosis as well as collateral veins on the thorax. Symptomatic thrombosis manifested by arm swelling can be treated conservatively with arm elevation, with heparin followed by oral anticoagulation, or more aggressively with thrombolytic drugs. Superior vena cava syndrome requires vascular consultation for possible surgical correction. The subclavian vein is occluded in about 30% of chronic cases.

Pulmonary embolism occurs rarely, but the incidence may be underestimated as it is usually unrecognized. The presence of a symptomatic pulmonary embolism (potentially life-threatening) in a patient with a device should raise the suspicion of a source from a pacing or ICD lead.

Brachial plexus injury may occur from the needle stick in the brachial plexus located close to the subclavian/axillary vein. This complication should be suspected postoperatively if the patient complains of pain or paresthesias of the upper extremity. There is usually complete recovery, but neural injury may result in permanent muscle atrophy and impairment of shoulder motion.

Lead-related complications

Lead malposition may occur during transvenous lead placement. In patients with atrial septal defect or a large patent foramen ovale, the ventricular lead may be advanced inadvertently into the left ventricle. This complication occurs because fluoroscopy is often limited to the AP projection during the procedure and LV placement may resemble RV placement. An LV lead should be suspected when the tip of the lead is posterior on fluoroscopy and ventricular pacing gives rise to an RBBB pattern in the ECG.

Lead dislodgment usually occurs in the first days after implantation, and may occur up to three months after initial implantation. RV lead dislodgment occurs in about 1% of cases, but atrial lead dislodgment is more common. Lead displacement may be due to improper initial lead positioning, poor lead fixation, or excessive arm–shoulder motions soon after surgery. Dislodgment of the lead may cause loss of capture and undersensing. The diagnosis is confirmed by device interrogation showing changes in the sensing and pacing thresholds compared to implantation data, and a chest x-ray in the case of macro-displacement. Immediate lead repositioning is mandatory.

Lead damage may occur during implantation. An insulation break may occur due to inadvertent placement of a suture around the lead without a protective sleeve, a too-tight suture on the sleeve, or an accidental cut during surgery.

Pocket-related complications

A pocket **seroma** is due to fluid accumulation and is usually benign when not accompanied by signs of inflammation. It is observed more commonly after pulse generator change when the new pulse generator is smaller than the previous one. Aspiration should be discouraged because of the risk of introducing infection by contamination.

Pocket **hematoma** is relatively common. A hematoma is usually managed conservatively unless it expands in size and becomes tense and painful, whereupon evacuation becomes necessary, with reoperation to identify and control the site of bleeding. Pocket aspiration should be avoided. The risk of postoperative bleeding is higher with heparin than with warfarin.

Erosion is characterized by deterioration of tissue over an implanted pulse generator or movement of a lead toward or through the skin. Risk factors include a too-small pocket with tension on the overlying tissue, and a too-superficial or lateral implantation of the pulse generator in thin adults or children. When erosion is recognized at an early stage, signaled by redness and thinning of the skin, elective re-operation can be considered to relocate the pulse generator to a submuscular site. If any portion of the pulse generator or lead completely erodes through the skin, the site should be considered infected.

Infection occurs in about 1–2% of primary implantations, but is more common after device replacement. The mortality is very high if the leads and the pulse generator are not removed. The manifestations range from local reactions (redness, tenderness, swelling, abscess around the device) to uncommon life-threatening systemic sepsis with positive blood cultures. Early infections are usually caused by *Staphylococcus aureus*. Late infections are commonly caused by *Staphylococcus epidermidis*, are more indolent, and may present months or years after implantation, sometimes with only pain at the pacemaker site. Vegetations may occur in the right atrium, right ventricle, and tricuspid valve. Vegetations are best visualized by transesophageal echocardiography. The presence of infection mandates complete lead and device removal followed by antibiotics. Partial removal is associated with a high recurrence rate.

Perforation

Cardiac perforation is a rare but potentially serious and often unrecognized complication of pacemaker lead implantation. It may occur at the time of implantation and cause hypotension from cardiac tamponade. Perforation usually does not lead to tamponade if the lead is withdrawn and repositioned, because the perforation is often self-sealing.

The reported incidence of symptomatic perforation after implantation is about 1%. The true incidence of perforation is not well known because it may be subclinical and asymptomatic. Indeed, CT scans in patients with uncomplicated pacing show a 5% incidence of right ventricular perforation and 10% in the case of atrial leads. Risk factors include female sex, increasing age, and the use of stiff stylets. Administration of oral steroid within 7 days preceding lead implantation predisposes to perforation.

After implantation, right ventricular perforation of the free wall may be recognized by pericardial pain, abdominal pain, dyspnea, syncope, friction rub, sinus tachycardia, increasing ventricular pacing threshold, poor sensing, diaphragmatic stimulation, intercostal muscle stimulation, pericardial effusion, and left hemothorax. Rarely, perforation occurs into the left ventricle through the ventricular septum. The ECG may show a right bundle branch pattern if the lead paces the left ventricle usually from the pericardial space. The chest x-ray may show the lead beyond the cardiac shadow. An echocardiogram and CT scan should be performed to document lead position. Transesophageal echocardiography is superior to transthoracic echocardiography in delineating the entire course of a pacing lead. The CT scan is particularly helpful when echocardiography is equivocal. Multidetector computed tomography is emerging as the imaging modality of choice in diagnosing atrial and ventricular lead perforation. The development of small-diameter active fixation pacing and implantable cardioverter-defibrillator (ICD) leads may be associated with increased risk for delayed right ventricular perforation. Subacute right ventricular perforation (several days or weeks after seemingly uncomplicated implantation and occasionally much later) is a rare but serious complication of lead implantation. The clinical presentation has changed, so that perforation currently occurs usually up to 60 days after implantation and rarely a few months later. The late presentation may create an important diagnostic problem, and the situation may become catastrophic if unrecognized.

These complications may lead to death if they are not recognized early. In most patients, the leads can safely be removed in the operating room under fluoroscopic guidance and continuous electrogram (EGM) monitoring to confirm the diagnosis, with surgical backup support and together with TEE. Simple withdrawal of the lead is successful in 80% of cases. A stable asymptomatic perforation can be left alone if pacing and sensing are satisfactory. If parameters are unsatisfactory, a stable asymptomatic perforated lead can be left in place and a new lead implanted.

The unipolar EGM may show an upright complex that looks like a standard precordial lead over the lateral chest. When the lead is gradually withdrawn, some ventricular ectopy may occur as the lead passes through the ventricular wall. Then, obvious ST elevation (current of injury) occurs. This disappears when endocardial contact is lost. The intracavitary EGM often shows a deep S wave followed by gradual reduction of its amplitude, and P waves eventually appear as the lead is further withdrawn.

Recording of an adequate unipolar ventricular electrogram from the proximal RV electrode but an atypical one from the distal electrode should raise the suspicion of lead perforation, as does the presence of ST elevation from the proximal electrode and its absence from the distal electrode.

Right atrial leads may perforate both pericardium and pleura, resulting in right-sided pneumothorax, pneumopericardium, and rarely aortic laceration.

Recurrent postcardiac injury syndrome in the absence of perforation should be considered in patients who, after pacemaker lead insertion, develop pericardial and pleural effusion associated with markers of inflammation.

Electrical complications

Accessory muscle stimulation

Accessory muscle stimulation may occur at several sites:

1. Contraction of the diaphragm. Left diaphragmatic stimulation by pacemaker stimuli may occur during traditional pacing with and without lead perforation of the RV. Perforation must always be excluded when diaphragmatic pacing is observed. Late appearance of diaphragmatic pacing suggests an insulation defect of the pacing lead. Left ventricular pacing from a coronary vein (in the absence of perforation) is an important and troublesome cause of left diaphragmatic pacing during biventricular pacing for the treatment of heart failure. Contraction of the right diaphragm is related to a malpositioned right atrial electrode.
2. Left intercostal muscle stimulation is invariably due to ventricular lead perforation.
3. Deltopectoral muscle stimulation (twitching) may be due to: (a) an extravascular lead insulation leak – in the case of a bipolar pacemaker, this always indicates an insulation problem; (b) a unipolar pacemaker that has flipped over in a

large pocket so that the anode faces the skeletal muscle; (c) a normally functioning unipolar pacemaker without any other problems – this is now rare with better pacemaker design but can occur at high voltage outputs.

Decreasing the output voltage with preservation of an adequate safety margin often minimizes or eliminates accessory muscle stimulation. Decreasing the pulse duration alone is usually ineffective.

Generator-related complications

Normal functioning of a pacing system depends on proper connection between the leads and the generator. Care should be exercised to avoid misconnection of the leads. A loose setscrew usually causes oversensing due to the generation of spurious signals, intermittent failure to pace, or increased pacing threshold and lead impedance.

Abnormalities involving pacemaker stimuli

Tables 8 and 9 list the causes of loss of capture by visible stimuli and the causes of absent stimuli.

Undersersensing

Table 10 lists the causes of undersensing.

Reminder: Occasionally undersensing with a small bipolar signal can be corrected by programming to unipolar sensing. Do not expect an appropriately programmed pacemaker to sense all kinds of VPCs, because they are associated with a variety of electrograms, some of which may not be sensed because of a low amplitude and/or slow slew rate. Attempting to increase sensitivity to sense all VPCs may cause oversensing.

Oversensing

Oversensing is not uncommon. Table 11 outlines the important causes of oversensing.

Afterpotential

The cathodal pacemaker stimulus charges the electrode–tissue interface to a large voltage (polarization voltage) which is subsequently dissipated over a relatively long time to electrical neutrality. The decay of the afterpotential (of lower amplitude, opposite polarity but longer duration than the output stimulus) creates a voltage that changes with time, and thus it can be sensed (like a changing spontaneous intracardiac signal) by a pacemaker coming out of its refractory period, when it will reset the lower rate interval. Sensing of the afterpotential should be suspected when the interval between two consecutive pacemaker stimuli lengthens to a

Table 8. Loss of capture by visible pacemaker stimuli.

1. Normal situation: stimuli in myocardial refractory period
2. Electrode–tissue interface
   - Early displacement or unstable position of pacing leads (commonest cause). Microdislodgment (a diagnosis of exclusion) causes a marked rise in capture threshold but displacement is not apparent on a chest x-ray
   - Elevated pacing threshold without obvious lead displacement (exit block): acute or chronic reaction at the electrode–tissue interface
   - Subcutaneous emphysema (see Table 7)
   - Twiddler's syndrome causing late displacement
   - Myocardial infarction or ischemia, hypoxia
   - Hypothyroidism
   - Elevation of pacing threshold after defibrillation or cardioversion. This is usually transient, for a few minutes or less
   - Electrolyte abnormalities, usually hyperkalemia, severe acidosis
   - Drug effect: flecainide and propafenone can elevate the pacing threshold with therapeutic doses
3. Electrode: fracture, short circuit, or insulation break
4. Pulse generator
   - Normal pacemaker with incorrect programming of parameters
   - Pacemaker failure from exhaustion or component failure
   - Iatrogenic causes: component failure after defibrillation, electrocautery, or therapeutic radiation

Table 9. Absence of pacemaker stimuli.

1. Normal situation: total inhibition of pacemaker when the intrinsic rate is faster than the preset pacemaker rate
2. Hysteresis with normal pacemaker function: escape interval after ventricular sensing is longer than the automatic interval during pacing
3. Pseudomalfunction: overlooking tiny bipolar stimuli in the ECG
4. Normal pulse generator with poor anodal contact:
   - Subcutaneous emphysema with air preventing contact of the anode of a unipolar pacemaker with the tissues. This occurs soon after subclavian vein puncture
   - Air entrapment in the pacemaker pocket preventing contact of the anode (on the can) of a unipolar pacemaker with the tissues. This may occur after battery replacement when a new and smaller pacemaker is inserted in a large pacemaker pocket
5. Lead problem: fracture, loose connection, or set-screw problem on the pacemaker itself
6. Abnormal pulse generator:
   - Total battery depletion
   - Component failure
   - Sticky reed-switch (magnet application produces no effect)
7. Extreme electromagnetic interference.
8. Oversensing of signals originating from outside or inside the pulse generator
9. Filter settings of ECG recorder masking pacing stimuli
10. Saturation of ECG amplifier

Table 10. Causes of undersensing.

Normal situations	Ventricular premature complexes with a small electrogram different from those of sensed conducted beats Beats falling inside blanking or refractory periods Oversensing can cause undersensing because an oversensed signal generates a refractory period into which a succeeding physiologic signal cannot be sensed *Note:* Ventricular pseudofusion beats should not be mistaken for undersensing
Abnormal situations	Poor lead position with low-amplitude electrogram Lead dislodgment: low amplitude electrogram Lead malfunction: insulation defect or partial fracture Hyperkalemia, severe metabolic disturbance, and toxic effects of antiarrhythmic drugs Transient undersensing after cardioversion or defibrillation Chronic fibrosis and scarring around the electrode Signal attenuation with the passage of time Development of new bundle branch block Myocardial infarction near the electrode Electronic component failure (rare) Jammed magnetic reed-switch (rare) Interference with reversion to the noise-reversion asynchronous rate Attenuation of adequate cardiac signal upon entry in the pacing system Mismatch between input and source impedance (e.g., combination of large-surface-area electrode with low-input-impedance pulse generator (rare with contemporary pacemakers)

Table 11. Causes of oversensing intracorporeal voltages.

Ventricular oversensing	T wave Afterpotential P wave (rare) Crosstalk: sensing of atrial stimulus Myopotentials False signals Triboelectric signals (static) in unipolar devices
Atrial oversensing	Far-field R wave (VA crosstalk) Myopotentials False signals Ventricular T wave (rare) Triboelectric signals (static) in unipolar devices

value approximately equal to the sum of the lower rate interval and the pacemaker refractory period. This form of oversensing is now rare, and it is easily controlled by prolonging the refractory period or decreasing the output or sensitivity.

False signals (voltage transients)

Abrupt changes in the resistance within a pacing system can produce large voltage changes between the poles used for pacing. Such signals are called false signals. False signals are almost always invisible on the surface ECG, so their presence must be assumed until they are revealed by a telemetered ventricular electrogram. Such "make–break" signals may occur with intermittent derangement of a pacemaker circuit from loose connections, wire fracture with otherwise well-apposed ends, insulation defect, short circuits, poorly designed active fixation leads, or the interaction of two leads in the heart (one active, the other inactive) lying side by side touching each other intermittently. Oversensing of false signals from a defective lead can cause erratic pacemaker behavior with pauses of varying duration. False signals often occur at random and can be demonstrated in the telemetered ventricular electrogram, often as large and irregular voltage deflections.

Remember that oversensing can be associated with undersensing, because the ventricular refractory period generated by a sensed false signal may contain a spontaneous QRS complex. This mixture of disturbances and the constantly changing pauses often create a chaotic pattern of pacing which is characteristic of a lead problem and must not be misinterpreted as pacemaker component failure. The characteristic pattern of false signals usually permits the exclusion of P-wave oversensing (rare), T-wave oversensing, and/or afterpotential oversensing, which can be identified by more regular manifestations. The telemetered ventricular electrogram can be diagnostic when oversensing of false signals (potentially serious) mimics T-wave sensing (less serious, as it causes only bradycardia).

Reminder: If false signals causing oversensing are suspected, move the pacemaker around in its pocket and evaluate the effect of deep respiration, arm movement, and changes in position to unmask an extravascular lead problem such an intermittent fracture. The lead impedance can be normal if the fracture is intermittent.

Myopotentials

Myopotentials represent electrical activity originating from skeletal muscles. A unipolar ventricular pacemaker may sense such myopotentials and cause ventricular inhibition. In a DDD pacemaker myopotentials sensed only by the atrial channel can be tracked, and they cause an increase in the ventricular pacing rate. Various maneuvers can bring out this interference during follow-up evaluation. This disturbance can often be controlled by a reduction in sensitivity, or programming to the bipolar mode if feasible.

Caveat: Lack of ventricular pacing during provocative maneuvers for myopotential oversensing may be due to myopotential inhibition (oversensing), but may sometimes be caused by an intermittent lead fracture which has become manifest during the testing procedure

Pacemaker response to oversensing interference

Pacemakers can be inhibited by low-frequency interference, which is uncommon. Pacemakers are designed to respond to rapidly occurring (high-frequency) extraneous signals by reverting temporarily to the protective asynchronous mode (interference mode), functioning usually at the programmed lower rate. A signal sensed in the unblanked portion of the ventricular refractory period (VRP) or in a part thereof (specifically called the noise sampling period) reinitiates a new VRP or noise sampling period respectively. This process repeats itself with each detected signal so that the "overlapping" effect of these special timing cycles

Table 12. Causes of changes in pacing rate.

Normal function	Application of the magnet Inaccurate speed of ECG machine Apparent malfunction in special situations such as hysteresis, sleep rate Reversion to interference rate in response to electromagnetic interference if the noise-reversion rate differs from the programmed lower rate
Abnormal function	Battery depletion with slowing of the rate Runaway pacemaker Component failure Permanent or temporary change in mode after electrocautery, therapeutic radiation, or defibrillation Phantom reprogramming (done without documentation) or misprogramming Oversensing (e.g., T-wave sensing) Crosstalk resulting in ventricular safety pacing causing an increase in the pacing rate

prevents the initiation of a lower rate interval because the entire pacemaker cycle consists of VRP or noise sampling periods. This repeated reinitiation or overlapping effect assures the delivery of a pacemaker stimulus at the interference rate. The pacemaker returns to its normal operating mode when noise is no longer detected.

Changes in pacemaker rate

Changes in pacemaker rate (Table 12) can be puzzling. The diagnosis should be relatively simple knowing the programmed parameters.

Lead malfunction

The lead is the weakest link in the pacing system. The manifestations of lead malfunction can be varied, and may be obvious or so subtle as to defy detection. Tables 13 and 14 list the manifestations of lead fracture and insulation defect.

Difficulties with atrial pacing and sensing

The diagnosis of atrial problems requires a thorough knowledge of pacemaker timing intervals,

Table 13. Manifestations of lead fracture.

- No stimuli because of an open circuit (markers may show normal emission of stimulus)
- Stimuli without capture
- Oversensing of false signals: the false signals are invisible on the ECG but can be demonstrated by telemetry of event markers and electrograms. Some devices record and count non-physiologic V–V intervals (< 140 ms) for storage in the pacemaker memory: a large number of abnormally short V–V intervals (reflecting false signals) is highly suggestive of lead dysfunction
- Oversensing can cause undersensing; occasionally the sensed signal itself can be attenuated
- Telemetry showing an abnormally high lead impedance, but the value can be normal if the fracture is intermittent or there is a concomitant insulation break; failure to secure the set screw can also cause a high impedance
- Maneuvers: if suspected, one should apply pressure along the course of the subcutaneous portion of the lead, extend the arm on the side of the pacemaker, place the arm behind the back, and rotate the shoulder backward to unmask a crush injury due to clavicle–first rib compression
- A fracture may or may not be detectable on an x-ray

Table 14. Manifestations of insulation defect.

- Extracardiac muscle stimulation if the defect is extravascular (twitching)
- Pacing may be preserved but loss of capture can occur when a large current is shunted from the electrodes; an insulation defect accelerates battery depletion
- Undersensing from signal attenuation
- Oversensing of false signals; oversensing can cause undersensing
- False signals are invisible on the ECG but telemetry with annotated markers can demonstrate false signals on the electrogram (also programming in the AAT or VVT mode may be of help). A large number of abnormally short V–V intervals (reflecting false signals) is highly suggestive of an insulation defect or lead fracture.
- Unipolarization of a bipolar lead
- Telemetry shows an abnormally low lead impedance, but the value can be normal if the insulation defect is intermittent
- The insulation is radiolucent, and abnormalities cannot be detected on an x-ray

especially when the ECG reveals only one stimulus, atrial or ventricular. In this respect Table 15 outlines the differential diagnosis of the presence of an atrial stimulus but no ventricular stimulus during DDD or DDDR pacing, and Table 16 deals with the presence of a ventricular stimulus but no atrial stimulus during DDD or DDDR pacing.

Never neglect determination of atrial capture in dual chamber pacemakers

The presence of atrial stimuli does not mean atrial capture. Unsuspected atrial fibrillation is a common cause of lack of atrial capture. Telemetered AP markers simply reflect release of AP, and cannot indicate successful atrial capture (Table 17).

Apparent atrial undersensing in dual chamber pacing (functional atrial undersensing)

True atrial undersensing is an important cause of prolongation of the interval from AS to VS beyond the programmed AV interval. Barring true atrial undersensing from a low-voltage atrial electrogram, other causes include the following:

1. Ventricular oversensing during the AV interval.
2. Long or extended PVARP. An atrial electrogram or P wave (with an adequate signal for sensing) may be forced into an excessively long PVARP sometimes due to automatic extension initiated by a pacemaker-defined VPC. If the patient's PR interval is quite long and the spontaneous rate is relatively fast, there is a greater likelihood that

Table 15. Presence of an atrial stimulus but no ventricular stimulus during DDD or DDDR pacing.

1. Atrial pacing followed by a conducted QRS complex before completion of the AV delay: apply the magnet for diagnosis
2. Isoelectric or tiny ventricular stimuli: use double standardization of the ECG machine
3. Concealed ventricular stimuli within the QRS complex (pseudofusion): marker channel confirms diagnosis
4. Disconnection of the ventricular circuit as in a lead fracture; this causes apparent AAI pacing: reprogram to the VVI mode, whereupon no stimuli will be seen in the VVI and VOO (magnet) modes
5. Crosstalk in devices without ventricular safety pacing: application of the magnet confirms diagnosis
6. Oversensing during the AV delay: apply magnet; use telemetry to demonstrate the electrogram and annotated markers

Table 16. Presence of a ventricular stimulus but no atrial stimulus during DDD or DDDR pacing.

1. In some devices, magnet application causes VOO pacing
2. Disconnection of the atrial circuit: VVI pacing in the DDD mode and no stimulation the AAI and AOO modes
3. Isoelectric or tiny atrial stimuli: use double standardization of the ECG machine
4. Concealed atrial stimuli within the QRS complex (pseudopseudofusion): use marker channel for diagnosis
5. DDI mode when the atrial channel is continually inhibited: apply magnet for diagnosis
6. Apparent VVI pacing: the atrial stimulus (occasionally because of atrial undersensing) is coincident with the onset of the spontaneous QRS complex with a left bundle branch block configuration

a P wave will fall closer to the preceding QRS complex and therefore in the PVARP, which need not be unduly long to cause "functional" atrial undersensing.

3. Upper rate response (pre-empted Wenckebach upper rate response). Prolongation of the AS–VS interval may result from failure of delivery of the ventricular stimulus if the URI has not timed out by the time the AVI has terminated. In this situation the interval between two consecutive QRS complexes must exceed the URI of the pulse generator.
4. Short but reinitiated PVARP. If the ventricular channel senses a signal other than the QRS (e.g., T wave), the PVARP is reinitiated by the oversensed signal and the P wave may fall in this new PVARP. In this situation, P-wave sensing may be restored by decreasing the sensitivity of the ventricular channel.

Table 17. How to test for atrial capture.

1. If the paced P wave is not discernible in the 12-lead ECG, record the ECG at double standardization to bring out P waves and tiny bipolar stimuli. Faster paper speed may help
2. In the presence of relatively normal AV conduction, program the AAI or AOO mode. Use several pacing rates to demonstrate the consistent relationship of the atrial stimulus to the succeeding spontaneous conducted QRS complex
3. In patients with AV block, reduce the pacing gradually to 30 ppm. This is often well tolerated. Then use the AAI or AOO at various fast rates to determine atrial capture by looking at the P-wave configuration and rate which must correspond to the pacing rate
4. A paced P wave may be difficult to see if the AV delay is too short. A relatively late P wave can be unmasked by prolonging the AV delay. A "late" P wave from the atrial stimulus usually indicates interatrial conduction delay and the risk of delivering the P wave too late to provide appropriate AV synchrony. In other words the atrial transport function provided by atrial pacing may be largely wasted if the P wave is too close to the paced QRS complex. In severe cases the paced P wave occurs inside the paced QRS complex. Such a patient requires careful programming of the AV delay under echocardiographic control and evaluation for pacemaker syndrome
5. Shorten the AV delay. If the paced QRS morphology changes, it means that there was ventricular fusion with the spontaneous QRS complex at the longer AV delay and therefore atrial capture giving rise to AV conduction
6. In patients with relatively fast sinus rhythm, program the DVI mode, which provides competitive atrial pacing beyond the atrial myocardial refractory period

Reminder: What looks like atrial undersensing may be functional in association with a atrial signal of sufficient size to be sensed.

Automatic mode switching

In the past, paroxysmal atrial arrhythmias constituted a contraindication to dual chamber pacing. Advances in pacemaker technology have now made it possible to use dual chamber pacemakers safely in this patient population. Dual chamber pacemakers equipped with automatic mode switching (AMS) can now protect the patient from rapid ventricular pacing by automatically functioning in a non-atrial tracking mode (VVI, VVIR, DDI, DDIR) during supraventricular tachycardia (SVT). AMS requires fundamental changes in the operation of pacemaker timing cycles to maximize SVT detection above the programmed upper rate. Although many of the AMS algorithms from a variety of manufacturers are device-specific, the actual timing cycles required for SVT detection are basically independent of AMS algorithm design. For appropriate SVT detection, the atrial signal should be of sufficient amplitude and the obligatory blanking periods (when the sensing amplifier is temporarily disabled), should be restricted to a small fraction of the pacing cycle. Blanking periods cannot be eliminated, because they prevent the oversensing of undesirable signals that are inherent to all pacing systems.

Appropriate AMS depends on several parameters:

(a) the programmed detection rate
(b) atrial sensing and the characteristics of the arrhythmia
(c) the characteristics of the AMS algorithm

AMS failure may occur if the amplitude of the atrial electrogram is intermittently or consistently too small to be sensed, or if an atrial signal occurs systematically during the atrial blanking period.

An AMS algorithm also provides important data about SVT: onset, AMS response, and resynchronization. Since AMS programs also provide data on the time of onset and duration of AMS episodes, AMS data may be considered a surrogate marker of SVT recurrence. Stored electrograms have enhanced the accuracy of AMS in detecting SVT. The total duration of atrial fibrillation (AF) is correctly represented by the total duration of AMS, which can be considered a reliable measure of total AF duration. Automatic mode switching algorithms, which provide data on the time of onset and duration of AMS episodes, allow a more accurate determination of the proportion of time a patient with AF is in AF, and have led to the concept of "AF burden." The extremely high sensitivity and specificity of AMS for AF is clinically useful for assessing the need for anticoagulation and/or the necessity or efficacy of antiarrhythmic therapy.

The prevalence of recurrent AF, particularly asymptomatic episodes, is easily underestimated. Asymptomatic AF is far more common than symptomatic AF. This has important implications for anticoagulation therapy. Furthermore, AMS events may serve as a valuable tool for studying the natural history and burden of SVT even in asymptomatic patients.

Timing cycles related to automatic mode switching

The unblanked portion of the AV interval (initiated by a paced or sensed atrial event) was designed to enhance sensing of AF during the AV interval to facilitate AMS. A ventricular paced or sensed event initiates the postventricular atrial refractory period (PVARP), the first portion of which is the postventricular atrial blanking period (PVAB). The second part of the PVARP is unblanked (PVARP-U), but sensing within it cannot initiate an AV delay. The PVARP initiated by ventricular pacing is almost always equal to the PVARP initiated by ventricular sensing. Far-field sensing of the R wave within the PVARP can be corrected by programming lower atrial sensitivity or the PVAB to a longer value. Programmability of the PVAB is a relatively new feature of pacemakers. A long PVAB predisposes to atrial undersensing of SVT, which is crucial for AMS activation. Sensing of SVT for AMS function is therefore possible during the unblanked refractory periods (AVI-U and PVARP-U) as well as during the cycle without atrial refractory periods, where atrial sensing initiates an AV delay.

VA crosstalk

The atrial channel cannot sense a signal associated with the ventricular stimulus because the atrial channel of all pacemakers is blinded or blanked by the relatively long PVAB that starts coincidentally with emission of the ventricular stimulus. Ventriculoatrial (VA) or reverse crosstalk refers to far-field sensing that occurs when ventricular signals in the atrial electrogram are sensed by the atrial channel in the PVARP beyond the PVAB (sensing the paced QRS complex) or in the unblanked terminal portion of the AV delay (sensing the spontaneous QRS complex). VA crosstalk occurs because the smaller atrial electrograms during SVT require higher atrial sensitivity for sensing than the normal rhythm. VA crosstalk can often be eliminated by reducing atrial sensitivity, but this carries the risk of atrial undersensing during SVT, when atrial signals become smaller. Far-field atrial sensing may be reduced by the use of bipolar sensing and improved pulse generator and lead technology.

Caveat: Detection of smaller signals during atrial tachyarrhythmias requires a high atrial sensitivity, which predisposes to VA crosstalk.

Testing for VA crosstalk

The propensity for VA crosstalk during the PVARP should be tested during ventricular pacing. The AS–VP interval is shortened to permit continual ventricular capture. The pacemaker is then programmed to the highest atrial sensitivity and the largest ventricular output (voltage and pulse duration). These settings should be evaluated at several pacing rates to at least 110–120 ppm, because faster ventricular pacing rates impair dissipation of the afterpotential or polarization voltage at the electrode–myocardial interface. Such parameters enhance the afterpotential and therefore generate a voltage superimposed on the tail end of the paced QRS complex. The combined voltage from these two sources may be sensed as a far-field signal by the atrial channel. VA crosstalk can be eliminated by decreasing atrial sensitivity provided one knows that the atrial signals during SVT can be sensed at the lower sensitivity. In devices with a programmable PVAB, the testing procedure if positive for VA crosstalk can be performed at various durations of the PVAB until VA crosstalk is eliminated. VA crosstalk within the AV interval is evaluated by programming a low lower rate and long AVI, to promote spontaneous sinus rhythm and AV conduction.

Mode switching algorithms

A "rate cut-off" criterion is commonly used to activate AMS, in the form of a sensed atrial rate exceeding a programmable value (for a defined period of time or number of cycles). The atrial rate is continuously monitored by increasing/decreasing counters or by consecutive rapid atrial event counters. AMS is activated when the count of the short atrial cycles exceeds the programmed cut-off criterion. Many Medtronic pacemakers activate AMS after detecting 4/7 atrial intervals shorter than the tachycardia detection interval. In one system (Boston Scientific), atrial events above the tachycardia detection rate increment the detection counter, whereas events below the tachycardia detection rate decrement the counter. Atrial tachyarrhythmia is detected when the counter reaches a fixed value. AMS then occurs over a programmable time between 1 and 5 minutes. Another algorithm uses a "running average" rate as a criterion to move towards AMS (Early Medtronic and current St. Jude devices). This mechanism ("mean, filtered, or matched atrial rate") is based on a moving value related to the duration of the prevailing sensed atrial cycle. AMS will occur when the "filtered" interval shortens to the tachycardia detection interval. It is faster for the filtered atrial interval to reach the tachycardia detection interval when atrial tachycardia starts in the setting of a higher resting sinus rate (shorter filtered atrial rate interval) than from a sinus bradycardia.

Detection of atrial flutter by dual chamber pacemakers

Patients with paroxysmal atrial flutter represent a challenge for AMS algorithms. AMS failure may occur during atrial flutter when alternate flutter waves coincide with the PVAB (lock-in phenomenon). Some devices provide additional algorithms to unmask the presence of "blanked" atrial flutter so as to activate AMS. In some designs, the duration of the blanking periods prevents the pacemaker from detecting atrial flutter, if the atrial cycle does not match the sensing window of the atrial channel. In other words, the duration of the PVAB imposes mathematical limits on the detection of atrial flutter. If AV interval + PVAB > atrial cycle length (P–P or f–f interval), the pacemaker will exhibit 2:1 atrial sensing of atrial flutter (2:1 lock-in). Sensing of alternate atrial signals will occur if AVI + PVARP < 2 atrial cycles. Abbreviation of the PVAB may solve the problem if far-field R-wave sensing does not occur. If PVAB is non-programmable, restoration of 1:1 atrial sensing would require programming of the AV interval to very short durations such as 50 ms. Restoration of AMS function by shortening of the AVI to circumvent a fixed PVAB produces unfavorable hemodynamics for long-term pacing if the AVI remains permanently short in the absence of SVT.

The detection of atrial signals can be ameliorated by reducing the blanked AV interval. Thus, a design that allows substantial shortening of the AS–VP interval only with increasing sensed atrial rates optimizes sensing of atrial flutter, and yet preserves a physiologic AV interval at rest and low levels of exercise. During SVT when (AS–VP interval) + PVAB = 30 + 150 = 180 ms, this combination allows sensing of atrial flutter with a cycle length up to 180 ms (333 bpm). Another algorithm, specifically designed for atrial flutter, automatically extends the PVARP for one cycle whenever the pacemaker detects an atrial cycle length less than twice (AV interval + PVAB) and the atrial rate is greater than half the tachycardia detection rate (or the atrial interval is less than twice the tachycardia detection interval). AMS occurs if an atrial event is sensed within the extended PVARP, thereby revealing the true atrial cycle.

Caveat: Troubleshooting automatic mode switching requires knowledge of the algorithm, blanking periods, atrial signal in sinus rhythm, and atrial sensitivity.

Retriggerable atrial refractory period

Some pacemakers with a retriggerable or resettable atrial refractory period revert to the DVI or DVIR mode upon sensing a fast atrial rate. In such a system, an atrial signal detected in the PVARP beyond the initial PVAB does not start an AV interval but reinitiates a new total atrial refractory period (TARP) or the sum of AVI + PVARP. This process repeats itself, so that SVT faster than the programmed upper rate (i.e., P–P interval < TARP) automatically converts the atrial channel to the asynchronous mode and the pacemaker to the DVI mode at the lower rate, or the DVIR mode, according to design and programmability.

Reminder: The concept of overlapping refractory periods is important in the ventricular channel of pacemakers, to prevent continuous inhibition due to rapidly recurring extraneous signals from interference.

Minimizing right ventricular pacing

Many studies in the last decade have shown that long-term RV apical pacing may produce substantial LV dysfunction and heart failure. At this juncture one cannot predict this risk in individual patients, though certain factors such as LV dysfunction at the time of implantation predispose to this complication (Table 18).

1. Do not pace if it is not necessary

The majority of patients treated with pacemakers for sick sinus syndrome, including those with dilated cardiomyopathy, reduced LV ejection fraction (LVEF), and congestive heart failure, have a normal ventricular activation sequence manifested as a QRS duration < 120 ms on the baseline electrocardiogram and therefore do not require continual ventricular pacing. Furthermore, most have reliable AV conduction that remains stable over time.

Avoidance of RV pacing is especially important in ICD patients without sinus or AV nodal dysfunction, where the VVI or DDI pacing mode (with a long AV delay) at a rate of 40 ppm may be appropriate for many patients equipped with ICDs incapable of providing automatic minimal ventricular pacing.

2. Alternative-site ventricular pacing

This includes the RV septum and RV outflow tract. Direct His bundle pacing may prevent the negative effects of RV apical pacing. However, it is a complex technique that cannot be achieved in all patients, and it is associated with high pacing thresholds and long implantation times. In contrast, paraHisian pacing, which produces physiologic ventricular activation similar to direct His bundle pacing, is easier to perform and more reliable than direct His bundle pacing. Preliminary data suggest that paraHisian pacing is superior to RV apical pacing in preserving LV function.

3. AAI and AAIR pacing

These pacing modes carry a small risk of AV block in a few patients (1–2% per year). These pacing modes are rarely used in the USA for fear of litigation. In Europe, AAI and AAIR modes are considered viable and acceptable in carefully screened patients with sick sinus syndrome without bundle branch block and delayed AV conduction.

4. Algorithms to minimize RV pacing

Much evidence has emerged recently about the harmful effects of chronic RV pacing (mostly apical) on LV function. Minimizing RV pacing may reduce chronic changes in cellular structure, changes in LV geometry that contribute to impaired hemodynamic performance, mitral regurgitation, and increased left atrial diameters, with the aim of reducing the risk of atrial fibrillation, congestive heart failure, and death. On this basis, strategies to minimize RV pacing have become important, especially in patients with sick sinus syndrome, where continual RV pacing may not be necessary.

(a) Long fixed AV delay

Using the DDDR (or DDIR) mode with a fixed long AV delay (250–300 ms) in patients with normal AV

Table 18. Methodology of pacing to minimize RV (apical) pacing.

Method	Comments
Do not pace if it is not necessary	Use the DDD(R) or DDI(R) mode with a long AV delay and slow lower rate according to behavior of the spontaneous rhythm
Alternative-site pacing away from the RV apex	**1.** RV septal and RVOT pacing **2.** Direct His bundle and paraHisian pacing **3.** Biventricular or monochamber ventricular pacing with LV lead: consider this approach in selected patients with LVEF ≤ 35% (even in the absence of HF) especially with mitral regurgitation and Cum%VP expected to be high (e.g., complete AV block) **4.** Bifocal RV pacing (2 RV sites): produces CRT of lesser magnitude than biventricular pacing in CRT candidates but may be useful in selected patients with poor LV function and narrow QRS complex. One of the sites may be paraHisian
Programming maneuvers (functional AAIR pacing)	**1.** Using the DDDR (or DDIR) mode with a fixed long AV delay (250–300 ms) in patients with normal AV conduction is of limited value **2.** AV search hysteresis (autointrinsic conduction search, Search AV+) in the DDDR mode
AAI and AAIR modes	By definition, AAI(R) pacing eliminates the possibility of RV pacing but carries a small risk of AV block
New pacing modes	A special algorithm maintains AAI or AAIR pacing. Return to AAIR from DDDR is achieved by periodic AV conduction checks. Occasional second-degree AV block is often well tolerated in the AAIR mode. Marked first-degree AV block may cause pacemaker syndrome. These new pacing modes are effective in minimizing RV pacing but long-term results on LV function are unknown. This pacing mode can reduce AF

conduction is of limited value in preventing RV pacing. During AV block, pacing must occur with the programmed long AV delay. A long atrial refractory period may cause atrial undersensing and limits the programmable upper rate. A long AV delay favors endless loop tachycardia or repetitive non-reentrant VA synchrony with functional loss of atrial capture and pacemaker syndrome.

(b) Dynamic AV delay (AV search hysteresis, autointrinsic conduction search, search AV+)

These algorithms in the DDDR mode promote spontaneous AV conduction by allowing the functional AV delay to be longer than the programmed AV delay as long as AV conduction remains intact. During AV block, the AV delay is physiologically shorter and more appropriate than with devices working with a fixed long AV delay (e.g., 200 vs. 300 ms). In this algorithm the device periodically extends the AV (AP-V and AS-V) delay (gradually or suddenly) to a programmable value to search for AV conduction. If a conducted ventricular event is sensed during this extended AV delay, the pacemaker inhibits the ventricular output and continues to function (in the functional AAI or AAIR mode) with such an extended AV delay until no ventricular event is sensed. If there is a single cycle with no intrinsic ventricular event within the extended AV delay, the AV extension is cancelled and the pacemaker reverts to the programmed (unextended) AV delay on the next cycle. The pacemaker then waits until the next search function (after a programmable time) is activated to look for the return of spontaneous AV conduction. This feature is particularly valuable in patients who would otherwise be suitable for permanent AAI or AAIR pacing.

(c) New pacing modes in which the algorithm maintains AAI or AAIR pacing (automatic mode switching DDDR → AAIR → DDDR)

The switch to AAIR from DDDR is achieved by periodic AV conduction checks by the device monitoring for a conducted ventricular sensed event. First- and second-degree AV block are tolerated in the AAIR mode up to a predetermined programmable limit. The permitted cycles of second-degree AV block are short, but an occasional patient may become symptomatic. Supraventricular tachyarrhythmias activate automatic mode switching to the DDIR mode (AAIR → DDIR or DDDR → DDIR).

Pacemakers with automatic mode switching DDDR → AAIR→ DDDR according to AV conduction are effective in minimizing RV pacing, especially in patients with ICDs, who often do not require rate support, but clinical benefit and long-term results (including impact on atrial fibrillation) are unknown at this time.

In this respect, Medtronic's Managed Ventricular Pacing™ (MVP) has no AV interval (ending in VS), so that no ventricular pacing will occur after a long PR (AS–VS or AP–VS) interval. Sustained marked first-degree AV block may be hemodynamically important and symptomatic, like retrograde VA conduction.

Effect of drugs and electrolyte imbalance

The class IA agents procainamide and disopyramide increase the pacing threshold only in toxic or supratherapeutic doses. Class IB drugs are safe. Class IC agents (flecainide and propafenone) can cause a marked increase in the pacing threshold in therapeutic doses. Beta-blockers generally do not increase the threshold. Despite the claim that sotalol can increase the threshold, the drug appears safe clinically. There is no convincing evidence that amiodarone increases the pacing threshold. Corticosteroids, epinephrine, and isoproterenol decrease the pacing threshold.

Hyperkalemia

In patients with pacemakers, hyperkalemia causes two important clinical abnormalities:

1. Widening of the paced QRS complex (and paced P wave) on the basis of delayed myocardial conduction. Other common causes of a wide paced QRS complex include amiodarone therapy and severe myocardial disease.
2. Increased atrial and ventricular pacing thresholds.

Pacing threshold

The level of hyperkalemia causing changes in the pacing threshold varies from patient to patient. When serum K > 7.0 mEq/L, there will almost always be an increase in the pacing threshold. A modest elevation of the K level (e.g., 6.5 mEq/L) may cause failure of atrial and/or ventricular capture, suggesting that other metabolic variables may influence the sensitivity of cardiac tissue to hyperkalemia. These include other types of electrolyte imbalance, acid–base abnormalities, oxygen saturation, the rate of change of plasma K level, the intracellular–extracellular gradient, and the etiology and severity of heart disease. For this reason, the cardiac manifestations of hyperkalemia in the clinical setting tend to occur at much lower K levels than those measured during an experimental infusion of potassium.

Latency

Hyperkalemia can cause prolonged latency, a condition also known as first-degree pacemaker exit block. Latency describes the delay from the pacing stimulus to the electrocardiographic onset of atrial or ventricular depolarization. The normal value for the RV is < 40 ms. First-degree ventricular pacemaker exit block can progress to second-degree Wenckebach (type I) exit block, characterized by gradual prolongation of the pacemaker stimulus to the onset of the paced QRS complex, ultimately resulting in an ineffectual stimulus. The pacing disturbance may then progress to 2 : 1, 3 : 1 exit block, etc., and eventually to complete exit block with total lack of capture. Total unresponsiveness to ventricular stimulation has been reported with a K level of only 6.6 mEq/L.

Hyperkalemia-induced ventricular pacemaker exit block (not uncommonly associated with drug toxicity, especially type 1A antiarrhythmic agents) is potentially reversible, unlike other causes of increased RV latency, which occur predominantly in severe or terminal myocardial disease. Wenckebach exit block can be produced experimentally in the laboratory by perfusion of cardiac tissue with a large concentration of antiarrhythmic agents and potassium, an effect that is often reversible. This phenomenon is rate- and output-dependent. Consequently, with first-degree exit block or prolonged latency, an increase in the pacing rate leads to prolongation of the latency interval. An increase in the amplitude of the stimulus may shorten the latency interval and convert type I second-degree to first-degree exit block.

Differential effect on atrial versus ventricular myocardium

In a dual chamber device, hyperkalemia may cause failure of atrial capture associated with preservation of ventricular pacing. This differential effect on atrial and ventricular excitability (pacing) correlates with the well-known clinical and experimental observations that the atrial myocardium is more sensitive to hyperkalemia than the ventricular myocardium. This situation should always be suspected in hospitalized patients who have severe heart failure with relatively sudden decompensation with hypotension and a wider paced QRS complex compared to previous recordings. In this situation, loss of atrial capture causing decompensation should be demonstrated at the maximum programmable AV delay to rule out increased latency, and at double ECG standardization to confirm the loss of atrial activity.

Magnet application

Magnet application is being used less and less nowadays, because telemetry offers more sensitive parameters of battery status. Magnet application is important in the evaluation of oversensing by eliminating the sensing function of pacemakers, and for assessing the presence of capture in the presence of a spontaneous rhythm faster than the lower rate of the pacemaker (Table 19).

Reminder: A magnet over an ICD eliminates its antitachycardia function but does not convert it to asynchronous pacing.

Table 19. Pacemaker magnet application.

1. Conversion to the asynchronous mode: VOO or DOO modes assess capture when the spontaneous rhythm is faster than the lower rate of the pacemaker
2. Assess capture during asynchronous pacing
3. Elective replacement indicator
4. Provides reed-switch activation as required for some programmers to function
5. Eliminates sensing: useful during electrocautery; provides diagnosis of oversensing
6. Patient can trigger electrogram storage during symptomatic episode
7. Termination of endless loop tachycardia
8. Competitive underdrive pacing for the termination of some reentrant tachycardias
9. May help identification of device, as some have typical magnet response

Capture verification algorithms

The longevity of an implantable pacemaker is determined by the capacity of the battery, its chemistry, and the current drain. Automatic capture verification aims at reducing the latter while maintaining safety. The pacing threshold may change according to physiologic conditions, disease conditions, and maturation of the lead–tissue interface. This has resulted in the traditional practice of programming pacing output voltages to at least twice as great as the measured pacing threshold (the so-called safety margin) to ensure consistent capture. This relatively high output voltage represents potential wastage of battery capacity.

The detection and evaluation of the cardiac depolarization (or evoked response, ER) of the pacing pulse is a reliable surrogate for myocardial systole. ER must be differentiated from polarization, which is the residual charge at the electrode–tissue interface that follows the output pulse. This voltage is normally blinded by the standard blanking period initiated upon delivery of the output pulse. The presence of a blanking period after the ventricular output therefore requires a special detection circuit for ER detection. As a rule, a large variety of capture verification systems work in > 90% of patients (Table 20).

St. Jude systems

The "traditional" St. Jude Ventricular AutoCapture™ feature or DMax is strictly dependent on lead type (low polarization) and configuration. It is mandatory to elicit ventricular stimulation tip to can, and to achieve ER detection tip to ring (bipolar leads are needed). Consequently, the pacing configuration has to be programmed to unipolar to use the original method.

The new Enhanced Ventricular AutoCapture™ system (PDI) from St. Jude can be used with either a unipolar or a bipolar lead, and, when a bipolar lead is implanted, the device can be programmed to either unipolar or bipolar ventricular pacing configuration. The original AutoCapture and the new enhanced AutoCapture feature are both predicated on analysis of the ER, but the methods of evaluating the ER are somewhat different. The availability of the two different analysis methods explains why the ventricular Enhanced AutoCapture feature can be used with leads and programmed configurations that the original method could not use. Although PDI should replace DMax, and this will probably happen in the future, it would be wise to keep DMax available until there is extensive experience

Table 20. Comparison of various capture verification systems.

Manufacturer	Beat-to-beat ER detection	Dedicated lead for ER detection	Configuration for ER detection	Fusion management
Right ventricle				
St. Jude DMax[a]	Yes	Low polarization	Bipolar	Yes
St. Jude PDI (Zephyr)[b]	Yes	No	Any	Yes
Boston Scientific	Yes	No	Any	Yes
Medtronic	No	No	Any	No
Atrium				
Medtronic[c]	No	No	N/A	No
St. Jude	No	Low polarization	Bipolar	No

[a] Traditional Autocapture system designated DMax.
[b] The Zephyr pacemaker permits the selection of either DMax or the new system (designated PDI) for Autocapture.
[c] The only system where ER detection is not involved. All the other listed systems use ER detection either on a beat-to-beat basis or strictly only at the time of periodic threshold determination.

with PDI. Both systems perform periodic threshold searches. Both versions of ventricular AutoCapture maintain a pacing output voltage of 0.25 V above the threshold determined by the system. In addition, a threshold search is triggered whenever the system detects a loss of capture as determined by the beat-to-beat capture verification analysis. Backup pacing pulses are delivered whenever the device detects a loss of capture with the primary ventricular pacing pulse.

Medtronic's Capture Management and Boston Scientific's Automatic Capture algorithms are the default algorithms in their respective devices: no special set-up is required, and they are on immediately upon implantation of the pulse generator. In contrast, St. Jude does not allow the autocapture algorithm to be the default setting in the pacemaker. The St. Jude system must be intentionally evaluated and then enabled. It is only in the post-implant phase that the patient can be evaluated to determine whether AutoCapture using either DMax or PDI can be utilized. For the ventricular Enhanced AutoCapture feature, the system automatically chooses between two evaluation methods based on the type of lead and programmed pacing configuration. With either the original or the new AutoCapture system, the AutoCapture Setup Test must be run, which automatically determines whether the ratio of evoked response to polarization is adequate to recommend activation of the AutoCapture feature. Consequently, the ability to use AutoCapture is assessed on a patient-by-patient basis, not on the type of lead per se. While setting up AutoCapture requires a few more steps, called the AutoCapture Setup Test, these initial steps will tell if the ER signal amplitude and polarization signal amplitudes are appropriate to allow AutoCapture to be enabled.

St. Jude automatic atrial capture verification

An atrial capture verification algorithm (Atrial Autocap) was recently introduced in the St. Jude Zephyr series of pacemakers. It requires a low polarization bipolar lead. The system works by detecting the atrial evoked response but does not function on a beat-to-beat basis like its ventricular counterpart. The atrial threshold is measured every 8–24 hours. The system can adjust the output, but with a larger margin than the 0.25 V working margin that is associated with the true AutoCapture algorithm, because between evaluations it does not monitor capture and cannot provide a higher-output backup pulse, which is only possible during the periodic evaluations. During threshold testing, the device emits a backup pulse only when there is loss of atrial capture. The safety margin cannot be programmed. After threshold determination the device increments the output voltage by a value according to a published table. The final atrial output voltage corresponds to a safety margin of approximately 1.7 : 1.

Keeping good records

Good records are essential, and they should include representative printouts of data and rhythm strips and stored electrograms. They should include a 12-lead ECG (Table 21).

Factors influencing pacemaker longevity

Battery current drain (expressed in μA) is the most important determinant of battery longevity. Pacing requires more current than sensing (Table 22).

Pacemaker longevity can be enhanced by careful programming, and by selecting steroid-eluting leads with a small-radius tip electrode (small surface area for stimulation), which provide low thresholds and

Table 21. Data required in pacemaker chart or computerized file.

Patient data	Name, age, address, phone number, etc.
Pacemaker data	Date of implantation Model and serial number of leads Model and serial number of pulse generator
Data from implantation	Pacing threshold(s) Sensing threshold(s) Intracardiac electrograms Lead impedance(s) Status of retrograde VA conduction Presence of diaphragmatic or accessory muscle stimulation with 5 and 10 V output
Technical specifications	Pacemaker behavior in the magnet mode Record of elective replacement indicator: magnet and/or free-running rate, mode change, telemetered battery data (impedance and voltage)
Data from pacemaker clinic	Programmed parameters from time of implantation and most recent changes 12-lead ECG and long rhythm strips showing pacing and inhibition of pacing to evaluate underlying rhythm 12-lead ECG upon application of the magnet Electronic rate intervals and pulse duration measured with a special monitor Interrogation and printout of telemetric data (always print a copy of the initial interrogation and measured data)
Systematic evaluation of pacing system	Atrial and ventricular pacing and sensing thresholds Retrograde VA conduction and propensity to endless loop tachycardia Evaluation of crosstalk Myopotential interference (record best way of reproducing abnormality) Special features: automatic mode switching parameters, ventricular safety pacing, non-competitive atrial pacing, etc. Evaluation of sensor function with exercise protocols, histograms, and other data to demonstrate heart rate response in the rate-adaptive mode Final telemetry printout at end of evaluation and date: check that any changes in parameters are intentional by comparing the final parameters with those obtained at the time of initial pacemaker interrogation; any discrepancy must be justified in the record
Ancillary data	Symptoms and potential pacemaker problems ECGs with event markers and electrograms mounted in the chart Intolerance of VOO pacing upon application of the magnet

Table 22. Causes of increased battery current drain.

1. The greater the percent pacing, the shorter the longevity
2. Increase in the pacing rate (cycle length)
3. Increase in output voltage
4. Increase in pulse duration
5. Change from single chamber to dual chamber mode
6. Use of rate-adaptive function with non-atrial sensor
7. Decrease in lead impedance (impedance, while not programmable, can be controlled by selecting a high-impedance lead at the time of implantation)
8. Programming, telemetering, storage of diagnostics

efficient high impedance (over 1000 Ω). The high impedance is at the electrode–tissue level, where the maximum voltage is available at the electrode tip for stimulation. The high impedance reduces current drain from the battery by Ohm's law. Thus, ideally one should implant small-surface-area, steroid-eluting, and porous electrodes. The porosity creates a complex surface structure which increases the effective surface area for sensing and improves the efficiency of sensing.

Caveat: Do not confuse battery current drain with current output (mA) at the electrode–myocardial interface with delivery of the pacemaker pulse. When trying to conserve battery life, monitor the battery current drain as you program various parameters.

Elective replacement indicator (ERI) versus reset situation: differential diagnosis when the mode of operation is identical

The reset mode, usually VVI or VOO, represents a normal protective response to high-intensity electromagnetic interference. A reset pacemaker does not represent malfunction, and it can easily be reprogrammed to its previous mode. The backup pacing circuit of certain DDD pacemakers can produce a similar situation when activated by low battery voltage as a mechanism to reduce the current requirement from the battery.

1. In ERI (or recommended replacement time, RRT), the battery voltage is low and the battery impedance is high. The ERI point is manufacturer-defined. Note that when the battery voltage of a dual chamber pacemaker reaches ERI, switching to the VVI mode automatically increases the battery voltage to a higher level than the specified ERI point. In reset, the battery voltage is high and the battery impedance has not yet reached the ERI points.
2. Battery stress test: program the pacemaker to dual chamber mode at a relatively fast rate and high output and watch for a while. If the pacemaker continues to function normally the diagnosis was reset (from EMI). If it switches back to VVI the diagnosis was ERI.

Caveat: From the ERI point, a pacemaker will reach end-of-life (EOL) or end-of-service (EOS) in about 3 months. At EOL, pacing becomes erratic and unreliable, with the possibility of total system failure.

Pacemaker follow-up

The frequency and type of follow-up depend on the projected battery life, type, mode, and programming of pacemakers, the stability of pacing and sensing, the need for programming change, the underlying rhythm (pacemaker dependency), travel logistics, type of third-party insurance, and alternative methods of follow-up such as remote monitoring via the Internet. Most centers follow the Medicare guidelines for pacemaker follow-up (for single chamber pacemakers, twice in the first 6 months after implant and then once every 12 months; for dual chamber pacemakers, twice in the first 6 months after implant and then once every 6 months).

Remote monitoring

Remote monitoring is recommended as part of a comprehensive and cost-effective pacemaker patient management program. Patients should be told of the availability of remote monitoring. Failure to inform patients may eventually cause medicolegal problems in the case of late discovery of an ICD problem. Furthermore, patient consent is advised as the data passes through a third party. Today, remote follow-up systems allow clinicians to monitor their pacemaker patients away from the device clinic or hospital. Follow-up done remotely uses specific equipment to interrogate and upload data to a secure web site via the patient's telephone line. These systems transmit device diagnostic data (from interrogation), stored electrograms, and the presenting rhythm. In this way, they provide the same information obtained at an office visit. Remote interrogations complement, and in some cases may even replace, in-clinic pacemaker follow-up visits. Remote follow-up is designed to supplement periodic visits to the pacemaker center, and should not replace comprehensive follow-up. Yet some workers use remote monitoring instead of visits on alternate follow-up sessions.

Remote monitoring may discover undocumented and asymptomatic arrhythmias, intermittent lead problems, and data helpful in optimizing device parameters and medical therapy. Remote monitoring should be considered as a form of intensified follow-up, especially in cases where an advisory mandates careful follow-up. Remote reprogramming of a pacemaker is not available. Medicare guidelines have also been published for this form of follow-up.

General approach

There is usually more than one correct way to evaluate and program a pacemaker for each patient. Using a systematic approach assures that no step is forgotten and no test unwittingly omitted. At the first visit, one examines the pacemaker and lead insertion sites for hematoma, seroma, increased warmth, or erythema for possible early infection.

In patients with recently or chronically implanted devices, arm swelling on the site of insertion or the presence of excessive superficial venous collaterals may indicate large vein thrombosis and the possible need for anticoagulation or thrombolytic therapy.

The minimum evaluation includes measurement of battery voltage, pacing threshold, impedance, and sensing functions. The degree of pacemaker dependence should be estimated. The session starts with device interrogation with a programmer wand or by wireless. Measured and diagnostic data are then examined. These capabilities include such features as real-time pacing, lead impedance, battery-life indicators, amplitudes of the atrial and ventricular signals, and real-time and stored ventricular EGMs.

Lead dislodgment usually occurs in the first days after implantation, and may occur up to 3 months after initial implantation. RV lead dislodgment occurs in 1–2% of cases. Lead displacement may be due to improper initial lead positioning, poor lead fixation, or excessive arm–shoulder motions soon after surgery. Dislodgment of the lead may cause loss of capture and undersensing. The diagnosis is confirmed by device interrogation showing changes in the sensing and pacing thresholds compared to implantation data, and the relatively long record of periodic automatic threshold measurements by the device itself. A chest x-ray confirms the diagnosis. Immediate lead repositioning is mandatory.

Real-time EGMs are recorded simultaneously with the surface ECGs, and annotated markers provide valuable information. The marker channel depicts how the device actually interprets cardiac activity. Annotations used by the marker channel vary according to the manufacturer, but there usually exists a legend key or description on the programmer screen or in the accompanying product manual.

Stored EGMs are recordings frozen in time and stored in the device memory for subsequent retrieval and analysis. The pacemaker records these electrograms automatically after a specific triggered event, typically arrhythmia detection, diagnosis, and outcome of therapy. A programmable pre-trigger interval immediately precedes the trigger; the longer the pre-trigger interval, the greater the likelihood of recording the initiating event of the tachyarrhythmia. The "pre-trigger" interval is programmable. Pacemakers possess a limited storage capacity, and a strategy of overwriting the oldest information means that only the most recent data may be retrievable (first in, first out). Obviously, with a finite memory capacity, single-channel EGM recording can store more episodes than dual-channel recordings that consume more memory. Representative strips of important stored electrograms should be printed and inserted into the patient's chart or electronic record.

Follow-up of lead impedance

The leads are the weakest part of the pacemaker system, and the mechanical stresses are responsible for fracture and insulation problems. The major lead complications include (in decreasing frequency) insulation defects, lead fractures, loss of ventricular capture, abnormal lead impedance, and sensing failure.

Lead impedance tends to fall in the first 2 weeks after implantation but then reaches a plateau and remains relatively stable at approximately 15% higher than the implantation value. Pacemakers automatically track the impedance over time by making periodic measurements. The trend data can be retrieved by standard pacemaker interrogation. However, such a change in an asymptomatic patient warrants closer follow-up.

The ventricular lead is evaluated for pacing impedance, R-wave amplitude, and pacing threshold, together with real-time recordings of the ventricular EGMs. The measured pacing impedance is compared to the chronic baseline value. Decreases of 30% or more or pacing impedances below 200–250 Ω may be indicative of insulation failure. Sudden and significant increases in pacing impedance may be indicative of conductor fracture. The atrial lead is evaluated in the same way.

Always print out the diagnostic data before programming. The therapy summary outlines the arrhythmic episodes since the last visit, and how the pacemaker interpreted them. These counters should be cleared after each visit to avoid confusion in the future. Diagnostic data offer invaluable information regarding the functional status of the device and leads. The device itself determines atrial and ventricular sensing data and lead impedances at regular intervals. The programmer measures the amplitude of the atrial and ventricular EGMs (as seen by the pacemaker) periodically and stores the values obtained automatically. Alternatively, one can determine the signals directly from the telemetered EGM by measuring from the upper peak to the lower peak. Significantly abnormal measurements of predetermined ranges, or deviations from previous measurements, are usually highlighted on the programmer upon interrogation of the device

Event counters

A heart-rate histogram shows the distribution of all recorded paced and sensed events by rate and other rate-related information recorded since the last patient session. Each bar represents the percentage of time the intrinsic or paced rate fell within a specific rate range. Each bar is divided into segments, which indicate the portion that was paced or sensed. Histograms are useful to evaluate the programmed sensor response by examining the breakdown of the heart rates into ranges. Careful analysis should enable an assessment of the appropriateness of the current rate sensor settings. If the sensor parameter is programmed "on" or "passive," a bar graph displays the percentage of paced events that would result if the rate were determined exclusively by response to the activity sensor (100% paced). Intermittent atrial fibrillation should be suspected if the atrial histogram shows a high rate event. If the spontaneous heart rate exceeds the sensor-indicated rate with inhibition of the pacemaker, the histogram will underestimate the actual heart rate.

Counter information will also indicate the number of atrial and ventricular extrasystoles, atrial/ventricular tachycardias, and will also indicate and display the number of times certain algorithms are activated – for example, mode switch, rate drop response, etc.

Like the rate histogram, the AV conduction histogram indicates the percentage of the total number of heart beats counted since the last patient session. It can also be displayed in rate groups. The AV conduction sequence categories are as follows:

AS – VS : atrial sense – ventricular sense
AS – VP : atrial sense – ventricular pace
AP – VS : atrial pace – ventricular sense
AP – VP : atrial pace – ventricular pace

The interpretation of many events requires knowledge of the integrity of pacing and sensing within the system. Many systems also report the number of ventricular premature complexes. Not all VPCs indicated by the pacemaker represent true VPCs, because a pacemaker-defined VPC is a sensed ventricular event that is not preceded by a detected atrial event. Atrial undersensing may falsely indicate a high percentage of VPCs. Loss of atrial or ventricular pacing cannot be determined by these recorded events. Histograms may enhance the programmability of the AV interval. The degree of ventricular pacing has become important to prevent LV dysfunction. It is estimated from the event histograms that record the cardiac activity. The data may lead to reprogramming to minimize RV pacing.

The pacemaker as an implantable Holter system: electrogram storage

It is questionable whether marker annotations alone stored in pacemaker memory are useful in assessing the number and duration of arrhythmic episodes. The development of electrogram storage and retrieval by pacemakers has added a new dimension to the diagnosis of spontaneous arrhythmias and device malfunction. Pacemakers store the data either automatically according to a detection algorithm or by a patient-activated system whenever a symptomatic patient applies a magnet or a special activator over the device. Annotated high-quality EGMs allow reliable assessment of stored episodes by visual inspection in practically 100% of cases. The final diagnosis of the retrieved data scrutinized by the physician may, of course, differ from the automatic interpretation by the detection algorithm of the device.

The EGM must be sampled at twice the minimal frequency component to register all the information contained in it. Sampling at 256 samples/second allows good reproduction, and a minimum rate of 128 samples/second is necessary to achieve a sufficiently diagnostic EGM quality. One byte of memory is generally required for each sample. Assuming a pacemaker with 8 kB of memory dedicated to EGM

Table 23. Special functions of pacemakers.

Function	Purpose	Details
Noncompetitive atrial pacing (NCAP) (Medtronic)	Intended to prevent initiation of atrial tachyarrhythmias by atrial stimulation in the relative refractory period of the atrial myocardium	An atrial event sensed in the unblanked PVARP starts a 300 ms NCAP interval, at the end of which the pacemaker emits an atrial stimulus. The resultant timing intervals may be altered
Autointrinsic conduction search (St. Jude); AV search hysteresis (Boston Scientific); search AV+ (Medtronic)	Determines the time the device periodically extends the paced/sensed AV delay to search for intrinsic conduction	The algorithm extends the paced/sensed AV delay periodically
Ventricular intrinsic preference (VIP) (St. Jude)	Upgraded autointrinsic conduction search, as above	As above
Sleep function	Intended to slow the pacing rate during sleep	Manual programming of sleep times or automatic detection of sleep by sensor activity
Rate smoothing (Boston Scientific)	Programmable feature designed to prevent sudden large changes in pacing cycle-to-cycle intervals	Prevents the pacing rate from changing by more than a programmable percentage from one cycle to the next. The pacemaker stores in memory the most recent R–R interval, either intrinsic or paced. Based on this R–R interval, and the rate smoothing value or percentage, the device determines the duration of the next pacing cycle involving atrium and ventricle
Ventricular rate stabilization (VRS) (Medtronic)	When VRS is enabled, it acts as a constant rate-smoothing algorithm. The VRS operates when the rate that corresponds to the R–R median interval (of the last 12 measured ventricular intervals) is less than or equal to a fixed rate of 85 bpm. It is intended as a response to VPCs	On each ventricular event, the device calculates a new ventricular interval as the sum of the previous ventricular interval plus the programmed interval increment value for VRS (or a predetermined minimum interval, if it is larger than this sum). This minimum interval is determined from the programmed maximum rate for VRS
Rate drop hysteresis (Medtronic); sudden Brady response (Boston Scientific)	Treatment of vasovagal syncope. Response to sudden decrease in intrinsic atrial rate by applying dual chamber pacing at an elevated rate	A programmable feature of some dual-pacemaker generators. Automatic acceleration of dual chamber pacing rate (e.g., to 100 ppm) for up to several minutes after detection of a sudden fall in intrinsic heart rate

continued

Table 23. Special functions of pacemakers (*continued*).

Function	Purpose	Details
Algorithms to prevent atrial fibrillation	Algorithms incorporated in antibradycardia pacemakers to control the atrial pacing rate or duration of atrial pacing cycles	Dynamic atrial overdrive pacing at a rate slightly faster than basic sinus rhythm, which results in an increase in pacing time and creates a consistent atrial activation sequence in the presence of an "irritable" atrium. Response to atrial premature complex (APC): (1) post-APC response to prevent short–long sequences (a form of rate smoothing); (2) APC suppression by increasing the basal pacing rate to suppress APCs. Post-exercise rate control to prevent abrupt drop in rate after exercise. Transient overdrive pacing after a mode-switch episode
Sinus preference (Medtronic)	Search function whereby the pacemaker looks for a sinus rate slightly below the sensor-indicated rate	Promotes sinus tracking (AV synchronization with an intrinsic P wave) within a programmable rate zone below the sensor-indicated rate
Sensing assurance (Medtronic); autosense (Boston Scientific)	Automatically adjusts atrial and ventricular sensitivities within defined limits	The pacemaker monitors the peak amplitude of sensed signals. The pacemaker automatically increases or decreases sensitivity to maintain an adequate sensing margin with respect to the patient's sensed P and R waves.
Conducted AF response (Medtronic); ventricular rate regularization (Boston Scientific)	Ventricular response pacing is designed to regularize the ventricular rate in patients with an irregular ventricular response during AF. A variant of rate-smoothing.	The pacing rate is modified on a beat-to-beat basis to pace at or just above the mean intrinsic ventricular rate. Long pauses and shorter cycles are suppressed, thereby reducing the ventricular rate irregularity
Sudden Brady response (Boston Scientific)	Designed to respond to sudden decreases in intrinsic atrial rates by applying dual chamber pacing at an elevated pacing rate	
Sensing integrity counter (Medtronic)	Diagnostic counter that stores the number of short unphysiologic ventricular intervals recorded between patient sessions	A large number of short intervals may indicate that the ventricular sensing lead is damaged and creates false signals. It may also indicate oversensing, a loose set-screw or VPCs

Table 23. Special functions of pacemakers (*continued*).

Function	Purpose	Details
Safety switch automatic lead configuration (Boston Scientific); lead monitor (Medtronic)	The safety switch feature allows the pacemaker to monitor lead integrity and to switch the pacing and sensing configuration from bipolar to unipolar if the impedance criteria indicate unacceptably high or low lead impedances. If very high-impedance leads are being used, this function should be turned off	The pacemaker monitors lead impedance during paced events. If the measured impedance falls outside a certain range (such as 200–2500 Ω) for any daily measurement, both pacing and sensing bipolar configurations will automatically be switched permanently to unipolar for that chamber
MRI-safe pacemaker	Specially designed for protection against MRI. About 50% of pacemaker patients eventually need an MRI	A number of circumstances must be addressed before programming the MRI-safe function

recording, and a sampling rate of 128 samples/second, the duration of (uncompressed) single-channel EGM recording is 8 kB × 1024 bytes/kB divided by 128 bytes/second, which is equal to 64 seconds. Compression algorithms can increase this duration further, because repeated sequences such as the baseline can be stored using far less memory. Thus the 64 seconds in the previous example can be expanded to 320 seconds with 5:1 average compression, yielding 320 seconds of EGM storage.

Pacemaker technology can now store electrograms with the following features:

1. Separate channels for atrial and ventricular EGMs of sufficient resolution and duration.
2. Onset and termination data: a programmable number of cardiac cycles before arrhythmia onset ("pre-trigger EGM") and some cycles after arrhythmia termination.
3. Simultaneous annotated markers are essential. Marker annotations and intervals may facilitate understanding of why and how the pacemaker detected and classified an event. An additional marker annotation (e.g., arrow, line) should indicate the exact moment when arrhythmia detection criteria are fulfilled.

The memory capability improves our understanding of a variety of electrophysiologic mechanisms that will enhance the diagnosis and treatment of atrial and ventricular tachyarrhythmias. The memory function will be especially useful to optimize programming of increasingly complex devices.

Most pacemakers can be programmed to record certain events such as high-rate atrial and ventricular events with stored electrograms, and to store other situations provided the device memory has not been fully utilized. The occurrence of abnormalities is recorded for retrieval even in the absence of electrograms. Stored episodes > 220 complexes per minute and > 5 minutes in duration have a high correlation with atrial fibrillation (AF) and flutter. Multiple episodes of AF with prolonged duration or rapid ventricular response may require anticoagulation and rate control. There is emerging evidence that strokes can be prevented by the early diagnosis and treatment of paroxysmal AF based on remote pacemaker monitoring. Atrial tachyarrhythmias (AT) are common in the general pacemaker population. Patients with prior history of AT show a higher arrhythmia burden, but the subsequent incidence is quite considerable even in those patients without any history of atrial arrhythmias. The majority of ATs in this patient population are asymptomatic, and symptoms do not correspond to an actual arrhythmic episode in most patients. Episodes of possible ventricular tachycardia can also be documented. Stored electrograms can reveal sensing problems, and other situations according to the manufacturer. These data contribute to optimal device programming and patient management. Triggers that activate the recording of representative electrograms include automatic mode switching, high atrial rates, high ventricular rates, ventricular premature beats under certain circumstances, pacemaker-mediated tachycardia, and magnet placement. Finally, stored electrograms may also help in defining whether the symptoms experienced by pacemaker patients are due to arrhythmias.

Special functions of pacemakers

Contemporary pacemakers are sophisticated devices with a multiplicity of functions, many of which are manufacturer-specific (Table 23). One must become familiar with these device refinements and apply them cautiously to pacemaker patients, and one must understand their behavior for troubleshooting what appears to be erratic pacemaker behavior or malfunction in the setting of manifestations according to pacemaker design.

Cardiac resynchronization (CRT)

Cardiac resynchronization hemodynamics

Dual-site or biventricular (RV and LV) pacing has emerged as an effective therapy for patients with dilated cardiomyopathy (severe systolic left ventricular dysfunction on the basis of ischemic or non-ischemic etiology) and congestive heart failure (CHF) associated with NYHA class III or IV symptoms and major left-sided intraventricular conduction delay such as left bundle branch block. The intraventricular conduction disorder causes an inefficient dyssynchronous or uncoordinated pattern of LV activation with segments contracting at different times. The erratic LV contraction causes a shorter diastole and/or overlapping systole/diastole with aggravation of functional mitral regurgitation. Biventricular pacing works by reducing the degree of electromechanical disparity. LV dyssynchrony typically arises from electrical delay resulting in mechanical delay between the septal and lateral walls. Thus the improved sequence of electrical activation (a process known as resynchronization) translates into beneficial acute and long-term hemodynamic effects by virtue of a more coordinated and efficient LV contraction associated with a reduction of functional mitral regurgitation. The target sites for LV pacing consist of the lateral and posterolateral coronary veins. There are virtually no data about the role of right ventricular outflow tract pacing as opposed to RV apical pacing during cardiac resynchronization therapy (CRT). The hemodynamic benefit of CRT occurs virtually with an on/off effect (with additional long-term reverse remodeling of the LV) and stems primarily from ventricular recoordination rather than optimization of the AV delay.

Patients for CRT are selected primarily on electrocardiographic criteria. However, the severity of LV mechanical systolic dyssynchrony is a much better predictor of a CRT response. Echocardiography has provided direct evidence of wall motion resynchronization in patients receiving CRT. In many studies the presence of ventricular dyssynchrony defined by various echocardiographic measurements appears to predict response to CRT, with the extent of improvement in the systolic function related to the degree of ventricular dyssynchrony. Although many workers have searched for the best echocardiographic index to identify LV dyssynchrony so as to predict responders to CRT before device implantation, this issue is still debatable. For this reason the American and European guidelines for CRT do not require echocardiographic proof of mechanical LV dyssynchrony.

Enrollment in most of the major CRT trials included: (1) CHF in NYHA functional class III or IV despite optimal pharmacologic therapy, (2) LVEF $<$ 35%, (3) LV end-diastolic diameter $>$ 55 mm, and (4) QRS duration $>$120 or specifically $<$ 150 ms. Many of the trials have shown benefit in patients with a QRS $\geq$ 120 ms. The American guidelines for biventricular pacing include medically refractory symptomatic NYHA class III or IV patients with idiopathic dilated or ischemic cardiomyopathy. The European guidelines are similar except that they require evidence of LV dilatation. Many CRT patients (almost all in the United States) also receive an ICD (CRT-D) device. The European guidelines (2007) recommend that the use of CRT without an ICD should be based on (1) the patient's expectation of survival less than 1 year, and (2) healthcare logistical constraints and cost considerations.

CRT with only left ventricular pacing

Initial investigations with monochamber LV pacing revealed similar hemodynamic benefit using either LV or biventricular pacing during acute CRT studies, and in some instances LV stimulation had even a greater positive hemodynamic effect than biventricular pacing. A prospective, multicenter, randomized, single-blind, parallel, controlled trial comparing biventricular versus monochamber LV pacing demonstrated that LV pacing alone resulted in a significant improvement of LV ejection fraction (LVEF), which was comparable in magnitude to the improvement in the biventricular group. Mortality and morbidity were also comparable in the two groups.

Indications for CRT with only left ventricular pacing

Proponents of single-lead LV pacing for CRT argue that the implantation technique is less challenging and less costly. In this respect the expanding use of the ICD in CRT patients for primary prevention of sudden death limits the applicability of monochamber LV pacing. Possible areas of clinical applicability might include CHF patients with important comorbidities associated with a dismal long-term prognosis. Thus the role for single-lead LV pacing is presently quite small. Single-lead LV pacing without an ICD may become important in the future if it is shown that primary prevention of LV dysfunction or heart failure with CRT is worthwhile in selected patients with LVEF > 35%.

Advantages of a right ventricular lead for CRT

Although RV pacing is not required for hemodynamic benefit in most CRT patients, the addition of an RV lead offers important advantages:

1. Many patients (almost all in the United States) receive an CRT-D device.
2. Programmability of the interventricular (V–V) interval between LV and RV stimulation may improve hemodynamics.
3. Sensing from only an LV lead runs the risk of left atrial sensing in case of lead displacement toward the left atrium. This may cause ventricular inhibition or inappropriate ICD discharge if there is an ICD in place.
4. Antitachycardia pacing (ATP) may be more effective with RV + LV ATP (with ICD) than physician-supervised LV ATP (with no ICD), because ventricular arrhythmias in patients with ischemic cardiomyopathy tend to originate from the septum.
5. Patients requiring antibradycardia pacing are best served with a biventricular system, because the dislodgment rate of LV leads is much higher than those of RV leads.
6. Theoretically, biventricular pacing may be less proarrhythmic than LV pacing alone, because it is associated with less temporal dispersion of repolarization. Finally, it is important to remember that turning off RV pacing may help a few patients refractory to biventricular pacing and those with marked latency of LV stimulation where V–V programmability cannot advance the LV output sufficiently ahead of the RV output.

NYHA class I and II patients with LBBB and depressed LV function

Recent studies in NYHA class I and II patients with QRS ≥ 120 ms and LVEF ≤ 35% have shown that CRT produces definite long-term improvement of LV function in the setting of minimal or no symptomatic changes. The REVERSE (Resynchronization Reverses Remodeling in Systolic Left Ventricular Dysfunction) trial involved asymptomatic or mildly symptomatic patients with QRS ≥ 120 ms and LVEF ≤ 40% for 24 months. Mean baseline LVEF was 28.0%. After 24 months of CRT, and compared with those of control subjects, clinical outcomes and LV function were improved and LV dimensions were decreased in this patient population. These observations suggest that CRT prevents the progression of disease in patients with asymptomatic or mildly symptomatic LV dysfunction. The MADIT III study involved patients with LVEF ≤ 30%, QRS ≥130 ms, and NYHA class I or II symptoms, but there was no change in mortality. CRT was associated with a significant reduction in LV volumes and improvement in the LVEF. CRT combined with ICD decreased the risk of heart-failure events. These findings may eventually find their way into the official guidelines.

Right bundle branch block

The incidence of LV dyssynchrony is much less in patients with RBBB than in those with an LBBB type of conduction disorder. CRT in patients with RBBB has generally been disappointing, although a few patients may improve. Some experts believe that CRT should not be used in patients with RBBB. If CRT is being considered in RBBB, significant LV dyssynchrony must be established before proceeding.

CRT in patients with a narrow QRS complex

Small non-controlled studies have demonstrated that heart-failure patients with a narrow QRS (< 120 ms) and evidence of LV dyssynchrony may benefit from CRT. Yet a recent trial showed no benefit. Despite the growing body of evidence suggesting that echocardiographic criteria may be reliable for the evaluation of mechanical LV dyssynchrony, CRT remains controversial in patients with a narrow QRS complex and is generally not recommended.

Impact of CRT

The improved sequence of electrical activation with CRT, which has no positive inotropic effect as such, improves cardiac efficiency by restoring the near-normal LV contraction pattern. This translates into beneficial acute and long-term hemodynamic effects by virtue of a more coordinated and efficient LV contraction and function. Long-term hemodynamic improvement by reverse LV remodeling causes an increase in LVEF (usually up to 6% in randomized trials) and a decrease in LV systolic and diastolic volumes. These changes occur progressively and may take 3–6 months or longer (> 1 year) to become established. CRT also reduces functional mitral regurgitation, with both an acute effect and further improvement on a long-term basis by superimposed LV reverse remodeling. Cardiac output increases, while LV filling pressure decreases without increasing myocardial oxygen consumption.

CRT improves NYHA functional class (0.5–0.8 in randomized trials), exercise tolerance (20% mean increase in distance walked in 6 minutes in randomized trials), quality of life, and morbidity. Long-term reverse remodeling of the failing LV results in reductions in CHF hospitalizations and mortality, independent of defibrillator therapy, when combined with optimal pharmacotherapy. There is also a reduction of sympathetic/parasympathetic imbalance, attenuating the chronic sympathetic activation of heart failure and of neurohumoral activation due to increased systolic blood pressure and improved LV filling time. The benefits of CRT are similar in magnitude to those of ACE inhibitors and beta-blockers, and are superimposed on the benefits of medical therapy. Despite the presence of LV reverse remodeling, interruption of CRT results in worsening of LV function and desynchronization.

Upgrading to a biventricular system in patients with advanced heart failure and continuous RV pacing results in significant reverse LV remodeling in the long-term follow-up, and improvement in overall synchronicity of LV function. The long-term risk of mortality and morbidity is similar to that in patients undergoing de novo CRT. Symptomatic improvements and degree of reverse remodeling are also comparable.

Percentage of biventricular pacing

One must ensure that biventricular pacing takes place 100% of the time. The percentage of biventricular pacing and ventricular sensing must be carefully checked in the stored memorized data retrieved from the device. Remote home monitoring is particularly helpful for this assessment. Devices must be programmed carefully to prevent "electrical" desynchronization. Troubleshooting loss of resynchronization may be difficult, and requires a thorough knowledge of biventricular pacemaker function, timing cycles, and complex algorithms.

Failure of CRT benefit

The transvenous implantation success rate is about 90–95%. About 30% of patients do not respond to CRT. A number of factors may be responsible for this failure. The two major causes are placement of LV lead at a suboptimal location and the limitation of ECG-based patient selection criteria. In about one-third of heart-failure patients with LBBB or left-sided intraventricular conduction delay, ECG patterns are not associated with significant LV mechanical dyssynchrony. This observation correlates with the incidence of the non-responder rate in clinical trials of CRT. Since retiming to recoordinate LV contraction is the primary goal of CRT, it is therefore unlikely, but not impossible, that CRT will benefit patients with wide QRS complexes in the absence of mechanical dyssynchrony. Echocardiography with tissue Doppler imaging (TDI) can detect the direction and velocity of the contracting or relaxing myocardium. TDI is a reproducible technique to detect regional myocardial function and timing of events by measuring the time to peak systolic velocity during ejection phase in several myocardial segments. TDI is emerging as a useful tool to improve the selection of patients for CRT.

Recent investigations (contrary to popular belief) suggest that in some patients an LV lead positioned in an anterior rather than a lateral or posterior LV location may not necessarily produce harmful or no effect. Hemodynamic measurement would be in order before considering lead revision.

Scar burden

Lack of adequate capture threshold and failure of response to CRT (in the presence of LV dyssynchrony) may be related to the presence of extensive scar tissue in the target region for LV pacing. Therefore, in patients with ischemic cardiomyopathy and history of previous infarction, the extent of scar tissue should be assessed before CRT implantation.

Alternative routes to left ventricular pacing

Constraints of coronary venous anatomy, diaphragmatic stimulation, and late LV lead dislodgements require alternative routes for LV pacing. Surgical techniques include minimally invasive surgical approaches (minithoracotomy, video-assisted thoracoscopic surgery, and robotically assisted placement of LV leads), and minimally invasive subxiphoid epicardial approach.

Only a few patients have received an endocardial LV lead for CRT implanted via a transseptal approach. LV endocardial pacing in a biventricular system provides more homogeneous intraventricular resynchronization and better hemodynamic performance than epicardial biventricular pacing (through the coronary venous system). The risks and benefits of this approach are unclear in view of insufficient experience. Major concerns include thromboembolism and mitral valve disruption.

Bifocal RV pacing consists of implantation of two RV leads: one placed at the RV apex, and the other in the RV outflow tract. This approach has been used when LV implantation is unsuccessful. It produces CRT of a lesser degree than biventricular pacing. Bifocal RV pacing must not be the first line of therapy, and should not be a substitute for cardiac surgery when LV pacing cannot be accomplished for technical reasons, except in patients who might not tolerate, or who refuse, a thoracotomy for LV lead placement.

Triventricular pacing (two leads in the RV and one in the LV) may produce important hemodynamic improvement in initial responders to biventricular pacing who eventually develop heart failure on a long-term basis. The question arises as to whether triangular ventricular pacing (a combination of bifocal RV pacing with LV pacing) might eventually prove more useful than regular biventricular pacing for primary CRT, rather than being presently considered a bail-out procedure. In contrast, systems with two LV leads and one RV lead do not appear useful.

What is a CRT responder?

There is no standardized definition of when a patient should be considered a non-responder. There is no consensus on whether indices of LV reverse remodeling or clinical status should be used as end points for assessing CRT response. This is compounded by the observations that CRT recipients may have clinical improvement without echocardiographic improvement and vice versa. Improvement in NYHA functional class or increased distance walked in 6 minutes, or improved heart-failure-related quality of life is considered by some workers as an adequate response, but these parameters may be influenced by spontaneous changes and/or a placebo effect. Others would consider an adequate response in terms of changes in oxygen uptake at anaerobic threshold during exercise or reduction of LV systolic and diastolic volumes along with improvement in NYHA functional class. Improved systolic function is assessed by the LVEF and LV end-systolic volume (LVESV), which are commonly used parameters of LV reverse remodeling. A change in LVESV (reduction of LVESV > 15%) after 6 months is the single best predictor of a good long-term prognosis, with lower long-term mortality and heart-failure events, and it is theoretically less subject to placebo effect. Some patients who have no or minimal acute changes in any assessment modality may show gradual and delayed improvement after a few months. As a rule, patients without reverse remodeling are more symptomatic, and there is clear evidence that reverse remodeling translates into reduced morbidity and mortality.

Complications of CRT implantation

Left ventricular lead dislodgment. The dislodgment rate for LV leads is higher (2–5%) than that for atrial or RV leads, and it tends to occur soon after implantation. Micro-dislodgment may cause a high pacing threshold.

Coronary venous lead complications. The incidence of short-term complications (displacement, high threshold, phrenic nerve stimulation) is about 5%. At 1 year another 5% of leads malfunction. Lead failure after 1 year is rare. The pacing threshold, R-wave amplitude from LV lead, and impedance do not change significantly on a long-term basis to produce a clinical problem.

Infection. The infection rate with a primary implantation should be 0.5–1%, but a long procedure for CRT increases the risk.

Coronary sinus dissection and perforation. Coronary sinus (CS) dissection may be caused by too vigorous advancement of the guiding catheter or by injection of the contrast medium through an angiography catheter with its tip pressed against the vessel wall. The incidence of coronary sinus dissection is 2–5%. CS dissection usually heals well, and CS perforation is rare. Some workers believe that lead placement should be abandoned if the dissection is distal in the coronary sinus, and implantation of the LV lead performed several weeks later. A lead can usually be passed through a proximal coronary sinus dissection by finding the true lumen of the coronary sinus for satisfactory passage of the LV lead. With a dissection, an echocardiogram should be performed to rule out a pericardial effusion.

Phrenic nerve stimulation and diaphragmatic pacing. Phrenic nerve stimulation is a common problem, and can be difficult to demonstrate during implantation in the sedated and supine patient. It may become evident only when the patient becomes active and changes body position. This complication is related to the anatomic vicinity of the left phrenic nerve to the LV pacing site, especially when the LV lead is implanted into a posterior or posterolateral coronary vein. It may also be related to LV lead dislodgment. Occasionally, after implantation, phrenic nerve stimulation can be controlled by lowering the LV voltage (maintaining capture), provided the capture threshold for phrenic nerve stimulation is much higher than that of LV capture. Special programmable options with bipolar LV leads allow programming of function in terms of true bipolar LV pacing as well as using the RV ring as an anode and the LV tip or ring as the cathode. The latter arrangement is available if there is an associated ICD. In the absence of an ICD, true unipolar pacing can also be performed from one or the other LV electrode to the device can as the anode. These manipulations alter the pacing vector non-invasively (electronic repositioning). This function enables more flexibility to overcome problems with high LV pacing thresholds and phrenic nerve stimulation.

Impact of comorbidities

After CRT, chronic renal failure, diabetes mellitus, and a history of atrial fibrillation are strong independent predictors of death.

Programming of CRT devices

Some of the CRT failures in randomized trials can be attributed to improper patient selection, suboptimal LV lead placement, inadequate medical therapy, and inappropriate device programming.

General considerations

The 12-lead ECG should be studied before any programming activity. The goal of CRT programming is to ensure ventricular resynchronization virtually 100% of the time and to optimize AV and interventricular (V–V) timing. As heart-failure patients represent a heterogeneous group, optimal CRT device performance can only be achieved by tailored programming on an individual basis(Table 24). It is important to evaluate the patient as well as the device. One should assess the patient's NYHA functional class, physical activity, current medications, heart-rate histograms, the percentage of atrial and ventricular pacing. and special problems such as phrenic nerve stimulation and any underlying atrial and ventricular rhythm abnormalities. Testing also includes evaluation of intrathoracic impedance data about pulmonary fluid status (in patients with a CRT-D device), and exercise testing in selected patients to look for abnormalities such as atrial undersensing or threshold problem not apparent at rest. CRT programming requires careful attention to the patient's hemodynamic problem, knowledge of CRT device technology, and the electrocardiographic manifestations of normal and abnormal device function.

Twelve-lead electrocardiography

Basic electrocardiography

A 12-lead ECG is essential for CRT evaluation. A single-channel rhythm strip from a pacemaker programmer is inappropriate. During evaluation of CRT devices the 12-lead ECG yields important information about the presence or absence of fusion with the intrinsic conducted QRS complex, the balance between RV and LV activation, and the presence of RV anodal capture in patients with unipolar LV leads. Complete assessment requires comparison of the QRS morphology during native conduction, single chamber RV, single chamber LV, and biventricular pacing.

QRS morphology during right ventricular apical pacing

Pacing from the RV, regardless of site, virtually always produces a left bundle branch block (LBBB) pattern in the precordial leads. RV apical pacing produces negative paced QRS complexes in the inferior leads (II, III, and aVF), because depolarization begins in the inferior part of the heart and travels superiorly away from the inferior leads. The mean paced QRS frontal-plane axis is always superior,

Table 24. Optimal programming of biventricular pacemakers.

AV delay	**1.** A long AV delay should not be used **2.** Optimize the AS–VP delay and avoid ventricular fusion with the spontaneous conducted QRS complex. Promote atrial sensing (VDD mode) because atrial pacing produces less favorable hemodynamics **3.** Consider promoting fusion of LV pacing with RBB activation (short AV delay) on a trial basis only if the absence of fusion yields suboptimal CRT **4.** Program rate-adaptive (dynamic) AV delay off during temporary pacing for testing (with VDD mode slower than sinus rate to sense atrial activity) **5.** Programming rate-adaptive AV delay for long-term pacing is controversial
V–V delay	Programming the interventricular delay may be important in patients with a suboptimal CRT response
Atrial sensing and PVARP	**1.** Short PVARP (aim for 250 ms); may have to use algorithms for the automatic termination of endless loop tachycardia. **2.** Program off the post-VPC PVARP extension and the pacemaker-mediated tachycardia termination algorithm based on one cycle of PVARP extension **3.** Automatic mode switching off in devices using a relatively long PVARP mandated by the mode-switching algorithm **4.** Program the PVAB to eliminate far-field R-wave sensing by the atrial channel
Upper rate	Relatively fast upper rate so the patient does not have "break- through" ventricular sensing within their exercise zone. Initial upper rate of 140 ppm or faster is often appropriate in the absence of myocardial ischemia during pacing at this rate
AV conduction	**1.** Use drugs that impair AV delay **2.** Consider ablation of the AV junction in patients with a long PR interval or intra- or interatrial conduction in case of difficult management

usually in the left, or less commonly in the right superior quadrant. Pacing from the RV outflow tract or septum shifts the frontal-plane paced QRS axis to the inferior quadrant. The inferior leads become positive.

QRS morphology during left ventricular pacing from the coronary venous system

Single-site LV pacing from the posterior or posterolateral coronary vein (the traditional sites for CRT) results in a right bundle branch block (RBBB) pattern (dominant R wave) in a correctly positioned lead V_1. Leads V_2 and V_3 may or may not be positive. With apical lead position, ECG leads V_4–V_6 are typically negative. With basal lead position, ECG leads V_4–V_6 are usually positive, as with the concordant positive R waves during overt pre-excitation in left-sided accessory pathway conduction in the Wolff–Parkinson–White syndrome. Pacing from the middle or the great (anterior) cardiac vein (unsatisfactory sites for CRT) produces an LBBB pattern of depolarization.

Thus, when lead V_1 during LV pacing shows a negative QRS complex during LV pacing, one should consider incorrect ECG lead placement, lead location in the middle or great (anterior) cardiac vein, or rarely an undefined mechanism involving a severe intra-myocardial conduction abnormality related to substantial scarring. The frontal-plane axis during LV pacing from the lateral and inferolateral wall often points to the right inferior quadrant (right axis deviation), less commonly to the right superior quadrant, and only occasionally the axis may point to the left inferior or left superior quadrant.

QRS morphology during biventricular pacing

Biventricular pacing with the RV lead located at the apex. Biventricular pacing often shifts the frontal-plane vector to the right superior quadrant in an anticlockwise fashion (as if starting with RV

Table 25. Lack of a dominant R wave in lead V_1 during biventricular pacing with apical right ventricular lead.

- Normal situation
- Right ventricular outflow tract and LV pacing
- Incorrect placement of lead V_1 (too high on the chest)
- Lack of LV capture
- LV lead displacement
- Marked LV latency (exit block, delay from the LV stimulation site with or without myocardial scar)
- Ventricular fusion with conducted QRS complex
- Pacing via the middle cardiac vein or anterior interventricular vein
- Unintended placement of two leads in the RV
- Reversal of RV and LV connections

pacing), although the frontal-plane axis may occasionally reside in the left superior quadrant during uncomplicated biventricular pacing. The QRS is often positive in lead V_1 during biventricular pacing when the RV is paced from the apex. A negative QRS complex in lead V_1 may occur during uncomplicated biventricular pacing with RV apical pacing, but its presence mandates a thorough investigation to rule out the following situations: incorrect placement of lead V_1 (too high on the chest), lack of LV capture, LV lead displacement, marked LV latency (exit block), major conduction delay from a scarred LV stimulation site, ventricular fusion with the conducted QRS complex, coronary venous pacing via the middle cardiac vein (also the anterior cardiac vein), or even unintended placement of two leads in the RV (Table 25). A negative QRS complex in lead V_1 during uncomplicated biventricular pacing probably reflects different activation of a heterogeneous biventricular substrate (ischemia, scar, His–Purkinje participation in view of the varying patterns of LV activation in spontaneous LBBB, etc.) and does not necessarily indicate a poor (electrical or mechanical) contribution from LV stimulation.

Biventricular pacing with the RV lead in the outflow tract. During biventricular pacing with the RV lead in the outflow tract, the paced QRS in lead V_1 is often negative, and the frontal-plane paced QRS axis is often directed to the right inferior quadrant (right axis deviation).

QRS duration

Measurement of QRS duration during follow-up is helpful in the analysis of appropriate biventricular capture and the presence of fusion with intrinsic conduction. Chronic studies have shown that the degree of narrowing of the paced QRS duration is a poor predictor of the mechanical CRT response. In this context, it is interesting that monochamber LV pacing with a paced QRS complex wider than that of biventricular pacing can produce CRT virtually as effective as that of biventricular pacing. Loss of capture in one ventricle will cause a change in the paced QRS morphology and duration in the 12-lead ECG similar to that of either single chamber RV or LV pacing. As the paced QRS during biventricular pacing is often narrower than that of monochamber RV or LV pacing, widening of the paced QRS complex may reflect loss of capture in one chamber with effectual capture in the other.

Paced QRS duration and status of mechanical ventricular resynchronization

The paced QRS during biventricular pacing is often narrower than that of monochamber RV or LV pacing. Thus, measurement of QRS duration during follow-up is helpful in the analysis of appropriate biventricular capture and fusion with the spontaneous QRS. If the biventricular ECG is similar to that recorded with RV or LV pacing alone and no cause is found, one should not automatically conclude that one of the leads does not contribute to biventricular depolarization without a detailed evaluation of the pacing system.

Chronic studies have shown that the degree of narrowing of the paced QRS duration is a poor predictor of the mechanical cardiac resynchronization response. In other words, the degree of QRS narrowing or its absence does not correlate with the long-term hemodynamic benefit of biventricular pacing, because the paced QRS does not reflect the underlying level of mechanical dyssynchrony. In this respect some patients with monochamber LV pacing exhibit an equal or superior degree of mechanical resynchronization compared to biventricular pacing despite a very wide paced QRS complex.

Long-term ECG changes

Many studies have shown that the paced QRS duration does not vary over time as long as the LV pacing lead does not move from its initial site. Yet surface ECGs should be performed periodically, because the LV lead may become displaced into a collateral branch of the coronary sinus. Dislodgement of the LV lead may result in loss of LV capture, with the ECG showing an RV-pacing QRS pattern with an increased QRS duration and superior axis deviation. Variation of QRS duration over time may play a determinant role if correlated with remodeling of the ventricles by echocardiography. Finally, the underlying spontaneous ECG should be exposed periodically to confirm the presence of an LBBB type of intraventricular conduction abnormality. In this respect, turning off the pacemaker could potentially improve LV function and heart failure in patients who have lost their intraventricular conduction delay or block through ventricular remodeling. In other words, a spontaneous narrow QRS is better than biventricular pacing.

Q, q, and QS configuration in lead I

A q wave in lead I is common during uncomplicated biventricular pacing. A q wave in lead I during uncomplicated RV apical pacing is rare. Loss of the q wave in lead I during biventricular pacing is 100% predictive of loss of LV capture. It therefore appears that analysis of the Q/q wave or a QS complex in lead I may be a reliable way to assess LV capture during biventricular pacing.

Ventricular fusion with native conduction

Ventricular fusion with the intrinsic conducted QRS complex may decrease the effectiveness of CRT in some patients, while others with a short PR interval may actually benefit from it. The clinical and hemodynamic impact of fusion in the individual patient can only be determined by trial and error. The presence of ventricular fusion should be suspected in the presence of marked QRS narrowing, especially in patients with a short spontaneous PR interval. It should be ruled out by observing the paced QRS morphology during progressive shortening of the AS–VP (atrial sensing – ventricular pacing) interval in the VDD mode or the AP–VP (atrial pacing – ventricular pacing) interval in the DDD mode.

In patients with sinus rhythm and a relatively short PR interval, ventricular fusion with competing native conduction during biventricular pacing may cause misinterpretation of the ECG, and this is a common pitfall in device follow-up. The AS–VP interval should be programmed (with rate-adaptive function) to ensure pure biventricular pacing under circumstances that might shorten the PR interval, such as increased circulating catecholamines. It is important to remember that a very narrow paced QRS complex may represent ventricular fusion (associated with a suboptimal hemodynamic response) with the conducted QRS complex rather than near-perfect electrical ventricular resynchronization. In this respect, remarkable narrowing of the paced QRS complex occurs with triventricular pacing (two RV sites + LV), as advocated for heart-failure patients who have become refractory to conventional biventricular pacing.

Upper rate response

Upper rate behavior of CRT devices differs from that of conventional pacemakers, because the majority of CRT patients have relatively normal sinus node function and AV conduction. When the atrial rate exceeds the programmed upper rate, biventricular pacemakers exhibit two forms of upper rate behavior according to the location of the P wave in the pacemaker cycle.

1. **Pre-empted Wenckebach upper rate response**. In the setting of a relatively short postventricular atrial refractory period (PVARP), when the spontaneous ventricular cycle shortens beyond the programmed upper rate interval, the AV interval of each pacemaker cycle becomes partially or incompletely extended (> programmed AS–VP interval), creating an attempted Wenckebach type upper rate response. There are no pacemaker stimuli because the P wave and the spontaneous QRS complex are both sensed by the device. This form of upper rate response, based on a sinus rate faster than the programmed (atrial-driven) upper rate, tends to occur in patients with relatively normal AV conduction, a short programmed AV delay, a short PVARP, and a relatively slow programmed (atrial-driven) upper rate.
2. **Upper rate limitation with P wave in the PVARP**. When the P–P interval during biventricular pacing becomes shorter than the total atrial refractory period (TARP) (in the setting of relatively normal sinus node function), spontaneous P waves fall into the PVARP, where they cannot be tracked. The conducted QRS complex (VS)

linked to the preceding P wave (in the PVARP) initiates a PVARP that will contain the succeeding P wave. This sequence ensures the perpetuation of functional atrial undersensing with loss of biventricular pacing. The prevailing AV delay (or the spontaneous PR interval or AR–VS) is longer than the programmed AS–VP. There are no pauses and no pacemaker stimuli. This form of upper response is therefore quite different from 2:1 fixed-ratio block produced by conventional pacemakers, because all the P waves remain in the PVARP.

Programming the upper rate

Because patients with heart failure are susceptible to sinus tachycardia (particularly during heart-failure exacerbation with elevated sympathetic tone), it is important to program a relatively fast upper rate to avoid an upper rate response manifested by the emergence of spontaneous conducted QRS complexes. In patients with normal sinus and AV nodal function, the risk of tracking rapid atrial rates with a biventricular device is not an important issue. Therefore, it is appropriate to program the upper rate to ≥ 140 bpm. If necessary the tendency towards sinus tachycardia may be attenuated by larger doses of beta-blockers, an important consideration in patients with an ICD and slow ventricular tachycardia (VT), where the VT detection rate must be faster then the programmed upper rate.

Loss of resynchronization below the programmed upper rate, and optimal programming of PVARP

Desynchronized fast AR–VS sequences containing trapped or locked P waves within the PVARP can occur in an upper rate response, but also in some circumstances below the programmed upper rate. There are numerous causes of electrical desynchronization at rates slower than the programmed upper rate, especially in association with a relatively long PVARP (Table 26). For example, during sinus

Table 26. Loss of cardiac resynchronization during DDD or DDDR pacing in the presence of preserved biventricular pacing.

(A) Intrinsic	**1.** Atrial undersensing from low-amplitude atrial potentials **2.** T-wave oversensing and other types of ventricular oversensing, such as diaphragmatic potentials. **3.** Long PR interval **4.** Circumstances that push the P wave into the PVARP, such as a junctional or idioventricular rhythm. **5.** New arrhythmia, such as atrial fibrillation with a fast ventricular rate **6.** Short runs of unsustained, often relatively slow, ventricular tachycardia; such arrhythmias are common and often asymptomatic **7.** First-generation devices with a common sensing channel: ventricular double counting and sensing of far-field atrial activity
(B) Extrinsic	**1.** Inappropriate programming of the AV delay or any function that prolongs the AV delay, such as rate smoothing, AV search hysteresis, etc. **2.** Low maximum tracking rate **3.** Slowing of the atrial rate upon exit from upper rate behavior **4.** Functional atrial undersensing below the programmed upper rate: (a) precipitated by an atrial premature beat or ventricular premature beat; (b) long PVARP including automatic PVARP extension after a VPC and single beat PVARP extension, related to algorithms for automatic termination of endless loop tachycardia **5.** Inappropriately slow programmed lower rate permitting junctional escape (cycle length < lower rate interval) in patients with periodic sinus arrest **6.** Intra-atrial conduction delay where sensing of AS is delayed in the right atrial appendage: a short AS–VP interval may not be able to achieve biventricular pacing

rhythm (below the upper rate), a sensed ventricular premature complex (or an oversensed T wave) initiates a regular PVARP. This event shifts pacemaker timing so that the succeeding undisturbed sinus P wave now falls into the PVARP. This refractory-sensed P wave inside the PVARP conducts to the ventricle, producing a spontaneous QRS complex sensed by the device. The sinus P waves will remain trapped in the PVARP as long as the P–P interval is shorter than the prevailing TARP (equal to (AR–VS) + PVARP). Hence, biventricular pacing will remain inhibited until either the occurrence of a non-refractory sensed atrial depolarization (when the P–P intervals becomes longer than the prevailing TARP) or delivery of an atrial pacing pulse outside the TARP.

Similarly, when a fast atrial rate (above the programmed upper rate) gradually drops below the programmed upper rate, biventricular pacing will remain inhibited for some time according to the above prevailing TARP formula. Based on these considerations, one should program a short PVARP of 250 ms or less. The PVARP extension after a ventricular premature complex should be turned off, as well as the pacemaker-mediated tachycardia termination algorithm based on PVARP prolongation for one cycle. A short PVARP is safe because endless loop tachycardia is rare in CRT patients without conduction system disease, apart from LBBB or its equivalent.

Some devices provide a programmable option to record ventricular sensing episodes. Such recordings are useful in reprogramming CRT devices. Many such episodes are due to AF or unsustained slow VT. The latter is very common and often of no important clinical significance. These ventricular sensing recordings may provide a clue to the mechanism of electrical desynchronization, such as an unsuspected upper rate response requiring reprogramming of the upper rate to a faster value.

Programming automatic unlocking of P waves from the PVARP

Locking of the P wave in the PVARP is facilitated by a long spontaneous PR interval, a long PVARP, and a relatively slow programmed upper rate. Special algorithms can be programmed to restore 1 : 1 atrial tracking when P waves are locked in the PVARP at rates slower than the programmed upper rate. A device can detect AR–VS sequences, a situation interpreted as electrical ventricular desynchronization whereupon temporary PVARP abbreviation (for one cycle) permits the device to sense a sinus P wave beyond the PVARP. This promotes atrial tracking and ventricular resynchronization. These algorithms do not function when the atrial rate is faster than the programmed upper rate, or during automatic mode switching. These algorithms are particularly useful in patients with sinus tachycardia and first-degree AV block, in whom prolonged locking of P waves inside the PVARP can be an important problem.

Programming the lower rate

The optimal lower rate in CRT patients is unknown and may exhibit great variability according to the presence and severity of heart failure. One should always aim for atrial sensing, which is hemodynamically more favorable than atrial pacing. There is evidence that atrial pacing may increase the risk of AF. Thus, the lower rate should be programmed to maintain sinus rhythm. In the occasional patient an accelerated idioventricular or junctional rhythm will compete with biventricular pacing, requiring an increase in the lower rate limit to overdrive and suppress the interfering rhythm.

Far-field R-wave oversensing

Far-field R-wave oversensing on the atrial channel impairs dual chamber SVT/VT discrimination but it does not cause inappropriate detection of VT (by an ICD) when the ventricular rate remains in the sinus zone. It may also cause inappropriate mode switching and loss of electrical desynchronization in the DDI mode. Far-field R-wave oversensing often shows a pattern of alternating short and long atrial cycle lengths, because the marker depicting the oversensed R wave remains close to the ventricular electrogram. Control of far-field R-wave sensing can be achieved by programmability in several ways:

1. Prolongation of the postventricular atrial blanking period, which carries the risk of undersensing AF.
2. Decrease of atrial sensitivity, which can also jeopardize sensing of AF.
3. Algorithmic rejection by identifying a specific pattern of atrial and ventricular events (Medtronic PR Logic).
4. Programmable automatic decrease of atrial sensitivity after ventricular events. This function is similar to the dynamic ventricular sensitivity in ICD devices.

Programming of left ventricular pacing output

Traditionally a safety margin of twice the voltage threshold is recommended for LV capture. Battery longevity is an important consideration in CRT devices, where two ventricles are being paced continuously and LV pacing may require a high output, as the pacing threshold is generally twice that of RV pacing. Thus, an LV safety margin of 1.5 × voltage threshold may be reasonable without increasing the risk of asystole. Such a lower safety margin must be individualized. Battery longevity may be enhanced by algorithms that automatically measure the LV threshold and may help maintain LV capture while reducing output.

Left ventricular automatic capture verification

Loss of LV capture and phrenic nerve stimulation (requiring a lower LV output for elimination) are two important causes of CRT interruption. To maintain effective LV capture with a minimal output, automatic algorithms for capture verification may be helpful. As an example, the Left Ventricular Capture Management (LVCM) algorithm of Medtronic measures the time from an atrial stimulus to the RV sensed event in one test cycle as the intrinsic AV interval (e.g. 200 ms). Thereafter, it measures the interval from LV pacing to the RV sensed event in another test cycle. Only if this V–V interval is significantly (at least 80 ms) shorter than the intrinsic AV interval, the algorithm assumes capture. Using this algorithm, LV output can be programmed (at a voltage safety margin < 2:1) to reduce battery current drain, improve resynchronization success, and decrease phrenic nerve stimulation

Anodal stimulation in biventricular pacemakers

Although anodal capture may occur with high-output traditional bipolar RV pacing, this phenomenon is almost always not discernible electrocardiographically. Biventricular pacing systems that utilize a unipolar lead for LV pacing via a coronary vein may create RV anodal pacing. The tip electrode of the LV lead is the cathode, and the proximal electrode of the bipolar RV lead often provides the anode for LV pacing. This arrangement creates a common anode for RV and LV pacing. A high current density (from two sources) at the common anode during biventricular pacing may cause anodal capture, manifested as a paced QRS complex with a somewhat different configuration from that derived from standard biventricular pacing.

A different form of anodal capture involving the proximal electrode of the bipolar RV lead can also occur with contemporary biventricular pacemakers with separately programmable ventricular outputs. During monochamber LV pacing at a relatively high output, RV anodal capture produces a paced QRS complex identical to that registered with biventricular pacing. Occasionally this type of anodal capture prevents electrocardiographic documentation of pure LV pacing if the LV pacing threshold is higher than that of RV anodal stimulation. Such anodal stimulation may complicate threshold testing and should not be misinterpreted as pacemaker malfunction. Furthermore, if the LV threshold is not too high, appropriate programming of the LV output should eliminate anodal stimulation in most cases. It is important to understand that in the presence of anodal capture it is impossible to advance LV activation by V–V interval programming because the effective V–V interval remains at zero. The use of true bipolar LV leads eliminates all forms of RV anodal stimulation.

Triggered ventricular pacing

The triggered ventricular pacing mode, available in some devices, is a programmable option that attempts resynchronization by triggering a biventricular output immediately when the CRT device senses a spontaneous QRS complex within the programmed AV delay, or when it senses a pacemaker-defined ventricular premature complex. Because ventricular sensing in modern CRT devices is limited to the RV channel, only rhythms arising from the RV will be sensed early enough to possibly allow resynchronization by triggered LV pacing. Ectopic rhythms arising remotely from the RV lead will be sensed relatively late and, therefore, the delivered triggered stimulus may occur too late for effective electrical resynchronization. There are little hemodynamic data about the efficacy of triggered biventricular pacing. Preliminary evidence suggests that this process may be helpful in some patients with improvement of the aortic VTI.

Programming verification by exercise testing

Exercise testing in CRT patients is now technically less difficult, with the advent of wireless device telemetry. Exercise testing is helpful in the overall evaluation of CRT, particularly in patients with a suboptimal CRT response where no obvious cause is found at rest. An exercise test may reveal loss of capture, atrial undersensing, various arrhythmias, and the development of spontaneous AV conduction because of PR shortening or upper rate limitation. In the latter, the upper rate should be reprogrammed to ensure consistent biventricular capture with effort.

Exercise testing is vital in CRT patients with permanent atrial fibrillation who have not undergone ablation of the AV junction.

In CRT patients with severe chronotropic incompetence (defined by the failure to achieve 85% of the age-predicted heart rate, determined as 220 minus the patient's age in years) rate-adaptive pacing DDDR may provide incremental benefit on exercise capacity. An exercise test facilitates programming the rate-adaptive mode and its related parameters.

Effect of interventricular timing on the electrocardiogram of biventricular pacemakers

Contemporary biventricular devices permit some degree of hemodynamic adjustment by programming the interventricular interval, usually in various steps from LV ahead of RV or RV ahead of LV. In the absence of anodal stimulation, increasing the V–V interval gradually from 0 to 80 ms (LV first) will progressively increase the duration of the paced QRS complex and alter its morphology, with a larger R wave in lead V_1 indicating more dominant LV depolarization. The varying QRS configuration in lead V_1 with different V–V intervals may correlate with the hemodynamic response, but this has not been established.

RV anodal stimulation during biventricular pacing interferes with a programmed interventricular (V–V) delay aimed at optimizing cardiac resynchronization (often programmed with the LV preceding the RV), because RV anodal capture causes simultaneous RV and LV activation (the V–V interval becomes zero). In the presence of anodal stimulation, the ECG morphology and its duration will not change if the device is programmed with V–V intervals of 80, 60, and 40 ms (LV before RV). The delayed RV cathodal output (80, 60, 40 ms) then falls in the myocardial refractory period initiated by the preceding anodal stimulation. At V–V intervals $\leq$ 20 ms, the paced QRS may change because the short LV–RV interval prevents propagation of activation from the site of RV anodal capture in time to render the cathodal site refractory. Thus, the cathode also captures the RV and contributes to RV depolarization, which then takes place from two sites: RV anode and RV cathode.

Programming the optimal AV delay

The atrioventricular (AV) interval during AV sequential pacing influences LV systolic performance by modulating preload. The influence of the AV delay appears to be less important than the proper choice of LV pacing site. The majority of the acute and long-term benefit from CRT is independent of the programmed AV interval. Nevertheless, programming of the left-sided AV delay is important in CRT patients. Appropriate AV interval timing can maximize CRT benefit, and if programmed poorly it has the potential to curtail the beneficial effects. Optimization will not convert a non-responder (according to strict definitions) to a responder, but may convert an under-responder to improved status.

The optimal AV delay in CRT patients exhibits great variability from patient to patient. This suggests that an empirically programmed AV delay interval is suboptimal in many patients. Thus, empiric programming of the AV delay is generally not recommended. One should always aim for atrial sensing, which is, as a rule, hemodynamically more favorable than atrial pacing. Thus the lower rate is often programmed to a relatively slow value. Optimized AV synchrony is achieved by the AV delay setting that provides the best left atrial contribution to LV filling, the maximum stroke volume, shortening of the isovolemic contraction time, and the longest diastolic filling time in the absence of diastolic mitral regurgitation (in patients with a long PR interval).

In clinical practice there are many techniques for optimizing the AV delay, as well as great variability in their use. The techniques include invasive (LV or aortic dP/dt max) and non-invasive techniques (largely echocardiography). AV optimization in DDD(R) pacemakers has traditionally been achieved using non-invasive Doppler echocardiography, which still remains widely used in CRT patients for acute and long-term hemodynamic assessment. However, Doppler echocardiographic methods for AV optimization in CRT patients vary substantially in performance. They include analysis of mitral, LV outflow tract, and aortic blood flow velocity profiles using conventional pulsed and continuous-wave Doppler techniques, and determination of dP/dt as derived from the continuous-wave Doppler profile of mitral regurgitation. Non-echocardiographic techniques include radionuclide angiography, impedance cardiography, plethysmography, and data from a peak endocardial acceleration sensor incorporated into a pacing lead.

Echocardiographic techniques for AV (and V–V) optimization require experienced personnel and are time-consuming. Furthermore, CRT optimization by echocardiography is sensitive to intra- and interobserver variability. The best method of measuring or assessing the effects of AV interval programming in terms of accuracy, cost, rapidity, ease, and perhaps full automaticity, remains to be defined, but a recently developed semi-automatic method holds great promise (discussed later).

Long-term evaluation of the AV delay

The optimal follow-up and long-term programming of the AV delay is uncertain. There is evidence suggesting that the optimal AV and V–V intervals change with time in patients undergoing CRT. Biventricular stimulation will result in LV reverse remodeling, with changes in LV end-diastolic and end-systolic volumes and pressures over time. This dynamic process also includes autonomic changes, and it may take several months before a new steady state of maximum improvement in LV function is reached. The status of AV interval optimization should therefore be assessed periodically. Further studies are needed to determine how often the AV interval needs to be optimized.

Intra- and interatrial conduction delay

Intra- and interatrial conduction delay are now being recognized as important abnormalities in patients with heart failure who are candidates for CRT. These abnormalities of conduction should be suspected in patients with extensive atrial myocardial disease, absent atrial electrical activity or low electrogram amplitudes, and in patients who underwent surgical procedures such as mitral valve replacement and a maze procedure.

Interatrial conduction delay

Interatrial conduction delay is characterized by a wide and notched P wave (> 120 ms), traditionally in ECG lead II, associated with a wide terminal negative deflection in lead V_1. The latter is commonly labeled left atrial enlargement, though it reflects left atrial conduction disease. Interatrial conduction time is also measured as the activation time from the high right atrium or onset of the P wave to the distal coronary sinus (60–85 ms). In the presence of interatrial conduction delay with late left atrial activation, left atrial contraction occurs late, and even during LV systole. Consequently, the need to program a long AV delay to adjust for delayed left atrial contraction can preclude ventricular resynchronization because of the emergence of competing spontaneous AV conduction. The incidence of interatrial conduction delay in patients who are candidates for CRT is unknown. When the ECG suggests interatrial conduction delay, it would be wise to look for delayed left atrial activation at the time of CRT implantation by showing that the conduction time from the right atrium to the left atrium is longer than the conduction time from the right atrium to the ventricles (onset of the QRS complex).

In the presence of interatrial conduction delay, one should consider placing the atrial lead in the high septum (Brachmann's bundle) or low interatrial septum or proximal coronary sinus where pacing produces a more simultaneous activation of both atria and abbreviates total atrial activation time judged by a decrease in P wave duration. In the presence of established CRT with an atrial lead in the right atrial appendage, restoration of mechanical left-sided AV synchrony requires simultaneous bi-atrial pacing performed by the implantation of a second atrial lead, either in the proximal coronary sinus or low atrium near the coronary sinus to preempt left atrial systole. Ablation of the AV junction permits control of the AV delay to promote mechanical left-sided AV synchrony.

Intra-atrial conduction delay (late atrial sensing)

In some patients with right intra-atrial conduction delay, conduction from the sinus node to the right atrial appendage (site of atrial sensing) is delayed in the absence of significant conduction delay from the sinus node to the AV junction or to the left atrium. The clinical incidence of this entity and its association with interatrial conduction delay are unknown. In this situation, left atrial activation may take place or may even be complete by the time the device senses the right atrial electrogram. The AS–VS interval (AS = atrial sensed event, VS = ventricular sensed event) becomes quite short because AS is delayed but VS is not. Thus, in CRT patients, it may be impossible to program an optimal AV delay without interference from a comparatively early VS event, because of the emergence of competing spontaneous conduction. In such a cases VS produces potentially harmful ventricular fusion or incomplete cardiac resynchronization. Thus, one is often forced to program unphysiologically short sensed AV delays, and possibly long paced AV delays, to adjust for the delay associated with first-degree pacemaker exit block. In a difficult situation, ablation of the fast pathway of the AV node or complete AV junctional ablation can be performed with satisfactory result. This approach is similar to the use of pacing in patients with hypertrophic obstructive cardiomyopathy and a short PR interval, where AV junctional ablation is the only way to ensure complete pacemaker-induced ventricular depolarization.

Fusion with the spontaneously conducted QRS complex: does it matter?

One study demonstrated that LV dP/dt max was higher with LV than with biventricular pacing, provided that LV pacing was associated with ventricular fusion caused by intrinsic activation via the right bundle branch. The clinical implications of this study are unclear. It is currently impossible to obtain sustained LV stimulation with a stable degree of fusion, because of perturbation of intrinsic conduction related to autonomic factors. As present, it is best to program the AV delay to minimize ventricular fusion with spontaneous ventricular activity until more data are available, and a reliable way is found to synchronize right bundle branch activity or unpaced RV sensed events with LV stimulation. The hemodynamic impact of fusion cannot as yet be predicted. It may be beneficial and inevitable in some patients with a short PR interval, but it may also carry the risk of incomplete resynchronization. Indeed, in some patients the elimination of fusion may be hemodynamically beneficial. In patients with a short PR interval, optimization of the AV interval may be suboptimal or impossible at short AV delays without fusion. Therefore, a relatively longer (possibly hemodynamically more favorable) AV interval associated with fusion may be programmed on a trial basis in a patient with a suboptimal CRT response.

Programming the interventricular (V–V) interval

The usefulness of programming the V–V interval is controversial, in view of two recent trials showing no benefit. Despite the negative results in these recent trials, V–V interval optimization may prove beneficial in some heart-failure patients with a suboptimal CRT response. In most patients, V–V interval optimization produces a rather limited improvement in LV function and/or stroke volume, but in individual patients it may lead to significant benefit. V–V interval optimization should decrease LV dyssynchrony, provide more simultaneous LV activation with faster LV emptying and longer diastolic filling, possibly increase LV ejection fraction, and reduce mitral regurgitation in some patients. V–V programmability may also partially compensate for less than optimal LV lead position by tailoring ventricular timing, and it may correct for individual heterogeneous ventricular activation patterns commonly found in patients with LV dysfunction and heart failure. V–V interval optimization can be viewed as the individual adjustment of left and right ventricular AV intervals, and its benefit is additive to AV interval optimization.

Programming of the V–V interval is guided by the same techniques as AV delay optimization. Determination of the extent of residual LV dyssynchrony after V–V programming requires more sophisticated echocardiographic techniques such as tissue Doppler imaging. Contemporary biventricular ICD devices permit programming of the V–V interval usually in steps from 0 to +80 ms (LV first) and from 0 to +80 ms (RV first), to optimize LV hemodynamics. The V–V interval is zero for simultaneous LV and RV pacing. Programmability of the V–V interval is based on evidence that CRT with sequential rather than simultaneous pacing of the two ventricles yields the best mechanical efficiency.

Optimized V–V intervals show great patient-to-patient variability and usually cannot be identified clinically in the majority of patients. Consequently, adjustment of the V–V interval, like the AV interval, must be individualized. The range of optimal V–V intervals is relatively narrow, most commonly involving LV pre-excitation by 20 ms. RV pre-excitation should be used cautiously, because advancing RV activation may cause a decline of LV function. Consequently, RV pre-excitation should be reserved for patients with LV dyssynchrony in the septal and inferior segments provided there is hemodynamic proof of benefit. Patients with ischemic cardiomyopathy (with slower conducting scars) may require more pre-excitation than those with idiopathic dilated cardiomyopathy. V–V programming is of particular benefit in patients with a previous myocardial infarction.

Prior to performing V–V interval optimization, consideration should be given to pacing lead configuration, the presence of anodal capture (which forces the V–V interval to 0), and manufacturer-related differences of V–V timing. Further, careful analysis of the 12-lead ECG during RV, LV, and biventricular pacing is crucial.

Impact of V–V interval programming on the effective AV delay: differences between device manufacturers

V–V interval programming allows separate programming of the RV and LV AV delays. In most devices (all American manufacturers except Boston Scientific/Guidant) the ventricular channel advanced by V–V interval programming will be paced at the programmed AS/AP delay. In Boston Scientific (Guidant) devices AS/AP timing seen on the programmer applies to the RV channel, and if LV activation is advanced by V–V interval programming, the LV/AV delay can be calculated by subtracting the V–V interval from the AS/AP delay.

Latency and delayed intra- and interventricular conduction

In some CRT patients, lack of hemodynamic improvement may be due to imbalance between RV and LV electrical activation related to variations of electrical excitability and impulse propagation such as electrical latency, slow impulse propagation in proximity of the lead (due to scar), or more globally delayed intra- and interventricular conduction.

The interval from the pacemaker stimulus to the onset of the earliest paced QRS complex on the 12-lead ECG is called latency, and during RV pacing this interval normally measures < 40 ms.

Prolonged LV latency intervals during stimulation from within epicardial cardiac veins may be due to interposed venous tissue and epicardial fat preventing direct contact between electrode and LV myocardium, and/or an overlying scar. Inferolateral akinesis or severe hypokinesis may be associated with prolonged LV latency intervals involving the area of the LV lead implantation site. This is concordant with recent reports about low response rates to CRT in patients with LV dyssynchrony and posterolateral scar, as demonstrated by echocardiography and contrast-enhanced magnetic resonance imaging. Delayed LV depolarization related to latency during simultaneous biventricular pacing (V–V = 0 ms) generates an ECG pattern dominated by RV stimulation. Advancing LV stimulation via a programmable interventricular (V–V) delay, or programming the device to monochamber LV pacing, can result in immediate hemodynamic and symptomatic improvement. Increasing the LV ventricular stimulus output decreases inter-ventricular conduction time in patients with biventricular pacing systems. Increasing output strength in all likelihood depolarizes larger volumes of myocardium by creating a larger virtual electrode, and this may be of particular importance during pacing of diseased myocardium.

Optimization of V–V timing using the electrocardiogram

RV and LV latency intervals on the ECG are measured at a speed of 50–100 mm/s and use the difference between LV and RV latency intervals as the value to program the V–V interval. In patients with long LV latency intervals, programming of incremental left-to-right ventricular (V–V) delays can unmask a dominant R wave in lead V_1 during biventricular pacing and may guide the selection of a V–V delay that yields balanced left and right ventricular depolarization. The accuracy and validity of these electrocardiographic methods for V–V interval optimization requires further investigation.

A simple ECG method was recently published which compares the time difference of the interval from the pacing spike to the beginning of the fast deflection of the QRS complex in leads V_1, V_2 during pacing from the LV (T_1), and from the RV (T_2). The T_2–T_1 interval was considered as a surrogate measurement of interventricular delay and defined as the best V–V, and this was compared to three echocardiographic measurements of LV synchrony at V–V interval setting of −30, 0, and +30 ms. Echo results had an 83% coincidence with the ECG method ($r = 0.81$, $P < 0.001$). The investigators concluded that the time difference in the fast ventricular depolarization observed between RV and LV stimulation on the surface ECG shows a good correlation with echocardiographic V–V optimization.

Semi-automatic optimization of AV and V–V intervals

QuickOpt Timing Cycle Optimization (St. Jude) runs an automatic sequence of intracardiac EGM measurements and displays on the programmer the optimal AV and V–V intervals in 90 seconds. The system uses an exclusive algorithm to calculate the optimal timing values. These values are then programmed manually into the CRT device. QuickOpt optimization was found to be consistently comparable to a traditional echocardiographic procedure for determining optimal AV and V–V delays. Another system (SmartAVDelay™), recently introduced by Boston Scientific (Guidant), also permits rapid programmer-based determination of the AV delay. The algorithm also uses a formula based on intracardiac electrograms that accurately predicts the AV delay associated with the maximum LV dP/dt. The device measures the sensed and paced AV delays (AS–VS and AP–VS). It also measures the interventricular conduction interval between the RV and LV electrograms in the case of a bipolar LV lead, whereupon the system provides the optimal AV delay automatically. The duration of the surface QRS complex is used in the semi-automatic function if the LV lead is unipolar. A further programming adjustment is required if the LV lead is not in the correct site. This system does not evaluate the V–V delay, which has to be programmed before determining the optimal AV delay. The sensed and paced AV delays are individually determined, in contrast to the St. Jude system, which calculates the paced AV delay by adding 50 ms to the optimal sensed AV delay.

Most CRT patients do not undergo AV and V–V optimization by traditional methods because echocardiographic optimization typically takes a long time and is expensive. These new systems based on intracardiac electrograms allow efficient and frequent optimization of AV and V–V intervals and can even be used when the device is being programmed before leaving the surgical suite. Although preliminary data are encouraging further study of these automatic or semi-automatic AV and V–V optimization based on intracardiac electrograms is needed.

Atrial fibrillation and atrial tachyarrhythmia

Many patients undergoing CRT have a history of paroxysmal atrial tachyarrhythmias, often associated with a rapid ventricular response that inhibits CRT delivery. Heart rate may be controlled at rest but not during exercise, and even if the mean heart rate is pharmacologically controlled, pronounced RR variability of conducted beats may decrease the number of resynchronized beats. Atrial fibrillation and atrial tachyarrhythmias should be aggressively treated, and if long-term sinus rhythm cannot be achieved, AV junctional ablation should be performed. In this respect, one should not be misled by what appears to be a satisfactory percentage of stored paced beats, because many could be fusion and/or pseudofusion beats unrelated to effective electrical resynchronization. Heart-failure patients with permanent AF treated with CRT show sustained long-term improvements of LV function and functional capacity similar to patients in sinus rhythm, but only if AV junctional ablation is performed.

Some devices have programmable algorithms that increase the percentage of biventricular pacing during AF so as to promote some degree of rate regularization and CRT (without an overall increase in the ventricular rate), by dynamic matching with the patient's own ventricular responses (up to the programmed maximum tracking rate). Activation of this algorithm does not result in ventricular rate control, and should not be a substitute for AV junctional ablation. Automatic mode switching should be activated, and is particularly important in patients with relatively slow conduction to the ventricle. Some devices have a lower rate interval that may be set separately during mode switching with the intention of increasing the percentage of biventricular pacing by virtue of a relatively fast pacing rate during the DDI mode. There is no need to program mode switching in patients without a history of atrial tachyarrhythmias, because possible far-field R-wave sensing may cause repeated automatic mode switching and electrical desynchronization in some devices when the base rate in the DDI mode is not particularly fast.

Congestive heart failure after CRT

Reduction of diuretics is important after CRT in patients with near-optimal LV filling pressures and an adequate diuresis to prevent prerenal azotemia, which may mask or delay the benefit of CRT. The dose of beta-blockers can be increased after CRT, and this may be successful in patients with previous intolerance. Few, if any, patients respond to CRT alone, and thus CRT cannot substitute for medical management. The combination of device therapy and optimal medical therapy provides synergistic effects to enhance reverse LV remodeling and long-term survival. The occurrence of CHF after CRT requires a comprehensive investigation (Table 27).

Table 27. Poor response to CRT.

- LV lead dislodgment or high threshold
- LV lead in the anterior cardiac vein
- LV lead on non-viable myocardium
- No LV dyssynchrony despite wide QRS
- Irreversible mitral regurgitation
- Long AV delay
- Suboptimal AV delay and/or V–V delay
- Atrial tachyarrhythmias with fast ventricular rate
- Frequent VPCs
- Severely impaired myocardial function
- Comorbidities
- Too strict a definition of positive response

Investigation of recurrent heart failure

1. A CRT non-responder should initially be evaluated for the development of atrial fibrillation, or cardiac ischemia, with a view to consider revascularization. Rate control, including AV node ablation or electrical cardioversion to restore normal sinus rhythm, is essential in patients who develop atrial fibrillation.
2. Evaluate LV lead for loss of capture.
3. Evaluate the percentage of biventricular paced beats from device memory.
4. Optimization of AV and V–V intervals may provide some improvement within a short period of time.
5. Echocardiographic evaluation of LV dyssynchrony. If significant intraventricular dyssynchrony is still present, then lead repositioning should be considered, using epicardial placement if necessary.
6. Persistent symptoms despite correction of LV dyssynchrony require evaluation for severe mitral regurgitation. Mitral valve surgery offers

symptomatic improvement to patients even with poor LV function, and should be considered in selected patients with persistent significant mitral regurgitation.

CRT device monitoring of heart failure

A variety of measurements by an ICD can be very useful in the management of CHF patients. It is believed that early diagnosis and treatment of impending CHF may reduce progression of LV dysfunction and mortality. Hence the importance of periodic remote monitoring. In this respect, it is interesting that patients may experience rather subtle symptoms 7–21 days before the clinical development of CHF. During this period, remote monitoring a number of parameters permits early diagnosis before clinical manifestations. One manufacturer provides the capability of remote transmission of blood pressure and weight.

Intrathoracic impedance

This function (not yet available in pacemakers) is pertinent to CRT patients, who often receive an ICD as part of a CRT system (CRT-D). Fluids conduct electricity more easily than solids. Fluid accumulation in the lungs leads to decreased intrathoracic impedance and increased conductivity. A Medtronic device can track thoracic fluid status by the emission of low-amplitude electrical pulses to measure transthoracic impedance between the coil of the RV lead and the can of a CRT device or ICD (OptiVol™). This measurement is made multiple times each day. The OptiVol fluid status monitoring system collects impedance signals between 12 pm and 6 pm, as this time period was shown earlier to best reflect fluid accumulation. Measures of LV end-diastolic pressure correlate inversely with impedance values.

This impedance level is averaged once a day to create a reference range, known as the OptiVol Fluid Index™, which is a surrogate of impedance. The fluid index represents the accumulation of consecutive day-to-day differences between daily and reference impedance. The physician can select a threshold for notification of decreased impedance for each patient, based on stored values. The fluid index rises as the impedance level drops from increased fluid in the lungs. An audible alert is available when the fluid index reaches a certain threshold. Abnormal values can occur 2 weeks before clinical deterioration. The cause of the abnormal findings must be investigated, as it may be due to recent-onset atrial fibrillation. Remote monitoring with the OptiVol feature can result in early treatment during the pre-clinical stage of heart-failure decompensation, and can lead to a significant reduction of hospital admissions for heart failure. The ICD provides a heart-failure management report with 14-month trends of AT/AF burden, ventricular rate during AF, heart-rate variability, patient activity, and night/day heart rates.

Heart-rate variability

Heart rate varies from heartbeat to heartbeat. Heart-rate variability (HRV) is the beat-to-beat variation in heart rate (between successive heartbeats, i.e., RR intervals), and provides an indirect indicator of autonomic status and neurohormonal activation, an important pathophysiologic factor in a number of cardiovascular disease states and heart failure. HRV of a well-conditioned heart is generally large at rest. During exercise, HRV decreases as the heart rate and exercise intensity increase. A reduction in HRV is a marker for reduced vagal activity. HRV reduction implies enhanced sympathetic activity, and it is lower in patients with high mortality and hospitalization risk. HRV software, which can record daily measures of HRV, is incorporated into many of the newer CRT devices. In a dual chamber device HRV is calculated from atrial sensed activity, while in a single chamber ICD it is derived from the RR intervals. As the neurohormonal system responds to detected changes in LV function before the patient experiences symptoms, HRV data may be useful for predicting a worsening condition and possibly preventing a hospital admission. Device-measured HRV parameters and patient outcomes improve significantly after CRT. Lack of HRV improvement 4 weeks after CRT identifies patients at higher risk for major cardiovascular events. One must remember that new AF can also cause abnormal HRV. At this time, HRV is not much used in the real world.

Activity

An activity sensor (piezoelectric or accelerometer) detects body movement and reflects patient daily physical activity. The data can be registered even if the rate-adaptive pacing mode is not programmed. The accuracy of using activity data to predict heart failure is dependent on the patient, and partly on the type of activities. The level of activity may not decrease early enough before the onset of decompensation, especially in patients with severe heart failure, who are mostly sedentary. In CRT patients, an increase in recorded activity represents a good symptomatic response and CRT efficiency, associated with a parallel improvement in the quality of life and NYHA class. Activity data may be important when deciding whether a patient can go back to work.

Nocturnal heart rate

Nocturnal heart rate is important in patients with CHF. An increase in nocturnal heart rate may be a sign of impeding decompensation. If the sinus rate is higher than expected (e.g., 90 bpm), a CHF patient requires more beta-blocker therapy. Nocturnal rate monitoring may also pick up unsuspected episodes of atrial fibrillation.

Arrhythmias after CRT

Atrial arrhythmias

A history of AF before CRT is associated with a higher risk of death. Spontaneous conversion of AF to sinus rhythm occurs in a minority of patients with permanent AF. CRT appears to reduce AF in patients with a prior AF history. This may be related to the significant improvement in LV systolic function and reduction in mitral regurgitation. In this respect, improvement in left atrial size and function after CRT is associated with a lower incidence of new AF. When compared to the patients who maintain sinus rhythm, patients with new-onset AF after CRT show less reverse remodeling, less improvement in LV function, more hospitalizations for heart failure, and increased mortality. Cardioversion of permanent AF should be done only 3–6 months after the initiation of CRT, when remodeling has stabilized. Cardioversion may be preceded by therapy with amiodarone or dofetilide.

Implantation of an atrial lead may be considered despite the presence of permanent AF for the following reasons: (1) it provides atrial monitoring capability, especially useful in patients with an ICD; (2) although CRT rarely induces spontaneous conversion of atrial fibrillation, electrical cardioversion may become an option after the establishment of significant LV and left atrial reverse remodeling. Lack of AV synchrony with the return of sinus rhythm carries the risk of pacemaker syndrome.

Ventricular arrhythmias

Ventricular proarrhythmia after CRT may present either as sustained monomorphic VT or rarely as polymorphic VT (torsades de pointes), precipitated mainly by epicardial (in the coronary venous system) LV and to a lesser degree by biventricular pacing. VT induced by LV pacing alone can be eliminated by turning off LV pacing, and some cases of LV-induced VT may sometimes be suppressed during biventricular pacing. In some patients, the induction of monomorphic VT by LV or biventricular pacing represents an exacerbation of a previously controlled arrhythmia, but in others it appears de novo. In contrast, torsades de pointes are caused by a different mechanism related to amplified transmural dispersion of repolarization associated with QT prolongation. This is due to enhanced transmural dispersion of repolarization (as in the long QT syndrome) induced by LV epicardial pacing. Fortunately, torsades de pointes are rare.

Appendix: guidelines

American guidelines for pacemaker implantation

Epstein AE, DiMarco JP, Ellenbogen KA, *et al.* ACC/AHA/HRS 2008 guidelines for device-based therapy of cardiac rhythm abnormalities: a report of the American College of Cardiology/American Heart Association Task Force on Practice Guidelines (Writing Committee to Revise the ACC/AHA/NASPE 2002 Guideline Update for Implantation of Cardiac Pacemakers and Antiarrhythmia Devices) developed in collaboration with the American Association for Thoracic Surgery and Society of Thoracic Surgeons. *J Am Coll Cardiol* 2008; **51**: e1–62.

The text that follows is an extract from the published guideline, reproduced with the permission of the American Heart Association. The full guideline, regularly updated, is available online at http://content.onlinejacc.org/cgi/content/full/51/21/e1.

Levels of evidence

Level A	Data derived from multiple randomized clinical trials or meta-analyses Multiple populations evaluated
Level B	Data derived from a single randomized trial or non-randomized studies Limited populations evaluated
Level C	Only consensus opinion of experts, case studies, or standard of care Very limited populations evaluated

Recommendations for permanent pacing in sinus node dysfunction

CLASS I

1. Permanent pacemaker implantation is indicated for sinus node dysfunction (SND) with documented symptomatic bradycardia, including frequent sinus pauses that produce symptoms. *(Level of evidence: C)*
2. Permanent pacemaker implantation is indicated for symptomatic chronotropic incompetence. *(Level of evidence: C)*
3. Permanent pacemaker implantation is indicated for symptomatic sinus bradycardia that results from required drug therapy for medical conditions. *(Level of evidence: C)*

Classification of recommendations

Class I	Class IIa	Class IIb	Class III
Benefit >>> Risk	Benefit >> Risk Additional studies with focused objectives needed	Benefit ≥ Risk Additional studies with broad objectives needed; Additional registry data would be helpful	Risk ≥ Benefit No additional studies needed
Procedure/ treatment SHOULD be performed/ administered	IT IS REASONABLE to perform procedure/administer treatment	Procedure/treatment MAY BE CONSIDERED	Procedure/treatment should NOT be performed/ administered SINCE IT IS NOT HELPFUL AND MAY BE HARMFUL

CLASS IIa

1. Permanent pacemaker implantation is reasonable for SND with heart rate less than 40 bpm when a clear association between significant symptoms consistent with bradycardia and the actual presence of bradycardia has not been documented. *(Level of evidence: C)*
2. Permanent pacemaker implantation is reasonable for syncope of unexplained origin when clinically significant abnormalities of sinus node function are discovered or provoked in electrophysiological studies. *(Level of evidence: C)*

CLASS IIb

1. Permanent pacemaker implantation may be considered in minimally symptomatic patients with chronic heart rate less than 40 bpm while awake. *(Level of evidence: C)*

CLASS III

1. Permanent pacemaker implantation is not indicated for SND in asymptomatic patients. *(Level of evidence: C)*
2. Permanent pacemaker implantation is not indicated for SND in patients for whom the symptoms suggestive of bradycardia have been clearly documented to occur in the absence of bradycardia. *(Level of evidence: C)*
3. Permanent pacemaker implantation is not indicated for SND with symptomatic bradycardia due to nonessential drug therapy. *(Level of evidence: C)*

Recommendations for acquired atrioventricular block in adults

CLASS I

1. Permanent pacemaker implantation is indicated for third-degree and advanced second-degree AV block at any anatomic level associated with bradycardia with symptoms (including heart failure) or ventricular arrhythmias presumed to be due to AV block. *(Level of evidence: C)*
2. Permanent pacemaker implantation is indicated for third-degree and advanced second-degree AV block at any anatomic level associated with arrhythmias and other medical conditions that require drug therapy that results in symptomatic bradycardia. *(Level of evidence: C)*
3. Permanent pacemaker implantation is indicated for third-degree and advanced second-degree AV block at any anatomic level in awake, symptom-free patients in sinus rhythm, with documented periods of asystole greater than or equal to 3.0 seconds or any escape rate less than 40 bpm, or with an escape rhythm that is below the AV node. *(Level of evidence: C)*
4. Permanent pacemaker implantation is indicated for third-degree and advanced second-degree AV block at any anatomic level in awake, symptom-free patients with AF and bradycardia with one or more pauses of at least 5 seconds or longer. *(Level of evidence: C)*
5. Permanent pacemaker implantation is indicated for third-degree and advanced second-degree AV block at any anatomic level after catheter ablation of the AV junction. *(Level of evidence: C)*
6. Permanent pacemaker implantation is indicated for third-degree and advanced second-degree AV block at any anatomic level associated with postoperative AV block that is not expected to resolve after cardiac surgery. *(Level of evidence: C)*
7. Permanent pacemaker implantation is indicated for third-degree and advanced second-degree AV block at any anatomic level associated with neuromuscular diseases with AV block, such as myotonic muscular dystrophy, Kearns–Sayre syndrome, Erb dystrophy (limb-girdle muscular dystrophy), and peroneal muscular atrophy, with or without symptoms. *(Level of evidence: B)*
8. Permanent pacemaker implantation is indicated for second-degree AV block with associated symptomatic bradycardia regardless of type or site of block. *(Level of evidence: B)*
9. Permanent pacemaker implantation is indicated for asymptomatic persistent third-degree AV block at any anatomic site with average awake ventricular rates of 40 bpm or faster if cardiomegaly or LV dysfunction is present or if the site of block is below the AV node. *(Level of evidence: B)*
10. Permanent pacemaker implantation is indicated for second- or third-degree AV block during exercise in the absence of myocardial ischemia. *(Level of evidence: C)*

CLASS IIa

1. Permanent pacemaker implantation is reasonable for persistent third-degree AV block with an escape rate greater than 40 bpm in asymptomatic adult patients without cardiomegaly. *(Level of evidence: C)*
2. Permanent pacemaker implantation is reasonable for asymptomatic second-degree AV block at intra- or infra-His levels found at electrophysiological study. *(Level of evidence: B)*

3. Permanent pacemaker implantation is reasonable for first- or second-degree AV block with symptoms similar to those of pacemaker syndrome or hemodynamic compromise. *(Level of evidence: B)*
4. Permanent pacemaker implantation is reasonable for asymptomatic type II second-degree AV block with a narrow QRS. When type II second-degree AV block occurs with a wide QRS, including isolated right bundle-branch block, pacing becomes a Class I recommendation. *(Level of evidence: B)*

CLASS IIb

1. Permanent pacemaker implantation may be considered for neuromuscular diseases such as myotonic muscular dystrophy, Erb dystrophy (limb-girdle muscular dystrophy), and peroneal muscular atrophy with any degree of AV block (including first-degree AV block), with or without symptoms, because there may be unpredictable progression of AV conduction disease. *(Level of evidence: B)*
2. Permanent pacemaker implantation may be considered for AV block in the setting of drug use and/or drug toxicity when the block is expected to recur even after the drug is withdrawn. *(Level of evidence: B)*

CLASS III

1. Permanent pacemaker implantation is not indicated for asymptomatic first-degree AV block. *(Level of evidence: B)* (See section on Chronic Bifascicular Block.)
2. Permanent pacemaker implantation is not indicated for asymptomatic type I second-degree AV block at the supra-His (AV node) level or that which is not known to be intra- or infra-Hisian. *(Level of evidence: C)*
3. Permanent pacemaker implantation is not indicated for AV block that is expected to resolve and is unlikely to recur (e.g., drug toxicity, Lyme disease, or transient increases in vagal tone or during hypoxia in sleep apnea syndrome in the absence of symptoms). *(Level of evidence: B)*

Recommendations for permanent pacing in chronic bifascicular block

CLASS I

1. Permanent pacemaker implantation is indicated for advanced second-degree AV block or intermittent third-degree AV block. *(Level of evidence: B)*
2. Permanent pacemaker implantation is indicated for type II second-degree AV block. *(Level of evidence: B)*
3. Permanent pacemaker implantation is indicated for alternating bundle-branch block. *(Level of evidence: C)*

CLASS IIa

1. Permanent pacemaker implantation is reasonable for syncope not demonstrated to be due to AV block when other likely causes have been excluded, specifically ventricular tachycardia (VT). *(Level of evidence: B)*
2. Permanent pacemaker implantation is reasonable for an incidental finding at electrophysiological study of a markedly prolonged HV interval (greater than or equal to 100 milliseconds) in asymptomatic patients. *(Level of evidence: B)*
3. Permanent pacemaker implantation is reasonable for an incidental finding at electrophysiological study of pacing-induced infra- His block that is not physiological. *(Level of evidence: B)*

CLASS IIb

1. Permanent pacemaker implantation may be considered in the setting of neuromuscular diseases such as myotonic muscular dystrophy, Erb dystrophy (limb-girdle muscular dystrophy), and peroneal muscular atrophy with bifascicular block or any fascicular block, with or without symptoms. *(Level of evidence: C)*

CLASS III

1. Permanent pacemaker implantation is not indicated for fascicular block without AV block or symptoms. *(Level of evidence: B)*
2. Permanent pacemaker implantation is not indicated for fascicular block with first-degree AV block without symptoms. *(Level of evidence: B)*

Acute phase of myocardial infarction

CLASS I

1. Permanent ventricular pacing is indicated for persistent second-degree AV block in the His–Purkinje system with alternating bundle-branch block or third-degree AV block within or

below the His–Purkinje system after ST-segment elevation MI. *(Level of evidence: B)*

2. Permanent ventricular pacing is indicated for transient advanced second- or third-degree infranodal AV block and associated bundle-branch block. If the site of block is uncertain, an electrophysiological study may be necessary. *(Level of evidence: B)*
3. Permanent ventricular pacing is indicated for persistent and symptomatic second- or third-degree AV block. *(Level of evidence: C)*

CLASS IIb

1. Permanent ventricular pacing may be considered for persistent second- or third-degree AV block at the AV node level, even in the absence of symptoms. *(Level of evidence: B)*

CLASS III

1. Permanent ventricular pacing is not indicated for transient AV block in the absence of intraventricular conduction defects. *(Level of evidence: B)*
2. Permanent ventricular pacing is not indicated for transient AV block in the presence of isolated left anterior fascicular block. *(Level of evidence: B)*
3. Permanent ventricular pacing is not indicated for new bundle-branch block or fascicular block in the absence of AV block. *(Level of evidence: B)*
4. Permanent ventricular pacing is not indicated for persistent asymptomatic first-degree AV block in the presence of bundle-branch or fascicular block. *(Level of evidence: B)*

Recommendations for permanent pacing in hypersensitive carotid sinus syndrome and neurocardiogenic syncope

CLASS I

1. Permanent pacing is indicated for recurrent syncope caused by spontaneously occurring carotid sinus stimulation and carotid sinus pressure that induces ventricular asystole of more than 3 seconds. *(Level of evidence: C)*

CLASS IIa

1. Permanent pacing is reasonable for syncope without clear, provocative events and with a hypersensitive cardioinhibitory response of 3 seconds or longer. *(Level of evidence: C)*

CLASS IIb

1. Permanent pacing may be considered for significantly symptomatic neurocardiogenic syncope associated with bradycardia documented spontaneously or at the time of tilt-table testing. *(Level of evidence: B)*

CLASS III

1. Permanent pacing is not indicated for a hypersensitive cardioinhibitory response to carotid sinus stimulation without symptoms or with vague symptoms. *(Level of evidence: C)*
2. Permanent pacing is not indicated for situational vasovagal syncope in which avoidance behavior is effective and preferred. *(Level of evidence: C)*

Recommendations for pacing after cardiac transplantation

CLASS I

1. Permanent pacing is indicated for persistent inappropriate or symptomatic bradycardia not expected to resolve and for other Class I indications for permanent pacing. *(Level of evidence: C)*

CLASS IIb

1. Permanent pacing may be considered when relative bradycardia is prolonged or recurrent, which limits rehabilitation or discharge after postoperative recovery from cardiac transplantation. *(Level of evidence: C)*
2. Permanent pacing may be considered for syncope after cardiac transplantation even when bradyarrhythmia has not been documented. *(Level of evidence: C)*

Recommendations for pacing to prevent tachycardia

CLASS I

1. Permanent pacing is indicated for sustained pause-dependent VT, with or without QT prolongation. *(Level of evidence: C)*

CLASS IIa

1. Permanent pacing is reasonable for high-risk patients with congenital long QT syndrome. *(Level of evidence: C)*

CLASS IIb

1. Permanent pacing may be considered for prevention of symptomatic, drug-refractory, recurrent AF in patients with coexisting SND. *(Level of evidence: B)*

CLASS III

1. Permanent pacing is not indicated for frequent or complex ventricular ectopic activity without sustained VT in the absence of the long-QT syndrome. *(Level of evidence: C)*
2. Permanent pacing is not indicated for torsade de pointes VT due to reversible causes. *(Level of evidence: A)*

Recommendation for pacing to prevent atrial fibrillation

CLASS III

1. Permanent pacing is not indicated for the prevention of AF in patients without any other indication for pacemaker implantation. *(Level of evidence: B)*

Recommendations for pacing in patients with hypertrophic cardiomyopathy

CLASS I

1. Permanent pacing is indicated for SND or AV block in patients with HCM. *(Level of evidence: C)*

CLASS IIb

1. Permanent pacing may be considered in medically refractory symptomatic patients with HCM and significant resting or provoked LV outflow tract obstruction. *(Level of evidence: A)* As for Class I indications, when risk factors for SCD are present, consider a DDD ICD.

CLASS III

1. Permanent pacemaker implantation is not indicated for patients who are asymptomatic or whose symptoms are medically controlled. *(Level of evidence: C)*
2. Permanent pacemaker implantation is not indicated for symptomatic patients without evidence of LV outflow tract obstruction. *(Level of evidence: C)*

Recommendations for permanent pacing in children, adolescents, and patients with congenital heart disease

CLASS I

1. Permanent pacemaker implantation is indicated for advanced second- or third-degree AV block associated with symptomatic bradycardia, ventricular dysfunction, or low cardiac output. *(Level of evidence: C)*
2. Permanent pacemaker implantation is indicated for SND with correlation of symptoms during age-inappropriate bradycardia. The definition of bradycardia varies with the patient's age and expected heart rate. *(Level of evidence: B)*
3. Permanent pacemaker implantation is indicated for postoperative advanced second- or third-degree AV block that is not expected to resolve or that persists at least 7 days after cardiac surgery. *(Level of evidence: B)*
4. Permanent pacemaker implantation is indicated for congenital third-degree AV block with a wide QRS escape rhythm, complex ventricular ectopy, or ventricular dysfunction. *(Level of evidence: B)*
5. Permanent pacemaker implantation is indicated for congenital third-degree AV block in the infant with a ventricular rate less than 55 bpm or with congenital heart disease and a ventricular rate less than 70 bpm. *(Level of evidence: C)*

CLASS IIa

1. Permanent pacemaker implantation is reasonable for patients with congenital heart disease and sinus bradycardia for the prevention of recurrent episodes of intra-atrial reentrant tachycardia; SND may be intrinsic or secondary to antiarrhythmic treatment. *(Level of evidence: C)*
2. Permanent pacemaker implantation is reasonable for congenital third-degree AV block beyond the first year of life with an average heart rate less than 50 bpm, abrupt pauses in ventricular rate that are 2 or 3 times the basic cycle length, or associated with symptoms due to chronotropic incompetence. *(Level of evidence: B)*

3. Permanent pacemaker implantation is reasonable for sinus bradycardia with complex congenital heart disease with a resting heart rate less than 40 bpm or pauses in ventricular rate longer than 3 seconds. *(Level of evidence: C)*
4. Permanent pacemaker implantation is reasonable for patients with congenital heart disease and impaired hemodynamics due to sinus bradycardia or loss of AV synchrony. *(Level of evidence: C)*
5. Permanent pacemaker implantation is reasonable for unexplained syncope in the patient with prior congenital heart surgery complicated by transient complete heart block with residual fascicular block after a careful evaluation to exclude other causes of syncope. *(Level of evidence: B)*

CLASS IIb

1. Permanent pacemaker implantation may be considered for transient postoperative third-degree AV block that reverts to sinus rhythm with residual bifascicular block. *(Level of evidence: C)*
2. Permanent pacemaker implantation may be considered for congenital third-degree AV block in asymptomatic children or adolescents with an acceptable rate, a narrow QRS complex, and normal ventricular function. *(Level of evidence: B)*
3. Permanent pacemaker implantation may be considered for asymptomatic sinus bradycardia after biventricular repair of congenital heart disease with a resting heart rate less than 40 bpm or pauses in ventricular rate longer than 3 seconds. *(Level of evidence: C)*

CLASS III

1. Permanent pacemaker implantation is not indicated for transient postoperative AV block with return of normal AV conduction in the otherwise asymptomatic patient. *(Level of evidence: B)*
2. Permanent pacemaker implantation is not indicated for asymptomatic bifascicular block with or without first-degree AV block after surgery for congenital heart disease in the absence of prior transient complete AV block. *(Level of evidence: C)*
3. Permanent pacemaker implantation is not indicated for asymptomatic type I second-degree AV block. *(Level of evidence: C)*
4. Permanent pacemaker implantation is not indicated for asymptomatic sinus bradycardia with the longest relative risk interval less than 3 seconds and a minimum heart rate more than 40 bpm. *(Level of evidence: C)*

Recommendations for cardiac resynchronization therapy in patients with severe systolic heart failure

CLASS I

1. For patients who have LVEF less than or equal to 35%, a QRS duration greater than or equal to 0.12 seconds, and sinus rhythm, CRT with or without an ICD is indicated for the treatment of NYHA functional Class III or ambulatory Class IV heart-failure symptoms with optimal recommended medical therapy. *(Level of evidence: A)*

CLASS IIa

1. For patients who have LVEF less than or equal to 35%, a QRS duration greater than or equal to 0.12 seconds, and AF, CRT with or without an ICD is reasonable for the treatment of NYHA functional Class III or ambulatory Class IV heart failure symptoms on optimal recommended medical therapy. *(Level of evidence: B)*
2. For patients with LVEF less than or equal to 35% with NYHA functional Class III or ambulatory Class IV symptoms who are receiving optimal recommended medical therapy and who have frequent dependence on ventricular pacing, CRT is reasonable. *(Level of evidence: C)*

CLASS IIb

1. For patients with LVEF less than or equal to 35% with NYHA functional Class I or II symptoms who are receiving optimal recommended medical therapy and who are undergoing implantation of a permanent pacemaker and/or ICD with anticipated frequent ventricular pacing, CRT may be considered. *(Level of evidence: C)*

CLASS III

1. CRT is not indicated for asymptomatic patients with reduced LVEF in the absence of other indications for pacing. *(Level of evidence: B)*
2. CRT is not indicated for patients whose functional status and life expectancy are limited predominantly by chronic non-cardiac conditions. *(Level of evidence: C)*

European guidelines for pacemaker implantation

Vardas PE, Auricchio A, Blanc JJ, *et al*. Guidelines for cardiac pacing and cardiac resynchronization therapy. The Task Force for Cardiac Pacing and Cardiac Resynchronization Therapy of the European Society of Cardiology. Developed in collaboration with the European Heart Rhythm Association. *Eur Heart J* 2007; **28**: 2256–95.

The information that follows is extracted from the published guideline, reproduced with the permission of Oxford University Press.

Recommendations for cardiac pacing in sinus node disease (European)

Clinical indication	Class	Level of evidence
1. Sinus node disease manifests as symptomatic bradycardia with or without bradycardia-dependent tachycardia. Symptom–rhythm correlation must have been: • spontaneously occurring • drug induced where alternative drug therapy is lacking **2.** Syncope with sinus node disease, either spontaneously occurring or induced at electrophysiological study **3.** Sinus node disease manifests as symptomatic chronotropic incompetence: • spontaneously occurring • drug induced where alternative drug therapy is lacking	Class I	C
1. Symptomatic sinus node disease, which is either spontaneous or induced by a drug for which there is no alternative, but no symptom rhythm correlation has been documented. Heart rate at rest should be < 40 bpm **2.** Syncope for which no other explanation can be made but there are abnormal electrophysiological findings (CSNRT > 800 ms)	Class IIa	C
1. Minimally symptomatic patients with sinus node disease, resting heart rate <40 bpm while awake, and no evidence of chronotropic incompetence	Class IIb	C
1. Sinus node disease without symptoms including use of bradycardia-provoking drugs **2.** ECG findings of sinus node dysfunction with symptoms not due directly or indirectly to bradycardia **3.** Symptomatic sinus node dysfunction where symptoms can reliably be attributed to non-essential medication	Class III	C

When sinus node disease is diagnosed, atrial tachyarrhythmias are likely even if not yet recorded, implying that serious consideration should be given to anticoagulant therapy.

Recommendations for cardiac pacing in acquired atrioventricular block (European)

Clinical indication	Class	Level of evidence
1. Chronic symptomatic third- or second-degree (Mobitz I or II) atrioventricular block	Class I	C
2. Neuromuscular diseases (e.g. myotonic muscular dystrophy, Kearns–Sayre syndrome, etc.) with third- or second-degree atrioventricular block		B
3. Third- or second-degree (Mobitz I or II) atrioventricular block: (i) after catheter ablation of the atrioventricular junction; (ii) after valve surgery when the block is not expected to resolve		C
1. Asymptomatic third- or second-degree (Mobitz I or II) atrioventricular block	Class IIa	C
2. Symptomatic prolonged first-degree atrioventricular block		C
1. Neuromuscular diseases (e.g. myotonic muscular dystrophy, Kearns–Sayre syndrome, etc.) with first-degree atrioventricular block	Class IIb	B
1. Asymptomatic first-degree atrioventricular block **2.** Asymptomatic second-degree Mobitz I with supra-Hisian conduction block **3.** Atrioventricular block expected to resolve	Class III	C

Recommendations for cardiac pacing in chronic bifascicular and trifascicular block (European)

Clinical indication	Class	Level of evidence
1. Intermittent third-degree atrioventricular block **2.** Second-degree Mobitz II atrioventricular block **3.** Alternating bundle branch block **4.** Findings on electrophysiological study of markedly prolonged HV interval (≥ 100 ms) or pacing-induced infra-His block in patients with symptoms	Class I	C
1. Syncope not demonstrated to be due to atrioventricular block when other likely causes have been excluded, specifically ventricular tachycardia	Class IIa	B
2. Neuromuscular diseases (e.g. myotonic muscular dystrophy, Kearns–Sayre syndrome, etc.) with any degree of fascicular block		C
3. Incidental findings on electrophysiological study of markedly prolonged HV interval (≥ 100 ms) or pacing-induced infra-His block in patients without symptoms		C
None	Class IIb	
1. Bundle branch block without atrioventricular block or symptoms **2.** Bundle branch block with first-degree atrioventricular block without symptoms	Class III	B

Recommendations for permanent cardiac pacing in conduction disturbances related to acute myocardial infarction (European)

Clinical indication	Class	Level of evidence
1. Persistent third-degree heart block preceded or not by intraventricular conduction disturbances **2.** Persistent Mobitz type II second-degree heart block associated with bundle branch block, with or without PR prolongation **3.** Transient Mobitz type II second- or third-degree heart block associated with new onset bundle branch block	Class I	B
None	Class IIa	
None	Class IIb	
1. Transient second- or third-degree heart block without bundle branch block **2.** Left anterior hemiblock newly developed or present on admission **3.** Persistent first-degree atrioventricular block	Class III	B

Recommendations for cardiac pacing in carotid sinus syndrome (European)

Clinical indication	Class	Level of evidence
1. Recurrent syncope caused by inadvertent carotid sinus pressure and reproduced by carotid sinus massage, associated with ventricular asystole of more than 3 s duration (patient may be syncopal or pre-syncopal), in the absence of medication known to depress sinus node activity	Class I	C
1. Recurrent unexplained syncope, without clear inadvertent carotid sinus pressure, but syncope is reproduced by carotid sinus massage, associated with a ventricular asystole of more than 3 s duration (patient may be syncopal or pre-syncopal), in the absence of medication known to depress sinus node activity	Class IIa	B
1. First syncope, with or without clear inadvertent carotid sinus pressure, but syncope (or pre-syncope) is reproduced by carotid sinus massage, associated with a ventricular asystole of more than 3 s duration, in the absence of medication known to depress sinus node activity	Class IIb	C
1. Hypersensitive carotid sinus reflex without symptoms	Class III	C

Recommendations for cardiac pacing in vasovagal syncope (European)

Clinical indication	Class	Level of evidence
None	Class I	C
1. Patients over 40 years of age with recurrent severe vasovagal syncope who show prolonged asystole during ECG recording and/or tilt testing, after failure of other therapeutic options and being informed of the conflicting results of trials	Class IIa	C
1. Patients under 40 years of age with recurrent severe vasovagal syncope who show prolonged asystole during ECG recording and/or tilt testing, after failure of other therapeutic options and being informed of the conflicting results of trials	Class IIb	C
1. Patients without demonstrable bradycardia during reflex syncope	Class III	C

Recommendations for cardiac pacing in hypertrophic cardiomyopathy (European)

Clinical indication	Class	Level of evidence
None	Class I	
1. Symptomatic bradycardia due to beta-blockade when alternative therapies are unacceptable	Class IIa	C
1. Patients with drug refractory hypertrophic cardiomyopathy with significant resting or provoked LVOT gradient and contraindications for septal ablation or myectomy	Class IIb	A
1. Asymptomatic patients **2.** Symptomatic patients who do not have left ventricular outflow tract obstruction	Class III	C

Cardiac resynchronization therapy in patients with heart failure

Recommendations (European guidelines) for the use of cardiac resynchronization therapy by biventricular pacemaker (CRT-P) or biventricular pacemaker combined with an implantable cardioverter defibrillator (CRT-D) in heart-failure patients

Heart failure patients who remain symptomatic in NYHA classes III–IV despite OPT [optimal pharmacological treatment], with LVEF ≤ 35%, LV dilatation [LV dilatation/different criteria have been used to define LV dilatation in controlled studies on CRT: LV end-diastolic diameter > 55 mm; LV end-diastolic diameter > 30 mm/m^2; LV end-diastolic diameter > 30 mm/m (height)], normal sinus rhythm and wide QRS complex (≥ 120 ms).

- *Class I: level of evidence A* for CRT-P to reduce morbidity and mortality.
- CRT-D is an acceptable option for patients who have expectancy of survival with a good functional status for more than 1 year. *(Class I: level of evidence B)*

Recommendations for the use of biventricular pacing in heart-failure patients with a concomitant indication for permanent pacing

Heart failure patients with NYHA classes III–IV symptoms, low LVEF ≤ 35%, LV dilatation and a concomitant indication for permanent pacing (first implant or upgrading of conventional pacemaker). *(Class IIa: level of evidence C)*

Recommendations for the use of an implantable cardioverter defibrillator combined with biventricular pacemaker (CRT-D) in heart-failure patients with an indication for an implantable cardioverter defibrillator

Heart-failure patients with a Class I indication for an ICD (first implant or upgrading at device change) who are symptomatic in NYHA classes III–IV despite OPT, with low LVEF ≤ 35%, LV dilatation, wide QRS complex (≥ 120 ms). *(Class I: level of evidence B)*

Recommendations for the use of biventricular pacing in heart-failure patients with permanent atrial fibrillation

Heart failure patients who remain symptomatic in NYHA classes III–IV despite OPT, with low LVEF ≤ 35%, LV dilatation, permanent AF and indication for AV junction ablation. *(Class IIa: level of evidence C)*

Commentary

Acquired AV block

There are many causes of atrioventricular (AV) block, but progressive idiopathic fibrosis of the conduction system related to an aging process of the cardiac skeleton is the most common cause of chronic acquired AV block. Barring congenital AV block, Lyme disease is the commonest cause of reversible third-degree AV block in young individuals, and it is usually AV nodal. Before implantation of a permanent pacemaker, reversible causes of AV block such as Lyme disease, hypervagotonia, athletic heart, sleep apnea, ischemia, and drug, metabolic, or electrolytic imbalance must be excluded. The indications for permanent pacing in second- or third-degree AV block unlikely to regress are often straightforward in *symptomatic* patients, but they are more difficult in *asymptomatic* patients.

Complete AV block

The 2008 ACC/AHA/HRS guidelines (Appendix 1) designate *asymptomatic* complete AV block with ventricular escape rates > 40 bpm as a class II indication for pacing. The rate criterion of > 40 bpm is arbitrary and unnecessary. It is not the escape rate that is critical to stability, but rather the site of origin of the escape rhythm (junctional or ventricular). Rate instability may not be predictable or obvious. Irreversible acquired complete AV block should be a class I indication for pacing. In neuromuscular disease such as myotonic dystrophy, pacing should be considered much earlier in the course of the disease and offered to the asymptomatic patient once any conduction abnormality is noted and subsequent follow-up shows progression even when second-degree AV block has not yet developed. Waiting for the development of complete AV block may expose patients to a significant risk of syncope or even sudden death.

Second-degree AV block

Type I block and type II second-degree AV block are electrocardiographic patterns, and as such should not be automatically equated with the anatomic site of block.

Type I block (Wenckebach or Mobitz type I)

Type I second-degree AV block is defined as the occurrence of a *single* non-conducted sinus P wave associated with inconstant PR intervals before and after the blocked impulse, provided there are at least two consecutive conducted P waves (i.e., 3 : 2 AV block) to determine behavior of the PR interval. The PR interval after the blocked impulse is always shorter if conducted to the ventricle. The term "inconstant" PR or AV intervals is important, because the majority of type I sequences are atypical and do not conform to the traditional teaching about the mathematical behavior of the PR intervals. The description of "progressive" prolongation of the PR interval is misleading, because PR intervals may shorten or stabilize and show no discernible or measurable change anywhere in a type I sequence. Indeed, atypical type I structures in their terminal portion can exhibit a number of consecutive PR intervals showing no discernible change before the single blocked beat. In such an arrangement the post-block PR interval is always shorter. Slowing or an increase of the sinus rate does not interfere with the diagnosis of type I block.

Increments in AV conduction: Increments in AV conduction (AH interval) in Type I AV nodal block are typically large, but they may occasionally be so tiny that they superficially mimic type II second-degree AV block. Type I infranodal block typically exhibits small increments in AV conduction (HV interval) and large increments in AV conduction occur uncommonly.

Site of block: In *narrow QRS type I block*, the block is in the AV node in almost all the cases. Type I block can be physiological, especially during sleep in normal individuals with high vagal tone, and these people need no treatment. Asymptomatic type I second-degree AV block present throughout the day is generally considered benign. However, some workers in Britain recommend permanent pacing in this setting for prognostic reasons, based on long-term mortality data from a single center. We believe that these observations need to be confirmed before recommending pacing for this situation.

IntraHisian narrow QRS type I block is rare. In practice, cases of narrow QRS intraHisian type I block due to chronic conduction system disease are not usually found, because virtually all narrow QRS type I blocks are dismissed as being AV nodal. IntraHisian block, although rare clinically, may be provoked by exercise, in contrast to type I AV nodal block, which generally improves with exercise. Improvement of AV block with exercise is highly suggestive of AV nodal second-degree AV block. His bundle recordings are unnecessary in an asymptomatic patient with narrow QRS type I block. However, if an electrophysiologic study (performed for other reasons) in such a patient reveals infranodal block, a pacemaker should be recommended as a class I indication because diffuse His–Purkinje disease is likely to be present.

Type I second-degree AV block with bundle branch block (which is far less common than narrow QRS type I block) must not be automatically labeled as AV nodal. Outside of acute myocardial infarction, type I block and bundle branch block (QRS ≥ 0.12 s) occurs in the His–Purkinje system in 60–70% of the cases. In such cases exercise is likely to aggravate the degree of AV block. Yet many still believe that type I blocks are all AV nodal and therefore basically benign. It is believed that the prognosis of infranodal type I block is as serious as that of type II block, and a permanent pacemaker is generally recommended in both types regardless of symptoms. On this basis, patients with type I block and bundle branch block should undergo an invasive study to determine the level of second-degree block in the conduction system.

However, it is unknown whether underlying right bundle branch block (unifascicular block) is prognostically different from underlying left bundle branch block (bifascicular block) in the setting of asymptomatic type I second-degree infranodal block.

Type II block (Mobitz type II)

The definition of type II second-degree AV block continues to be problematic in clinical practice. Type II second-degree AV block is defined as the occurrence of a *single* non-conducted sinus P wave associated with constant PR intervals before and *after* the blocked impulse, provided the sinus rate or the PP interval is constant and there are at least two consecutive conducted P waves (i.e., 3 : 2 AV block) to determine behavior of the PR interval. The pause encompassing the blocked P wave should equal two (PP) cycles. The PR interval is either normal or prolonged but remains constant. Type II block cannot be diagnosed whenever a single blocked impulse is followed by a shortened post-block PR interval or no P wave at all. In this situation it is either a type I pattern or an unclassifiable sequence. Stability of the sinus rate is a very important criterion because a vagal surge can cause simultaneous sinus slowing and AV nodal block, generally a benign condition that can superficially resemble type II second-degree AV block. In the presence of sinus arrhythmia, the diagnosis of type II block may not be possible if there is sinus slowing, especially if the block occurs in one of the longer cycles. In contrast, the diagnosis of type II block is possible with an increasing sinus rate.

The 2002 and 2008 ACC/AHA/HRS guidelines use a new classification of type II second-degree AV block: wide QRS type II block (which makes up 65–80% of type II blocks) with a class I indication for pacing, and narrow QRS type II block with a class II indication for permanent pacing. This differentiation is strange, because there is no evidence that narrow QRS type II block is less serious than wide QRS type II block. The statement that "type II block is usually infranodal especially when the QRS is wide" may be the basis for this potentially misleading distinction. Type II block according to the strict definition is always infranodal and should be a class I indication regardless of QRS duration, symptoms, or whether it is paroxysmal or chronic.

The literature on the diagnosis of type II block is replete with errors, because the diagnostic importance of the rate criterion and need for an unchanged PR interval *after* a single blocked impulse are often ignored. A constant PR after the blocked beat is a *sine qua non* of type II block. The diagnosis of type II cannot be made if the P wave after a blocked impulse is not conducted with the same PR interval as all the other conducted P waves. The shorter PR interval after a single blocked P wave may caused either by improved conduction (type I block) or by AV dissociation due to an escape AV junctional beat that bears no relationship to the preceding P wave. In other words, type II second-degree AV block cannot be diagnosed whenever shortened AV interval occurs after the blocked P wave. In such a situation the pattern is either type I or unclassifiable. Type II block is sometimes described as having all the conducted PR intervals constant. There is an important loophole in this statement. It could be interpreted to mean that the behavior of the first P wave after the blocked impulse can be disregarded in the diagnosis. If the P wave is absent there is no opportunity to determine the behavior of the first PR interval after the blocked impulse, and the diagnosis of type II block cannot be established.

Site of block: Type II according to the strict definition occurs in the His–Purkinje system and rarely above the site of recording of the His bundle potential in the proximal His bundle or nodo-Hisian junction. Type II block has not yet been convincingly demonstrated in the N zone of the AV node. Most if not all the purported exceptions involve reports where type I blocks (shorter PR interval after the blocked beat) are claimed to be type II blocks by using loopholes in the definitions of second-degree AV block. Because type II invariably occurs in the His–Purkinje system, it should be a class I indication for pacing.

Type II second-degree AV block: true or false?

When confronted with a pattern that appears to be type II with a narrow QRS complex (especially in Holter recordings), one must consider the possibility of type I block without discernible or measurable increments in the PR intervals. Sinus slowing with AV block rules out type II block. Vagal AV block (discussed later) rarely involves more than block of two consecutive P waves. Difficulty arises when the sinus rate is stable. When a type II-like pattern with a narrow QRS complex occurs in association with type I sequences, true type II block can be safely excluded, because the coexistence of both types of block in the His bundle is almost unknown. True narrow QRS type II block occurs without sinus slowing and is typically associated with sustained advanced second-degree AV block far more commonly than type I block in association with true type II block. In other words, AV conduction ratios > 2 : 1 (3 : 1, 4 : 1) are rare in vagal block.

Fixed-ratio AV block

A 2 : 1 AV block can be AV nodal or in the His–Purkinje system. It cannot be classified as type I or type II block because there is only one PR interval to examine before the blocked P wave. A 2 : 1 AV block is best labeled simply as 2 : 1 block. For the purpose of classification according to the World Health Organization and the ACC, it is considered as "advanced block," as are 3 : 1, 4 : 1 and other AV blocks. Confusion arises when the term "advanced AV block" (defined in the ACC/AHA/HRS guidelines as a form of second-degree AV block of two or more P waves) is used to describe both second- and third-degree AV block.

The site of the lesion in 2 : 1 AV block can often be determined by seeking the company the 2 : 1 AV block keeps. An association with either type I or type II second-degree AV block helps localization of the lesion according to the correlations already discussed. Outside of acute myocardial infarction, sustained 2 : 1 and 3 : 1 AV block with a wide QRS complex occurs in the His–Purkinje system in 80% of cases, with 20% in the AV node. It is inappropriate to label AV nodal 2 : 1 or 3 : 1 AV block as type I block and infranodal 2 : 1 or 3 : 1 AV block as type II block, because the diagnosis of type I and type II blocks is based on electrocardiographic patterns and not on the anatomical site of block.

When stable sinus rhythm and 1 : 1 AV conduction is followed by sudden AV block of several impulses (> 1), and all the PR intervals before and after the block remain constant, this strongly suggests infranodal block and the need for a pacemaker. This arrangement is sometimes called type II block, although it does not conform to the accepted contemporary definition of type II block. The purist will insist on calling this pattern (3 : 1, 4 : 1 AV block) type II AV block by citing the original description by Mobitz in 1924, despite the accepted contemporary definitions that such patterns should not be labeled type II AV block. When the first PR interval after the blocked P waves (in 3 : 1, 4 : 1 AV block) is not equal to previous PR intervals the block can be either in the AV node or in the His–Purkinje system.

Paroxysmal AV block has been defined as the abrupt occurrence or repetitive block of the atrial impulses with a relatively long (approximately 2 seconds or more) ventricular asystole before the return of conduction or escape of a subsidiary ventricular pacemaker. We believe that this form of AV block does not represent a separate entity and is best considered simply as advanced or complete block.

First-degree AV block

It is now recognized that even an isolated markedly long PR interval can cause symptoms similar to the pacemaker syndrome, especially in the presence of normal left ventricular function. During markedly prolonged anterograde AV conduction, the close proximity of atrial systole to the preceding ventricular systole produces the same hemodynamic consequences as continual retrograde ventriculoatrial conduction during VVI pacing. This is why symptomatic marked first-degree AV block has been called "pacemaker syndrome without a pacemaker," but we believe that the term "pacemaker-like syndrome" is more appropriate. An AV junctional rhythm with retrograde ventriculoatrial conduction may also produce the same pathophysiology. The 2008 ACC/AHA/HRS guidelines for pacemaker implantation now advocate pacing in acquired marked first-degree AV block (> 0.30 s) as a Class IIa indication. Patients with a long PR interval may or may not be symptomatic at rest. They are more likely to become symptomatic with mild or moderate exercise when the PR interval does not shorten appropriately and atrial systole shifts progressively closer towards ventricular systole. The class II recommendation does not really apply to patients with congestive heart failure, dilated cardiomyopathy, and marked first-degree AV block, where biventricular pacing would be more beneficial than conventional dual chamber pacing. The clinician must decide in the individual patient whether there is a net benefit provided by two opposing factors: a positive effect from AV delay optimization and a negative impact of reduced LV function from aberrant pacemaker-controlled depolarization. A recent study suggests that improvement with dual chamber pacing becomes evident with a PR interval > 0.28 seconds.

Intraventricular conduction and provocable AV blocks

Although the meaning of *bifascicular block* is obvious, that of *trifascicular block* is not as simple. The term trifascicular block is often used rather loosely. Bilateral bundle branch block, despite 1 : 1 AV conduction, carries a poor prognosis and should be a class I indication for pacing, even in an asymptomatic patient.

Exercise: Permanent pacing is recommended as a class I indication in symptomatic or asymptomatic patients with exercise-induced AV block (absent at rest), because the vast majority is due to tachycardia-dependent block in the His–Purkinje system and carry a poor prognosis. This form of AV block is often reproducible in the electrophysiology laboratory by rapid atrial pacing, because it is tachycardia-dependent and rarely due to AV nodal disease. Exercise-induced AV block secondary to myocardial ischemia is rare and does not require pacing unless ischemia cannot be alleviated.

During an electrophysiologic study: When an electrophysiologic study is performed for the evaluation of syncope, many workers believe that AV block or delay in the following circumstances constitutes an indication for permanent pacing:

(a) A markedly prolonged HV (from His bundle potential to earliest ventricular activation) interval (≥ 100 ms; normal = 35–55 ms) identifies patients with a higher risk of developing complete AV block and need for a pacemaker. A study can define by a process of exclusion which patients might benefit from pacing in the presence of HV prolongation (≥ 70 ms) and no other electrophysiologic abnormality such as inducible ventricular tachycardia.

(b) The development of second- or third-degree His–Purkinje block in an electrophysiological "stress test" performed by gradually increasing the atrial rate by pacing is an insensitive sign of conduction system disease but constitutes a class I indication for pacing because it correlates with a high incidence of third-degree AV block or sudden death.

(c) Bradycardia-dependent (phase 4) block (not bradycardia-associated, as in vagally induced AV block) is rare and always infranodal. It can be evaluated with His bundle recordings by producing bradycardia and pauses by the electrical induction of atrial or ventricular premature beats.

(d) A drug challenge with procainamide that depresses His–Purkinje conduction may be used to provoke HV interval prolongation or actual His–Purkinje block (according to published criteria) in susceptible patients and define the need for a pacemaker.

Permanent pacing for AV block after acute myocardial infarction

The requirement for temporary pacing in acute myocardial infarction (MI) does not by itself constitute an indication for permanent pacing. Unlike many other indications, the need for permanent pacing after acute MI does not necessarily depend on the presence of symptoms

Acute inferior myocardial infarction

Permanent pacing is almost never needed in inferior MI and narrow QRS AV block. Pacemaker implantation should be considered only if second- or third-degree AV block persists for 14–16 days. The use of permanent pacing is required in only 1–2% of all the patients who develop acute second or third-degree AV block regardless of thrombolytic therapy. Narrow QRS type II second-degree AV block has not yet been reported in acute inferior MI.

Acute anterior myocardial infarction

Patients who develop bundle branch block and transient second- and third-degree AV block during anterior MI have a high in-hospital mortality rate and are at a high risk of sudden death after hospital discharge. Sudden death usually is due to malignant ventricular tachyarrhythmias, and less commonly related to the development of complete AV block with prolonged ventricular asystole. The use of permanent pacing in patients with transient trifascicular AV block or bilateral (alternating) bundle branch block is still controversial, but most workers recommend it with the aim of preventing sudden death from asystole despite the return of 1 : 1 AV conduction. Permanent pacing is not indicated in patients with acute anterior MI and residual bundle branch or bifascicular block without documented transient second- or third-degree AV block because there is no appreciable risk of late development of complete AV block. Measurement of the HV interval does not predict which patients will develop progressive conduction system disease.

Patients with an anterior MI who require permanent pacing often have a low LV ejection fraction that makes them potential candidates for a prophylactic implantable cardioverter-defibrillator. A recent study in patients who suffered an acute MI suggests waiting 3–6 months before implanting a defibrillator. Despite this recommendation, it makes sense to implant a cardioverter-defibrillator (which contains a pacemaker component) in patients who actually require only a permanent pacemaker at that juncture. Such patients are also at risk for sudden death from a ventricular tachyarrhythmia. It makes no sense to wait 3–6 months without permanent protection for bradycardia until a cardioverter-defibrillator can be implanted on the basis of a poor LV ejection fraction according to the recommendations of a recent trial of ICD after MI.

Vagally mediated AV block

Vagally mediated AV block is generally a benign condition that can superficially resemble type II block. This phenomenon has been called "apparent type II block," because it simulates type II block, but it is generally considered a type I variant. Vagally mediated AV block occurs in the AV node and differs from neurally mediated (malignant vasovagal) syncope where head-up tilt testing causes sinus arrest and rarely predominant AV block. Vagally induced AV block can occur in otherwise normal individuals, and also in patients with cough, swallowing, hiccups, micturition, etc. when vagal discharge is enhanced. Electrophysiologic studies in vagally mediated AV block are basically normal. Vagally mediated AV block is characteristically paroxysmal and often associated with sinus slowing. As a rule, AV nodal block is associated with obvious irregular and longer PP intervals, and is bradycardia-associated (not bradycardia-dependent), i.e., both AV block and sinus slowing result from vagal effects.

An acute increase in vagal tone may occasionally produce AV block without preceding prolongation of the AH interval (constant PR), giving the superficial appearance of a type II AV block mechanism, i.e., no PR prolongation before the blocked beat. In this situation, AH prolongation may occur during the initial several beats when AV conduction resumes. Vagally induced block is occasionally expressed in terms of constant PR intervals before and after the blocked impulse, an arrangement that may lead to an erroneous diagnosis of the more serious type II block if sinus slowing is ignored. Sinus slowing can sometimes be subtle because the P–P interval may increase by as little as 0.04 s.

AV block in athletes

Severe sinus bradycardia and third-degree AV block can occur at rest or after exercise in athletes and lead to symptoms such as lightheadedness, syncope, or even Stokes–Adams attacks. These changes are considered secondary to increased parasympathetic (hypervagotonia) and decreased sympathetic tone on the sinus and AV node related to physical training. Most patients become asymptomatic after physical deconditioning. If the latter produces no response or the patient refuses to decrease athletic activities, a permanent pacemaker becomes indicated. Some of the so-called "athletic patients" improved by pacing represent individuals who would otherwise benefit from pacing, i.e., subjects with sinus node disease rendered symptomatic by increased vagal tone related to training or athletes with spontaneous or exercise-induced infranodal block.

Atrioventricular block in athletes is most probably an expression of hypervagotonia. This form of AV block may or may not be associated with sinus bradycardia, because the relative effects of sympathetic and parasympathetic systems on the AV and sinus node may differ. AV block in athletes responds to exercise or atropine. A number of authors have indicated that Mobitz type II second-degree AV block (sometimes called Mobitz AV block as opposed to Wenckebach AV block) can occur in young athletes. The diagnosis of type II AV block immediately raises the question of a permanent pacemaker, especially in symptomatic patients. We believe that Mobitz type II second-degree AV block (always infranodal) does not occur in otherwise healthy athletes. The purported occurrence of type II AV block in some reports (with ECGs) appears related to failure to apply the correct definition of type II second-degree AV block (Table 28).

Hypertrophic cardiomyopathy

The benefits of pacing in hypertrophic cardiomyopathy (HCM) have been the subject of significant and ongoing debate. Pacing is not primary therapy for HCM. Dual chamber right ventricular apical (DDD) pacing is supposed to reduce LV outflow tract gradients by a form of cardiac desynchronization by altering the regional pattern of ventricular contraction. Pacing should only be considered when the resting left ventricular outflow gradient is greater than 30 mm Hg, or greater than 50 mm Hg when provoked. In uncontrolled and observational studies, chronic dual chamber pacing was associated with amelioration of symptoms and reduction of outflow gradient in many HCM patients. Pacing often reduces the gradient by about 50%. However, several

Table 28. Pitfalls in the diagnosis and treatment of AV block.

- Mobitz type I AV block can be physiological in athletes resulting from heavy physical training
- Mobitz type I AV block can be physiological during sleep in individuals with high vagal tone
- Failure to suspect vagally induced AV block, e.g., vomiting
- Failure to recognize reversible causes of AV block:
  (1) Lyme disease
  (2) Electrolyte abnormalities
  (3) Inferior myocardial infarction
  (4) Sleep apnea
- Poor correlation between narrow QRS type I block and symptoms
- Beliefs that all type I blocks with a wide QRS complex are AV nodal
- Non-conducted atrial premature beats masquerading as AV block
- What appears to be narrow QRS type II block may be a type I variant
- Atypical type I sequence mistaken for type II block
- Making the diagnosis of type II block without seeing a truly conducted post-block P wave (shortage of PR intervals)
- A recording that appears to show both types I and II and a narrow QRS complex may in fact represent only type I block
- Concealed extrasystoles causing pseudo-AV block (look for associated unexpected sudden PR prolongation, combination of what appears to be type I and type II and isolated retrograde P waves from retrograde conduction of the concealed extrasystole)
- Relying solely on a computer-rendered ECG diagnosis: computer interpretations are notoriously error-prone

randomized crossover clinical trials reported that subjective symptomatic benefit during pacing frequently occurs with little objective evidence of improved exercise capacity, and can be largely explained as a placebo effect. Symptomatic relief does not correlate with gradient reduction.

Although it is not a primary treatment, there is evidence to support utilizing a trial of dual chamber pacing without an ICD in selected patient subgroups such as elderly patients (older than 65 years) with modest hypertrophy and no risk factors, who may exhibit both subjective and objective symptomatic benefit with pacing. Pacing, in this subgroup, provides an alternative more desirable than surgery. Producing and maintaining a reduction in gradient (and presumably in symptoms) requires that pre-excitation of the right ventricular apex and distal septum be established and that there is complete ventricular capture (at rest and during exercise) without compromising ventricular filling and cardiac output. In this respect, it is important for the right ventricular lead to be positioned way out at the apex for apical preexcitation. Programming of the AV interval is vital to guarantee complete ventricular capture. This may require slowing of AV nodal conduction with a beta-blocker or verapamil, or possibly ablation of the AV node in selected cases. Pacing alone does not reduce the risk of sudden death. Patients with well-known risk factors should be considered for an ICD. Even a single risk marker is often considered an indication for an ICD.

Vasovagal syncope

Vasovagal syncope carries a benign prognosis in the majority of patients. Pacing is not a first-line treatment and should really be considered therapy of last resort. Pacing can only treat the consequences of bradycardia; it plays no role in preventing vasodilatation and hypotension, frequently the dominant mechanism leading to syncope. Indeed, a study using implantable loop recorders revealed that that only half the patients had a recorded asystolic pause at the time of spontaneous vasovagal syncope. The result of tilt testing is not predictive of outcome with pacing. Furthermore, the mechanism of tilt-induced syncope is frequently different from that during spontaneous syncope recorded with an implantable loop recorder. The effectiveness of pacing has been studied in five multicenter randomized controlled trials. Three gave a positive result and two gave negative results. The decision to implant a pacemaker must consider the fact that vasovagal syncope is basically a benign condition that frequently affects young patients, in whom a pacemaker means potential complications over several decades of pacing.

VVI pacing may aggravate hemodynamics during an episode and is contraindicated. Dual chamber pacing should be used with rate hysteresis or a rate drop algorithm that allows an increased pacing rate when the device detects a decrease in heart rate. Pacing may have a role for some patients, specifically those who have little or no prodrome (no warning symptoms), those in whom other forms of therapy fail (refractory to at least three medication attempts), those with unacceptable injuries, those with potential occupational hazard, and those who have profound bradycardia or asystole during syncope. The recommendation should favor the elderly. Patients selected on the basis of asystole and syncope recorded by an implanted loop recorder are more likely to benefit from pacing. For such patients, cardiac pacing may reduce the frequency of syncope and increase the amount of time from the onset of symptoms to a loss of consciousness, thereby providing time for the patient to take evasive action (i.e., lie down) and avoid injuries.

Atrial fibrillation

Clinical trials have reported that in patients with conventional pacemaker indications, atrial-based "physiologic" pacing is associated with a lower incidence of paroxysmal and permanent atrial fibrillation (AF) than single chamber ventricular pacing. This benefit is not particularly striking despite the maintenance of AV synchrony. This is most likely due to unnecessary ventricular pacing, which is frequent in dual chamber pacing. At nominal values, dual chamber devices usually do not permit intrinsic AV conduction but promote ventricular pacing. Whether atrial pacing itself is antiarrhythmic remains uncertain. A pacemaker should never be implanted with the sole purpose of treating paroxysmal AF in the absence of bradycardia.

Advanced atrial pacing algorithms for AF prevention may be classified as follows:

1. dynamic sinus rhythm overdrive
2. premature atrial beat reaction (short–long cycle prevention and ectopy overdrive)
3. post-tachycardia overdrive to prevent early recurrence of atrial fibrillation
4. prevention of inappropriate rate fall after exercise

These algorithms for AF prevention in patients with indications for device implantation have shown mixed and inconsistent benefits. These contradictory results and recently demonstrated very limited benefit were possibly due to different trial designs, end points and patient populations. These algorithms are safe and not costly. A trial of these algorithms may be warranted in an occasional patient. Importantly, AF can be prevented or reduced by minimizing RV pacing.

A number of clinical trials have investigated the impact of site-specific atrial pacing on secondary prevention of AF. Multisite pacing (dual-site right atrial or biatrial pacing) was demonstrated to add only minimal benefit for AF prevention. By contrast, in some studies septal pacing was reported to reduce AF recurrence in selected patients. Atrial septal pacing (high atrium, low atrium and proximal coronary sinus) can produce important beneficial effects in patients with paroxysmal AF and interatrial conduction delay.

Atrial antitachycardia pacing (ATP) therapies are effective in treating organized atrial tachyarrhythmias (which precede AF), mainly when delivered early after the onset, particularly if the tachycardia is relatively slow. Despite this capability of terminating atrial tachycardia, devices with atrial ATP in combination with atrial pace-prevention algorithms do not suppress atrial tachycardia/AF over long-term follow-up compared with DDD/R pacing. However, there are subsets of patients, e.g., those with atrial flutter, who are likely to benefit from this therapy. However, the treatment of choice is radiofrequency ablation of the cavotricuspid isthmus for isthmus-dependent atrial flutter.

Further reading

Books

Barold SS, Ritter P. *Devices for Cardiac Resynchronization: Technologic and Clinical Aspects*. New York, NY: Springer, 2008.

Ellenbogen KA, Auricchio A. *Device Therapy for Congestive Heart Failure*. Hoboken, NJ: Wiley-Blackwell, 2008.

Ellenbogen KA, Wood MA. *Cardiac Pacing and ICDs*, 5th edn. Hoboken, NJ: Wiley-Blackwell, 2008.

Hayes DL, Friedman PA. *Cardiac Pacing, Defibrillation, and Resynchronization: a Clinical Approach*, 2nd edn. Hoboken, NJ: Wiley-Blackwell, 2008.

Timperley J, Leeson P. *Pacemakers and ICDs*. Oxford: Oxford University Press, 2008.

Yu CM, Hayes DL, Auricchio A. *Cardiac Resynchronization Therapy*, 2nd edn. Hoboken, NJ: Wiley-Blackwell, 2008.

Kusumoto FM, Goldschlager NF. *Cardiac Pacing for the Clinician*, 2nd edn. New York, NY: Springer, 2007.

Moses HW, Mullin JC. *A Practical Guide to Cardiac Pacing*, 6th edn. Hagerstown, MD: Lippincott Williams & Wilkins, 2007.

Chow A, Buxton A. *Implantable Cardiac Pacemakers and Defibrillators: All You Wanted to Know*. London: BMJ Publishing Group, 2006.

Ellenbogen KA, Kay GN, Lau CP, Wilkoff BL. *Clinical Cardiac Pacing, Defibrillation, and Resynchronization Therapy*, 3rd edn. Philadelphia, PA: Saunders, 2006.

Love CJ. *Cardiac Pacemakers and Defibrillators*, 2nd edn. Austin, TX: Landes Bioscience, 2006.

Mond HG, Karpawich PP. *Pacing Options in the Adult with Congenital Heart Disease*. Hoboken, NJ: Wiley-Blackwell, 2006.

Conventional pacing

Basics

Crick JC, Rokas S, Sowton E. Identification of pacemaker dependent patients by serial decremental rate inhibition. *Eur Heart J* 1985; **6**: 891–6.

Gillis AM, Willems R. Controversies in pacing: indications and programming. *Curr Cardiol Rep* 2005; **7**: 336–41.

Kaszala K, Huizar JF, Ellenbogen KA. Contemporary pacemakers: what the primary care physician needs to know. *Mayo Clin Proc* 2008; **83**: 1170–86.

Kindermann M, Berg M, Pistorius K, Schwerdt H, Fröhlig G. Do battery depletion indicators reliably predict the need for pulse generator replacement? *Pacing Clin Electrophysiol* 2001; **24**: 945–9.

Mortensen K, Rudolph V, Willems S, Ventura R. New developments in antibradycardic devices. *Expert Rev Med Devices* 2007; **4**: 321–33.

Platia EV, Brinker JA. Time course of transvenous pacemaker stimulation impedance, capture threshold, and electrogram amplitude. *Pacing Clin Electrophysiol* 1986; **9**: 620–5.

Reynolds DW, Murray CM. New concepts in physiologic cardiac pacing. *Curr Cardiol Rep* 2007; **9**: 351–7.

Roberts PR. Follow up and optimisation of cardiac pacing. *Heart* 2005; **91**: 1229–34.

Trohman RG, Kim MH, Pinski SL. Cardiac pacing: the state of the art. *Lancet* 2004; **364**: 1701–19

Indications

Barold SS. Optimal pacing in first-degree AV block. *Pacing Clin Electrophysiol* 1999; **22**: 1423–4.

Fananapazir L, McAreavey D. Therapeutic options in patients with obstructive hypertrophic cardiomyopathy and severe drug-refractory symptoms. *J Am Coll Cardiol* 1998; **31**: 259–64.

Kalahasty G, Ellenbogen K. The role of pacemakers in the management of patients with atrial fibrillation. *Med Clin North Am* 2008; **92**: 161–78.

Knight BP, Gersh BJ, Carlson MD, *et al.* Role of permanent pacing to prevent atrial fibrillation: science advisory from the American Heart Association Council on Clinical Cardiology (Subcommittee on Electrocardiography and Arrhythmias) and the Quality of Care and Outcomes Research Interdisciplinary Working Group, in collaboration with the Heart Rhythm Society. *Circulation* 2005; **111**: 240–3.

Maggi R, Brignole M. Update in the treatment of neurally-mediated syncope. *Minerva Med* 2007; **98**: 503–9.

Villain E. Indications for pacing in patients with congenital heart disease. *Pacing Clin Electrophysiol* 2008; **31** (Suppl 1): S17–20.

Ventriculoatrial conduction

Ausubel K, Gabry MD, Klementowicz PT, Furman S. Pacemaker-mediated endless loop tachycardia at rates below the upper rate limit. *Am J Cardiol* 1988; **61**: 465–7.

Barold SS. Repetitive reentrant and non-reentrant ventriculoatrial synchrony in dual chamber pacing. *Clin Cardiol* 1991; **14**: 754–63.

Barold SS, Levine PA. Pacemaker repetitive nonreentrant ventriculoatrial synchronous rhythm: a review. *J Interv Card Electrophysiol* 2001; **5**: 45–58.

Hariman RJ, Pasquariello JL, Gomes JA, Holtzman R, el-Sherif N. Autonomic dependence of ventriculoatrial conduction. *Am J Cardiol* 1985; **56**: 285–91.

Klementowicz P, Ausubel K, Furman S. The dynamic nature of ventriculoatrial conduction. *Pacing Clin Electrophysiol* 1986; **9**: 1050–4.

Timing cycles

Barold SS. Ventricular- versus atrial-based lower rate timing in dual chamber pacemakers: does it really matter? *Pacing Clin Electrophysiol* 1995; **18**: 83–96.

Barold SS, Falkoff MD, Ong LS, Heinle RA. All dual-chamber pacemakers function in the DDD mode. *Am Heart J* 1988; **115**: 1353–62.

Stroobandt RX, Barold SS, Vandenbulcke FD, Willems RJ, Sinnaeve AF. A reappraisal of pacemaker timing cycles pertaining to automatic mode switching. *J Interv Card Electrophysiol* 2001; **5**: 417–29.

Wang PJ, Al-Ahmed A, Hayes DL. Pacemaker timing cycles. In: Ellenbogen KA, Wood MA (eds), *Cardiac Pacing and ICDs*, 5th edn. Hoboken, NJ: Wiley-Blackwell, 2008: 282–343.

12-lead electrocardiography

Barold SS, Giudici MC, Herweg B, Curtis AB. Diagnostic value of the 12-lead electrocardiogram during conventional and biventricular pacing for cardiac resynchronization. *Cardiol Clin* 2006; **24**: 471–90.

Barold SS, Herweg B, Curtis AB. Electrocardiographic diagnosis of myocardial infarction and ischemia during cardiac pacing. *Cardiol Clin* 2006; **24**: 387–99.

Firschke C, Zrenner B. Images in clinical medicine. Malposition of dual-chamber pacemaker lead. *N Engl J Med* 2002; **346**: e2.

Kistler PM, Mond HG, Vohra JK. Pacemaker ventricular block. *Pacing Clin Electrophysiol* 2003; **26**: 1997–9.

Klein HO, Di Segni E, Kaplinsky E, Schamroth L. The Wenckebach phenomenon between electric pacemaker and ventricle. *Br Heart J* 1976; **38**: 961–5.

Kleinfeld M, Barold SS, Rozanski JJ. Pacemaker alternans: a review. *Pacing Clin Electrophysiol* 1987; **10**: 924–33.

Miyoshi F, Kobayashi Y, Itou H, *et al.* Prolonged paced QRS duration as a predictor for congestive heart failure in patients with right ventricular apical pacing. *Pacing Clin Electrophysiol* 2005; **28**: 1182–8.

Patberg KW, Shvilkin A, Plotnikov AN, *et al.* Cardiac memory: mechanisms and clinical implications. *Heart Rhythm* 2005; **2**: 1376–82.

Sgarbossa EB, Pinski SL, Gates KB, Wagner GS, for the Gusto-1 Investigators. Early electrocardiographic diagnosis of acute myocardial infarction in the presence of a ventricular paced rhythm. *Am J Cardiol* 1996; **77**: 423–4

Shvilkin A, Ho KK, Rosen MR, Josephson ME. T-vector direction differentiates postpacing from ischemic T-wave inversion in precordial leads. *Circulation* 2005; **111**: 969–74.

Sweeney MO, Hellkamp AS, Lee KL, Lamas GA; Mode Selection Trial (MOST) Investigators. Association of prolonged QRS duration with death in a clinical trial of pacemaker therapy for sinus node dysfunction. *Circulation* 2005; **111**: 2418–23.

van Gelder BM, Bracke FA, Oto A, *et al.* Diagnosis and management of inadvertently placed pacing and ICD leads in the left ventricle: a multicenter experience and review of the literature. *Pacing Clin Electrophysiol* 2000; **23**: 877–83.

Complications

Bailey SM, Wilkoff BL. Complications of pacemakers and defibrillators in the elderly. *Am J Geriatr Cardiol* 2006; **15**: 102–7.

Barold SS, Falkoff MD, Ong LS, Heinle RA. Oversensing by single-chamber pacemakers: mechanisms, diagnosis, and treatment. *Cardiol Clin* 1985; **3**: 565–85.

Barold SS, Ong LS, Falkoff MD, Heinle RA. Inhibition of bipolar demand pacemaker by diaphragmatic myopotentials. *Circulation* 1977; **56**: 679–83.

Exner DV, Rothschild JM, Heal S, Gillis AM. Unipolar sensing in contemporary pacemakers: using myopotential testing to define optimal sensitivity settings. *J Interv Card Electrophysiol* 1998; **2**: 33–40.

Henrikson CA, Leng CT, Yuh DD, Brinker JA. Computed tomography to assess possible cardiac lead perforation. *Pacing Clin Electrophysiol* 2006; **29**: 509–11.

Hirschl DA, Jain VR, Spindola-Franco H, Gross JN, Haramati LB. Prevalence and characterization of asymptomatic pacemaker and ICD lead perforation on CT. *Pacing Clin Electrophysiol* 2007; **30**: 28–32.

Inama G, Santini M, Padeletti L, *et al.* Far-field R wave oversensing in dual chamber pacemakers designed for atrial arrhythmia management: effect of pacing site and lead tip to ring distance. *Pacing Clin Electrophysiol* 2004; **27**: 1221–30.

Kowalski M, Huizar JF, Kaszala K, Wood MA. Problems with implantable cardiac device therapy. *Cardiol Clin* 2008; **26**: 441–58.

Laborderie J, Barandon L, Ploux S, *et al.* Management of subacute and delayed right ventricular perforation with a pacing or an implantable cardioverter-defibrillator lead. *Am J Cardiol* 2008; **102**: 1352–5.

Ortega DF, Sammartino MV, Pellegrino GM, *et al.* Runaway pacemaker: a forgotten phenomenon? *Europace* 2005; **7**: 592–7.

Sun Q, Chen K, Zhang S. Crosstalk triggered safety standby pacing associated with an improperly seated ventricular lead. *Europace* 2008; **10**: 75–6.

van Gelder LM, el Gamal MI, Tielen CH. P-wave sensing in VVI pacemakers: useful or a problem? *Pacing Clin Electrophysiol* 1988; **11**: 1413–18.

Waxman HL, Lazzara R, El-Sherif N. Apparent malfunction of demand pacemakers due to spurious potentials generated by contact between two endocardial electrodes. *Pacing Clin Electrophysiol* 1978; **1**: 531–4.

Effects of drugs and electrolyte imbalance

Barold SS, Falkoff MD, Ong LS, Heinle RA. Hyperkalemia-induced failure of atrial capture during dual-chamber cardiac pacing. *J Am Coll Cardiol* 1987; **10**: 467–9.

Barold SS, McVenes R, Stokes K. Effect of drugs on pacing threshold in man and canines: old and new facts. In: Barold SS, Mugica J (eds), *New Perspectives in Cardiac Pacing 3*. Mount Kisco, NY: Futura, 1993: 57–83.

Bianconi L, Boccadamo R, Toscano S, *et al.* Effects of oral propafenone therapy on chronic myocardial pacing threshold. *Pacing Clin Electrophysiol* 1992; **15**: 148–54.

Fornieles-Perez H, Montoya-Garcia M, Levine PA, Sanz O. Documentation of acute rise in ventricular capture thresholds associated with flecainide acetate. *Pacing Clin Electrophysiol* 2002; **25**: 871–2.

Ortega-Carnicer J, Benezet J, Benezet-Mazuecos J. Hyperkalaemia causing loss of atrial capture and extremely wide QRS complex during DDD pacing. *Resuscitation* 2004; **62**: 119–20.

Atrial pacing and sensing

Daubert JC, Pavin D, Jauvert G, Mabo P. Intra- and interatrial conduction delay: implications for cardiac pacing. *Pacing and Clin Electrophysiol* 2004: **27**: 507–25.

Hakacova N, Velimirovic D, Margitfalvi P, Hatala R, Buckingham TA. Septal atrial pacing for the prevention of atrial fibrillation. *Europace* 2007; **9**: 1124–8.

Huang CY, Tuan TC, Lee WS, *et al.* Long-term efficacy and stability of atrial sensing in VDD pacing. *Clin Cardiol* 2005; **28**: 203–7.

Ovsyshcher IE, Crystal E. VDD pacing: under evaluated, undervalued, and underused. *Pacing Clin Electrophysiol* 2004; **27**: 1335–8.

Padeletti L, Michelucci A, Pieragnoli P, Colella A, Musilli N. Atrial septal pacing: a new approach to prevent atrial fibrillation. *Pacing Clin Electrophysiol* 2004; **27**: 850–4.

Automatic mode switching

Goethals M, Timmermans W, Geelen P, Backers J, Brugada P. Mode switching failure during atrial flutter: the '2 : 1 lock-in' phenomenon. *Europace* 2003; **5**: 95–102.

Israel CW. Analysis of mode switching algorithms in dual chamber pacemakers. *Pacing Clin Electrophysiol* 2002; **25**: 380–93.

Lau CP. Pacing technology and its indications: advances in threshold management, automatic mode switching and sensors. In: Saksena S, Camm AJ (eds), *Electrophysiological Disorders of the Heart*. Philadelphia, PA: Elsevier, 2005: 731–63.

Rate-responsive pacing

Lamas GA, Knight JD, Sweeney MO, *et al.* Impact of rate-modulated pacing on quality of life and exercise capacity: evidence from the Advanced Elements of Pacing Randomized Controlled Trial (ADEPT). *Heart Rhythm* 2007; **4**: 1125–32.

Lau W, Corcoran SJ, Mond HG. Pacemaker tachycardia in a minute ventilation rate-adaptive pacemaker induced by electrocardiographic monitoring. *Pacing Clin Electrophysiol* 2006; **29**: 438–40.

Lau CP, Tse HF, Camm J, Barold SS. Evolution of pacing for bradycardias: sensors. *Eur Heart J Suppl* 2007; **9**: I11–22.

Southorn PA, Kamath GS, Vasdev GM, Hayes DL. Monitoring equipment induced tachycardia in patients with minute ventilation rate-responsive pacemaker. *Br J Anaesth* 2000; **84**: 508–9.

Weiss DN, Gold MR, Peters RW. Rate-responsive pacing mimicking ventricular tachycardia. *J Invasive Cardiol* 1996; **8**: 228–30.

Wills AM, Plante DT, Dukkipati SR, Corcoran CP, Standaert DG. Pacemaker-induced tachycardia caused by inappropriate response to parkinsonian tremor. *Neurology* 2005; **65**: 1676–7.

Pacemaker syndrome

Ellenbogen KA, Stambler BS, Orav EJ, *et al.* Clinical characteristics of patients intolerant to VVIR pacing. *Am J Cardiol* 2000; **86**: 59–63.

Link MS, Hellkamp AS, Estes NA, *et al.*; MOST Study Investigators. High incidence of pacemaker syndrome in patients with sinus node dysfunction treated with ventricular-based pacing in the Mode Selection Trial (MOST). *J Am Coll Cardiol* 2004; **43**: 2066–71.

Sulke N, Dritsas A, Bostock J, *et al.* "Subclinical" pacemaker syndrome: a randomised study of symptom free patients with ventricular demand (VVI) pacemakers upgraded to dual chamber devices. *Br Heart J* 1992; **67**: 57–64.

Alternative site pacing and left ventricular function

Barold SS. Adverse effects of ventricular desynchronization induced by long-term right ventricular pacing. *J Am Coll Cardiol* 2003; **42**: 624–6.

Barold SS, Stroobandt RX. Harmful effects of long-term right ventricular pacing. *Acta Cardiol* 2006; **61**: 103–10.

Chen L, Hodge D, Jahangir A, *et al.* Preserved left ventricular ejection fraction following atrioventricular junction ablation and pacing for atrial fibrillation. *J Cardiovasc Electrophysiol* 2008; **19**: 19–27.

Deshmukh P, Casavant DA, Romanyshyn M, Anderson K. Permanent, direct His-bundle pacing: a novel approach to cardiac pacing in patients with normal His–Purkinje activation. *Circulation* 2000; **101**: 869–77.

Deshmukh PM, Romanyshyn M. Direct His-bundle pacing: present and future. *Pacing Clin Electrophysiol* 2004; **27**: 862–70.

Gammage MD. Base over apex: does site matter for pacing the right ventricle? *Europace* 2008; **10**: 572–3.

Hayes JJ, Sharma AD, Love JC, *et al.*; DAVID Investigators. Abnormal conduction increases risk of adverse outcomes from right ventricular pacing. *J Am Coll Cardiol* 2006; **48**: 1628–33.

Hillock RJ, Stevenson IH, Mond HG. The right ventricular outflow tract: a comparative study of septal, anterior wall, and free wall pacing. *Pacing Clin Electrophysiol* 2007; **30**: 942–7.

Kim JJ, Friedman RA, Eidem BW, *et al.* Ventricular function and long-term pacing in children with congenital complete atrioventricular block. *J Cardiovasc Electrophysiol* 2007; **18**: 373–7.

Manolis AS. The deleterious consequences of right ventricular apical pacing: time to seek alternate site pacing. *Pacing Clin Electrophysiol* 2006; **29**: 298–315.

Manolis AS, Sakellariou D, Andrikopoulos GK. Alternate site pacing in patients at risk for heart failure. *Angiology* 2008; **59** (2 Suppl): 97S–102S.

McGavigan AD, Roberts-Thomson KC, Hillock RJ, Stevenson IH, Mond HG. Right ventricular outflow tract pacing: radiographic and electrocardiographic correlates of lead position. *Pacing Clin Electrophysiol* 2006; **29**: 1063–8.

Medi C, Mond HG. Right ventricular outflow tract septal pacing: long-term follow-up of ventricular lead performance. *Pacing Clin Electrophysiol* 2009; **32**: 172–6.

Mond HG. Right ventricular septal lead implantation: new site, new risks? *J Cardiovasc Electrophysiol* 2008; **19**: E38.

Mond HG, Hillock RJ, Stevenson IH, McGavigan AD. The right ventricular outflow tract: the road to septal pacing. *Pacing Clin Electrophysiol* 2007; **30**: 482–91.

Muto C, Ottaviano L, Canciello M, *et al.* Effect of pacing the right ventricular mid-septum tract in patients with permanent atrial fibrillation and low ejection fraction. *J Cardiovasc Electrophysiol* 2007; **18**: 1032–6.

Nothroff J, Norozi K, Alpers V, *et al.* Pacemaker implantation as a risk factor for heart failure in young adults with congenital heart disease. *Pacing Clin Electrophysiol* 2006; **29**: 386–92.

Occhetta E, Bortnik M, Magnani A, *et al.* Prevention of ventricular desynchronization by permanent para-Hisian pacing after atrioventricular node ablation in chronic atrial fibrillation: a crossover, blinded, randomized study versus apical right ventricular pacing. *J Am Coll Cardiol* 2006; **47**: 1938–45.

Parekh S, Stein KM. Selective site pacing: rationale and practical application. *Curr Cardiol Rep* 2008; **10**: 351–9.

Siu CW, Wang M, Zhang XH, Lau CP, Tse HF. Analysis of ventricular performance as a function of pacing site and mode. *Prog Cardiovasc Dis* 2008; **51**: 171–82.

Sweeney MO. Minimizing right ventricular pacing: a new paradigm for cardiac pacing in sinus node dysfunction. *Am Heart J* 2007; **153** (4 Suppl): 34–43.

Sweeney MO, Hellkamp AS, Ellenbogen KA, *et al.*; Mode Selection Trial Investigators. Adverse effect of ventricular pacing on heart failure and atrial fibrillation among patients with normal baseline QRS duration in a clinical trial of pacemaker therapy for sinus node dysfunction. *Circulation* 2003; **107**: 2932–7.

Sweeney MO, Prinzen FW. A new paradigm for physiologic ventricular pacing. *J Am Coll Cardiol* 2006; **47**: 282–8.

Tops LF, Schalij MJ, Bax JJ. The effects of right ventricular apical pacing on ventricular function and dyssynchrony implications for therapy. *J Am Coll Cardiol* 2009; **54**: 764–76.

Tse HF, Wong KK, Siu CW, *et al.* Upgrading pacemaker patients with right ventricular apical pacing to right ventricular septal pacing improves left ventricular performance and functional capacity. *J Cardiovasc Electrophysiol* 2009; **20**: 901–5.

Vanagt WY, Prinzen FW, Delhaas T. Physiology of cardiac pacing in children: the importance of the ventricular pacing site. *Pacing Clin Electrophysiol* 2008; **31** (Suppl 1): S24–7.

van Geldorp IE, Vanagt WY, Bauersfeld U, *et al.* Chronic left ventricular pacing preserves left ventricular function in children. *Pediatr Cardiol* 2009; **30**: 125–32.

Vernooy K, Dijkman B, Cheriex EC, Prinzen FW, Crijns HJ. Ventricular remodeling during long-term right ventricular pacing following His bundle ablation. *Am J Cardiol* 2006; **97**: 1223–7.

Zanon F, Bacchiega E, Rampin L, *et al.* Direct His bundle pacing preserves coronary perfusion compared with right ventricular apical pacing: a prospective, cross-over mid-term study. *Europace* 2008; **10**: 580–7.

Zhang XH, Chen H, Siu CW, *et al.* New-onset heart failure after permanent right ventricular apical pacing in patients with acquired high-grade atrioventricular block and normal left ventricular function. *J Cardiovasc Electrophysiol* 2008; **19**: 136–41.

Algorithms to minimize right ventricular pacing

Fröhlig G, Gras D, Victor J, *et al.* Use of a new cardiac pacing mode designed to eliminate unnecessary ventricular pacing. *Europace* 2006; **8**: 96–101.

Gillis AM, Pürerfellner H, Israel CW, *et al.*; Medtronic Enrhythm Clinical Study Investigators. Reducing unnecessary right ventricular pacing with the managed ventricular pacing mode in patients with sinus node disease and AV block. *Pacing Clin Electrophysiol* 2006; **29**: 697–705.

Kaltman JR, Ro PS, Zimmerman F, *et al.* Managed ventricular pacing in pediatric patients and patients with congenital heart disease. *Am J Cardiol* 2008; **102**: 875–8.

Melzer C, Sowelam S, Sheldon TJ, *et al.* Reduction of right ventricular pacing in patients with sinus node dysfunction using an enhanced search AV algorithm. *Pacing Clin Electrophysiol* 2005; **28**: 521–7.

Olshansky B, Day J, McGuire M, Pratt T. Inhibition of unnecessary RV pacing with AV search hysteresis in ICDs (INTRINSIC RV): design and clinical protocol. *Pacing Clin Electrophysiol* 2005; **28**: 62–6.

Pürerfellner H, Brandt J, Israel C, *et al.* Comparison of two strategies to reduce ventricular pacing in pacemaker patients. *Pacing Clin Electrophysiol* 2008; **31**: 167–76.

Quesada A, Botto G, Erdogan A, *et al.*; PreFER MVP Investigators. Managed ventricular pacing vs. conventional dual-chamber pacing for elective replacements: the PreFER MVP study: clinical background, rationale, and design. *Europace* 2008; **10**: 321–6.

Sweeney MO, Bank AJ, Nsah E, *et al.*; Search AV Extension and Managed Ventricular Pacing for Promoting Atrioventricular Conduction (SAVE PACE) Trial. Minimizing ventricular pacing to reduce atrial fibrillation in sinus-node disease. *N Engl J Med* 2007; **357**: 1000–8.

Sweeney MO, Ellenbogen KA, Casavant D, *et al.*; The Marquis MVP Download Investigators. Multicenter, prospective, randomized safety and efficacy study of a new atrial-based managed ventricular pacing mode (MVP) in dual chamber ICDs. *J Cardiovasc Electrophysiol* 2005; **16**: 811–17.

Electromagnetic interference

Dyrda K, Khairy P. Implantable rhythm devices and electromagnetic interference: myth or reality? *Expert Rev Cardiovasc Ther* 2008; **6**: 823–32.

Sutton R, Kanal E, Wilkoff BL, *et al.* Safety of magnetic resonance imaging of patients with a new Medtronic EnRhythm MRI SureScan pacing system: clinical study design. *Trials* 2008: **9**: 68.

Tondato F, Ng DW, Srivathsan K, *et al.* Radiotherapy-induced pacemaker and implantable cardioverter defibrillator malfunction. *Expert Rev Med Devices* 2009; **6**: 243–9.

Yerra L, Reddy PC. Effects of electromagnetic interference on implanted cardiac devices and their management. *Cardiol Rev* 2007; **15**: 304–9.

Capture verification

Biffi M, Bertini M, Saporito D, *et al.* Automatic management of left ventricular stimulation: hints for technologic improvement. *Pacing Clin Electrophysiol* 2009; **32**: 346–53.

Biffi M, Spertzel J, Martignani C, Branzi A, Boriani G. Evolution of pacing for bradycardia: Autocapsure. *Eur Heart J Suppl* 2007; **9** (Suppl I): I23–32.

Roelke M, Simonson J, Englund J, Farges E, Compton S. Automatic measurement of atrial pacing thresholds in dual-chamber pacemakers: clinical experience with atrial capture management. *Heart Rhythm* 2005; **2**: 1203–10.

Pacemaker memory and stored electrograms

Cheung JW, Keating RJ, Stein KM, *et al.* Newly detected atrial fibrillation following dual chamber pacemaker implantation. *J Cardiovasc Electrophysiol* 2006; **17**: 1323–8.

Defaye P, Leclercq JF, Guilleman D, *et al.* Contributions of high resolution electrograms memorized by DDDR pacemakers in the interpretation of arrhythmic events. *Pacing Clin Electrophysiol* 2003; **26**: 214–20.

Glotzer TV, Hellkamp AS, Zimmerman J, *et al.* Atrial high rate episodes detected by pacemaker diagnostics predict death and stroke: report of the Atrial Diagnostics Ancillary Study of the MOde Selection Trial (MOST). *Circulation* 2003; **107**: 1614–19.

Israel CW, Barold SS. Pacemaker systems as implantable cardiac rhythm monitors. *Am J Cardiol* 2001; **88**: 442–5.

Israel CW, Grönefeld G, Ehrlich JR, Li YG, Hohnloser SH. Long-term risk of recurrent atrial fibrillation as documented by an implantable monitoring device: implications for optimal patient care. *J Am Coll Cardiol* 2004; **43**: 47–52.

Mandava A, Mittal S. Clinical significance of pacemaker-detected atrial high-rate episodes. *Curr Opin Cardiol* 2008; **23**: 60–4.

Mittal S, Stein K, Gilliam FR, *et al.* Frequency, duration, and predictors of newly-diagnosed atrial fibrillation following dual-chamber pacemaker implantation in patients without a previous history of atrial fibrillation. *Am J Cardiol* 2008; **102**: 450–3.

Nowak B, McMeekin J, Knops M, *et al.*; Stored EGM in PulsarMax II and Discovery II Study Group. Validation of dual-chamber pacemaker diagnostic data using dual-channel stored electrograms. *Pacing Clin Electrophysiol* 2005; **28**: 620–9.

Orlov MV, Ghali JK, Araghi-Niknam M, *et al.*; Atrial High Rate Trial Investigators. Asymptomatic atrial fibrillation in pacemaker recipients: incidence, progression, and determinants based on the atrial high rate trial. *Pacing Clin Electrophysiol* 2007; **30**: 404–11.

Paraskevaidis S, Giannakoulas G, Polymeropoulos K, *et al.* Diagnostic value of stored electrograms in pacemaker patients. *Acta Cardiol* 2008; **63**: 59–63.

Remote monitoring

Burri H, Senouf D. Remote monitoring and follow-up of pacemakers and implantable cardioverter defibrillators. *Europace* 2009; **11**: 701–9.

Boriani G, Diemberger I, Martignani C, *et al.* Telecardiology and remote monitoring of implanted electrical devices: the potential for fresh clinical care perspectives. *J Gen Intern Med* 2008; **23** (Suppl 1): 73–7.

Jung W, Rillig A, Birkemeyer R, Miljak T, Meyerfeldt U. Advances in remote monitoring of implantable pacemakers, cardioverter defibrillators and cardiac resynchronization therapy systems. *J Interv Card Electrophysiol* 2008; **23**: 73–85.

Lazarus A. Remote, wireless, ambulatory monitoring of implantable pacemakers, cardioverter defibrillators, and cardiac resynchronization therapy systems: analysis of a worldwide database. *Pacing Clin Electrophysiol* 2007; **30** (Suppl): S2–S12.

Ricci RP, Morichelli L, Gargaro A, Laudadio MT, Santini M. Home monitoring in patients with implantable cardiac devices: is there a potential reduction of stroke risk? results from a computer model tested through Monte Carlo simulations. *J Cardiovasc Electrophysiol* 2009; **20**: 1244–51.

Ricci RP, Morichelli L, Santini M. Remote control of implanted devices through home monitoring technology improves detection and clinical management of atrial fibrillation. *Europace* 2009; **11**: 54–61.

Cardiac resynchronization

Overview

Abraham WT. Cardiac resynchronization therapy. *Prog Cardiovasc Dis* 2006; **48**: 232–8.

Auricchio A, Prinzen FW. Update on the pathophysiological basics of cardiac resynchronization therapy. *Europace* 2008; **10**: 797–800.

Barold SS. What is cardiac resynchronization therapy? *Am J Med* 2001; **111**: 224–32.

Hasan A, Abraham WT. Cardiac resynchronization treatment of heart failure. *Annu Rev Med* 2007; **58**: 63–74.

Herre J. Keys to successful cardiac resynchronization therapy. *Am Heart J* 2007; **153** (4 Suppl): 18–24.

Kashani A, Barold SS. Significance of QRS complex duration in patients with heart failure. *J Am Coll Cardiol* 2005; **46**: 2183–92.

McAlister FA, Ezekowitz J, Hooton N, *et al.* Cardiac resynchronization therapy for patients with left ventricular systolic dysfunction: a systematic review. *JAMA* 2007; **297**: 2502–14.

Trials and indications

Abraham WT, Fisher WG, Smith AL, *et al.*; MIRACLE Study Group. Multicenter InSync Randomized Clinical Evaluation. Cardiac resynchronization in chronic heart failure. *N Engl J Med* 2002; **346**: 1845–53.

Bristow MR, Saxon LA, Boehmer J, *et al.*; Comparison of Medical Therapy, Pacing, and Defibrillation in Heart Failure (COMPANION) Investigators. Cardiac-resynchronization therapy with or without an implantable defibrillator in advanced chronic heart failure. *N Engl J Med* 2004; **350**: 2140–50.

Byrne MJ, Helm RH, Daya S, *et al.* Diminished left ventricular dyssynchrony and impact of resynchronization in failing hearts with right versus left bundle branch block. *J Am Coll Cardiol* 2007; **50**: 1484–90.

Cazeau S, Leclercq C, Lavergne T, *et al.*; Multisite Stimulation in Cardiomyopathies (MUSTIC) Study Investigators. Effects of multisite biventricular pacing in patients with heart failure and intraventricular conduction delay. *N Engl J Med* 2001; **344**: 873–80.

Cleland JG, Daubert JC, Erdmann E, *et al.*; Cardiac Resynchronization-Heart Failure (CARE-HF) Study Investigators. The effect of cardiac resynchronization on morbidity and mortality in Heart failure. *N Engl J Med* 2005; **352**: 1539–49.

Cleland JG, Freemantle N, Daubert JC, *et al.* Long-term effect of cardiac resynchronisation in patients reporting mild symptoms of heart failure: a report from the CARE-HF study. *Heart* 2008; **94**: 278–83.

Daubert C, Gold MR, Abraham WT, *et al.*; REVERSE Study Group. Prevention of disease progression by cardiac resynchronization therapy in patients with asymptomatic or mildly symptomatic left ventricular dysfunction: insights from the European cohort of the REVERSE (Resynchronization Reverses Remodeling in Systolic Left Ventricular Dysfunction) trial. *J Am Coll Cardiol* 2009; **20**: 1837–46.

Gasparini M, Auricchio A, Metra M, *et al.*; Multicentre Longitudinal Observational Study (MILOS) Group. Long-term survival in patients undergoing cardiac resynchronization therapy: the importance of performing atrio-ventricular junction ablation in patients with permanent atrial fibrillation. *Eur Heart J* 2008; **29**: 1644–52.

Herweg B, Barold SS. When is it too late for cardiac resynchronization therapy? *Pacing Clin Electrophysiol* 2008; **31**: 525–8.

Khoo M, Kelly PA, Lindenfeld J. Cardiac resynchronization therapy in NYHA class IV heart failure. *Curr Cardiol Rep* 2009; **11**: 175–83.

Moss AJ, Hall WJ, Cannom DS, *et al.*; MADIT-CRT Trial Investigators. Cardiac-resynchronization therapy for the prevention of heart-failure events. *N Engl J Med* 2009; **361**: 1329–38.

Strickberger SA, Conti J, Daoud EG, *et al.* Patient selection for cardiac resynchronization therapy: from the Council on Clinical Cardiology Subcommittee on Electrocardiography and Arrhythmias and the Quality of Care and Outcomes Research Interdisciplinary Working Group, in collaboration with the Heart Rhythm Society. *Circulation* 2005; **111**: 2146–50.

Imaging

Abraham T, Kass D, Tonti G, *et al.* Imaging cardiac resynchronization therapy. *JACC Cardiovasc Imaging* 2009; **2**: 486–97.

Anderson LJ, Miyazaki C, Sutherland GR, Oh JK. Patient selection and echocardiographic assessment of dyssynchrony in cardiac resynchronization therapy. *Circulation* 2008; **117**: 2009–23.

Bax JJ, Gorcsan J. Echocardiography and noninvasive imaging in cardiac resynchronization therapy: results of the PROSPECT (Predictors of Response to Cardiac Resynchronization Therapy) study in perspective. *J Am Coll Cardiol* 2009; **53**: 1933–43.

Becker M, Franke A, Breithardt OA, *et al.* Impact of left ventricular position on the efficacy of cardiac resynchronisation therapy: a two-dimensional strain echocardiography study. *Heart* 2007; **93**: 1197–203.

Bleeker GB, Mollema SA, Holman ER, *et al.* Left ventricular resynchronization is mandatory for response to cardiac resynchronization therapy: analysis in patients with echocardiographic evidence of left ventricular dyssynchrony at baseline. *Circulation* 2007; **116**: 1440–8.

Chung ES, Leon AR, Tavazzi L, *et al.* Results of the Predictors of Response to CRT (PROSPECT) trial. *Circulation* 2008; **117**: 2608–16.

Hawkins NM, Petrie MC, Burgess MI, McMurray JJ. Selecting patients for cardiac resynchronization therapy: the fallacy of echocardiographic dyssynchrony. *J Am Coll Cardiol* 2009; **53**: 1944–59.

Kass DA. An epidemic of dyssynchrony: but what does it mean? *J Am Coll Cardiol* 2008; **51**: 12–17.

Krishnan SC, Tops LF, Bax JJ. Cardiac resynchronization therapy devices guided by imaging technology. *JACC Cardiovasc Imaging* 2009; **2**: 226–30.

Sanderson JE. Echocardiography for cardiac resynchronization therapy selection: fatally flawed or misjudged? *J Am Coll Cardiol* 2009; **53**: 1960–4.

Sutton MG, Plappert T, Hilpisch KE, *et al.* Sustained reverse left ventricular structural remodeling with cardiac resynchronization at one year is a function of etiology: quantitative Doppler echocardiographic evidence from the Multicenter InSync Randomized Clinical Evaluation (MIRACLE). *Circulation* 2006; **113**: 266–72.

Yu CM, Bax JJ, Gorcsan J. Critical appraisal of methods to assess mechanical dyssynchrony. *Curr Opin Cardiol* 2009; **24**: 18–28.

Ypenburg C, Westenberg JJ, Bleeker GB, *et al.* Noninvasive imaging in cardiac resynchronization therapy–part 1: selection of patients. *Pacing Clin Electrophysiol* 2008; **31**: 1475–99.

Follow-up

Aktas MK, Jeevanantham V, Sherazi S, *et al.* Effect of biventricular pacing during a ventricular sensed event. *Am J Cardiol* 2009; **103**: 1741–5.

Barold SS, Herweg B, Giudici M. Electrocardiographic follow-up of biventricular pacemakers. *Ann Noninvasive Electrocardiol* 2005; **10**: 231–55.

Castellant P, Fatemi M, Bertault-Valls V, Etienne Y, Blanc JJ. Cardiac resynchronization therapy:

"nonresponders" and "hyperresponders". *Heart Rhythm* 2008; **5**: 193–7.

Fish JM, Brugada J, Antzelevitch C. Potential proarrhythmic effects of biventricular pacing. *J Am Coll Cardiol* 2005; **46**: 2340–7.

Fung JW, Yu CM. Leveraging cardiac resynchronization therapy devices to monitor patients with heart failure. *Curr Heart Fail Rep* 2008; **5**: 44–50.

Gras D, Böcker D, Lunati M, *et al.* Implantation of cardiac resynchronization therapy systems in the CARE-HF trial: procedural success rate and safety. *Europace* 2007; **9**: 516–22.

Gurevitz O, Nof E, Carasso S, *et al.* Programmable multiple pacing configurations help to overcome high left ventricular pacing thresholds and avoid phrenic nerve stimulation. *Pacing Clin Electrophysiol* 2005; **28**: 1255–9.

Johnson WB, Abraham WT, Young JB, *et al.*; InSync Registry Investigators. Long-term performance of the attain model 4193 left ventricular lead. *Pacing Clin Electrophysiol* 2009; **32**: 1111–16.

Knight BP, Desai A, Coman J, Faddis M, Yong P. Long-term retention of cardiac resynchronization therapy. *J Am Coll Cardiol* 2004; **44**: 72–7.

Lin G, Anavekar NS, Webster TL, *et al.* Long-term stability of endocardial left ventricular pacing leads placed via the coronary sinus. *Pacing Clin Electrophysiol* 2009; **32**: 1117–22.

Sitges M, Vidal B, Delgado V, *et al.* Long-term effect of cardiac resynchronization therapy on functional mitral valve regurgitation. *Am J Cardiol* 2009; **104**: 383–8.

Thibault B, Roy D, Guerra PG, *et al.* Anodal right ventricular capture during left ventricular stimulation in CRT-implantable cardioverter defibrillators. *Pacing Clin Electrophysiol* 2005; **28**: 613–19.

Turitto G, El-Sherif N. Cardiac resynchronization therapy: a review of proarrhythmic and antiarrhythmic mechanisms. *Pacing Clin Electrophysiol* 2007; **30**: 115–22.

Wang L. Fundamentals of intrathoracic impedance monitoring in heart failure. *Am J Cardiol* 2007; **99**: 3G–10G.

Ypenburg C, Lancellotti P, Tops LF, *et al.* Acute effects of initiation and withdrawal of cardiac resynchronization therapy on papillary muscle dyssynchrony and mitral regurgitation. *J Am Coll Cardiol* 2007; **50**: 2071–7.

Yu CM, Wang L, Chau E, *et al.* Intrathoracic impedance monitoring in patients with heart failure: correlation with fluid status and feasibility of early warning preceding hospitalization. *Circulation* 2005; **112**: 841–8.

Yu CM, Wing-Hong Fung J, Zhang Q, Sanderson JE. Understanding nonresponders of cardiac resynchronization therapy: current and future perspectives. *J Cardiovasc Electrophysiol* 2005; **16**: 1117–24.

Optimization of AV and V–V intervals

Baker JH, McKenzie J, Beau S, *et al.* Acute evaluation of programmer-guided AV/PV and VV delay optimization comparing an IEGM method and echocardiogram for cardiac resynchronization therapy in heart failure patients and dual-chamber ICD implants. *J Cardiovasc Electrophysiol* 2007; **18**: 185–91.

Barold SS, Ilercil A, Herweg B. Echocardiographic optimization of the atrioventricular and interventricular intervals during cardiac resynchronization. *Europace* 2008; **10** (Suppl 3): iii88–95.

Gold MR, Niazi I, Giudici M, *et al.* A prospective comparison of AV delay programming methods for hemodynamic optimization during cardiac resynchronization therapy. *J Cardiovasc Electrophysiol* 2007; **18**: 490–6.

Gras D, Gupta MS, Boulogne E, Guzzo L, Abraham WT. Optimization of AV and VV delays in the real-world CRT patient population: an international survey on current clinical practice. *Pacing Clin Electrophysiol* 2009; **32** (Suppl 1): S236–9.

Mokrani B, Lafitte S, Deplagne A, *et al.* Echocardiographic study of the optimal atrioventricular delay at rest and during exercise in recipients of cardiac resynchronization therapy systems. *Heart Rhythm* 2009; **6**: 972–7.

Rao RK, Kumar UN, Schafer J, *et al.* Reduced ventricular volumes and improved systolic function with cardiac resynchronization therapy: a randomized trial comparing simultaneous biventricular pacing, sequential biventricular pacing, and left ventricular pacing. *Circulation* 2007; **115**: 2136–44.

van Gelder BM, Bracke FA, Meijer A. The effect of anodal stimulation on V–V timing at varying V–V intervals. *Pacing Clin Electrophysiol* 2005; **28**: 771–7.

Programmability

Barold SS, Ilercil A, Leonelli F, Herweg B. First-degree atrioventricular block: clinical manifestations, indications for pacing, pacemaker management and consequences during cardiac resynchronization. *J Interv Card Electrophysiol* 2006; **17**: 139–52.

Burri H, Sunthorn H, Shah D, Lerch R. Optimization of device programming for cardiac resynchronization therapy. *Pacing Clin Electrophysiol* 2006; **29**: 1416–25.

Gassis S, Leon AR. Cardiac resynchronization therapy: strategies for device programming, troubleshooting and follow-up. *J Interv Card Electrophysiol* 2005; **13**: 209–22.

Hasan A, Abraham WT. Optimization of cardiac resynchronization therapy after implantation. *Curr Treat Options Cardiovasc Med* 2008; **10**: 319–28.

Stanton T, Hawkins NM, Hogg KJ, *et al.* How should we optimize cardiac resynchronization therapy? *Eur Heart J* 2008; **29**: 2458–72.

Vidal B, Sitges M, Marigliano A, *et al.* Optimizing the programation of cardiac resynchronization therapy devices in patients with heart failure and left bundle branch block. *Am J Cardiol* 2007; **100**: 1002–6.

Index

Note: page numbers in **bold** refer to tables